SEVENTH EDITION

PHARMACEUTICAL DOSAGE FORMS AND DRUG DELIVERY SYSTEMS

Howard C. Ansel, Ph.D.
Professor and Dean Emeritus
College of Pharmacy
The University of Georgia

Loyd V. Allen, Jr., Ph.D.
Professor Emeritus
College of Pharmacy
University of Oklahoma, and
Editor-in-Chief
International Journal of Pharmaceutical Compounding

Nicholas G. Popovich, Ph.D.
Professor and Associate Head
Department of Pharmacy Practice
School of Pharmacy and Pharmacal Sciences
Purdue University

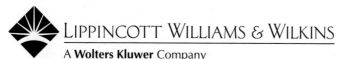

LIPPINCOTT WILLIAMS & WILKINS
A **Wolters Kluwer** Company
Philadelphia · Baltimore · New York · London
Buenos Aires · Hong Kong · Sydney · Tokyo

Editor: Donna Balado
Managing Editor: Jennifer Schmidt
Marketing Manager: Christine Kushner

Copyright © 1999 Lippincott Williams & Wilkins

351 West Camden Street
Baltimore, Maryland 21201–2436 USA

227 East Washington Square
Philadelphia, PA 19106

The publisher is not responsible (as a matter of product liability, negligence, or otherwise) for any injury resulting from any material contained herein. This publication contains information relating to general principles of medical care which should not be construed as specific instructions for individual patients. Manufacturers' product information and package inserts should be reviewed for current information, including contraindications, dosages, and precautions.

Printed in the United States of America

Library of Congress Cataloging-in-Publication Data

Ansel, Howard C., 1933–
 Pharmaceutical dosage forms and drug delievery systems / Howard C.
Ansel, Loyd V. Allen, Jr., Nicholas G. Popovich. — 7th ed.
  p. cm.
 Includes bibliographical references and index.
 ISBN 0–683–30572–7
 1. Drugs—Dosage forms. 2. Drug delivery systems. I. Allen, Loyd V.
II. Popovich, Nicholas G. III. Title.
 [DNLM: 1. Dosage Forms. 2. Drug Delivery Systems. QV 785 A618i 1999]
RS200.A57 1999
615'.1—dc21
DNLM/DLC
for Library of Congress   99–17498
                       CIP

The publishers have made every effort to trace the copyright holders for borrowed material. If they have inadvertently overlooked any, they will be pleased to make the necessary arrangements at the first opportunity.

The use of portions of the text of USP23/NF18, copyright 1994, is by permission of the USP Convention, Inc. The Convention is not responsible for any inaccuracy of quotation or for any false or misleading implication that may arise from separation of excerpts from the original context or by obsolescence resulting from publication of a supplement.

To purchase additional copies of this book call our customer service department at **(800) 638–3030** or fax orders to **(301) 824–7390**. International customers should call **(301) 714–2324**.

                        03
                   4 5 6 7 8 9 10

Preface

The purpose of this text is to introduce pharmacy students to the basic pharmaceutic principles and technologies applied in the preparation of pharmaceutical dosage forms and drug delivery systems. An integrated presentation is used to demonstrate the interrelationships which exist between pharmaceutic and biopharmaceutic principles, product design, formulation, manufacture, and the clinical application of the various dosage forms in patient care.

As has been the hallmark of this textbook since its first edition some thirty years ago, each chapter is written at a level consistent with the requirements of students being introduced to this academic area of study. Because this textbook often is used early in the professional curriculum, important introductory topics are included as the historical development of drugs and pharmacy; the role of the pharmacist in contemporary practice; standards of the *United States Pharmacopeia/National Formulary;* systems and techniques of pharmaceutical measurement; basic pharmaceutic and biopharmaceutic principles applicable to drug product development; current good manufacturing practice and current good compounding practice standards; and the regulatory process by which pharmaceuticals are approved for marketing by the federal Food and Drug Administration.

The Seventh Edition represents a complete rewrite of the previous edition and the reorganization of the various chapters into seven divisions based upon traditional pharmaceutic pedagogy. This allows the systematic presentation of dosage forms according to their physical form and characteristics. The "Physical Pharmacy Capsules," introduced in the Sixth Edition to emphasize important underlying pharmaceutic principles have been expanded in the new edition. Other important changes include enhanced considerations of dosage form design and formulation, a new section on current good compounding practices, expanded clinical considerations in the use of each dosage form, and a new chapter on "Novel Dosage Forms and Drug Delivery Technologies." Also new with this edition is the "chapter-at-a-glance" format at the beginning of each chapter.

Acknowledgments

I acknowledge with grateful appreciation the major contributions of co-authors Loyd V. Allen, Jr. and Nicholas G. Popovich in sustaining the vitality of this work. Their respective expertise in the fields of physical pharmacy and formulation technology and in clinical pharmacy and pharmacy practice has allowed the integrated approach utilized in this work. Together, we extend our gratitude to students and colleagues who have shared their thoughts with us on this revision and trust that we have been successful in responding to their suggestions. We also acknowledge with appreciation, our colleagues in industry who generously have provided scientific and technical information and updated figures for our use. We especially thank our friends at Lippincott Williams & Wilkins who have contributed so expertly to the planning, preparation, and production of this new edition, namely Donna Balado, Acquisitions Editor; Jennifer Schmidt, Managing Editor; Karen Gulliver, Freelance Managing Editor, and Susan Rockwell, Production Manager, Copyediting.

HOWARD C. ANSEL
Athens, Georgia

Contents

INTRODUCTION TO DRUGS AND PHARMACY

Chapter at a Glance

A DRUG is defined as an agent intended for use in the diagnosis, mitigation, treatment, cure, or prevention of disease in humans or in other animals. One of the most astounding qualities of drugs is the diversity of their actions and effects on the body.

This quality enables their selective use in the treatment of a range of common and rare conditions involving virtually every body organ, tissue, and cell.

Some drugs selectively stimulate the cardiac muscle, the central nervous system, or the gastrointestinal tract, whereas other drugs have the opposite effect. Mydriatic drugs dilate the pupil of the eye, and miotics constrict or diminish pupillary size. Drugs can render blood more coagulable or less coagulable; they can increase the hemoglobin content of the erythrocytes, reduce serum cholesterol, or expand blood volume.

Drugs termed emetics induce vomiting, whereas antiemetic drugs prevent vomiting. Diuretic drugs increase the flow of urine; expectorant drugs increase respiratory tract fluid; and cathartics or laxatives evacuate the bowel. Other drugs decrease the flow of urine, diminish body secretions, or induce constipation.

Drugs may be used to reduce pain, fever, thyroid activity, rhinitis, insomnia, gastric acidity, motion sickness, blood pressure, and mental depression. Other drugs can elevate mood, blood pressure, or activity of the endocrine glands. Drugs can combat infectious disease, destroy intestinal worms, or act as antidotes against the poisoning effects of other drugs. Drugs can assist in smoking cessation, alcohol withdrawal, or modify obsessive compulsive disorders.

Drugs are used to treat common infections, AIDS, benign prostatic hyperplasia, cancer, cardiovascular disease, asthma, glaucoma, Alzheimer's disease, and male impotence. They can protect against the rejection of transplanted tissues and organs and reduce the incidence of measles and mumps. Antineoplastic drugs provide one means of attacking the cancerous process; radioactive pharmaceuticals provide another.

Drugs may be used to diagnose diabetes, liver malfunction, tuberculosis, or pregnancy. They can replenish a body deficient in antibodies, vitamins, hormones, electrolytes, protein, enzymes, or blood. Drugs can prevent pregnancy, assist fertility, and sustain life itself.

Certainly the vast array of effective medicinal agents available today represents one of our greatest scientific accomplishments. It is difficult to conceive our civilization devoid of these remarkable and beneficial agents. Through their use, many of the diseases that have plagued humans throughout history, such as smallpox and poliomyelitis, are now virtually extinct. Illnesses such as diabetes, hypertension, and mental depression are now effectively controlled with modern drugs. Today's surgical procedures would be virtually impossible without the benefit of anesthetics, analgesics, antibiotics, blood transfusions, and intravenous fluids.

New drugs may be derived from plant or animal sources, as byproducts of microbial growth, through chemical synthesis, molecular modification, or biotechnology. Computer libraries or data banks of chemical compounds and sophisticated methods of screening for potential biological activity assist the process of drug discovery.

The process of drug discovery and development is complex. It involves the collective contributions of many scientific specialists including organic, physical, and analytical chemists, biochemists, molecular biologists, bacteriologists, physiologists, pharmacologists, toxicologists, hematologists, immunologists, endocrinologists, pathologists, biostatisticians, pharmaceutical scientists, clinical pharmacists, physicians, and many others.

After a potential new drug substance is discovered and has undergone definitive chemical and physical characterization, a great deal of biological information must be gathered. The basic pharmacology or the nature and mechanism of action of the drug on the biological system must be determined including toxicologic features. A study must be made of the drug's site and rate of absorption, its pattern of distribution and concentration within the body, its duration of action, and the method and rate of its elimination or excretion. Information must be obtained on the drug's metabolic degradation and the activity of any of its metabolites. A comprehensive study must be made of the short-term and long-term effects of the drug on various body cells, tissues, and organs. Highly specific information may be obtained, as the effect of the drug on the fetus of a pregnant animal or its ability to pass to a nursing baby through the breast milk of its mother. Many a promising new drug has been abandoned because of its potential to cause excessive or hazardous adverse effects.

The most effective routes of administration (e.g., oral, rectal, parenteral) must be determined, and guidelines have to be established concerning the dosages recommended for persons of varying ages (e.g., neonates, children, adults, geriatrics), weights, and states of illness. To facilitate administration of the drug by the selected routes, appropriate dosage forms as tablets, capsules, injections, suppositories, ointments, aerosols, and others are formulated and prepared. Each of these dosage units is designed to contain a specified quantity of medication for ease and accuracy of dosage administration. These dosage forms are highly sophisticated pharmaceutical drug delivery systems. Their design, development, production, and utilization represent the application of the pharmaceutical sciences—the blending of the basic, applied, and clinical sciences with pharmaceutical technology.

Each particular pharmaceutical product is a formulation unique unto itself. In addition to the active therapeutic ingredients, a pharmaceutical formulation also contains a number of nontherapeutic or pharmaceutic ingredients. It is through their use that a formulation achieves its unique composition and characteristic physical appearance. Pharmaceutic ingredients include such materials as fillers, thickeners, solvents, suspending agents, tablet coatings and disintegrants, stabilizing agents, antimicrobial preservatives, flavors, colorants, and sweeteners.

To ensure the stability of a drug in a formulation and the continued effectiveness of the drug product throughout its usual shelf life, the principles of chemistry, physical pharmacy, microbiology, and pharmaceutical technology must be applied. The formulation must be such that all components are physically and chemically compatible, including the active therapeutic agents, the pharmaceutic ingredients, and the packaging materials. The formulation must be preserved against decomposition due to chemical degradation and protected from microbial contamination and the destructive influences of excessive heat, light, and moisture. The therapeutic ingredients must be released from the dosage form in the proper quantity and in such a manner that the onset and duration of the drug's action is that which is desired. The pharmaceutical product must lend itself to efficient administration and must possess attractive features of flavor, odor, color, and texture that enhance patient acceptance. Finally, the product must be effectively packaged and clearly and completely labeled according to existing legal regulations.

Once prepared, the pharmaceutical product must be properly administered if the patient is to receive maximum benefit. The medication must be taken in sufficient quantity, at specified intervals, and for an indicated duration of time to achieve the desired therapeutic outcomes. The effectiveness of the medication in achieving the prescriber's objectives should be reevaluated at regular intervals and necessary adjustments made in the dosage, dosage regimen or dosage schedule, dosage form, or indeed, in the choice of the drug administered. Patient expressions of disappointment in his or her rate of progress or complaints of side effects to the prescribed drug should be evaluated and decisions made as to the continuance, adjustment, or major change in drug therapy. Before initially taking a medication, a patient should be advised of any expected side effects, and of foods, beverages, and/or other drugs that may interfere with the effectiveness of the medication.

Through professional interaction and communication with other health professionals the pharmacist is able to contribute greatly to patient care. An intimate knowledge of drug actions, pharmacotherapeutics, formulation and dosage form design, available pharmaceutical products, and drug information sources makes the pharmacist a vital member of the health care team. The pharmacist is entrusted with the legal responsibility for the procurement, storage, control, and distribution of effective pharmaceutical products and for the compounding and filling of prescription orders. Utilizing extensive training and knowledge, the pharmacist serves the patient as an advisor on drugs and encourages their safe and proper utilization. The pharmacist delivers pharmaceutical services in a variety of community and institutional health care environments and effectively utilizes medication records, patient monitoring, and assessment techniques in safeguarding the public health.

To appreciate the progress that has been made in drug discovery and development and to provide background for the study of modern drugs and pharmaceutical dosage forms, it is important to examine pharmacy's heritage.

The Heritage of Pharmacy

Drugs, in the form of vegetation and minerals, have existed longer than humans. Human disease and the instinct to survive have, through the ages, led to their discovery. The use of drugs, crude though they may have been, undoubtedly dates back long before recorded history, for the instinct of primitive man to relieve the pain of a wound by bathing it in cool water or by soothing it with a fresh leaf or protecting it with mud is within the realm of belief. From experience, primitive humans would learn that certain therapy was more effective than others, and from these beginnings, came the practice of drug therapy.

Among many early races, disease was believed to be caused by the entrance of demons or evil spirits into the body. The treatment naturally involved ridding the body of the supernatural intruders. From the earliest records, the primary methods of removing spirits were through the use of spiritual incantations, the application of noisome materials, and the administration of specific herbs or plant materials.

The First Apothecary

Before the days of the priestcraft, the wise man or woman of the tribe, whose knowledge of the healing qualities of plants had been gathered through experience or handed down by word of mouth, was called upon to attend to the sick or wounded and prepare the remedy. It was in the preparation of the medicinal materials that the art of the apothecary originated.

The art of the apothecary has always been associated with the mysterious, and its practitioners were believed to have connection with the world of spirits and thus performed as intermediaries between the seen and the unseen. The belief that a drug had magical associations meant that its action, for good or for evil, did not depend upon its natural qualities alone. The compassion of a god, the observance of ceremonies, the absence of evil spirits, and the healing intent of the dispenser were individually and collectively needed to make the drug therapeutically effective. Because of this, the tribal apothecary was one to be feared, respected, trusted, sometimes mistrusted, worshiped, and revered, for it was through his potions that spiritual contact was made and upon which the cures or failures depended.

Throughout history, the knowledge of drugs and their application to disease has always meant power. In the Homeric epics, the term pharmakon (Gr.) from which our word pharmacy was derived connotes a charm or a drug that can be used for good or for evil purposes. Many of the tribal apothecary's failures were doubtless due to impotent or inappropriate medicines, underdosage, overdosage, and even poisoning. Successes may be attributed to experience, mere coincidence of appropriate drug selection, natural healing, inconsequential effect of the drug, or placebo effects, successful treatment due to psychologic rather than therapeutic effects. Even today, placebo therapy with nonpotent or inconsequential chemicals is used successfully to treat individual patients and is a routine practice in the clinical evaluation of new drugs, in which subjects' responses to the effects of the actual drug and the placebo are compared and evaluated.

As time passed, the art of the apothecary became combined with priestly functions, and among the early civilizations, the priest-magician or priest-physician became the healer of the body as well as of the soul. Pharmacy and medicine are indistinguishable in their early history because their practice was the combined function of the tribal religious leaders.

Early Drugs

Due to the patience and intellect of the archeologist, the types and specific drugs used in the early history of drug therapy are not as indefinable as one might suspect. Numerous ancient tablets, scrolls, and other relics dating as far back as 3000 BC have been uncovered and deciphered by archaeologic scholars to the delight of historians of both medicine and pharmacy; these ancient documents are specific associations with our common heritage (Fig. 1.1).

Perhaps the most famous of these surviving memorials is the Papyrus Ebers, a continuous scroll

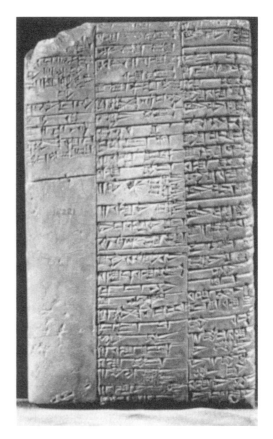

Fig. 1.1 *Sumerian clay tablet from the third millennium* BC *on which are believed to be the world's oldest written prescriptions. Among them are a preparation of the seed of "carpenter plant," gum resin of markhazi, and thyme, all pulverized and dissolved in beer, and a combination of powdered roots of "Moon plant," and white pear tree, also dissolved in beer. (Courtesy of the University Museum, University of Pennsylvania.)*

some 60 feet long and a foot wide dating back to the 16th century before Christ. This document, which is now preserved at the University of Leipzig, is named for the noted German Egyptologist, Georg Ebers, who discovered it in the tomb of a mummy and partly translated it during the last half of the nineteenth century. Since that time, many scholars have participated in the translation of the document's challenging hieroglyphics, and although they are not unanimous in their interpretations, there is little doubt that by 1550 BC, the Egyptians were using some drugs and dosage forms that are still used today.

The text of the Ebers Papyrus is dominated by drug formulas, with more than 800 formulas or prescriptions being described and over 700 different drugs being mentioned. The drugs referred to are chiefly botanic, although mineral and animal drugs are also noted. Such botanic substances as acacia, castor bean (from which we express castor oil), and fennel are mentioned along with apparent references to such minerals as iron oxide, sodium carbonate, sodium chloride, and sulfur. Animal excrements were also used in drug therapy.

The formulative vehicles of the day were beer, wine, milk, and honey. Many of the pharmaceutical formulas employed two dozen or more different medicinal agents, a type of preparation later referred to as a "polypharmacal." Mortars, hand mills, sieves, and balances were commonly used by the Egyptians in their compounding of suppositories, gargles, pills, inhalations, troches, lotions, ointments, plasters, and enemas.

Introduction of the Scientific Viewpoint

Throughout history, many individuals have contributed to the advancement of the health sciences. Notable among those whose genius and creativeness had a revolutionary influence on the development of pharmacy and medicine were Hippocrates (ca. 460–377 BC), Dioscorides (1st century AD), Galen (ca. 130–200 AD), and Paracelsus (1493–1541 AD).

Hippocrates was a Greek physician who is credited with the introduction of scientific pharmacy and medicine. He rationalized medicine, systematized medical knowledge, and put the practice of medicine on a high ethical plane. His thinking on the ethics and science of medicine dominated the medical writings of his and successive generations, and his concepts and precepts are embodied into the now renowned Hippocratic Oath of ethical behavior for the healing professions. His works included the descriptions of hundreds of drugs, and it was during this period that the term pharmakon came to mean a purifying remedy for good only, transcending the previous connotation of a charm or drug for good or for evil purposes. Because of his pioneering work in medical science and his inspirational teachings and advanced philosophies that have become a part of modern medicine, Hippocrates is honored by being called the "Father of Medicine."

Dioscorides, a Greek physician and botanist, was the first to deal with botany as an applied science of pharmacy. His work, De Materia Medica, is considered a milestone in the development of pharmaceutical botany and in the study of naturally occurring medicinal materials. This area of study is today known as pharmacognosy, a term formed from two Greek words, *pharmakon*, drug, and *gnosis*, knowledge. Some of the drugs described by Dioscorides, as opium, ergot, and hyoscyamus, continue to have use in medicine. His descriptions of the art of identifying and collecting natural drug products, the methods of their proper storage, and the means of detecting adulterants or contaminants were the standards of the period, established the need for additional work, and set guidelines for future investigators.

Claudius Galen, a Greek pharmacist-physician who attained Roman citizenship, aimed to create a perfect system of physiology, pathology, and treatment and formulated doctrines that were followed for 1500 years. He was one of the most prolific authors of his or any other era, having been credited with 500 treatises on medicine and some 250 others on subjects of philosophy, law, and grammar. His medical writings include descriptions of numerous drugs of natural origin with a profusion of drug formulas and methods of compounding. He originated so many preparations of vegetable drugs by mixing or melting the individual ingredients that the area of pharmaceutical preparations was once commonly referred to as "Galenic pharmacy." Perhaps the most famous of his formulas is one for a cold cream, called Galen's Cerate, which has similarities to some in use today.

Pharmacy remained a function of medicine until the increasing variety of drugs and the growing complexity of compounding demanded specialists who could devote full attention to the art. Pharmacy was officially separated from medicine for the first time in 1240 AD when a decree of the German Emperor Frederick II regulated the practice of pharmacy within that part of his kingdom called the Two Sicilies. His edict separating the two professions acknowledged that pharmacy required special knowledge, skill, initiative, and responsibility if adequate care to the medical needs of the people was to be guaranteed. Pharmacists were obligated by oath to prepare reliable drugs of uniform quality according to their art. Any exploitation of the patient through business relations between the pharmacist and the physician was strictly forbidden. Between that time and the evolution of chemistry as an exact science, pharmacy and chemistry became united as pharmacy and medicine had been.

Perhaps no person in history exercised such a revolutionary influence on pharmacy and medicine as did Aureolus Philippus Theophrastus Bombastus von Hohenheim, a Swiss physician and chemist who called himself Paracelsus. He influenced the transformation of pharmacy from a profession based primarily on botanic science to one based on chemical science. Some of his chemical observations were astounding for his time and for their anticipation of later discoveries. He believed it was possible to prepare a specific medicinal agent to combat each specific disease and introduced a host of chemical substances to internal therapy.

Early Research

As the knowledge of the basic sciences increased, so did their application to pharmacy. The opportunity was presented for the investigation of medicinal materials on a firm scientific basis, and the challenge was accepted by numerous pharmacists who conducted their research in the back rooms and basements of their pharmacies. Noteworthy among them was Karl Wilhelm Scheele (1742–1786), a Swedish pharmacist who is perhaps the most famous of all pharmacists because of his scientific genius and dramatic discoveries. Among his discoveries were the chemicals lactic acid, citric acid, oxalic acid, tartaric acid, and arsenic acid. He identified glycerin, invented new methods of preparing calomel and benzoic acid, and discovered oxygen a year before Priestley.

The isolation of morphine from opium by the German pharmacist Friedrich Sertürner (1783–1841) in 1805 prompted a series of isolations of other active materials from medicinal plants by a score of French pharmacists. Joseph Caventou (1795–1877) and Joseph Pelletier (1788–1842) combined their talents and isolated quinine and cinchonine from cinchona, and strychnine and brucine from nux vomica. Pelletier together with Pierre Robiquet (1780–1840) isolated caffeine, and Robiquet independently separated codeine from opium. Methodically one chemical after another was isolated from plant drugs and identified as an agent responsible for the plants' medicinal activity. Today we are still engaged in this fascinating activity as we probe nature for more useful and more specific therapeutic agents. Contemporary examples of drugs isolated from a natural source include paclitaxel (Taxol), an agent with antitumor activity derived from the Pacific yew tree (Taxus baccata) and employed in the treatment of metastatic carcinoma of the ovary; vincaleukoblastine, another antineoplastic drug, from Vinca rosea; and digoxin, a cardiac glycoside, from Digitalis lanata.

Throughout Europe during the late 18th century and the beginning of the 19th century, pharmacists like Pelletier and Sertürner were held in great es-

teem because of their intellect and technical abilities. They applied the art and the science of pharmacy to the preparation of drug products that were of the highest standards of purity, uniformity, and efficacy possible at that time. The extraction and isolation of active constituents from crude (unprocessed) botanic drugs led to the development of dosage forms of uniform strength containing singly effective therapeutic agents of natural origin. Many pharmacists of the period began to manufacture quality pharmaceutical products on a small but steadily increasing scale to meet the growing drug needs of their communities. Some of today's largest pharmaceutical research and manufacturing companies developed from these progressive prescription laboratories of two centuries ago.

Although many of the drugs indigenous to America and first used by the American Indian were adopted by the settlers, the vast majority of drugs needed in this country before the 19th century were imported from Europe, either as the raw materials or as finished pharmaceutical products. With the Revolutionary War, however, it became more difficult to import drugs, and the American pharmacist was stimulated to acquire the scientific and technologic expertise of his European contemporary. From this period until the Civil War, pharmaceutical manufacture was in its infancy in this country. A few of the pharmaceutical firms established during the early 1800s are still in operation. In 1821, the Philadelphia College of Pharmacy was established as the nation's first school of pharmacy.

Drug Standards

As the scientific basis for drugs and drug products developed, so did the need for uniform standards to ensure quality. This need led to the development and publication of monographs and reference books containing such standards to be utilized by those involved in the production of drugs and pharmaceutical products. Organized sets of monographs or books of these standards are referred to as "pharmacopeias" or "formularies."

The United States Pharmacopeia and The National Formulary

The term pharmacopeia comes from the Greek, *pharmakon,* meaning "drug," and *poiein,* meaning "make," and the combination indicates any recipe or formula or other standards required to make or prepare a drug. The term was first used in 1580 in connection with a local book of drug standards in Bergamo, Italy. From that time on there were countless city, state, and national pharmacopeias published by various European pharmaceutical societies. As time passed, the value of a uniform set of national drug standards became apparent. In England, for example, three city pharmacopeias—the London, the Edinburgh, and the Dublin—were official throughout the kingdom until 1864, when they were replaced by the British Pharmacopoeia (BP).

In the United States, drug standards were first provided on a national basis in 1820, when the first United States Pharmacopeia (USP) was published. However, the need for drug standards was recognized in this country long before the first USP was published. For convenience and because of their familiarity with them, colonial physicians and apothecaries used the pharmacopeias and other references of their various homelands. The first American pharmacopeia was the so-called "Lititz Pharmacopeia," published in 1778 at Lititz, Pennsylvania, for use by the Military Hospital of the United States Army. It was a 32-page booklet containing information on 84 internal and 16 external drugs and preparations.

During the last decade of the 18th century, several attempts were made by various local medical societies to collate drug information, set appropriate standards, and prepare an extensive American pharmacopeia of the drugs in use at that time. In 1808, the Massachusetts Medical Society published a 272-page pharmacopeia containing information or monographs on 536 drugs and pharmaceutical preparations. Included were monographs on many drugs indigenous to America, which were not described in the European pharmacopeias of the day.

On January 6, 1817, Dr. Lyman Spalding, a physician from New York City, submitted a plan to the Medical Society of the County of New York for the creation of a national pharmacopeia. Dr. Spalding's efforts were later to result in his being recognized as the "Father of the United States Pharmacopeia." He proposed dividing the United States as then known into four geographic districts—Northern, Middle, Southern, and Western. The plan provided for a convention in each of these districts, to be composed of delegates from all medical societies and medical schools within them. Where there was as yet no incorporated medical society or medical school, voluntary associations of physicians and surgeons were invited to assist in the undertaking. Each district's convention was to draft a pharmacopeia and appoint delegates to a general convention to be held later in Washington, D.C. At the general convention, the four district pharma-

copeias were to be compiled into a single national pharmacopeia.

Draft pharmacopeias were submitted to the convention by only the Northern and Middle districts. These were reviewed, consolidated, and adopted by the first United States Pharmacopeial Convention assembled in Washington, D.C., on January 1, 1820. The first United States Pharmacopeia (USP) was published on December 15, 1820, in English and also in Latin, then the international language of medicine, to render the book more intelligible to physicians and pharmacists of any nationality. Within its 272 pages were listed 217 drugs considered worthy of recognition; many of them were taken from the Massachusetts Pharmacopeia, which is considered by some to be the precursor to the USP. The objective of the first USP was stated in its preface and remains important. It reads in part: (1)

It is the object of a Pharmacopeia to select from among substances which possess medicinal power, those, the utility of which is most fully established and best understood; and to form from them preparations and compositions, in which their powers may be exerted to the greatest advantage. It should likewise distinguish those articles by convenient and definite names, such as may prevent trouble or uncertainty in the intercourse of physicians and apothecaries.

Before adjourning, the Convention adopted a Constitution and Bylaws, with provisions for subsequent meetings of the Convention leading to a revised United States Pharmacopeia every 10 years. As many new drugs entered into drug therapy, the need for more frequent issuance of standards became increasingly apparent. In 1900, the Pharmacopeial Convention granted authority to issue supplements to the currently official USP whenever necessary to maintain satisfactory standards. At the 1940 meeting of the Convention, it was decided to revise the Pharmacopeia every 5 years while maintaining the use of periodic supplements.

The first United States Pharmacopeial Convention was composed exclusively of physicians. In 1830, and again in 1840, prominent pharmacists were invited to assist in the revision, and recognition of their contributions pharmacists were awarded full membership in the Convention of 1850 and have participated regularly ever since. By 1870, the Pharmacopeia was so nearly in the hands of pharmacists that vigorous efforts were required to revive interest in it among physicians. The present Constitution and Bylaws of The United States Pharmacopeial Convention provide for accredited delegates representing educational institutions, professional and scientific organizations, divisions of governmental bodies, non-United States international organizations and pharmacopeial bodies, persons who possess special scientific competence or knowledge of emerging technologies, and public members.(3) Of the seven elected members of the Board of Trustees, at least two must be representatives of the medical sciences, two others must be representatives of the pharmaceutical sciences, and at least one must be a public member.

After the appearance of the first USP, the art and science of both pharmacy and medicine changed remarkably. Before 1820, drugs to treat disease were the same for centuries. The Pharmacopeia of 1820 reflected the fact that the apothecary of that day was competent at collecting and identifying botanic drugs and preparing from them the mixtures and preparations required by the physician. The individual pharmacist seemed fulfilled as he applied his total art to the creation of elegant pharmaceutical preparations from crude botanic materials. It was a time that would never be seen again because of the impending upsurge in technologic capabilities and the steady development of the basic sciences, particularly synthetic organic chemistry.

The second half of the 19th century brought great and far-reaching changes. The United States was now under the full impact of the industrial revolution. The steam engine, which used water power to turn mills that powdered crude botanic drugs, was replaced by the gas, diesel, or electric motor. New machinery was substituted for the old whenever possible, and often machinery from other industries was adapted to the special needs of pharmaceutical manufacturing. Mixers from the baking industry, centrifugal machines from the laundry industry, and sugarcoating pans from the candy industry were a few examples of the type of improvisations made. Production increased rapidly, but the new industry had to wait for the scientific revolution before it could claim newer and better drugs for mankind. A symbiosis was needed between science and the advancing technology.

By 1880, the industrial manufacture of chemicals and pharmaceutical products had become well established in this country, and the pharmacist was relying heavily on commercial sources for drug supply. Synthetic organic chemistry began to have its influence on drug therapy. The isolation of some active constituents of plant drugs had led to knowledge of their chemical structure. From this arose methods of synthetically duplicating the same structures, as well as manipulating molecular structure to produce organic chemicals yet undiscovered in nature. In 1872, the synthesis of salicylic acid from phenol inaugurated the synthesis of a group of analgesic compounds including acetylsalicylic acid (aspirin), which was introduced into medicine in 1899. Among other chemicals synthesized for the first time were sleep-producing derivatives of barbituric acid called "barbiturates." This new source of drugs—synthetic organic chemistry—welcomed the turn into the 20th century.

Until this time, drugs created through the genius of the synthetic organic chemist relieved a host of maladies, but none had been found to be curative—none, that is, until 1910, when arsphenamine, a specific agent against syphilis, was introduced to medical science. This was the start of an era of chemotherapy, an era in which the diseases of humans became curable through the use of specific chemical agents. The concepts, discoveries, and inspirational work that led mankind to this glorious period are credited to Paul Ehrlich, the German bacteriologist who together with a Japanese colleague, Sahachiro Hata, discovered arsphenamine. Today most of our new drugs, whether they are curative or palliative, originate in the flask of the synthetic organic chemist.

The advancement of science, both basic and applied, led to drugs of a more complex nature and to more of them. The drug standards advanced by the USP were more than ever needed to protect the public by ensuring the purity and uniformity of the drugs administered.

When the American Pharmaceutical Association (APhA) was organized in 1852, the only authoritative and recognized book of drug standards available was the third revision of the United States Pharmacopeia. To serve as a therapeutic guide to the medical profession, its scope, then as now, was restricted to drugs of established therapeutic merit. Because of strict selectivity, many drugs and formulas that were accepted and used by the medical profession were not granted admission to early revisions of the Pharmacopeia. As a type of a protest, and in keeping with the original objectives of the American Pharmaceutical Association to establish standardization of drugs and formulas, certain pharmacists, with the sanction of their national organization, prepared a formulary containing many of the popular drugs and formulas denied admission to the Pharmacopeia. The first edition was published in 1888 under the title National Formulary of Unofficial Preparations. The designation Unofficial Preparations reflected the protest mood of the authors, since the Pharmacopeia had earlier adopted the term "official" as applying to the drugs for which it provided standards. The title was changed to National Formulary (NF) on June 30, 1906 when President Theodore Roosevelt signed into law the first federal Pure Food and Drug Act, designating both the USP and NF as establishing legal standards for medicinal and pharmaceutic substances. Thus the two publications became official compendia. Among other things, the law required that whenever the designations "USP" or "NF" were used or implied on drug labeling, the products must conform to the physical and chemical standards set forth in the compendium monograph.

The early editions of the National Formulary served mainly as a convenience to practicing pharmacists by providing uniform names of drugs and preparations and working directions for the small-scale manufacture of popular pharmaceutical preparations prescribed by physicians. Before 1940, the NF, as the USP, was revised every 10 years. After that date, new editions appeared every 5 years, with supplements issued periodically as necessary.

In 1975, the United States Pharmacopeial Convention, Inc. purchased the National Formulary, unifying the official compendia and thereby provided the mechanism for a single, national compendium.

The first combined compendium, representing the USPXX and NFXV became official on July 1, 1980. All monographs on therapeutically active drug substances appeared in the USP section of the volume, whereas all monographs on pharmaceutic agents appeared in the NF section. This format has been continued in subsequent revisions. The United States Pharmacopeia 23/National Formulary 18, which became official in 1995 was the first edition to drop the use of roman numerals in favor of arabic numerals to indicate the edition. The most recent edition of the USP-NF contains over 3,400 drug monographs and is published both in print and on CD-ROM.

The standards advanced by the United States Pharmacopeia and the National Formulary are put to active use by all members of the health care industry who share the responsibility and enjoy the public's trust for assuring the availability of quality drugs and pharmaceutical products. Included in this group are pharmacists, physicians, dentists, veterinarians, nurses, producers, and suppliers of bulk chemicals for use in drug production, large and small manufacturers of pharmaceutical products, drug procurement officers of various private and public health agencies and institutions, drug regulatory and enforcement agencies, and others.

USP and NF Monographs

The United States Pharmacopeia and the National Formulary adopt standards for drug substances, pharmaceutic ingredients, and dosage forms reflecting the best in the current practices of medicine and pharmacy and provide suitable tests and assay procedures for demonstrating compliance with these standards. In fulfilling this function, the compendia become legal documents, every statement of which must be of a high degree of clarity and specificity.

Many pharmaceutical products on the market, especially those which are combinations of therapeutic ingredients, are not represented by formulation or dosage form monographs in the official compendia. However, the individual components in these products are either represented by monographs in the compendia, in supplements to the compendia, or in drug applications for marketing approved by the Food and Drug Administration.

An example of a typical monograph for a drug substance appearing in the USP is shown in Figure 1.2. This monograph demonstrates the type of information that appears for organic medicinal agents.

The initial part of the monograph consists of the official title (generic or nonproprietary name) of the drug substance. This is followed by its graphic or structural formula, its empirical formula, molecular weight, established chemical names, and the drug's Chemical Abstracts Service (CAS) Registry Number. The CAS Registry Number identifies each compound uniquely in the CAS computer-oriented information retrieval system. Appearing next in the monograph is a statement of chemical purity, a cautionary statement that reflects the toxic nature of the agent, packaging and storage recommendations, and chemical and physical tests and the prescribed method of assay to substantiate the identification and purity of the chemical.

In each monograph, the standards set forth are specific to the individual therapeutic agent, pharmaceutic material, or dosage form preparation to assure purity, potency, and quality.

The USP Drug Research and Testing Laboratory provides direct laboratory assistance to the United States Pharmacopeia and the National Formulary. The Laboratory's main functions are the evaluation of USP Reference Standards and the evaluation and development of analytical methods to be used in the compendia.

Other Pharmacopeias

In addition to the USP and the NF, other references to drug standards such as the Homeopathic Pharmacopeia of the United States (HPUS) and the International Pharmacopeia (IP) provide additional

Chlorambucil

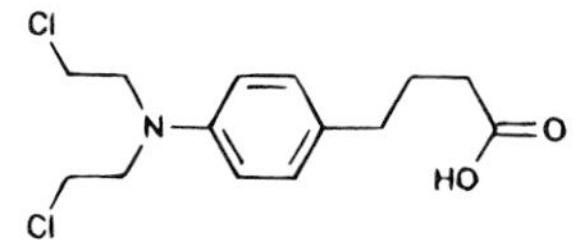

$C_{14}H_{19}Cl_2NO_2$ **304.22 Benzenebutanoic acid, 4-[bis(2-chloroethyl)amino]-4-[p[Bis(2-chloroethyl)amino]phenyl]butyric acid** [305-03-3].

▶ Chlorambucil contains not less than 98.0% and not more than 101.0% of $C_{14}H_{19}Cl_2NO_2$, calculated on the anhydrous basis.

Caution—Great care should be taken to prevent inhaling particles of Chlorambucil and exposing the skin to it.

Packaging and storage—Preserve in tight, light-resistant containers.

Reference standard—*USP Chlorambucil Reference Standard—[Caution—Avoid contact]*—Dry over silica gel for 24 hours before using.

Identification—

A: The infrared absorption spectrum of a 1 in 125 solution in carbon disulfide, in a 1-mm cell, exhibits maxima only at the same wavelengths as that of a similar solution of USP Chlorambucil RS.

B: Dissolve 50 mg in 5 mL of acetone, and dilute with water to 10 mL. Add 1 drop of 2 N sulfuric acid, then add 4 drops of silver nitrate TS: no opalescence is observed immediately *(absence of chloride ion)*. Warm the solution on a steam bath: opalescence develops *(presence of ionizable chlorine)*.

Melting range (741): between 65° and 69°.

Water, *Method I* (921): not more than 0.5%.

Assay—Dissolve about 200 mg of Chlorambucil, accurately weighed, in 10 mL of acetone, add 10 mL of water, and titrate with 0.1 N sodium hydroxide VS, using phenolphthalein TS as the indicator. Each mL of 0.1 N sodium hydroxide is equivalent to 30.42 mg of $C_{14}H_{19}Cl_2NO_2$.

Fig. 1.2   *Chlorambucil.*

guidelines for drug quality required by certain practitioners and agencies. The Homeopathic Pharmacopeia is used by pharmacists and homeopathists as well as by law enforcement agencies that must ensure the quality of homeopathic drugs. The term homeopathy was coined by Samuel Hahnemann (1755–1843) from the Greek homoios, meaning similar, and pathos, meaning disease. In essence, the basic tenet of homeopathy is the "law of similars" or that like cures like: that is, a drug that produces symptoms of the illness in healthy persons will also be capable of treating those same symptoms and curing the disease. Embodied in the homeopathic approach are 1) the testing of a drug on healthy persons to find the drug's effects so that it may be employed against the same symptoms manifesting a disease in an ill person, 2) the use of only minute doses of drugs in therapy, employed in dilutions expressed as "1x" (a 1:10 dilution), "2x" (a 1:100 dilution), etc., 3) the administration of not more than one drug at a time, and 4) the treatment of the entire symptom complex of the patient, not just one symptom (4–6). The Homeopathic Pharmacopeia is essential for pharmacists who prepare drugs to be used in the practice of homeopathy.

The Pharmacopeia Internationalis, or International Pharmacopeia is published by the World Health Organization (WHO) of the United Nations with the cooperation of member countries. It is intended as a recommendation to national pharmacopeial revision committees to modify their respective pharmacopeias according to the international standards adopted. It has no legal authority, only the mutual respect and recognition accorded it by the participating countries in their effort to provide acceptable drug standards on an international basis. The first volume of the Pharmacopeia Internationalis was published in 1951. It has been revised periodically since that time.

Over the years, a number of countries have published their own pharmacopeias, including Great Britain, France, Italy, Japan, India, Mexico, Norway, and the former Union of Soviet Socialist Republics. These pharmacopeias and the European Pharmacopeia (EP or Ph Eur) are used within the respective legal jurisdictions and by multinational pharmaceutical companies that develop and market products internationally. Countries not having a national pharmacopeia frequently adopt one of another country in setting and regulating drug standards. The pharmacopeia selected is usually based on geographic proximity, a common heritage or language, or a similarity of drugs and pharmaceutical products used. For example, Canada, which does not have its own national pharmacopeia, has traditionally used USP/NF standards. The Mexican Pharmacopeia [Farmacopea de los Estados Unidos Mexicanos (FEUM)] is the only other actively maintained pharmacopeia in this hemisphere (7).

Standards Set Forth in FDA-Approved New Drug Applications

In the United States, in addition to the official compendia, some initial drug and drug product standards and assay methods are established as set forth in New Drug and Antibiotic Applications approved by the Food and Drug Administration (see Chapter 2). These initial standards must be rigidly adhered to by the manufacturer to maintain product quality and continued FDA-approval for marketing. Ultimately, these or subsequently developed standards, are adopted as new monographs by the USP/NF.

International Organization for Standardization (ISO)

The International Organization for Standardization (ISO) is an international consortium of representative bodies constituted to develop and promote uniform or harmonized international standards. Representing the United States in the consortium is the American National Standards Institute.

Among the various ISO-standards used in the pharmaceutical industry are those in the series ISO 9000-ISO 9004. Included here are standards pertaining to development, production, quality assurance (QA), quality control (QC), detection of defective products, quality management (QM), and other issues as product safety and liability. Industry compliance with the standards is voluntary. However, many firms find it advantageous to their business to comply with ISO-standards and to be identified within their industry as having an internationally recognized quality-management system. Some companies choose to become ISO-certified through a rigorous evaluation and accreditation process (8).

Drug Regulation and Control

The first Federal law in the United States designed to regulate drug products manufactured domestically was the Food and Drug Act of 1906. The law required drugs marketed through interstate commerce to comply with their claimed standards for strength, purity, and quality. Manufacturers' claims of therapeutic benefit were not regulated until 1912, when the passage of the Sherley Amendment specifically prohibited false claims of therapeutic effects, declaring such products "misbranded."

The Federal Food, Drug, and Cosmetic Act of 1938

The need for additional drug standards was tragically demonstrated in 1938. The then-new wonder drug, sulfanilamide, which was not soluble in most common pharmaceutical solvents of the day, was prepared and distributed by an otherwise reputable manufacturer as an elixir using as the solvent diethylene glycol, a highly toxic agent used in antifreeze solutions. Before the product could be removed from the market, more than 100 persons lost their lives due to the toxic effects of diethylene glycol. The necessity for proper product formulation and thorough pharmacologic and toxicologic testing of the therapeutic agent, pharmaceutic ingredients, and the completed product was painfully recognized. Congress responded with passage of the Federal Food, Drug, and Cosmetic Act of 1938 and the creation of the Food and Drug Administration (FDA) to administer and enforce it. Included in the Act is a provision that prohibits the distribution and use of any new drug or drug product without the prior filing of a New Drug Application (NDA) and approval of the FDA. It became the responsibility of the FDA to either grant or deny permission to distribute a new product after reviewing the applicant's filed data on the product's ingredients, methods of assay and quality standards, formulation and manufacturing processes, preclinical (animal, tissue- or cell-culture) studies including pharmacology and toxicology, and clinical trials on human subjects. Although the Act of 1938 required pharmaceutical products to be safe for human use, it did not require them to be efficacious.

Durham-Humphrey Amendment of 1952

Drugs approved for marketing by the Food and Drug Administration are categorized according to the manner in which they may be legally obtained by the patient. Drugs deemed safe enough for use by the layman in the self-treatment of simple conditions for which competent medical care is not sought are classified as "over-the-counter" (OTC) or non-prescription drugs and may be sold without the requirement of a physician's or other legally authorized prescriber's prescription. The over-the-counter status of a drug product may be changed if more stringent control over the drug's distribution and use is warranted later. Other drugs that are considered useful only after expert diagnosis or too dangerous for use in self-medication are made available to the patient only by prescription. These drugs must bear the symbol "Rx-only" or the legend: "Caution: Federal Law Prohibits Dispensing Without Prescription." New drug substances are limited to prescription-only dispensing. However, their legal status may be changed to OTC, albeit usually at lower recommended dosage, should they later be considered useful and safe enough for the layperson's discretionary use. Examples of such drugs include ibuprofen, ketoprofen, cimetidine, and ranitidine.

According to the Durham-Humphrey Amendment, prescriptions for Legend drugs may not be refilled (dispensed again after the initial filling of the prescription) without the express consent of the prescriber. The refill status of prescriptions for certain Legend drugs known to be subject to public abuse was further regulated with the passage of the Drug Abuse Control Amendments of 1965 and then by the Comprehensive Drug Abuse Prevention and Control Act of 1970.

Kefauver-Harris Amendments of 1962

A major drug tragedy that occurred in 1960 led to the passage of the Kefauver-Harris Amendments to the Federal Food Drug and Cosmetic Act of 1938. A new synthetic drug, thalidomide, recommended as a sedative and tranquilizer, was being sold in Europe without the requirement of a physician's prescription. It was a drug of special interest due to its apparent lack of toxicity even at extreme dosage levels. It was hoped that it would replace the barbiturates as a sedative and therefore prevent the frequent deaths caused from accidental and intentional barbiturate overdosage. A pharmaceutical company was awaiting FDA approval for marketing in the United States when reports of a toxic effect of the drug's use in Europe began to appear. Thalidomide given to women during pregnancy produced birth defects, most notably phocomelia, an arrested development of the limbs of the affected newborn. Thousands of children were affected to various extents (9). Some were born without arms or legs; others, with partially formed limbs. The more fortunate were born with only disfigurations of the nose, eyes, and ears. Those more severely afflicted died—the result of internal malformation of the heart or gastrointestinal tract. This drug catastrophe spurred Congress to strengthen the existing laws regarding new drugs. Without dissent, on October 10, 1962, the Kefauver-Harris Drug Amendments to the Food, Drug, and Cosmetic Act of 1938 were passed by both houses of Congress. The purpose of the enactment was to ensure a greater degree of safety for approved drugs and manufacturers were now required to prove a drug both safe and effective before it would be granted FDA approval for marketing.

Under the Food, Drug, and Cosmetic Act as amended, the sponsor of a new drug is required to file an Investigational New Drug Application (IND) with the FDA before the drug may be clinically tested on human subjects. Only after carefully designed and structured human clinical trials, in which the drug is evaluated for safety and effectiveness, may the drug's sponsor file a New Drug Application seeking approval for marketing. The requirements for these and other submissions to the FDA are presented in Chapter 2.

Interestingly, thalidomide is now considered by the World Health Organization to be the standard treatment for the fever and painful skin lesions associated with erythema nodosum leprosum (ENL) in patients with leprosy and has been used for this purpose worldwide for many years (10). In 1997, an FDA Advisory Committee recommended that the agency approve thalidomide for the treatment of ENL in the United States under strict distribution controls and with appropriate patient education programs (11). The potential usefulness of thalidomide in other conditions, as rheumatoid arthritis, multiple sclerosis, AIDs- and cancer-related cachexia, HIV/AIDS progression, and aphthous ulcers, is under current investigation (12).

Comprehensive Drug Abuse Prevention and Control Act of 1970

The Comprehensive Drug Abuse Prevention and Control Act of 1970 served to consolidate and codify control authority over drugs of abuse into a single statute. Under its provisions, the Drug Abuse Control Amendments of 1965, the Harrison Narcotic Act of 1914, and other related laws governing stimulants, depressants, narcotics and hallucinogens were repealed and replaced by regulatory framework now administered by the Drug Enforcement Administration (DEA) in the Department of Justice.

The Comprehensive Drug Abuse Prevention and Control Act of 1970 established five "schedules" for the classification and control of drug substances that are subject to public abuse. These schedules provide for decreasing levels of control from Schedule I drugs to those classified as Schedule V drugs. The drugs in the five schedules may be described as follows:

Schedule I—Drugs with no accepted medical use, or other substances, with a high potential for abuse. In this category are agents as heroin, LSD, mescaline, peyote, methaqualone, and similar items. Any non-medical substance that is being abused can be placed in this category.

Schedule II—Drugs with accepted medical uses and a high potential for abuse which, if abused, may lead to severe psychological or physical dependence. In this category are morphine, cocaine, methamphetamine, amobarbital, and other such drugs.

Schedule III—Drugs with accepted medical uses and a potential for abuse less than those listed in Schedules I and II which, if abused, may lead to moderate psychological or physical dependence. In this category are specified quantities of codeine, hydrocodone, and similar agents.

Schedule IV—Drugs with accepted medical uses and low potential for abuse relative to those in Schedule III which, if abused, may lead to limited physical dependence or psychological dependence relative to drugs in Schedule III. In this category are specified quantities of diphenoxin, diazepam, oxazepam, and similar agents.

Schedule V—Drugs with accepted medical uses and low potential for abuse relative to those in Schedule IV and which, if abused, may lead to limited physical dependence or psychological dependence relative to drugs in Schedule IV. Included in this category are specified quantities of dihydrocodeine, diphenoxylate, and similar agents.

In all instances, local and state laws may strengthen the Federal drug laws but may not be used to weaken them.

Drug Listing Act of 1972

The Drug Listing Act was enacted to provide the Food and Drug Administration with the legislative authority to compile a list of currently marketed drugs to assist the Agency in the enforcement of Federal laws requiring that drugs be safe and effective and not adulterated or misbranded. Under the regulations of the Act, each firm that manufactures or repackages drugs for ultimate sale or distribution to patients or consumers must register with the FDA and submit appropriate information for listing. All foreign drug manufacturing and distributing firms whose products are imported into the United States are also included in this regulation. Exempt from the registration and listing requirements are hospitals, clinics, and the various health practitioners who prepare pharmaceutical products for use in their respective institutions and practices. Also exempt are research and teaching institutions in which drug products are prepared for purposes other than sale. Each registrant is assigned a permanent registration number, following the format of the National Drug Code (NDC) numbering system. Under this system, the first 4 numeric characteristics of 10-character code identify the manufacturer or distributor and are referred to as the "Labeler Code." The last 6 numeric characters of the 10-character code identify the drug formulation and the trade package size and type. The segment that identifies the drug formulation is known as the "Product Code," and the segment that identifies the trade package size and type is called the "Package Code." The manufacturer or distributor determines the ratio of use of the last 6 digits for the two codes, as a 3-to-3 digit Product-Code-Package Code configuration (e.g., 542-112) or a 4-to-2 digit configuration (e.g., 5421-12). Only one such type of configuration may be selected for use by a manufacturer or distributor who then assigns a code number to each product to be included in the drug listing. A final code number is presented as the example: NDC 0081-5421-12.

The National Drug Code numbers appear on all manufacturer's drug labeling. In some instances, manufacturers imprint the NDC number directly on the dosage units, as capsules and tablets, for rapid and positive identification when the number is matched in the National Drug Code Directory or against a decoding list provided by the manufacturer. Once a number is assigned to a drug product, it is a permanent assignment. Even in instances in which a drug manufacturer discontinues the manufacture and distribution of a product, the number may not be used again. If a drug product is substantially changed, as through an alteration in the active ingredients, dosage form, or product name, a new NDC number is assigned to the product by the registrant and the FDA advised accordingly.

The product information received by the FDA from each registrant is processed and stored in computer files to provide easy access to the following types of information:

1. List of all drug products.
2. List of all drug products broken down by labeled indications or pharmacologic category.

3. List of all drug products, broken down by manufacturer.
4. List of a drug product's active ingredients.
5. List of a drug product's inactive ingredients.
6. List of drug products containing a particular ingredient.
7. List of drug products newly marketed or re-marketed.
8. List of drug products discontinued.
9. All labeling of drug products.
10. All advertising of drug products.

The drug listing program enables the FDA to monitor the quality of all drugs on the market in the United States.

In a continuing effort to ensure the standards for drug quality control, the FDA's regulations provide not only for the inspection and certification of pharmaceutical manufacturing procedures and facilities, but also for the field surveillance and assay of products obtained from the shelves of retail distributors.

In instances in which a manufacturer is not meeting the established standards for drug product quality, that manufacturer will be denied permission to continue to produce products for distribution until compliance with the standards is attained.

Drug Price Competition and Patent Term Restoration Act of 1984

Changes to speed FDA approval of generic drugs and the extension of patent life for innovative new drugs were the major components of the Drug Price Competition and Patent Restoration Act of 1984.

Under the provisions of the legislation applications for generic copies of an originally approved new drug can be filed through an Abbreviated New Drug Application (ANDA) and not require the extensive animal and human studies of an NDA. This reduces considerably the time and expense of bringing a generic version of the drug to market. The FDA evaluates the chemistry, manufacturing, control standards and the drug's bioavailability in determining that the generic version is sufficiently equivalent to the originally approved drug.

For holders of patented drugs, the legislation provides an extension of patent life, equal to the time required for FDA review of the NDA, plus half the time spent in the testing phase, up to a maximum of 5 years and not to exceed the usual 20-year patent term. This extends the effective patent life and exclusive marketing period for innovative new

drug product thereby encouraging pioneering research and development.

Prescription Drug Marketing Act of 1987

The Prescription Drug Marketing Act of 1987 established new safeguards on the integrity of the nation's supply of prescription drugs. Because of its author, Representative John Dingell, and its purpose to prevent drug diversion, the Act has often been referred to as the Dingell Bill, and the Drug Diversion Act. The Act is intended to reduce the risks of adulterated, misbranded, repackaged, or mislabeled drugs entering the legitimate marketplace through "secondary sources." The primary sections of the Act are summarized as follows:

1. Reimportation. Prohibits the reimportation of drug products manufactured in the United States except by the manufacturer of the product.
2. Sales Restrictions. Prohibits selling, trading, purchasing, or the offer to sell, trade or purchase a drug sample. It also prohibits resales by health care institutions of pharmaceuticals purchased explicitly for the use of the institution. Charitable institutions that receive drugs at reduced prices or no cost cannot resell the drugs.
3. Distribution of Samples. Samples may only be distributed to: (a) practitioners licensed to prescribe such drugs and, (b) at the written request of the practitioner, to pharmacies of hospitals or other health care institutions. Sample distribution must be made through mail or common carrier and not directly by employees or agents of the manufacturer.
4. Wholesale Distributors. Manufacturers are required to maintain a list of their authorized distributors. Wholesalers who desire to distribute a drug for which they are not authorized distributors must inform their wholesale customers, prior to the sale, the name of the person from whom they obtained the goods and all previous sales.

Dietary Supplement Health and Education Act of 1994

In passing the Dietary Supplement Health and Education Act (DSHEA) of 1994, Congress recognized the growing interest in the use of various herbs and dietary supplements and addressed the need to regulate the labeling claims made for these products. These products, which include vitamins, minerals, amino acids and botanicals, legally are not considered drugs if they have not been submitted for review on New Drug Applications and thus have not been evaluated for safety and efficacy by the Food and Drug Administration. However, like drugs, their safe use is of concern to the FDA.

The Act forbids manufacturers or distributors of these products to make any advertising or labeling claims that indicate that the use of the product can prevent or cure a specific disease. In fact, a disclaimer must appear on the product that states: "This product is not intended to diagnose, treat, cure, or prevent any disease." However, the law does permit claims of benefit as they may properly relate to a nutrient deficiency disease; or, based on scientific evidence, how an ingredient may affect the body's "structure or function," (as increase circulation or lower cholesterol); or, how use of the product can affect a persons general well-being. But, before any promotional or labeling claims may be made, they first must be submitted to the FDA as being truthful and not misleading (13).

The use of herbs and nutritional supplements are part of today's milieu of "alternative" therapies and as such are receiving increased attention on the part of the scientific community and the FDA. Many of these agents, as ginseng, ginkgo, saw palmetto, St. John's wort, and echinacea are used worldwide and have been the subject of literature reports and research conducted in Europe and Asia. In 1997, a report of the U.S. Presidential Commission on Dietary Supplement Labels called for more research in this country on the health benefits of dietary supplements. In response, academic and NIH-sponsored studies are being undertaken to assess the therapeutic usefulness of some of these agents and to determine their safety.

The Food and Drug Administration (FDA) and the Food and Drug Administration Modernization Act of 1997

As noted previously, the Food and Drug Administration was established in 1938 to administer and enforce the Federal Food Drug and Cosmetic Act. Starting with this initial authority, today the FDA is responsible for enforcing many additional pieces of legislation.

The mission of the FDA is to protect the public health against risks associated with the production, distribution, and sale of food and food additives, human drugs and biologics, radiological and medical devices, animal drugs and feeds, and cosmetics.

In carrying out the intent of legislation it is mandated to enforce, the FDA:

- Sets policies, establishes standards, issues guidelines, and promulgates and enforces rules and regulations governing the affected industries and their products;
- Monitors for regulatory compliance through reporting requirements, product sampling and testing, and establishment inspections;
- Establishes product labeling requirements, disseminates product use and safety information, issues product warnings, and directs product recalls; and,
- Acts as the government's gatekeeper in making safe and effective new drugs, clinical laboratory tests, and medical devices available through a carefully conducted application and review process.

Within the federal organizational structure, the FDA is an agency of the Department of Health and Human Services (HHS). The FDA is organized into appropriate units to support its various responsibilities and functions (e.g., new drug evaluation, regulatory compliance). The Center for Drug Evaluation and Research (CDER) and the Center for Biologics Evaluation and Research (CBER), are responsible for the drug/biologics approval process as described in Chapter 2. The FDA is headquartered in Rockville, MD, with employees throughout the United States in six geographic regions, each with district offices and resident inspection posts.

The FDA Modernization Act of 1997 was enacted to streamline FDA policies and to codify many of the agency's newer regulations (14). The bill expanded patient access to investigational treatments for AIDS, cancer, Alzheimer's disease and other serious or life-threatening illnesses. It also provided for faster new drug approvals by using drug sponsor's fees to hire additional internal reviewers, by the authorized use of external reviewers, and by changes in the requirements demonstrating a drug's clinical effectiveness. It also provided incentives for investigations of drugs for pediatric patient use.

The legislation included provisions to track clinical trial data in a joint program with the National Institutes of Health (NIH); established a system to follow and review studies of the safety and efficacy of marketed drug products; established a program for the dissemination of information on "off-label uses" of marketed drugs and encouraged applications for additional therapeutic indications; and fostered the expansion of the FDA's information management system and the agency's progress toward paperless systems for human drug applications.

Of special importance to pharmacists, the legislation contains a section on pharmaceutical compounding that recognizes and defines this component of professional practice. Standards for Good Compounding Practices are presented in Chapter 5.

To codify, enable, and enforce legislative authority, the FDA develops relevant guidelines and regulations. These are first published in the Federal Register for public comment, and when finalized, in the Code of Federal Regulations.

Code of Federal Regulations and The Federal Register

Title 21 of the Code of Federal Regulations (CFR) consists of eight volumes containing all regulations issued under the Federal Food, Drug and Cosmetic Act and other statutes administered by the FDA. A ninth volume contains regulations issued under statutes administered by the Drug Enforcement Administration. The volumes are updated each year to incorporate all regulations issued during the preceding 12-month period. The Federal Register (FR), is issued each workday by the Superintendent of Documents, U.S. Government Printing Office (GPO), and contains proposed and final regulations and legal notices issued by Federal agencies, including the Food and Drug Administration and the Drug Enforcement Administration. These publications provide the most definitive information on Federal laws and regulations pertaining to drugs. The Federal Register and the Code of Federal Regulations are available in print and online through GPO Access (http://www.access.gpo.gov/nara/cfr).

Drug Product Recall

In instances in which the FDA or a manufacturer finds that a marketed product presents a threat or a potential threat to consumer safety, that product may be "recalled" or sought for return to the manufacturer from its depth of distribution. The pharmaceutical manufacturer is legally bound to report serious unlabeled adverse reactions to the FDA within 15 working days of learning of an adverse drug reaction. The FDA/USP Drug Product Problem Reporting (DPPR) Program, which began in 1970, is designed to protect the public health, to monitor manufacturer compliance with Current Good Manufacturing Practices (CGMP) and to detect product defects in the marketplace. A practitioner can report a problem with any drug product

or medical device by telephone or written report form, using the FDA's Medical Products Reporting Program, termed "MedWatch." Reported problems may include product defects, product adulteration, container leakage, improper labeling, unexpected adverse reactions, and others.

A drug product recall may be initiated by the FDA or by the manufacturer, the latter case being termed a "voluntary recall."' A numerical classification, as follows, indicates the degree of consumer hazards associated with the product being recalled:

Class I is a situation in which there is a reasonable probability that the use of, or exposure to, a violative product will cause serious, adverse health consequences or death.

Class II is a situation in which the use of, or exposure to, a violative product may cause temporary or medically reversible adverse health consequences or where the probability of serious adverse health consequences is remote.

Class III is a situation in which the use of, or exposure to, a violative product is not likely to cause adverse health consequences.

The "depth of recall,"' or the level of market removal or correction (as wholesaler, retailer, consumer), depends on the nature of the product, the urgency of the situation, and depth to which the product has been distributed. The lot numbers of packaging control numbers on the containers or labels of the products help in identifying the product to be recalled.

The Pharmacist's Contemporary Role

Pharmacy graduates holding the Bachelor of Science in Pharmacy (BS) degree or the Doctor of Pharmacy (PharmD) degree practice in a variety of settings in which the basic pharmaceutical sciences, the clinical sciences, and professional training and experiences are applied. This includes practice in community pharmacies, patient-care institutions, managed care, home health care, military and government service, academic settings, professional associations, and the pharmaceutical research and manufacturing industry as well as in other positions requiring the pharmacist's expertise.

The majority of pharmacists practice within an ambulatory care/community pharmacy setting. In this setting, the pharmacist plays an active role in the patient's use of prescription and nonprescription medication, diagnostic agents, durable medical equipment and devices, and other health-related products. The pharmacist develops individualized patient medication profiles, issues patient information leaflets (PILS), counsels patients on their health status, and provides information on the use of drug and nondrug measures. As members of the health care team, pharmacists serve as a source of drug information and participate in the selection, monitoring, and assessment of drug therapy.

A substantial number of pharmacists practice in institutional settings as hospitals, clinics, extended care facilities and Health Maintenance Organizations (HMOs). In these settings, pharmacists manage drug distribution and control systems and provide a variety of clinical services as drug utilization reviews (DUR), drug use evaluations (DUE), therapeutic drug monitoring, intravenous admixture programs, pharmacokinetic consult service, investigational drug supplies, and poison control and drug information.

The Board of Pharmaceutical Specialties certifies practice specialties in nuclear pharmacy, nutrition support pharmacy, pharmacotherapy, psychiatric pharmacy, and oncology pharmacy.

In recent years, managed health care programs have grown extraordinarily. Managed health care organizations have enrolled a large and rapidly growing base of patients and thus have assumed major responsibilities in the delivery of health care, including the delivery of pharmaceutical services. Many new positions have evolved for pharmacists within the managed care industry, including positions for pharmacy benefits managers, disease management specialists, drug formulary managers, therapeutic outcomes researchers, drug utilization review specialists, and others (15–16). In these functions, managed care pharmacists apply administrative, epidemiological, clinical, financial, research, information technology systems, and communication skills to their practice.

A number of pharmacy graduates, particularly those having an interest in institutional practice, participate in postgraduate residency and/or fellowship programs to enhance their practice and/or research skills. A pharmacy residency is: an organized, directed postgraduate training program in a defined area of practice. The chief purpose is to train pharmacists in professional practice and management skills. Residency programs are conducted primarily in institutional practice settings. A fellowship, to develop skill in research, is: a directed, highly individualized postgraduate program designed to prepare the participant to become an independent researcher. Both pharmacy residencies

and fellowships last 12 months or longer and require the close direction of a qualified preceptor.

Pharmacists working for pharmaceutical research, development, and manufacturing firms can participate in a range of activities, including drug discovery, drug analysis and quality control, product development and production, clinical studies and drug evaluation, labeling and drug literature, marketing and sales, and management. The pharmacist's knowledge of the basic chemical, biological and pharmaceutical sciences along with technical knowledge of product formulation, dosage form design and clinical use meshes well with the requirements of the pharmaceutical industry. Pharmacists with advanced degrees (Master's degrees or Doctor of Philosophy [PhD]) in the basic or pharmaceutical sciences or in areas of health care administration are highly sought within the pharmaceutical industry.

In government service, pharmacists perform professional and administrative functions in the development and implementation of pharmaceutical care delivery programs and in the design and enforcement of regulations involving drug distribution and drug quality standards. Career opportunities for pharmacists in government service at the Federal level include positions in the military service, in the Public Health Service, and in such Civil Service agencies as the Food and Drug Administration, Veterans Administration, Department of Health and Human Services, Drug Enforcement Administration of the Department of Justice, National Institutes of Health, and others. At the state and local levels, many pharmacists find rewarding careers in health departments, family and children's services, drug investigation and regulatory control, clinics and other health-care institutions, and with state boards of pharmacy.

Schools of pharmacy hire pharmacists, some with and some without advanced degrees, to serve as preceptors within the practice setting, to teach specific courses and/or laboratories within the academic institution, to participate in extramural research, and to contribute to the service and continuing education mission of the school. Some pharmacists work full-time in the academic setting, whereas many others provide part-time professional instruction in community or hospital pharmacies, teaching hospitals and clinics, drug information centers, nursing homes and extended care facilities, health departments, home health care, managed care, and in other areas in which pharmaceutical services are delivered.

A number of pharmacists serve their profession

in volunteer or professional positions with local, state and national pharmaceutical associations.

Pharmacists exercise a vital health education role in their communities through participation in drug/health education community forums, by speaking on drug-related issues in schools, by conducting in-service education programs in patient-care settings, and by providing input on drug/health issues to legislators and other community leaders and officials.

The Mission of Pharmacy

In 1990, the Board of Trustees of the American Pharmaceutical Association (APhA) adopted the following mission statement for pharmacy (17):

The mission of pharmacy is to serve society as the profession responsible for the appropriate use of medications, devices, and services to achieve optimal therapeutic outcomes.

The elements of the statement were defined as follows:

Pharmacy is the health profession that concerns itself with the knowledge system that results in the discovery, development, and use of medications and medication information in the care of patients. It encompasses the clinical, scientific, economic, and educational aspects of the profession's knowledge base and its communication to others in the health-care system.

Society encompasses patients, other health-care providers, health-policy decision makers, corporate health benefits managers, the healthy public, and other individuals and groups to whom health care and medication use are important.

Appropriate refers to the pharmacist's responsibility to ensure that a medication regimen is specifically tailored for the individual patient, based on accepted clinical and pharmacological parameters. Further, the pharmacist should evaluate the regimen to assure maximum safety, cost effectiveness, and compliance by the patient.

Medications refers to legend and nonlegend agents used in the diagnosis, treatment, prevention, and/or cure of disease. The term is specifically and purposefully used and is distinguished from the term drug, which has a negative and nontherapeutic public image.

Devices refers to the equipment, process, biotechnological entities, diagnostic agents, or other products that are used to assist in effective management of the medication regimen.

Services refers to patient, health professional and public education services, screening and monitoring programs, medication-regimen management, and related activities that contribute to effective medication use by patients.

Optimal therapeutic outcomes declares the profession's ultimate contribution to public health. Pharmacy

asserts it unique rights, privileges, and responsibilities—and accepts the attendant liabilities—associated with medication use. Pharmacy recognizes the need effectively to integrate its healthcare role with the complementary roles of the patient and other health care professionals.

Definition of Pharmaceutical Care

Today, the primary role of the pharmacist in contemporary practice is the delivery of pharmaceutical care. The term pharmaceutical care was first proposed in 1975 by Mikeal and others, as "the care that a given patient requires and receives which assures rational drug usage" (18). Since then, the term has been redefined by many authors, including Strand and others who, in 1992, stated (19):

Pharmaceutical care is that component of pharmacy practice which entails the direct interaction of the pharmacist with the patient for the purpose of caring for that patient's drug-related needs.

The American Society of Health-System Pharmacists (ASHP), a national organization that represents pharmacists who practice in hospitals, health maintenance organizations (HMOs), long-term care facilities, home care agencies, and other components of health care systems, advanced the following statement on pharmaceutical care in 1993 (20):

The mission of the pharmacist is to provide pharmaceutical care. Pharmaceutical care is the direct, responsible provision of medication-related care for the purpose of achieving definite outcomes that improve a patient's quality of life.

The American Pharmaceutical Association, in 1996, issued its Principles of Practice for Pharmaceutical Care including the following general statement (21):

Pharmaceutical care is a patient-centered, outcomes oriented pharmacy practice that requires the pharmacist to work in concert with the patient and the patient's other healthcare providers to promote health, to prevent disease, and to assess, monitor, initiate, and modify medication use to assure that drug therapy regimens are safe and effective.

The goal of pharmaceutical care is to optimize the patient's health-related quality of life and achieve positive clinical outcomes, within realistic economic expenditures.

Implicit in all of these statements is the requirement of pharmacists to participate fully in all aspects of medication provision and their appropriate clinical use to achieve optimal therapeutic outcomes. The contemporary pharmacy literature is replete with research papers and articles in support of the concept and practice of pharmaceutical care, including: clinical skill development (22), pharmaceutical care databases (23), information technology (24) and literature retrieval (25), therapeutic drug monitoring and outcomes assessment (26–29), drug utilization review (30), pharmacotherapy and disease management (31–32), drug treatment protocols (33), adverse drug reaction monitoring (34), pharmacokinetic services (35), and strategies to implement pharmaceutical care (36).

In 1997, the American Association of Colleges of Pharmacy's (AACP) Janus Commission issued a report titled "Approaching the Millennium," which stated that to provide pharmaceutical care, the successful pharmacy graduate must be (37):

- A problem solver, capable of adapting to changes in health care;
- Able to achieve health outcomes through effective medication use that are valued by the health care system;
- Able to collaborate with and be a resource to physicians, nurses, and other health care team members; and,
- A committed life-long learner.

Pharmacy Practice Standards

The scope and standards of pharmacy practice are established in each state through laws and regulations promulgated by the state's Board of Pharmacy. Together with applicable Federal laws, they constitute the basis for the legal practice of pharmacy.

Over the years, various professional associations in pharmacy have developed documents termed standards of practice. One such document, "Practice Standards of the American Society of Health-System Pharmacists," is updated and published annually. In 1991, the American Pharmaceutical Association, the American Association of Colleges of Pharmacy, and the National Association of Boards of Pharmacy engaged a study of the scope of pharmacy practice to revalidate the Standards of Practice for the Profession of Pharmacy (which were published in 1979 and updated in 1986 as Competency Statements for Pharmacy Practice (38). They can be summarized as follows.

General Management and Administration of the Pharmacy: Selects and supervises pharmacists and non-professionals for pharmacy staff; establishes a pricing structure for pharmaceutical services and products; ad-

ministers budgets and negotiates with vendors; develops and maintains a purchasing and inventory system for all drugs and pharmaceutical supplies; initiates a formulary system. In general, establishes and administers pharmacy management, personnel and fiscal policy.

Activities Related to Processing the Prescription: Verifies prescription for legality, and physical and chemical compatibility; checks patient record before dispensing prescription; measures quantities needed to dispense prescription; performs final check of finished prescription; dispenses prescription.

Patient Care Functions: Clarifies patient's understanding of dosage; integrates drug-related with patient-related information; advises patient of potential drug-related conditions; refers patient to other health care resources; monitors and evaluates therapeutic response of patient; reviews and/or seeks additional drug-related information.

Education of Health Care Professionals and Patients: Organizes, maintains and provides drug information to other health care professionals; organizes and/or participates in "in pharmacy" education programs for other pharmacists; makes recommendations regarding drug therapy to physician or patient; develops and maintains system for drug distributions and quality control.

In 1998, a "Pharmacy Practice Activity Classification" project was undertaken by a consortium of ten pharmacy organizations to develop uniform language in describing practice activities in areas as pharmacotherapy, monitoring and therapeutic outcomes, dispensing medications, health promotion and disease prevention, and health systems management (39). The developed classification is intended to provide the common language to be used and understood within and without the profession in describing the practice activities of pharmacists.

The Omnibus Budget Reconciliation Act of 1990

The Omnibus Budget Reconciliation Act of 1990 (OBRA 90), which became effective on January 1, 1993, established a requirement for each state to develop and mandate drug use review (DUR) programs to improve the quality of pharmaceutical care provided to patients covered by the Federal medical assistance (Medicaid) program (40–41). The statute was designed to ensure that prescriptions are appropriate, medically necessary, and not likely to result in adverse medical effects. The statute required that each state's plan provide for a review of drug therapy before each prescription is filled and delivered to an eligible patient.

The regulations required patient medication monitoring for therapeutic appropriateness, therapeutic duplication, overutilization, underutilization, drug–disease contraindications, drug–drug interactions with other prescribed and OTC medications, drug–allergy interactions, correct drug dosage, duration of treatment, and clinical abuse or misuse. They also required that pharmacists offer therapeutic counseling to each recipient of a prescription, or the recipient's caregiver, regarding the drug, dosage and duration of use, route of administration, side effects, contraindications, techniques for self-monitoring drug therapy, proper storage, refill information, and action to be taken in the event of a missed dose. Pharmacists are to maintain patient medication profiles and therapeutic counseling records.

In designing the DUR programs, state boards of pharmacy commonly included the Federal requirements in the state's pharmacy practice regulations, thereby applying them to each recipient of a prescription—not only to patients receiving benefits under the Medicaid program. Many states used the model regulations for the practice of pharmaceutical care developed by the National Association of Boards of Pharmacy (NABP).

Code of Ethics for Pharmacists— American Pharmaceutical Association*

By definition, a profession is founded on an art, built on specialized intellectual training, and has as its primary objective the performing of a service. The principles on which the professional practice of pharmacy is based are embodied in the Code of Ethics of the American Pharmaceutical Association (APhA).

The APhA Code of Ethics has been revised over the years to reflect dynamic changes in the profession. The current version, revised in 1994, is as follows.

Preamble

Pharmacists are health professionals who assist individuals in making the best use of medications. This Code, prepared and supported by pharmacists, is intended to state publicly the principles that form the fundamental basis of the roles and responsibilities of pharmacists. These principles, based on moral obligations and virtues, are established to guide pharmacists in relationships with patients, health professionals, and society.

I. A pharmacist respects the covenantal relationship between the patient and pharmacist.

Considering the patient-pharmacist relationship as a covenant means that a pharmacist has moral obligations in response to the gift of trust received from society. In return for this gift, a pharmacist promises to help individuals achieve optimum benefit from their medications, to be committed to their welfare, and to maintain their trust.

II. A pharmacist promotes the good of every patient in a caring, compassionate, and confidential manner.

A pharmacist places concern for the well-being of the patient at the center of professional practice. In doing so, a pharmacist considers needs stated by the patient as well as those defined by health science. A pharmacist is dedicated to protecting the dignity of the patient. With a caring attitude and a compassionate spirit, a pharmacist focuses on serving the patient in a private and confidential manner.

III. A pharmacist respects the autonomy and dignity of each patient.

A pharmacist promotes the right of self-determination and recognizes individual self-worth by encouraging patients to participate in decisions about their health. A pharmacist communicates with patients in terms that are understandable. In all cases, a pharmacist respects personal and cultural differences among patients.

IV. A pharmacist acts with honesty and integrity in professional relationships.

A pharmacist has a duty to tell the truth and to act with conviction of conscience. A pharmacist avoids discriminatory practices, behavior or work conditions that impair professional judgment, and actions that compromise dedication to the best interests of patients.

V. A pharmacist maintains professional competence.

A pharmacist has a duty to maintain knowledge and abilities as new medications, devices, and technologies become available and as health information advances.

VI. A pharmacist respects the values and abilities of colleagues and other health professionals.

When appropriate, a pharmacist asks for the consultation of colleagues or other health professionals or refers the patient. A pharmacist acknowledges that colleagues and other health professionals may differ in the beliefs and values they apply to the care of the patient.

VII. A pharmacist serves individual, community, and societal needs.

The primary obligation of a pharmacist is to individual patients. However, the obligations of a pharmacist may at times extend beyond the individual to the community and society. In these situations, the pharmacist recognizes the responsibilities that accompany these obligations and acts accordingly.

VIII. A pharmacist seeks justice in the distribution of health resources.

When health resources are allocated, a pharmacist is fair and equitable, balancing the needs of patients and society.

Code of Ethics— American Association of Pharmaceutical Scientists

Like pharmacy practitioners, pharmaceutical scientists recognize their special obligation to society and to the public welfare. Members of the American Association of Pharmaceutical Scientists (AAPS) adopted the following Code of Ethics in 1991 (42).

In their scientific pursuits, they:

- Conduct their work in a manner that adheres to the highest principles of scientific research so as to merit the confidence and trust of peers and the public in particular regarding the rights of human subjects and concern for the proper use of animals involved and provision for suitable safeguards against environmental damage.
- Avoid scientific misconduct and expose and condemn it when recognized. This includes: knowingly misrepresenting data, experimental procedures or data analysis; plagiarism, improper inclusion or exclusion of authors, and willful exclusion of acknowledgments for previous contributions.
- Recognize latitude for differences of scientific opinion in the interpretation of scientific data and that such differences of opinion do not constitute unethical conduct.
- Disclose sources of external financial support for, or significant financial interests in the content of, research reports/publications and avoid the ma-

nipulation of the release of such information for illegal financial gain.
- Report results accurately, stating explicitly any known or suspected bias, opposing efforts to improperly modify data or conclusions and offering professional advice only on those subjects concerning which they themselves regard themselves competent through scientific education, training, or experience.
- Respect the known ownership rights of others in scientific research and seek prior authorization from the owner before disclosure or use of such information including the contents of manuscripts submitted for pre-publication review.
- Support in their research and among their employers the participation and employment of all qualified persons regardless of race, gender, creed, or national origin.

References

1. History of the Pharmacopeia of the United States. In: United States Pharmacopeia, 23rd rev. Rockville, MD: United States Pharmacopeial Convention, Inc., 1995;xlii–xlv.
2. History of the National Formulary. In: National Formulary, 18th ed. Rockville, MD: United States Pharmacopeial Convention, Inc., 1995;2196–2200.
3. Constitution and Bylaws. The United States Pharmacopeial Convention, Inc., Rockville, MD, 1990.
4. Chavez ML. Homeopathy. Hosp Pharm 1998;33:41–49.
5. Der Marderosian AH. Understanding homeopathy. J Am Pharm Assoc 1996;NS36:317–321.
6. Pray WS. The challenge to professionalism presented by homeopathy. Am J Pharm Ed 1996;60:198–204.
7. The United States Pharmacopeia, 23rd rev. Rockville, MD: United States Pharmacopeial Convention, Inc., 1995:liv.
8. Hassler J, Yankowsky, A. An overview of ISO 9001 certification. BioPharm 1995;19:48–50.
9. FDA. The thalidomide tragedy—25 years ago. FDA Consumer 1987;21:14–17.
10. Safety issues raised as thalidomide is considered for approval. Pharm Today 1997;3:1.
11. FDA talk paper. Rockville, MD: Food and Drug Administration 1997;T97–43:1–4.
12. Levien T, Baker DE, Ballasiotes, AA. Reviews of dexrazoxane and thalidomide. Hosp Pharm 1996;31:487–510.
13. Bonnell L. Packaging nutritional supplements. Pharmaceut Med Packaging News 1997;5:42–50.
14. Wechsler J. Congress modernizes FDA. Pharm Tech 1997;21:16–26.
15. Wynn P. New directions in pharmacy careers. Managed Care Pharm Prac 1996;3:14–19.
16. Vogenberg FR. Managed health care: a review. Hosp Pharm 1997;32:975–982.

17. The mission of pharmacy. Washington DC: American Pharmaceutical Association, 1990.
18. Mikeal RL, Brown TP, Lazarus HL, Vinson MC. Quality of pharmaceutical care in hospitals. Am J Hosp Pharm 1975;32:567–574.
19. Strand LM, Cipolle RJ, Morley PC. Pharmaceutical care: an introduction. Current Concepts. Kalamazoo MI: The Upjohn Co, 1992.
20. ASHP statement on pharmaceutical care. Bethesda MD: American Society of Health-System Pharmacists, 1993.
21. Principles of practice for pharmaceutical care. Washington DC: American Pharmaceutical Association, 1996.
22. Barnette DJ, Murphy CM, Carter BL. Clinical skill development for community pharmacists. JAPhA 1996; NS36:573–579.
23. Rodriquez de Bittner M, Michocki R. Pharmaceutical care databases. JAPhA 1997;NS37:595–596.
24. West DS, Szeinbach S. Information technology and pharmaceutical care. JAPhA 1997;NS37:497–501.
25. Grant KL, Herrier RN, Armstrong EP. Teaching a systematic search strategy improves literature retrieval skills of pharmacy students. Am J Pharm Ed 1996;60: 281–286.
26. Madan, PL. Therapeutic drug monitoring. US Pharm 1996;21:92–105.
27. McDonough RP. Interventions to improve patient pharmaceutical care outcomes. JAPhA 1996;NS36: 453–459.
28. Grainger-Rousseau TJ, Miralles MA, Hepler CH, et al. Therapeutic outcomes monitoring: application of pharmaceutical care guidelines to community pharmacy. JAPhA 1997;NS37:647–661.
29. Mullins, CD, Baldwin R, Perfetto, EM. What are outcomes? JAPhA 1996;NS36:39–49.
30. Kubacka RT. A primer on drug utilization review. JAPhA 1996;NS36:257–261.
31. Armstrong EP, Langley PC. Disease management programs. Am J Health-Syst Pharm 1996;53:53–58.
32. Rodriques de Bittner M, Haines ST. Pharmacy-based diabetes management: a practical approach. JAPhA 1997;NS37:443–455.
33. APhA Guide to drug treatment protocols. Washington DC: American Pharmaceutical Association, 1997.
34. ASHP guidelines on adverse drug reaction monitoring and reporting. Bethesda MD: American Society of Health-System Pharmacists, 1995.
35. ASHP statement on the pharmacist's role in clinical pharmacokinetic services. Bethesda MD: American Society of Health-System Pharmacists, 1989.
36. Chrymko MM. Strategies for implementing pharmaceutical care in a community health system. Hosp Pharm 1996;31:1567–1576.
37. Approaching the millennium: the report of the AACP Janus Commission. Alexandria VA: American Association of Colleges of Pharmacy, 1997.
38. Pancorbo SA, Campagna KD, Davenport JK, et al. Task force report of competency statements for pharmacy practice. Am J Pharm Ed 1987;51:196–206.
39. Pharmacy Practice Classification. JAPhA 1998;38: 139–148.
40. Medicaid program: drug use review program and electronic claims management system for outpatient drug claims. Washington DC: Health Care Financing Administration, Department of Health and Human Services, 1992; Federal Register 57:49397–49412.
41. Brushwood DB, Catizone CA, Coster J M. OBRA 90: what it means to your practice. US Pharm 1992;17: 64–73.
42. American Association of Pharmaceutical Scientists, Alexandria, VA.

2

NEW DRUG DEVELOPMENT AND APPROVAL PROCESS

Chapter at a Glance

THE FEDERAL Food, Drug, and Cosmetic Act, as regulated through Title 21 of the U.S. Code of Federal Regulations, requires a new drug to be approved by the Food and Drug Administration (FDA) before it may be legally introduced in interstate commerce (1). The regulations apply to drug products manufactured domestically as well as those imported into the United States.

To gain approval for marketing, a drug's sponsor (e.g., a pharmaceutical company) must demonstrate, through supporting scientific evidence, that the new drug/drug product is safe and effective for its proposed use. The sponsor must also demonstrate that the various processes and controls used in producing the drug substance and in manufacturing, packaging, and labeling the drug product are properly controlled and validated, to ensure the production of a product that meets established standards of quality.

The process and time-course from drug discovery to approval for marketing can be lengthy and tedious, but are well defined and understood within the pharmaceutical industry. A schematic representation of the process for new drug development is shown in Figure 2.1 and the usual time-course is depicted in Figure 2.2. After the discovery (e.g., synthesis) of a proposed new drug, the agent is biologically characterized for pharmacologic and toxicologic effects and for potential therapeutic application. Preformulation studies are initiated to define the physical and chemical properties of the agent. Formulation studies follow, to develop the initial features of the proposed pharmaceutical product or dosage form. To obtain the required evidence that will demonstrate the drug's safety and effectiveness for its proposed use, a carefully designed and progressive sequence of preclinical (e.g., cell culture, whole animal) and clinical (human) studies are undertaken.

Only when the preclinical studies demonstrate adequate safety and the new agent shows promise as a useful drug will the drug's sponsor file an Investigational New Drug Application (IND) with the FDA for initial testing in humans. If the drug demonstrates adequate safety in these initial human studies, termed Phase 1, progressive human trials through Phases 2 and 3 are undertaken to assess both safety and efficacy. As the clinical trials progress, laboratory work continues toward defining the agent's basic and clinical pharmacology and toxicology, product design and development, manufacturing scale-up and process controls, analytical methods development, proposed labeling and package design, and initial plans for marketing. At the completion of the carefully designed preclinical and clinical studies, the drug's sponsor may file a New Drug Application (NDA) seeking approval to market the new product.

The FDA's approval of an NDA indicates that the body of scientific evidence submitted sufficiently demonstrates that the drug/drug product is safe and effective for the proposed clinical indications; that there is adequate assurance of its proper manufacture and control; and that the final labeling accurately presents the necessary information for its proper use.

The content of a product's approved labeling, represented by the package insert, is a summary of the entire drug development process because it contains the essential chemistry, pharmacology, toxicology, indications and contraindications for use, adverse effects, formulation composition, dosage, and storage requirements, as ascertained during the research and development process.

In addition to the general new drug approval process, special regulations apply for the approval of certain new drugs to treat serious or life-threatening illnesses, as AIDS and cancer. These may be placed on an accelerated or "fast track" program for approval. Also, in instances in which there are no satisfactory approved-drug or treatment alternatives to treat a serious medical condition, special protocols may be issued permitting use of an investigational drug to treat some patients prior to approval of the NDA. This type of protocol is termed a "Treatment IND." Treatment INDs often are sought for "orphan drugs," which are targeted for small numbers of patients who have rare conditions or diseases for which there are no satisfactory alternative treatments.

For certain changes in a previously approved NDA, such as a labeling or formulation change, a manufacturer is required to submit for approval a Supplemental New Drug Application (SNDA).

An Abbreviated New Drug Application (ANDA) is used to gain approval to market a duplicate product (usually a competing generic product) to one that had been approved previously and marketed by the pioneer, or original sponsor, of the drug. In these instances, the sponsor of the ANDA provides documentation on the chemistry, manufacturing, controls, and bioavailability of the proposed product to demonstrate biologic equivalency to the original product (2). Clinical data on the drug's safety and efficacy are not required because clinical studies were previously provided by the pioneer sponsor.

Federal regulations are varied and specific for antibiotic drugs (3); for biologics, such as human blood products and vaccines, which require approval of a Biologics Licensing Application (BLA) for distribution (4); for OTC drugs (5); and for animal drugs, which may require an Investigational New Animal Drug Application (INADA), a New Animal Drug Application (NADA) or a Supplemental New Animal Drug Application (SNADA) (6). Medical devices, such as catheters and cardiac pacemakers, follow a separate premarket approval process as defined in the Code of Federal Regulations (7).

The following sections are intended to serve as an overview of the new drug development and approval process. More specific and detailed information may be obtained directly from the referenced sections of the Code of Federal Regulations (1–7), from relevant entries in the Federal Register (8), and from other treatises on the topic (9–13).

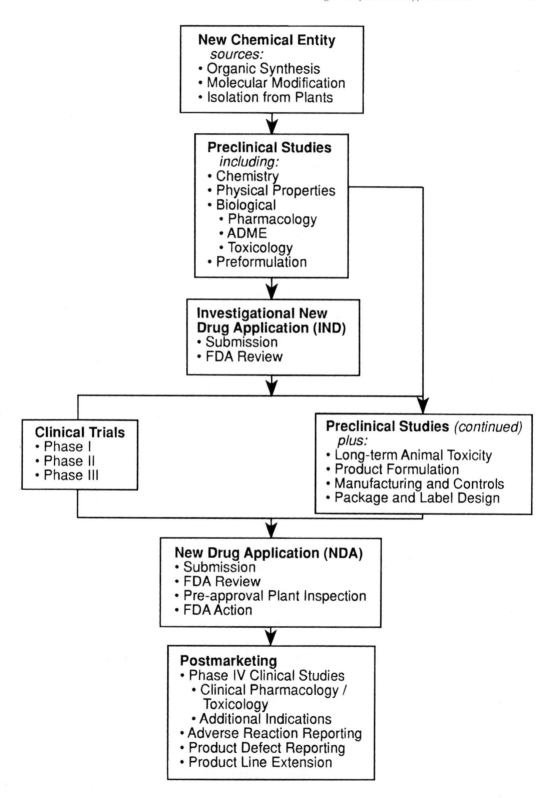

Fig. 2.1 *Schematic representation of the new drug development process, from drug discovery, through preclinical and clinical studies, FDA review of the new drug application, and postmarketing activities.*

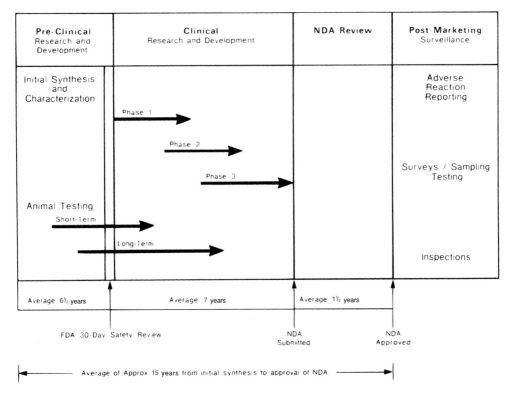

Fig. 2.2 *Time course for the development of a new drug. (Adapted from FDA Consumer, 21:5, 1987 and New Drug Approvals in 1997, Pharmaceutical Research and Manufacturers Association, January, 1998.)*

Drug Discovery and Drug Design

The discovery of new drugs and their development into commercial products takes place across the broad scope of the pharmaceutical industry. The basic underpinning for this effort is the cumulative body of scientific and biomedical information generated worldwide in research institutes, academic centers, and industry. The combined efforts of chemists, biologists, molecular biologists, pharmacologists, toxicologists, statisticians, physicians, pharmacists and pharmaceutical scientists, engineers, and many others are involved in the drug discovery and development process.

Some pharmaceutical firms focus their research and development (R&D) activities on new prescription drugs for human use, whereas other firms concentrate on the development of OTC medications, generic drugs, biotechnology products, animal health-care drugs, diagnostic products, and/or medical devices. Many of the large pharmaceutical companies develop and manufac-

ture products of various types, with some firms having subsidiary companies for specialized functions and products.

The pharmaceutical industry in the United States grew rapidly during World War II and in the years immediately following. The upsurge in the domestic production of drugs and pharmaceutical products stemmed in part from the wartime hazards and consequent undependability of overseas shipping, the unavailability of drugs from previous sources, and the increased need for drugs of all kinds, but especially those with life-saving capabilities. One such drug is penicillin, the antibiotic which became commercially available in 1944, 15 years after its discovery in England by Sir Alexander Fleming and 1 year before the end of the war.

After the war, other antibiotics were developed and today there is a host of them, with effectiveness against a range of pathogens. The postwar boom in drug discovery continued with the development of many new agents, as vaccines to protect against poliomyelitis, measles, and influenza, and new pharmacologic categories of drugs including oral hypoglycemic drugs effective against certain types of diabetes mellitus, antineoplastic or anticancer drugs, immunosuppressive agents which assist the body's acceptance of organ transplants, oral contraceptives to prevent pregnancy, and a host of tranquilizers and antidepressant drugs to treat the emotionally distressed.

In recent years, many new and important innovative therapeutic agents have been developed and approved by the FDA, including drugs to treat: acquired immune deficiency syndrome, AIDS (indinavir, Crixivan); refractory benign prostatic hyperplasia (finasteride, Proscar); migraine headaches (sumatriptan, Imitrex); ovarian carcinoma (paclitaxel, Taxol); gastric ulcers (cimetidine, Tagamet); hyperlipidemia (gemfibrozil, Lopid); hypertension (enalapril, Vasotec); congestive heart failure (carvedilol, Coreg); coronary artery disease (fluvastatin, Lescol); obsessive compulsive disorders (fluoxetine, Prozac); arthritis (nedocromil, Tilade); osteoporosis (alendronate, Fosamax); male impotence (sildenafil citrate, Viagra), infectious disease (ciprofloxacin, Cipro); and other diseases and conditions, with literally hundreds of potential therapeutic agents in various stages of clinical evaluation. Annually, approximately 40 new molecular entities (NME) receive FDA approval for marketing. In addition, many new dosage strengths and dosage forms of previously approved drugs, new generic products, and new biologics are approved each year.

Not all drugs are discovered, developed, and first approved in the United States. There are many pharmaceutical companies involved in drug research and development in other countries and many drugs are first marketed abroad. Many of the world's largest pharmaceutical companies are multinational firms and have facilities for research and development, manufacturing, and distribution in countries around the world. Irrespective of country of origin, a drug may be proposed by its sponsor for regulatory approval for marketing in the United States and/or in other countries. These approvals do not occur simultaneously, as they are subject to the laws, regulations, and requirements peculiar to each country's governing authority. However, the international effort to harmonize regulations through the work of the International Conference on Harmonization (ICH) as described at the end of this chapter fosters multinational drug approvals.

Sources of New Drugs

New drugs may be discovered from a variety of natural sources or created synthetically in the laboratory. They may be discovered by accident or as the result of many years of tireless pursuit.

Throughout history, plant materials have served as a reservoir of potential new drugs. Yet, only a small portion of the approximate 270,000 known plants thus far have been investigated for medicinal activity. Certain major contributions to modern drug therapy may be attributed to the successful conversion of botanic folklore remedies into modern wonder drugs. The chemical reserpine, a tranquilizer and hypotensive agent, is an example of a medicinal chemical isolated by design from the folklore remedy *Rauwolfia serpentina*. Another plant drug, periwinkle or *Vinca rosea*, was first scientifically investigated as a result of its reputation in folklore as an agent useful in the treatment of diabetes mellitus. Plant extractives from *Vinca rosea* yielded two potent drugs, which when screened for pharmacologic activity surprisingly exhibited antitumor capabilities. These two materials, vinblastine and vincristine, since have been used successfully in the treatment of certain types of cancer including acute leukemia, Hodgkin's disease, lymphocytic lymphoma, and other malignancies. Another example, paclitaxel (Taxol), prepared from an extract from the Pacific yew tree, is used in the treatment of ovarian cancer.

After the isolation and structural identification of active plant constituents, organic chemists may recreate them by total synthesis in the laboratory or more importantly use the natural chemical as the starting material in the creation of slightly different chemical structures through molecule manipulation procedures. The new structures, termed semisynthetic drugs, may have a slightly or vastly different pharmacologic activity than the starting substance, depending on the nature and extent of chemical alteration. Other plant constituents that in themselves may be inactive or rather unimportant therapeutically may be chemically modified to yield important drugs with profound pharmacologic activity. For example, the various species of *Dioscorea*, popularly known as Mexican yams, are rich in the chemical *steroid structure* from which cortisone and estrogens are semisynthetically produced.

Animals have served humans in their search for drugs in a number of ways. They not only have yielded to drug testing and biologic assay procedures but also have provided drugs that are mannered from their tissues or through their biologic processes. Hormonal substances such as thyroid extract, insulin, and pituitary hormone obtained from the endocrine glands of cattle, sheep, and swine are lifesaving drugs used daily as replacement therapy in the human body. The urine of pregnant mares is a rich source of estrogens. Knowledge of the structural architecture of the individual hormonal substances has produced a variety of synthetic and semisynthetic compounds with hormone-like activity. The synthetic chemicals used as oral contraceptives are notable examples.

The use of animals in the production of various biologic products, including serums, antitoxins, and vaccines, has been of lifesaving significance ever since the pioneering work of Dr. Edward Jenner on the smallpox vaccine in England in 1796. Today, the poliomyelitis vaccine is prepared in cultures of renal monkey tissue, the mumps and influenza vaccines in fluids of chick embryo, the rubella (German measles) vaccine in duck embryo, and the smallpox vaccine from the skin of bovine calves inoculated with vaccinia virus. New vaccines for diseases as AIDS and cancer are being developed through the use of cell and tissue cultures.

Today, we are witnessing a new era in the development of pharmaceutical products due to the advent of genetic engineering, the sub-microscopic manipulation of the "double helix," the spiral DNA chain of life. Through this process, will come more abundant and vastly purer antibiotics, vaccines, and yet unknown chemical and biological products to combat human disease.

There are two basic technologies that drive the genetic field of drug development; they are recombinant DNA (rDNA) and monoclonal antibody (MoAB) production (14–16). Common to each technique is the ability to manipulate and produce proteins, the building blocks of living matter. Proteins represent an almost infinite source of drugs. Made up of long chains of amino acids, their sequence and spatial configuration offer a staggering number of possibilities. Both recombinant DNA and monoclonal antibody production techniques influence cells in their ability to produce proteins.

The more fundamental of the two techniques is recombinant DNA. It can potentially produce almost any protein. Genetic material can be transplanted from higher species, such as humans, into a lowly bacterium. This so-called "gene splicing" can induce the lower organism to make proteins, it would not otherwise have made. Such drug products as human insulin, human growth hormone, hepatitis B vaccine, epoetin alpha, and interferon are being produced in this manner.

Whereas recombinant DNA techniques involve the manipulation of proteins within the cells of lower animals, monoclonal antibody production is conducted entirely within the cells of higher animals, including the patient. The technique exploits the ability of cells that have the potential to produce a desired antibody and stimulates an unending stream of pure antibody production. These antibodies then have the capacity to combat the specific target.

Monoclonal antibodies have an enormous potential to change the face of medicine and pharmacy in the next decade and applications for their use are already in progress. Diagnostically, for example, monoclonal antibodies are used in home pregnancy testing products. Their use ensures that a woman can perform the test easily, in a short period, with high reproducibility, and in an inexpensive manner. In these tests, the monoclonal antibody is highly sensitive to binding on one site on the human chorionic gonadotropin (HCG) molecule, a specific marker to pregnancy because in healthy women, HCG is synthesized exclusively by the placenta. In medicine, monoclonal antibodies are being used to stage and to localize malignant cells of cancer, and it is anticipated that they will be used in the future to combat disease such as lupus erythematosus, juvenile-onset diabetes, and myasthenia gravis.

Human gene therapy, used to prevent, treat, cure, diagnose, or mitigate human disease caused by genetic disorders, represents another promising new technology. The human body contains up to 100,000 genes. Genes that are aligned on a double strand of DNA in the nucleus of every cell control all of the body's functions. Base pairs of adenine (A) and thymine (T), and cytosine (C), and guanine (G), constitute the instructions on a gene. Only those genes necessary for a specific cell's function are active or expressed. When a gene is expressed, a specific type of protein is produced. In genetic-based diseases, gene expression may be altered and/or gene sequences may be mismatched, partly missing, or repeated too many times, causing cellular malfunction and disease.

Gene therapy is a medical intervention based on the modification of the genetic material of living cells. Cells may be modified outside the body (ex vivo) for subsequent administration, or they may be modified within the body (in vivo) by gene therapy products given directly to the patient. In either case, gene therapy involves the transfer of new genetic material to the cells of a patient afflicted with a genetic disease. The genetic material, usually cloned DNA, may be transferred into the patient's cells physically, as through microinjection, through chemically mediated transfer procedures, or through disabled retroviral gene transfer systems that integrate genetic material directly into the host cell chromosomes (17–19)

The first human gene therapy used was to treat adenosine deaminase (ADA) deficiency, a condition that results in abnormal functioning of the immune system. Therapy consisted of the administration of genetically modified cells capable of producing ADA (18). Many emerging biopharmaceutical companies are exploring the application of gene therapy to treat sickle cell anemia, malignant melanoma, renal cell cancer, heart disease, familial hypercholesteremia, cystic fibrosis, lung and colorectal cancer, and AIDS. The first commercialized gene therapy product is expected to reach the market soon after the publication date of this textbook (20).

Although there is justified excitement and great expectation for the potential of the new biotechnologies in the development of advanced therapies, the work of the synthetic organic chemist remains today's most usual source of new drugs. The modern chemists's work is enhanced by computer-based molecular modeling, access to hugh chemical libraries, and through the use of high throughput screening in discovering compounds having an affinity for specific biological target sites (21–22).

A "Goal Drug"

In theory, a "goal drug" would produce the specifically desired effect, be administered by the most desired route (generally orally) at minimal dosage and dosing frequency, have optimal onset and duration of activity, exhibit no side effects, and following its desired effect would be eliminated from the body efficiently, completely, and without residual effect. It would also be easily produced at low cost, be pharmaceutically elegant, and physically and chemically stable under various conditions of use and storage. Although not completely attainable in practice, these qualities and features are sought in drug and dosage form design.

Methods of Drug Discovery

Although some drugs may be the result of fortuitous discovery, most drugs are the result of carefully designed research programs of screening, molecular modification, and mechanism-based drug design (23).

Random or nontargeted screening involves the testing of large numbers of synthetic organic compounds or substances of natural origin for biologic activity. Random screens may be used initially to detect an unknown activity of the test compound or substance or to identify the most promising compounds to be studied by more sophisticated *nonrandom* or targeted screens to determine a specific activity.

Although random and nonrandom screening programs can examine a host of new compounds for activity, sometimes promising compounds may be overlooked if the screening models are not sensitive enough to reflect accurately the specific disease against which the agent, or its metabolites, may be useful (24).

To detect and evaluate biological activity, *bioassays* are used to differentiate the effect and potency (strength of effect) of the test agent compared with controls of known action and effect. The initial bioassays may be performed in vitro using cell cultures to test the new agent's effect against enzyme systems or tumor cells, whereas subsequent bioassays may be performed in vivo and involve more expensive and disease-specific animal models.

Newer methods, as high throughput screening, are capable of examining 15,000 chemical compounds a week using 10–20 biological assays (22). To be effective, this requires a sizeable and chemically diverse collection of compounds to examine, which many pharmaceutical and chemical companies have in "chemical libraries." Frequently these libraries, which may contain hundreds of thousands of compounds, are purchased or licensed from academic or commercial sources. With the advent of techniques as combinatorial chemistry, it has become feasible to increase substantially the size and diversity of a chemical library (22).

Molecular modification involves the chemical alteration of a known and previously characterized organic compound (frequently a *lead compound;* see next section) for the purpose of enhancing its usefulness as a drug. This could mean—enhancing its specificity for a particular body target site; increasing its potency; improving its rate and extent of absorption; modifying to advantage its time-course in the body; reducing its toxicity; or changing its physical or chemical properties (e.g., solubility) to provide pharmaceutically desired features (23). The molecular modifications may be slight or substantial, involving changes in functional groups, ring structures, or configuration. Knowledge of chemical structure-pharmacologic activity relationships (SAR) plays an important role in designing new drug molecules. Through molecular modification, new chemical entities and improved therapeutic agents result. Figures 2.3A and 2.3B present the

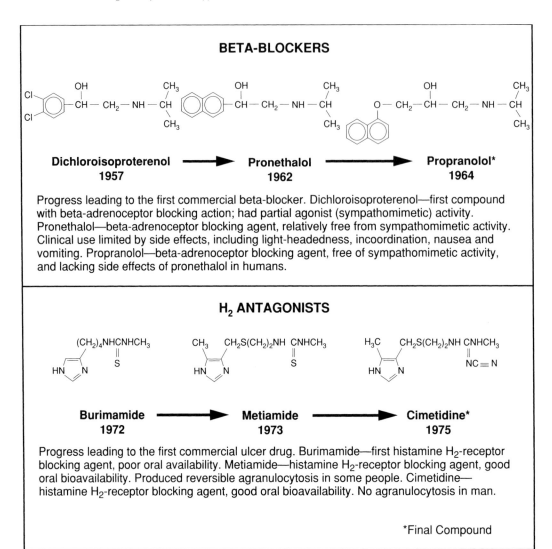

Fig. 2.3 *Molecular modifications leading to the development of the first commercial beta blocker, propranolol, and the first commercial histamine H₂-receptor blocking agent, cimetidine. (Reprinted with permission from Maxwell RA. The state of the art of the science of drug discovery. Drug Development Research 1984;4:375–389; through Pharmaceutical Research: Therapeutic and Economic Value of Incremental Improvements, 1990, p. 12. Courtesy of National Pharmaceutical Council, Reston, VA).*

molecular modifications that led to the discoveries of the first commercial beta blocker, propranolol, and the first commercial histamine H_2-receptor blocking agent, cimetidine.

Mechanism-based drug design involves molecular modification in designing a drug that interferes specifically with the known or suspected biochemical pathway or mechanism of a disease process. The intention is the interaction of the drug with specific cell receptors, enzyme systems, or the metabolic processes of pathogens or tumor cells,

resulting in a blocking, disruption, or reversal of the disease process. In designing drugs on this basis, it is essential to understand the biochemical pathway of the disease process and the manner in which it is regulated. *Molecular graphics,* the use of computer graphics to represent and manipulate the structure of the drug molecule to "fit" the simulated molecular structure of the receptor site, is a useful and complementary tool in drug molecule design.

An example of mechanism-based drug design is the compound enalaprilat (Vasotec), which inhibits the angiotensin-converting enzyme that catalyzes the conversion of angiotensin I to the vasoconstrictor substance angiotensin II. Inhibition of the enzyme results in decreased plasma angiotensin II leading to decreased vasopressor effects and the drug's use in lowering blood pressure in treating hypertension. Another example is ranitidine (Zantac), an inhibitor of histamine at the histamine H_2-receptors including receptors on the gastric cells. This inhibits gastric acid secretion making the drug effective in the treatment of gastric ulcers and other gastrointestinal conditions related to the production of gastric acid. A third example is sertraline (Zoloft), which inhibits the central nervous system neuronal uptake of serotonin, making the drug useful in the treatment of depression.

A "Lead Compound"

A "lead compound" is a prototype chemical compound that has a fundamental desired biologic or pharmacologic activity. Although active, the lead compound may not possess all of the features desired; i.e., potency, absorbability, solubility, low toxicity, and so forth. Thus, the medicinal chemist may seek to modify the lead compound's chemical structure to achieve the desired features while reducing the undesired ones. The chemical modifications produce analogs that have additional or different functional chemical groups, altered ring structures, or different chemical configurations. The results are modified chemical compounds capable of having different interactions with the body's receptors, thereby eliciting different actions and intensities of action.

The synthesis of derivatives of the prototype chemical may ultimately lead to successive "generations" of new compounds of the same pharmacologic type. This may be exemplified by the development of new generations of cephalosporin antibiotics; additional H_2 antagonists from the pioneer drug cimetidine; and the large series of antianxiety drugs derived from the benzodiazepine structure and the innovator drug chlordiazepoxide (Librium).

Most drugs exhibit activities secondary to their primary pharmacologic action. It is not uncommon to take advantage of a secondary activity by developing new compounds, through molecular modification, that amplify the secondary use of the drug, or by gaining approval to market the drug for a secondary indication. For example, the drug finasteride (Proscar) was originally developed and approved to treat benign prostatic hyperplasia. Later, the same drug, at a lower recommended dosage, was approved (as Propecia) to treat male pattern baldness.

Prodrugs

Prodrug is a term used to describe a compound that requires metabolic biotransformation after administration to produce the desired pharmacologically active compound. The conversion of an inactive prodrug to an active compound occurs primarily through enzymatic biochemical cleavage. Depending on the specific prodrug-enzyme interaction, the biotransformation may occur anywhere along the course of drug transit or at the body site where the requisite enzymes are sufficiently present. An example of a prodrug is enalapril (enalapril maleate, Vasotec) which, after oral administration, is bioactivated by hydrolysis to enalaprilat, an ACE inhibitor used in the treatment of hypertension. Prodrugs may be designed preferentially for the following reasons (23).

Solubility

A prodrug may be designed to possess solubility advantages over the active drug, enabling the use of specifically desired dosage forms and routes of administration. For example, if an active drug is insufficiently soluble in water to prepare a desired intravenous injection, a water-soluble prodrug could be prepared through the addition of a functional group that later would be detached by the metabolic process to yield, once again, the active drug molecule.

Absorption

A drug may be made more water- or lipid-soluble, as desired, to facilitate absorption via the intended route of administration.

Biostability

If an active drug is prematurely destroyed by biochemical or enzymatic processes, the design of a prodrug may protect the drug during its transport in the body. In addition, the use of a prodrug could result in site-specific action of greater potency.

Prolonged Release

Depending on a prodrug's rate of metabolic conversion to active drug, it may provide prolonged drug release and extended therapeutic activity.

FDA's Definition of a New Drug

According to the FDA, any drug that is not recognized among experts, qualified by scientific training and experience, as being safe and effective under the conditions recommended for its use is termed a"new drug"(1).

A drug need not be a new chemical entity to be considered a new drug by the FDA. A change in a previously approved drug product's formulation or method of manufacture constitute's"newness"under the law since such changes can alter the therapeutic efficacy and/or safety of a product.

A new combination of two or more old drugs or a change in the usual proportions of drugs in an established combination product would be considered "new" if a question of safety or efficacy is introduced by the change.

A proposed new use for an established drug, a new dosage schedule or regimen, a new route of administration, or a new dosage form all cause a drug or drug product to be"new"and reconsidered for safety and efficacy.

Drug Nomenclature

When first synthesized, or identified from a natural source, an organic compound is represented by an *empirical formula*, as $C_{14}H_{19}Cl_2NO_2$ for chlorambucil, which indicates the number and the relationship of the atoms comprising the molecule. As knowledge of the relative locations of these atoms is gained, the compound receives a *systematic chemical name*, as 4-[bis(2-chloroethyl)amino] − 4 − [*p*-[Bis(2-chloroethyl)amino]phenyl]butyric acid. To be adequate and fully specific, the name must reveal every part of the compound's molecular structure, so that it describes only that compound and no other. The systematic name is generally so formidable that it soon is replaced in scientific communication by a shortened name, which, although less descriptive chemically, is understood to refer only to that chemical compound. This shortened name is the chemical's *nonproprietary* (or generic) name (e.g., chlorambucil; see Fig. 1.2).

Today many companies give their new compounds *code numbers* before the assignment of a nonproprietary name. These code numbers take the form of an identifying prefix letter or letters that identify the drug's sponsor, followed by a number that further identifies the test compound (for example, SQ 14,225, the investigational code number for the drug captopril, initially developed by Squibb). The code number frequently stays with a compound from its initial preclinical laboratory investigation through human clinical trials.

When the results of testing indicate that a compound shows sufficient promise of becoming a drug, the sponsor may formally propose a nonproprietary name and may also apply to the U.S. Patent Office (and foreign agencies as well) for a proprietary or trademark name. Should the drug receive recognition in an official compendium, the nonproprietary name established during the period of the drug's early usage is adopted. Nonproprietary names are issued only for single agents whereas proprietary or trademark names may be associated with a single chemical entity or with a mixture of chemicals comprising a specific proprietary product.

The task of designating appropriate nonproprietary names for chemical agents rests primarily with the United States Adopted Names Council (USAN Council). This organized effort at coining nonproprietary names for drugs was inaugurated in 1961 as a joint project of the American Medical Association and the United States Pharmacopeial Convention. They were joined in 1964 by the American Pharmaceutical Association to form the USAN Council; in 1967, the Food and Drug Administration was invited to take part in the work of the Council.

The United States Pharmacopeial Convention publishes the USAN and the *USP Dictionary of Drug Names*. In addition to listing the US Adopted Names, the reference also includes brand names of research-oriented firms, investigational drug code designations, official names of USP and NF articles with their chemical names and graphic formulas, and international nonproprietary names (INN) published by the World Health Organization (WHO). This reference of drug names now includes more than 18,000 entries.

A proposal for a USAN usually originates from a firm or an individual who has developed a substance of potential therapeutic usefulness to the point where there is a distinct possibility of its being marketed in the United States. Occasionally, the initiative is taken by the USAN Council in the form of a request to parties interested in a substance for which a nonproprietary name appears to be lacking. Proposals are expected to conform to the Council's guidelines for coining nonproprietary names. The name should: 1) be short and distinctive in sound and spelling and not be such that it is easily confused with existing names, 2) indicate the general pharmacologic or therapeutic class into which the substance falls or the general chemical nature of the substance if the latter is associated with the specific pharmacologic activity, and 3) embody the syllable or syllables characteristic of a related group of compounds.

When general agreement on a name has been reached between the Council and the drug's sponsor, it is announced as a "Proposed USAN." This indicates the Council's intention to adopt the name and serves notice on those who wish to protest the selection. The tentatively adopted USAN is then submitted for consideration by various American and foreign drug regulatory agencies, including the World Health Organization, the British Pharmacopoeia Commission, the French Codex, the Nordic Pharmacopeia, the United States Pharmacopeia and National Formulary, and the U.S. Food and Drug Administration. Under the 1962 Drug Amendments, the Secretary of the Department of Health and Human Services has authority to designate the nonproprietary name for any drug in the interest of usefulness or simplicity. The authority is delegated to the Commissioner of the Food and Drug Administration within the Department. If no objections are raised, adoption is considered final, and the USAN is published in the various literature of the medical and pharmaceutical professions. On rare occasion, a USAN-adopted name is changed to foster clarity or uniformity. With the creation of the USAN Council and the cooperation of the interested parties on a worldwide basis, nonproprietary drug nomenclature has become standardized.

Biological Characterization

Prospective drug substances must undergo preclinical testing for biologic activity to assess their potential as useful therapeutic agents. These studies fall into the general areas of pharmacology, drug metabolism, and toxicology, and involve many types of scientists including general biologists, microbiologists, molecular biologists, biochemists, geneticists, pharmacologists, physiologists, pharmacokineticists, pathologists, toxicologists, statisticians, and others. Their work leads to the determination of whether a chemical agent possesses adequate features of safety and sufficient promise of usefulness to pursue as a prospective new drug.

To judge whether a drug is safe and effective, information must be gained on how it is absorbed, distributed throughout the body, stored, metabolized, excreted, and how it affects the action of the body's cells, tissues, and organs. Scientists have developed studies that may be conducted outside the living body by using cell and tissue culture and computer programs that simulate human and animal systems. Cell cultures are being used increasingly to screen for toxicity before progressing to whole-animal testing. Computer models help to predict the properties of substances and their probable actions in living systems. Although these non-animal systems have reduced dependence on the use of animals in drug studies, they have not completely replaced the need to study drugs in whole animals as a safeguard before their administration to humans.

Pharmacology

Within its broad definition, *pharmacology* embraces the physical and chemical properties, biochemical and physiological effects, mechanisms of action, absorption, distribution, biotransformation, excretion, and useful applications of drugs (25). From this basic field of study come such subareas as *pharmacodynamics,* which is the study of the biochemical and physiological effects of drugs and their mechanisms of action; *pharmacokinetics,* which deals with the absorption, distribution, metabolism or biotransformation, and excretion (ADME) of drugs; and *clinical pharmacology,* which applies pharmacologic principles to the study of the effects and actions of drugs in humans.

Today's emphasis in the development of new drugs is directed toward identifying the cause and process of a disease and then designing drug molecules capable of interfering with that process. Although the precise cause of each disease is not yet known, what is known is that most diseases arise from a biochemical imbalance, an abnormal proliferation of cells, an endogenous deficiency, or an exogenous chemical toxin or invasive pathogen.

The biochemical processes within the body's cells involve intricate enzymatic reactions. An understanding of the role of a particular enzyme system in the body's healthy state and disease state can lead to the design of drugs that affect the enzyme system with positive results, as exemplified earlier in this chapter for the drug enalaprilat (Vasotec).

Different drug substances produce different effects on the biological system due to the specific interactions between a drug's chemical structure and specific cells or cellular components of a particular tissue or organ, termed receptor sites (Fig. 2.4). The action of most drugs takes place at the molecular level with the drug molecules interacting with the molecules of the cell structure or its contents. The selectivity and specificity of drugs for a certain body tissue—for example, drugs that act primarily on the nerves, heart, or kidney—are related to specific sites on or within the cells, receptive only to chemicals of a particular chemical structure and configuration. This is the basis for *structure–activity*

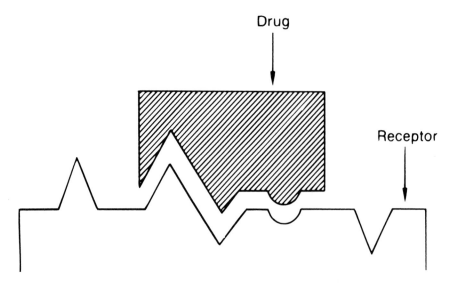

Fig. 2.4   *Schematic drawing of receptor site and substrate (drug). (Reprinted with permission from Clark FH, ed. How Modern Medicines are Discovered. Courtesy of Futura Publishing Company, Inc.)*

relationships (SAR) established for drugs and for families of drugs within therapeutic categories. Studies of the pharmacologic activities of a series of analogs with varied functional groups and side chains can reveal the most specific structure for a given drug–cell or drug–enzyme interaction.

Although receptors for many drugs have yet to be identified, they, like the active centers of enzymes, are considered to be carboxyl, amino, sulfhydryl, phosphate, and similar reactive groups oriented on or in the cell in a pattern complementary to that of the drugs with which they react. The binding of a drug to the receptor is thought to be accomplished mainly by ionic, covalent, and other relatively weak reversible bonds. Occasionally, firm covalent bonding is involved, and the drug effect is then slowly reversible.

There is a relationship between the *quantity* of drug molecules available for interaction and the capacity of the specific receptor site. For instance, after a dose of drug and its transit to the site of action, the cell's receptors may or may not become fully saturated with interacting drug. When the receptors *are* saturated, the effects of the specific interaction are maximized. Any additional drug present (as in the circulation) and not participating in the interaction may serve as a reservoir to replace drug molecules that become released from the complex. Two drugs, when present in a biologic system, may compete for the same binding sites, with the drug having the stronger bonding attraction for the site

generally prevailing. Already-bound molecules of the more weakly bound drug may be replaced from the binding site and left free in the circulation as unbound drug.

Certain cells within the body are capable of binding drugs without eliciting a drug effect. These cells act as carriers and may be important to a drug's transport to active sites or to sites of the drug's biotransformation and elimination.

The process of evaluating chemical compounds for biologic activity and the determination of their mechanisms of action is the responsibility of the pharmacologist. In vitro cultures of cells and enzymes systems, and in vivo animal models are used to define a chemical's *pharmacologic profile.*

To define a pharmacologic profile, pharmacologists progress stepwise through increasingly sophisticated levels of evaluation, based on the test compound's success in prior studies. Whole-animal studies are reserved for test compounds that have demonstrated reasonable potential as a drug candidate.

Among the early studies undertaken are the determination of a compound's selectivity for various receptors and its activity against select enzyme systems. Studies of the compound's effects on cell function are then performed to detect evidence of efficacy and to determine whether the compound is an agonist or antagonist. These are followed by studies with isolated animal tissues to define further the compound's activity and selectivity. Then whole-animal studies are used to evaluate the pharmacologic effects of the agent on specific organ systems. Finally, studies are undertaken using animal models of human disease for which the compound is considered a drug candidate.

The majority of animal testing is done using small animals, usually rodents (mouse, rat) for a number of reasons including cost, availability, the small amount of drug required for a study, the ease of administration by various routes (oral, inhalation, intravenous), and experience with drug testing in these species. However, in final pharmacologic and toxicologic studies, two or more animal species are used as required by the FDA, including a rodent and a nonrodent. Drugs are studied at various dose levels to determine effect, potency, and toxicity.

The primary objective of the animal studies is to obtain basic information on the drug's effects that may be used to predict safe and effective use in humans. This is a difficult task because of species variation and the fact that animals are not absolute predictors of human response. However, a number of animal models have been developed to mimic certain human diseases, and these are used effectively. For instance, there are animal models for type I diabetes and hypertension, using genetically diabetic and hypertensive animals, respectively, and for tumor growth, using tumor transplants into various species. Certain animal species have been determined to be best for certain studies of organ systems, or as human disease models, including: the dog and rat for hypertension; the dog and guinea pig for respiratory effects; the dog for diuretic activity; the rabbit for blood coagulation; and the mouse and rat for central nervous system studies (26–27). Unfortunately, useful animal models are not available for every human disease. As a drug candidate progresses in its preclinical pharmacologic evaluation, drug metabolism and toxicity tests are initiated.

Drug Metabolism

A series of animal studies of a proposed drug's absorption, distribution, metabolism, and elimination (ADME) are undertaken to determine: 1) the *extent* and *rate* of drug absorption from various routes of administration, including the one intended for human use; 2) the rate of distribution of the drug through the body, and the site(s) and duration of the drug's residence; 3) the rate, primary and secondary sites, and mechanism of the drug's metabolism in the body, and the chemistry and pharmacology of any metabolites; and 4) the proportion of administered dose eliminated from the body, and its rate and route of elimination. In these studies, a minimum of two animal species are employed (generally the same as used in the pharmacologic and toxicologic studies), a rodent and a nonrodent, usually a dog.

The biochemical transformation or metabolism of drug substances is the body's means of transforming nonpolar drug molecules into polar compounds, which are more readily eliminated. Specific and nonspecific enzymes participate in drug metabolism, primarily in the liver, but also in the kidneys, lung, and gastrointestinal tract. Drugs that enter the hepatic circulation after absorption from the gut, as after oral administration, are particularly exposed to rapid drug metabolism. This transit through the liver and exposure to hepatic enzyme system is termed the *first-pass effect*. If the first-pass effect is to be avoided, other routes of administration (buccal, rectal) may be used that allow the drug to be absorbed into the systemic circulation through blood vessels other than hepatic.

Drug metabolism or biotransformation frequently results in the production of one or more metabolites of the administered drug, some of which may be pharmacologically active compounds, others not. As noted previously, drug metabolism may be essential to convert prodrugs to active compounds. For reasons of drug safety, it is important to determine whether a drug's metabolic products are toxic or nontoxic to the animal, and later, to the human. When metabolites are found, they are chemically and biologically characterized for activity and toxicity. Some new drugs have been discovered as metabolic byproducts or metabolites of parent compounds.

ADME studies are performed through the timely collection and analysis of urine, blood, and feces samples, and through a careful examination of animal tissues and organs upon autopsy. In addition, special studies are undertaken to determine: the presence, if any, of a test drug or its metabolites in the milk of lactating animals; the ability of the drug to cross the placental barrier and enter the fetal blood supply; and, the long-term retention of drug or metabolites in the body. In studying the formation and disposition of metabolites, a radioactive label is commonly incorporated into the administered compound and traced in the animal's waste products and tissues.

The relationship between ADME and drug product development is discussed in Chapter 4.

Toxicology

Toxicology is the area of pharmacology that deals with the adverse, or undesired, effects of drugs (25). Although the ability to predict the safe use of a new drug in humans based on preclinical animal studies is desirable, it is not entirely achievable. The direct extrapolation of preclinical animal safety data to humans is difficult because of species variation, different dose—response relationships, immunologic differences, subjective reactions nondeducible in animals (such as headache), and for other reasons (27). Although many adverse reactions that occur in humans cannot be predicted in advance through animal studies, the greater the number of animal species tested which demonstrate a toxic effect, the greater the likelihood the effect will also be seen in humans.

In drug development programs, preclinical drug safety evaluation (DSE) or toxicity studies are undertaken to determine: 1) the substance's potential for toxicity with short-term (acute effects) or long-term use (chronic effects); 2) the substance's potential for specific organ toxicity; 3) the mode, site, and degree of toxicity; 4) dose—response relationships, for low- high- and intermediate doses over a specified time course; (5) gender, reproductive, or teratogenic toxicities; and 6) the substance's carcinogenic and genotoxic potential.

Initial toxicology studies are conducted on rodents. After successful initial testing, a nonrodent species, usually a dog, is added to the testing program to develop the FDA-required two species toxicology profile. The toxicology profile includes acute or short-term toxicity; subacute or subchronic toxicity; chronic toxicity; carcinogenicity testing; reproduction studies; and mutagenicity screening (9, 28–29). Figure 2.1 shows that short-term and long-term toxicity studies span the entire program of drug development, from preclinical studies through clinical trials and into postmarketing surveillance.

Acute or Short-Term Toxicity Studies

These studies are designed to determine the toxic effects of a test compound when administered in a single dose and/or in multiple doses over a short period, usually a single day. Although various routes of administration may be used (such as lavage dosing via gastric tube), the studies should be conducted to represent the intended route for human use.

The test compound is administered at various dose levels, with toxic signs observed for onset, progression or reversal, severity, mortality, and rates of incidence. Doses are ranged, to find the largest single dose of the test compound that will not produce a toxic effect; the dose level at which severe toxicity occurs; and intermediate toxicity levels. The animals are observed and compared with controls for eating and drinking habits, weight change, toxic effects, psychomotor changes, and any other signs of untoward effects, usually over a 30-day postdose period. Feces and urine specimens are collected and clinical laboratory tests performed to detect changes in clinical chemistry and other changes that could indicate toxicity. When they occur, animal deaths are recorded, studied by histology and pathology, and statistically evaluated on the basis of dose–response, gender, age, intraspecies, interspecies, and against laboratory controls.

Subacute or Subchronic Studies

In designing an animal toxicology program, relationships to projected human clinical studies for safety must be considered. For example, animal toxicity studies of a minimum of 2 weeks duration of daily drug administration at three or more dosage levels to two animal species are required to support the initial administration of a single dose in human clinical testing (8). These studies are termed *subacute* or *subchronic*. The initial human dose is usually one-tenth of the highest nontoxic dose (based on a milligram-per-kilogram weight basis) shown during the animal studies. For drugs intended to be given to humans for a week or more, animal studies of 90 to 180 days in length must demonstrate safety. These are termed *chronic toxicity* studies. And, if the drug is to be used for a chronic human illness, long-term animal studies of 1 year or longer must be undertaken to support human use. Some animal toxicity studies last 2 years or longer and may be used to corroborate findings obtained during the course of human clinical trials.

Included in the subchronic and chronic studies are comparative data of test and control animal species, strain, sex, age, dose levels and ranges, routes of administration, duration of treatment, observed effects, mortality, body weight changes, food/water consumption, physical examinations (e.g., ECG, ophthalmic), hematology, clinical chemistry, organ weights, gross pathology, neoplastic pathology, histopathology, urinalysis, ADME data, and other (28). Figure 2.5 shows a toxicologist examining research data of body weight changes during preclinical rodent studies.

Carcinogenicity Studies

Carcinogenicity testing is usually a component of chronic testing and is undertaken when the compound has shown sufficient promise as a drug to enter human clinical trials. Carcinogenicity stud-

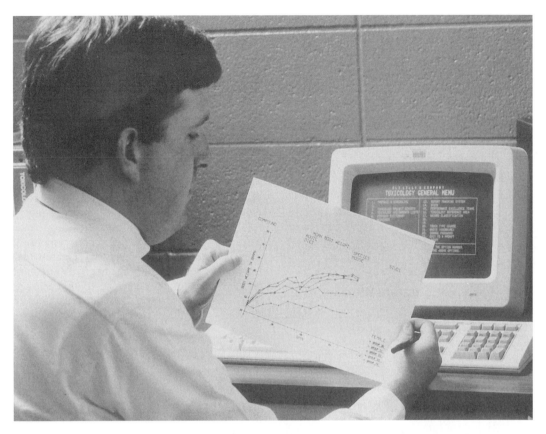

Fig. 2.5 *A toxicologist examining research data of body weight changes during preclinical studies in mice. (Courtesy of Toxicology Research Laboratories, Lilly Research Laboratories, Division of Eli Lilly and Co.)*

ies are usually carried out in a limited number of rat and mouse strains for which there is reasonable information on spontaneous tumor incidence.

Dose-ranging studies are done with female and male animals using high, intermediate, and low doses over a 90-day period. For carcinogenicity studies, the high dose should be only high enough (the maximum tolerated dose) to elicit signs of minimal toxicity without significantly altering the animal's normal lifespan due to effects other than carcinogenicity (30).

Carcinogenicity studies are long term (18–24 months), with surviving animals sacrificed and studied at defined weeks during the test period. Data are collected and evaluated on the causes of animal death (other than sacrifice), tumor incidence, type and site, and necropsy findings. The occurrence of preneoplastic lesions and/or tissue-specific proliferative effects are important findings.

Reproduction Studies

These studies are undertaken to reveal *any* effect of an active ingredient on mammalian reproduc-

tion. Included in these studies are fertility and mating behavior, early embryonic and pre- and postnatal development, multigenerational effects, and teratology. The combination of studies allows exposure from conception to sexual maturity and allows immediate and latent effects to be detected through complete life cycles and through successive generations.

In these studies, the maternal parent, fetus, neonates, and weaning offspring are evaluated for anatomical abnormalities, growth, and development. The same species of animal used in other toxicity studies are used in reproductive studies, usually the rat. In *embryotoxicity* studies only, a second mammalian species traditionally has been required. The rabbit is the preferred choice due to practicality and the extensive background knowledge accumulated on this species.

In reproductive studies, as is the case for other toxicity studies, the doses selected and the routes of administration used are critical. A high-dose, based on previous acute and chronic toxicity and pharmacokinetic studies, is selected with lower dosages chosen in descending sequence. Setting close dosage intervals is useful to reveal trends in dose-related toxicity. Although once daily dosing is usual, the drug's pharmacokinetics may influence the frequency of dosing (31). The route or routes of administration used should be similar to that intended for human use. A single route of administration may be acceptable if it can be shown that a similar drug distribution (kinetic profile) results from different routes of administration.

Genotoxicity or Mutagenicity Studies

These studies are performed to determine if the test compound can affect gene mutation, or cause chromosome or DNA damage. Strains of *Salmonella typhimurium* are routinely used in assays to detect mutations (9,32).

Early Formulation Studies

As a promising compound is characterized for biological activity, it is also evaluated with regard to those chemical and physical properties that have a bearing on its ultimate and successful formulation into a stable and effective pharmaceutical product. This is the area of responsibility of pharmaceutical scientists and formulation pharmacists trained in the field of *pharmaceutics*. When sufficient information is gleaned on the compound's physical and chemical properties, initial formulations of the dosage form are developed for use in human clinical trials. During the course of the clinical trials, the proposed product is developed further, from initial formulation to final formulation, and from pilot plant (or small-scale production) to scale-up, in preparation for large-scale manufacturing.

To provide sufficient quantities of the bulk chemical (drug) compound for the sequence of preclinical studies, clinical trials, and small-scale and large-scale dosage form production, the careful planning, scheduling, and implementation of the bulk chemical's production must be undertaken by chemical engineers. Quality control and validation must be built into each step of the process.

Full documentation of the chemistry, manufacturing, and controls (CMC) is an essential part of all drug applications filed with the FDA (1, 33).

Preformulation Studies

Each drug substance has intrinsic chemical and physical characteristics that must be considered before the development of a pharmaceutical formulation. Among these are the drug's solubility, parti-

tion coefficient, dissolution rate, physical form, and stability. These and other factors are considered more fully in Chapter 3 and throughout the text, but are briefly noted here as an introduction to their importance in the preparation of dosage forms for drug evaluation in human clinical trials, and, in the development of a final product submitted to the FDA for marketing approval.

Drug Solubility

A drug substance administered by any route must possess some aqueous solubility for systemic absorption and therapeutic response. Poorly soluble compounds (e.g., less than 10 mg/mL aqueous solubility) may exhibit either incomplete or erratic absorption and thus produce a minimal response at desired dosage. Enhanced aqueous solubility may be achieved through the preparation of more soluble derivatives of the parent compound, such as salts or esters, through chemical complexation, or through drug particle-size reduction.

Partition Coefficient

To produce a pharmacologic response, a drug molecule must first cross a biologic membrane of protein and lipid, which acts as a lipophilic barrier to many drugs. The ability of a drug molecule to penetrate this barrier is based, in part, on its preference for lipids (lipophilic) versus its preference for an aqueous phase (hydrophilic). A drug's partition coefficient is a measure of its distribution in a lipophilic/hydrophilic phase system, and is indicative of its ability to penetrate biologic multiphase systems.

Dissolution Rate

The speed, or rate, at which a drug substance dissolves in a medium is called its *dissolution rate.* Dissolution rate data, when considered along with data on a drug's solubility, dissolution constant, and partition coefficient, can provide an indication of the drug's absorption potential following administration. For a chemical entity, its acid, base, or salt forms, as well as its physical form (e.g., particle size), may result in substantial differences in the dissolution rate.

Physical Form

The crystal or amorphous forms and/or the particle size of a powdered drug can affect the dissolution rate, and thus the rate and extent of absorption, for a number of drugs. For example, by increasing powder fineness and therefore the surface area of a poorly soluble drug, its dissolution rate in the gut is enhanced (through greater drug/gastrointestinal fluid exposure) and its biologic absorption increased. Small and controlled particle size is also critical for drugs administered to the lung by inhalation. The smaller the particle, the deeper is the penetration into the alveoli. Thus, by selective control of the physical parameters of a drug, biologic response may be optimized.

Stability

The chemical and physical stability of a drug substance alone, and when combined with formulation components, is critical in preparing a successful pharmaceutical product. For a given drug, one type of crystal structure may provide greater stability than other structures and may therefore be preferred. For drugs susceptible to oxidative decomposition, the addition of antioxidant stabilizing agents to the formulation may be required to protect potency. For drugs destroyed by hydrolysis, protection against moisture in formulation, processing, and packaging may be required to prevent decomposition. In every case, drug stability testing at various temperatures, conditions of relative humidity (RH)—as 40°C 75% RH/30°C 60% RH—durations, and environments of light, air, and packaging is essential in assessing drug and drug product stability. Such information is vital in developing label instructions for use and storage, assigning product expiration dating, and packaging and shipping.

Initial Product Formulation and Clinical Trial Materials (CTM)

An initial product is formulated using the information gained during the preformulation studies and with consideration of the dose(s), dosage form, and route of administration desired for the clinical studies and for the proposed marketed product. Thus, depending upon the design of the clinical protocol and desired final product, formulation pharmacists are called upon to develop a specific dosage form (e.g., capsule, suppository, solution) of one or more dosage strengths for administration by the intended route of administration (e.g., oral, rectal, intravenous). Additional dosage forms for other than the initial route of administration may later be developed, depending on patient requirements, therapeutic utility, and marketing assessments.

The initial formulations prepared for Phase 1 and Phase 2 of the clinical trials, although not as sophisticated and elegant as the final formulation, should be of high pharmaceutical quality, meet analytical specifications for composition, manufacturing, and control, and be sufficiently stable for the period of use.

Often during Phase 1 studies, for orally administered drugs, capsules are employed containing the active ingredient alone, without pharmaceutical excipients. Excipients are included in the formulation for Phase 2 trials. During the course of the human trials, studies of the drug's absorption, distribution, metabolism, and excretion are undertaken to obtain a profile of the drug's human pharmacokinetics and biologic availability from the formulation administered. Different formulations may be prepared and examined to develop the one having the desired characteristics (see Chapter 4). During Phase 2, the final dosage form is selected and developed for Phase 3 trials and represents the formulation that is submitted to the FDA for marketing approval.

Clinical supplies or clinical trial materials (CTM), refer to all dosage formulations used in the clinical evaluation of a new drug. This includes the proposed new drug, *placebos* (nonmedicated forms for controlled studies) and drug products against which the new drug is to be compared (*comparator* drugs or drug products). They all must be prepared in indistinguishable dosage forms (look alike, taste alike, etc.) and packaged with coded labels to reduce possible bias when *blinded* studies are called for in the clinical protocol. Blinded studies are controlled studies in which at least one of the parties (e.g., patient, physician) is not knowledgeable of which product is being administered. At the conclusion of the clinical study, the codes for the products administered are broken and the clinical results statistically evaluated. Some studies are *open label* in which all parties may be aware of the products administered.

Some pharmaceutical companies have special units for the preparation, analytical control, coding, packaging, labeling, shipping, and record maintenance of clinical supplies. Other companies integrate this activity within their existing drug product development and production operations. Still other companies employ contract firms specializing in this field to prepare and manage their clinical trial materials program.

In all clinical study programs, the package label of the investigational drug must bear the statement "Caution: New Drug—Limited by Federal (or United States) Law to Investigational Use." Once received by the investigator, the clinical supplies may be administered only to subjects included in the study. Blister packaging is commonly used in clinical studies, with immediate labels containing the clinical study or protocol number, patient identification number, sponsor number, directions for use, code number to distinguish between investigational drug, placebo, and/or comparator product, and other relevant information. Records of the disposition of the drug must be maintained by patient number, dates, and quantities administered. When there is a department of pharmacy at the site of the clinical study (e.g., university teaching hospital) pharmacists frequently assist in the control and management of clinical supplies. When an investigation is terminated, suspended, discontinued, or completed, all unused clinical supplies must be returned to the sponsor and an accounting made of used and unused product.

All formulations, from those developed initially through the final marketed version, must be prepared under the conditions and procedures set out by the FDA in its Current Good Manufacturing Practice (CGMP) guidelines (34), as outlined in Chapter 5.

The Investigational New Drug (IND) Application

Under the Food, Drug, and Cosmetic Act as amended, the sponsor of a new drug is required to file with the FDA an *Investigational New Drug Application* (*IND*) before the drug may be given to human subjects (1). This is to protect the rights and safety of the subjects and to ensure that the investigational plan is sound and is designed to achieve the stated objectives. The *sponsor* of an IND takes responsibility for and initiates a clinical investigation. The sponsor may be an individual (a sponsor-investigator), a pharmaceutical company, governmental agency, academic institution, or other private or public organization. The sponsor may actually conduct the study or employ, designate, or contract other qualified persons to do so. Nowadays there are many *contract research organizations* (*CROs*) that conduct all or designated portions of clinical studies or clinical drug trials for others through contractual arrangements.

After submission of the IND, the sponsor must delay use of the drug in human subjects for not less than 30 days from the date the FDA acknowledges receipt of the application. An IND automatically goes into effect following this period unless the FDA notifies the sponsor that, based on its review of the submission, the period is waived (and the sponsor may initiate the study early), or the investigation is being placed on a *clinical hold.*

A *clinical hold* is an order issued by the FDA to delay the start of a clinical investigation or, in the case of an ongoing investigation, to suspend the study. During a clinical hold, the investigational drug may not be administered to human subjects (unless specifically permitted by the FDA for individual patients in an ongoing study). A clinical hold is issued when there is concern that human subjects will be exposed to unreasonable and significant risk of illness or injury; where there is question over the qualifying credentials of the clinical investigators; or in instances in which the IND is considered incomplete, inaccurate, or misleading. If the concerns raised are addressed to the FDA's satisfaction, a clinical hold may be lifted and clinical investigations resumed; if not, an IND may be maintained in a clinical hold position, declared inactive, withdrawn by the sponsor, or terminated by the FDA.

Content of the IND

The content of an IND is prescribed in the *Code of Federal Regulations* and is submitted under a cover sheet (*Form FDA-1571*) (1).

Among the items required are:

- Name and address and telephone number of the sponsor of the drug;
- Name and title of the person responsible for monitoring the conduct and progress of the investigation;
- Name(s) and title(s) of the person(s) responsible for the review and evaluation of information relevant to the safety of the drug;
- Name and address of any contract research organization involved in the study;
- Identification of the phase or phases of the clinical investigation to be conducted;
- Introductory statement and general investigational plan, including: the name of the drug and all active ingredients, the drug's structural formula and pharmacological class, the formulation of the dosage form and route of administration, the broad objectives and planned duration of the study;
- Description of the investigational plan, including: the rationale for the drug/research study, the indication(s) to be studied, the approach in evaluating the drug, the types of studies to be conducted, the estimated number of subjects to be given the drug, and any serious risks anticipated based on animal studies or other human experiences with the drug;
- Brief summary of previous human experience

with the drug (domestic or foreign), including reasons if the drug has been withdrawn from any other investigation and/or marketing;

- Chemistry, manufacturing and control information, including: a complete description of the drug substance including its physical, chemical, and biological characteristics, its method of preparation, and analytical methods to assure its identity, strength, quality, purity and stability, a quantitative list of the active and inactive components of the dosage form to be administered, the methods, facilities, and controls employed in the manufacture, processing, packaging and labeling of the new drug to assure appropriate qualitative and quantitative standards and product stability during the clinical investigation;
- Pharmacology and toxicology information, including: the drug's mechanism of action (if known), information on the drug's absorption, distribution, metabolism, and excretion, and acute, subacute, chronic and reproductive and developmental toxicity studies;
- If the new drug is a combination of previously investigated components, a complete preclinical and clinical summary of these components when administered singly and any data or expectations relating to the effect when combined;
- *Clinical protocol* for each planned study (discussed in the next section);
- Commitment that an *Institutional Review Board* (*IRB*) has approved the clinical study and will continue to review and monitor the investigation (discussed in the next section);
- *Investigator Brochure* (discussed in the next section); and,
- Commitment not to begin clinical investigations until the IND is in effect, the signature of the sponsor or authorized representative, and the date of the signed application.

The Clinical Protocol

As a part of the IND application, a *clinical protocol* must be submitted to ensure the appropriate design and conduct of the investigation. Clinical protocols include:

- Statement of the purpose and objectives of the study;
- Outline of the investigational plan and study design, including the kind of control group and methods to minimize bias on the part of the subjects, investigators, and analysts;

- Estimate of the number of patients to be involved;
- Basis for subject selection, including inclusion and exclusion criteria;
- Description of the dosing plan, including dose levels, route of administration, and duration of patient exposure;
- Description of the patient observations, measurements, and tests to be used;
- Clinical procedures, laboratory tests and monitoring to be used in minimizing patient risk;
- Names, addresses and credentials of the principal investigators and subinvestigators;
- Locations and descriptions of the clinical research facilities to be used; and,
- Approval of the authorized Institutional Review Board.

Once an IND is in effect, a sponsor must submit an amendment for approval of any proposed changes. This may involve changes of dosing levels, testing procedures, the addition of new investigators, additional sites for the study, and so on.

For many years, women and the elderly were included only rarely in clinical drug investigations. Women of child-bearing age were excluded from early drug tests out of fear that the subject would become pregnant during the investigation with possible harm to the fetus. Exceptions were made only in cases of potentially life-saving drugs. However, in recognition that the general exclusion of women from drug investigations results in inadequate data on any gender-based differences in a drug's effects, the FDA now calls for the inclusion of women in numbers adequate to allow detection of clinically significant differences in drug response.

The FDA "Guideline for the Study and Evaluation of Gender Differences in the Clinical Evaluation of Drugs" issued in 1993 states the agency's gender inclusion policy (35). Although the guideline does not require participation of women in any particular trial, it sets forth FDA's general expectations regarding the inclusion of both women and men in drug development, analysis of clinical data by gender, and assessment of potential pharmacokinetic differences between genders. In 1994, the National Institutes of Health (NIH) similarly issued its policy that women (and minorities) be included in all NIH-supported biomedical and behavioral research projects involving human subjects "unless there is a clear and compelling rationale and justification that their inclusion is inappropriate with respect to the health of the subjects or the purpose of the research" (36).

Pregnancy is a concern in drug investigations because drugs are readily transported from the maternal to the fetal circulation (37). Because of undeveloped drug detoxication and excretion mechanisms in the fetus, concentrations of drugs may actually reach a higher level in the fetus than in the maternal circulation with toxic levels resulting. To reduce the risk of fetal exposure to investigational drugs in child-bearing age women, the FDA guideline calls for pregnancy testing, use of contraception, and full information disclosure of potential fetal risks to prospective study subjects. The FDA has made a special effort to ensure that women who have a life-threatening disease (e.g., AIDS-related) are not *automatically* excluded from investigational trials of drug products for that disease due to a perceived risk of reproductive or developmental toxicity from use of the investigational drug (38). There are other instances in which drug studies/use during pregnancy are justified, as for example, agents intended to prevent Rh immunization and subsequent hemolytic disease of the newborn (39).

When a proposed drug is likely to have significant use in the elderly, elderly patients are required to be included in clinical studies to yield age-related data of a drug's effectiveness and the occurrence of adverse effects. Older people handle a drug differently, not because of age itself, but because of altered body functions such as diminished liver and kidney function, reduced circulation, and changes in drug absorption, distribution, metabolism, and excretion. Further, compared with younger adults, the elderly have a greater incidence of chronic illness and multiple disease states, and as a result, take multiple medications daily increasing the potential for drug–drug interactions. This potential is studied and defined.

Recognition of the need to examine in children new drugs intended for the pediatric patient has a similar requirement to ensure a drug's safe and effective use in this patient population. Also, differentiation in a drug's activity in minority groups and their subpopulations is important in the full assessment of a drug's potential. It is well known that there are interethnic variations both in disease incidence and in biologic response to some medications and these factors need to be considered in the clinical evaluation of drug substances.(40)

Each IND submission must have the prior approval of the *Institutional Review Board* (*IRB*) having jurisdiction over the site of the proposed clinical investigation. An IRB is a body of professional and public members that has the responsibility for reviewing and approving any study involving human subjects within the institution they serve. The purpose of the IRB is to protect the safety of human subjects by assessing a proposed clinical protocol, evaluating the benefits against potential risks, and ensuring that the plan includes all needed measures for subject protection. By law, the IRB shall be constituted to include persons competent to review clinical research proposals and be diverse in membership with consideration of race, gender, cultural background, and sensitivity to issues affecting the subjects and the community (41). Any substantive change or an amendment to an originally approved clinical protocol must be submitted, reviewed and approved by the IRB and the FDA before implementation.

Each clinical investigator must receive from the sponsor an *Investigator's Brochure,* which contains all of the pertinent information developed during the preclinical studies, including summary information on the drug's chemistry, pharmacology, toxicology, pharmacokinetics; formulation of the clinical trial materials; any known information related to the drug's safety and effectiveness; a description of possible risks and side effects that may be anticipated and special monitoring required; the clinical protocol and study design; criteria for patient inclusion and exclusion; laboratory and clinical tests to be performed; and drug control and record keeping information.

Each study has defined criteria for *subject inclusion or exclusion.* These criteria may relate to age, sex (as qualified above), smoking, health status, and other factors deemed necessary in a given phase of investigation. Each subject in a clinical investigation must participate willingly and with full knowledge of the benefits and risks associated with the investigation.

The sponsor of the study must certify that each person who will receive the investigational drug has given *informed consent*—that is, has been informed of the following: participation in the study is voluntary; the purpose and nature of the study; the procedures involved; a description of any foreseeable risks or discomforts; the potential benefits (for patients); disclosure of alternative procedures or courses of treatments, if any (for patients); the extent of confidentiality of records; conditions under which the subject's participation in the study may be terminated; consequences of a patient's decision to withdraw from the study; the approximate number of subjects to be enrolled; and, whom to contact to answer pertinent questions and/or in case of research-related illness or injury. These elements of informed consent, and additional protections that apply to prisoners involved in clinical investigations, must be in conformance with the *Code of Federal Regulations* (42). Individuals who agree to be subjects in an investigation indicate their consent by signing the form or document containing the above-information.

Investigator(s) selected by the sponsor to conduct a clinical investigation must be qualified as experts by training and experience to investigate a particular drug. Each investigator's qualifications are submitted to the FDA as a part of the IND application. To participate in an investigation, each investigator signs a form agreeing to comply with and to be responsible for: ensuring that the study is conducted according to the IND's investigational plan and clinical protocol; protecting their rights, safety, and welfare of the human subjects; control of the investigational drug; written records of case histories and clinical observations; and, for the timely submission of progress reports, safety reports and a final report. It is the responsibility of the sponsor to monitor the progress of all clinical investigations under its IND. If a sponsor discovers that an investigator is not in compliance with the investigational plan, it is the sponsor's responsibility to gain compliance or to terminate the investigator's participation in the study.

Any serious, unexpected, life-threatening, or fatal adverse experience that may be associated with the use of the drug during a clinical investigation must be reported promptly to the sponsor and, subsequently, to the FDA for investigation. Depending on the severity and assessment of the adverse experience, an alert notice may be sent to other investigators, a clinical hold may be placed on the study for further evaluation and assessment, or the IND may be withdrawn by the sponsor, placed on inactive status, or terminated by the FDA.

Pre-IND Meetings

On request, the FDA will advise a sponsor on scientific, technical, or formatting concerns relating to the preparation and submission of an IND. This may include advice on the adequacy of data to support an investigational plan, the design of a clinical trial, or whether the proposed investigation is likely to produce the data needed to meet the requirements of the next step, the filing of a New Drug Application to gain approval for marketing.

FDA Review of an IND Application

The FDA's objectives in reviewing an IND are to protect the safety and rights of the human subjects and to help ensure that the study allows the evaluation of the drug's safety and effectiveness. These objectives are best met by the accuracy and completeness of the IND submission, the design and conduct of the investigational plan, and the expertise and diligence of the investigators.

When received by the FDA, the IND submission is stamped with the date of receipt, assigned an application number, and forwarded to either the Center for Drug Evaluation and Research (CDER) or the Center for Biologics Evaluation and Research (CBER) for review. Applications for chemical agents are sent to CDER and applications for biologics to CBER.

Within CDER, applications are forwarded to the appropriate Office of Drug Evaluation and then to one of its divisions for review as follows:

Office of Drug Evaluation I
  Division of Neuropharmacological Drug Products
  Division of Oncology Drug Products
  Division of Cardio-Renal Drug Products
Office of Drug Evaluation II
  Division of Metabolic and Endocrine Drug Products
  Division of Pulmonary Drug Products
  Division of Reproductive and Urologic Drug Products
Office of Drug Evaluation III
  Division of Gastro-Intestinal and Coagulation Drug Products
  Division of Anesthetic, Critical Care, and Addiction Drug Products
  Division of Medical Imaging and Radiopharmaceutical Drug Products
Office of Drug Evaluation IV
  Division of Anti-Viral Drug Products
  Divsion of Anti-Infective Drug Products
  Division of Special Pathogen and Immunologic Drug Products
Office of Drug Evaluation V
  Division of Anti-Inflammatory, Analgesic, and Ophthalmologic Drug Products
  Division of Dermatologic and Dental Drug Products
  Division of Over-The-Counter Drug Products

After assignment to one of the divisions, the content of the application is thoroughly reviewed to determine whether the preclinical data indicate that the drug is sufficiently safe for administration to human subjects and that the proposed clinical studies are designed to provide the desired data on drug safety and efficacy while not exposing the human subjects to unnecessary risks.

AUTHOR'S NOTE: *although the discussion in this chapter is based principally on the evaluation and approval of new chemical entities and products, for biologic products, there is a similar but necessarily distinct procedure of application review and product licensing through CBER and its divisions* (4):

Division of Allergenic Products and Parasitology
Division of Bacterial Products
Division of Viral products
Division of Vaccines and Related Products
Division of Hematologic Products
Division of Blood Establishment and Products
Division of Cellular and Gene Therapy
Division of Monoclonal Antibodies Applications

FDA Drug Classification System

Upon receipt and examination of an IND or NDA application, the FDA classifies the drug by chemical type and therapeutic potential, as shown in Table 2.1. The classification system allows the FDA to set review priorities based on the level of therapeutic advance or need (43).

Phases of a Clinical Investigation

An IND may be submitted for one or more *phases* of a clinical investigation, namely Phase 1, Phase 2 or Phase 3 (Fig. 2.2, Table 2.2). Although the phases are conducted sequentially, certain studies may overlap.

Phase 1 includes the initial introduction of an investigational drug into humans and is primarily for the purpose of assessing safety. The studies are closely monitored by clinicians expert in such investigations. The human subjects are usually healthy volunteers, although in certain protocols they may be patients. The total number of subjects included in Phase 1 studies varies with the drug, but is usually in the range of 20 to 100. The initial dose of the drug is usually low, usually one-tenth of the highest "no-effect dose" observed during the animal studies. If the first dose is well tolerated, the investigation is continued with the administration of progressively greater doses (to new subjects) until some evidence of the drug's effects are observed.

Phase 1 studies are designed to determine the human pharmacology of the drug, structure-activity

Table 2.1.   FDA Drug Classification System*

By chemical type

Type 1	New molecular entity; not marketed in the U.S.
Type 2	New ester, new salt, or other derivative of an approved active moiety
Type 3	New formulation of a drug marketed in the U.S.
Type 4	New combination of two or more compounds
Type 5	New manufacturer of a drug marketed in U.S.
Type 6	New therapeutic indication for an approved drug

Note: a drug may receive a single or multiple classification, as "3,4"

By therapeutic classification

Type P	Priority review; a therapeutic gain
Type S	A standard review; similar to other approved drugs

Additional classifications

Type AA	For treatment of AIDS or HIV-related disease
Type E	For life-threatening or severely debilitating disease
Type F	Review deferred pending data validation
Type G	Data validated, removal of "F" rating
Type N	Nonprescription drug
Type V	Drug having orphan drug status

Note: a drug may receive a single or multiple classification, as "Type P, AA, V"

*Adapted from information from Mathieu M. New drug development: a regulatory overview, 3rd ed. Cambridge, MA: PAREXEL International Corporation, 1994, and Hunter JR, Rosen DL, DeChristoforo R. How FDA expedites evaluation of drugs for AIDS and other life-threatening illnesses. Wellcome Programs in Hospital Pharmacy, No. 67930093009, 1993.

relationships, side effects associated with increasing doses, and, if possible, early evidence on effectiveness. Among the basic data collected are: the rate of the drug's absorption; the concentration of drug in the blood versus time; the rate and mechanism of drug metabolism and elimination; toxic effects, if any, in body tissues and major organs; and, changes in physiologic processes from baseline. The subjects' ability to tolerate the drug and any unpleasant effects of the drug are observed and recorded. Phase 1 studies are often useful in selecting from among different chemical analogs of a lead compound. As noted previously, capsules without excipients, are used for orally administered drugs in Phase 1 studies. If the studies demonstrate sufficient merit and if the order of drug toxicity is low, *Phase 2* is begun, using up to several hundred patients.

Phase 2 trials involve controlled clinical studies to

Table 2.2. Phases of Clinical Testing

	Number of Patients	Length	Purpose	Percent of Drugs Successfully Completing*
Phase 1:	20–100	Several months	Mainly safety	67
Phase 2:	Up to several hundred	Several months to 2 years	Some short-term safety, but mainly effectiveness	45
Phase 3:	Several hundred to several thousand	1–4 years	Safety, effectiveness, dosage	5–10

*For example, of 20 drugs entering clinical testing, 13 or 14 will successfully complete Phase 1 trials and go on to Phase 2; about nine will complete Phase 2 and go to Phase 3; only one or two will clear Phase 3 and, on average, about one of the original 20 will ultimately be approved for marketing. (Reference: FDA Consumer, 1987; 21: 12.)

evaluate the effectiveness of a drug in patients with the condition for which the drug is intended, and to assess side effects and risks that may be revealed. Because this phase involves the use of patients as subjects, side effects or toxicity symptoms that were not shown in the preclinical animal studies or in Phase 1 studies with healthy volunteers may be revealed for the first time. Only clinicians expert in the disease being treated are used as investigators during Phase 2 studies (Fig. 2.6). During this phase, additional data are collected on the drug's pharmacokinetics and studies undertaken to determine dose–response and dose ranging (often called *Phase 2a studies*). Each patient is monitored for the appearance of the drug's effects while the dose is carefully increased to determine the minimal effective dose. Then, the dose is extended beyond the minimally effective dose to the level at which a patient reveals extremely undesirable or intolerable toxic or adverse effects. The greater the range between the dose of drug determined to be minimally effective and that which causes severe side effects, the greater is the drug's safety margin. These dose–determination studies (often called *Phase 2b studies*) result in the specific doses and the dose range to be used in *Phase 3* studies. During Phase 2 trials, the drug product is refined with the final formulation developed for use during late Phase 2 and Phase 3 trials.

If the clinical results of Phase 2 trials indicate continued promise for the new drug and if the margin of safety appears to be good, *end-of-Phase 2* meetings between the drug's sponsor and the FDA's review division are held to analyze the data from Phases 1 and 2, to resolve any questions and issues, and to establish investigational plans for Phase 3 studies.

Phase 3 studies may include several hundred to several thousand patients in controlled and uncontrolled trials. The objective is to determine the usefulness of the drug in an expanded patient base. Many additional clinicians having patients with the condition for drug's intended use are recruited to participate in this trial. Several dosage strengths of the proposed drug may be evaluated during this phase, using formulations intended to be proposed in the NDA and for marketing. Sufficient information on the drug's effectiveness and safety is expected to be gathered during Phase 3 to evaluate the overall benefit–risk relationship of the drug and to file a complete NDA.

It is not uncommon for certain Phase 3 studies to be continued after an NDA is filed but *prior to* approval. In these instances, the completed studies (referred to as *Phase 3a* studies) are considered sufficient for the NDA. The additional studies (referred to as *Phase 3b* studies) are used to gather supplemental information which may support certain labeling requests, provide information on patients' quality of life issues, reveal product advantages over already marketed competing drugs, provide evidence in support of possible additional drug indications, or provide other clues for prospective postmarketing studies (*Phase 4*).

Clinical Study Controls and Designs

As indicated, Phase 2 and some Phase 3 studies are *controlled,* that is, the effects of the investigational drug are compared with another agent. The second agent may be a placebo (*placebo control*) or an active drug (*positive control*) as a standard drug or comparator drug product. Both a placebo and an active drug may be used as controls in the same study. For studies that are *blinded,* the identities of the investigational drug and the control(s) are not revealed to

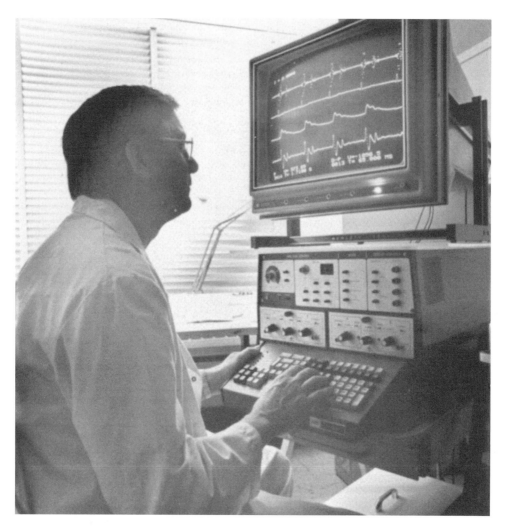

Fig. 2.6   *Monitoring the effects for cardiac function of an uninvestigational drug as a part of its clinical evaluation. (Courtesy of Eli Lilly and Company.)*

certain participants to decrease bias. In *single blind* studies, the patient is unaware of the agent administered. In *double blind* studies, neither the patient nor the clinician is aware of the agent administered. In preparing dosage forms for blinded studies, all of the agents administered, investigational drug, placebo, and/or comparator drug, must be indistinguishable to the blinded individuals. This requires the preparation of clinical trial materials of the same dosage form, having the same size, shape, color, flavor, texture, and so forth. Indistinguishable clinical trial materials are not necessary for *open label* studies in which all parties are aware of the identities of the agents administered.

In designing a clinical trial, many additional factors are considered, including the scheme of the study design and the duration of the treatment period. Before treatment, *baseline data* are obtained on each subject through physical examination and appropriate laboratory tests and procedures. Subjects randomly are assigned to different treatment groups to allow treatment comparisons. Some common parallel and crossover study designs are depicted in Figure 2.7 (44). These studies may be blinded or non-blinded using placebo and/or active drug controls. The parallel designs are applicable to most clinical trials. Crossover designs are useful in comparing different treatments within individuals since following one treatment a patient is "crossed over" to a different treatment. Between treatment periods, subjects may be given no drugs as a *washout* period to allow return to baseline.

SOME CLINICAL TRIAL PARALLEL STUDY DESIGNS

1. COMMON PARALLEL DESIGNS

A.
——————— Treatment Group I
——————— Treatment Group II

B.
——————— Treatment Group I
——————— Treatment Group II
——————— Treatment Group III

2. TWO PART PARALLEL DESIGN

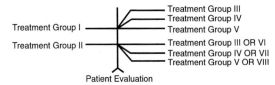

Treatment Group I ——————— Treatment Group III
Treatment Group IV
Treatment Group V

Treatment Group II ——————— Treatment Group III OR VI
Treatment Group IV OR VII
Treatment Group V OR VIII

Patient Evaluation

3. INTRODUCTION OF PLACEBO DURING TREATMENT

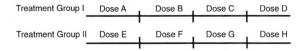

Treatment Group I	Placebo	Treatment Group I
Treatment Group II	Placebo	Treatment Group II
Treatment Group III	Placebo	Treatment Group III

4. MULTIPLE DOSES WITHIN EACH TREATMENT GROUP

Treatment Group I | Dose A | Dose B | Dose C | Dose D

Treatment Group II | Dose E | Dose F | Dose G | Dose H

SOME CLINICAL TRIAL CROSSOVER STUDY DESIGNS

1. SINGLE CROSSOVER WITH NO INTERVENING BASELINE

Tr. A   Tr. A
BL   BL
Tr. B   Tr. B

2. SINGLE CROSSOVER WITH INTERVENING BASELINE

Tr. A   Tr. A
BL   BL   BL
Tr. B   Tr. B

3. EXTRA PERIOD CROSSOVER

Tr. A   Tr. A   Tr. A
BL   BL
Tr. B   Tr. B   Tr. B

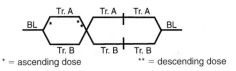

* = ascending dose   ** = descending dose

Fig. 2.7 *Some common clinical study designs.(Reprinted with permission from Spilker B. Guide to Clinical Trials, New York: Raven Press, 1991).*

Drug Dosage and Terminology

A major part of any clinical drug study is the determination of a drug's safe and effective dose. As noted earlier, dose and dose ranging studies are conducted during Phase 2 and concluded during Phase 3 clinical trials.

The safe and effective dose of a drug depends on a number of factors, including characteristics of the drug substance, the dosage form and its route of administration and a variety of patient factors including a patient's age, body weight, general health status, pathologic condition(s), and concomitant drug therapy. All of these factors and others are integral to clinical drug trials.

For convenience of dosage administration, most products are formulated to contain a drug's usual dose within a single dosage unit (e.g., capsule), or within a specified volume (e.g., 5 mL or a teaspoonful) of a liquid dosage form. To serve varying dosage requirements, manufacturers often formulate a drug into more than one dosage form and in more than a single strength.

The dose of a drug may be described as an amount that is "enough but not too much"; the idea being to achieve the drug's optimum therapeutic effect with safety but at the lowest possible dose. The effective dose of a drug may be different for different patients. The familiar bell-shaped curve, presented in Figure 2.8 shows that in a normal distribution sample, a drug's dose will provide what might be called an average effect in the majority of

individuals. However, in a portion of the population the drug will produce little effect and in another portion the drug will produce an effect greater than average. The amount of drug that will produce the desired effect in the majority of adult patients is considered the drug's *usual adult dose* and would likely be the starting dose for a patient. From this initial dose the physician may, if necessary, increase or decrease subsequent doses to meet the particular requirements of the patient. Certain drugs may produce more than one effect depending on the dose administered. For example, a low dose of a barbiturate produces sedation, whereas a larger dose produces hypnotic effects. The *usual dosage range* indicates the quantitative range or amounts of the drug that may be prescribed safely within the framework of usual medical practice. Doses falling outside of the usual dosage range may result in drug underdosage or overdosage or may reflect a patient's special requirements. For drugs administered to children, a *usual pediatric dose* may be determined as discussed later in this section.

The schedule of dosage, or the *dosage regimen,* is determined during the clinical investigation and is based largely on a drug's inherent duration of action, its pharmacokinetics, and the characteristics of the dosage form (e.g., instant drug release or modified-release). Due to these factors, some drugs are recommended for once a day dosage and others more frequently.

For certain drugs, an *initial, priming or loading*

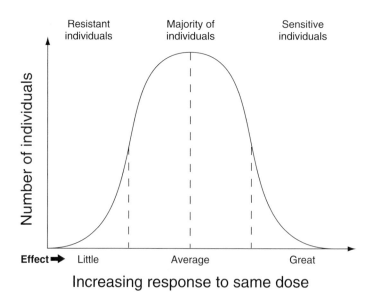

Fig. 2.8   *Drug effect in a population sample.*

dose may be required to attain the desired concentration of the drug in the blood or tissues, after which the blood level may be maintained through the subsequent administration of regularly scheduled *maintenance doses.*

Certain biological products, as Tetanus Immune Globulin, may have two different usual doses, one the *prophylactic dose,* or that amount administered to protect the patient from contracting the illness, and the second, the *therapeutic dose,* which is administered to a patient after exposure or contraction of the illness. The doses of vaccines and other biological products, as insulin, sometimes are expressed in *units of activity* rather than in specific quantitative amounts of the drug substance. This is due to the unavailability of suitable chemical assay methods for the active biologic component necessitating the use of biological assays to determine a product's potency.

To provide systemic effects, a drug must be absorbed from its route of administration at a suitable rate, be distributed in adequate concentration to the receptor sites, and remain there for a sufficient period. One measure of a drug's absorption characteristics is its blood serum concentration at various time intervals after administration. For certain drugs, a correlation can be made between blood serum concentration and the presentation of drug effects. For these drugs, an average blood serum concentration can be determined which represents the minimum concentration that can be expected to produce the drug's desired effects in a patient. This concentration is referred to as the *minimum effective concentration* (*MEC*). As shown in Figure 2.9, for a hypothetical drug, the serum concentration of the drug reaches the MEC 2 hours after its administration, achieves a peak concentration in 4 hours and decreases below

the MEC in 10 hours. If it would be desired to maintain the drug serum concentration above the MEC for a longer period, a second dose of the drug would be required at approximately the 8-hour time frame. The time-blood level curve presented in Figure 2.9 is hypothetical. In practice, the curve would vary, depending on the nature of the drug substance, its chemical and physical characteristics, the dosage form administered as well as individual patient factors. The second level of serum concentration of drug refers to the *minimum toxic concentration* (*MTC*). Drug serum concentrations above this level would be expected to produce dose-related toxic effects in the average individual. Ideally, the serum drug concentration in a well-dosed patient would be maintained between the MEC and the MTC (the "therapeutic window" for the drug) for the period that drug effects are desired. Table 2.3 presents examples of therapeutic, toxic, and considered lethal concentrations for some drug substances.

The *median effective dose* of a drug is that amount which will produce the desired intensity of effect in 50 percent of the individuals tested. The *median toxic dose* is that amount which will produce a defined toxic effect in 50 percent of the individuals tested. The relationship between the desired and undesired effects of a drug is commonly expressed as the *therapeutic index* and is defined as the ratio between a drug's median toxic dose and its median effective dose, TD50/ED50. Thus, a drug with a therapeutic index of 15 would be expected to have a greater margin of safety in its use than a drug with a therapeutic index of 5. For certain drugs, the therapeutic index may be as low as 2 and extreme caution must be exercised in their administration. Examples of therapeutic indices for same drugs are shown in Table 2.4.

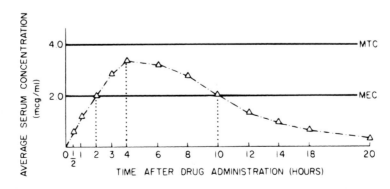

Fig. 2.9 *Example of a blood level curve for a hypothetical drug as a function of time following oral administration. MEC stands for minimum effective concentration and MTC for minimum toxic concentration.*

Table 2.3. Examples of Therapeutic and Toxic Blood Level Concentrations of Some Drug Substances*

Drug Substance	Drug Substance Concentration, mg/liter		
	Therapeutic	Toxic	Lethal
Acetaminophen	10–20	400	1500
Amitriptyline	0.5–0.20	0.4	10–20
Barbiturates:			
short acting	1	7	10
intermediate acting	1–5	10–30	30
long acting	~10	40–60	80–150
Dextropropoxyphene	0.05–0.2	5–10	57
Diazepam	0.5–2.5	5–20	>50
Digoxin	0.0006–0.0013	0.002–0.009	—
Imipramine	0.05–0.16	0.7	2
Lidocaine	1.2–5.0	6	—
Lithium	4.2–8.3	13.9	13.9–34.7
Meperidine	0.6–0.65	5	30
Morphine	0.1	—	0.05–4
Phenytoin	5–22	50	100
Quinidine	3–6	10	30–50
Theophylline	20–100	—	—

*Adapted from Winek CL. Clin Chem 1976;22:832; and Goth A. Medical Pharmacology, 11th ed. St. Louis: C.V. Mosby Co., 1984;757–759.

Some patient factors considered in determining a drug's dose in clinical investigations and in medical practice include the following.

Age

The age of the patient may be a consideration in the determination of drug dosage. Age is particularly important in the treatment of neonatal, pediatric, and geriatric patients. Infants, especially newborn and those born prematurely, have immature hepatic and renal function by which drugs are normally inactivated and eliminated from the body. A reduced capacity to detoxify and eliminate drugs can result in drug accumulation in the tissues to toxic levels. Often, drug blood levels are determined in these patients and carefully monitored.

Before there was sufficient understanding of the capacity of the pediatric patient to detoxify and eliminate drugs, infants and children were dosed by fractions of the adult dose determined by an age-based formula. Age alone is no longer considered to be a singularly valid criterion in the determination of pediatric dosage. Today, doses for many drugs are determined through pediatric clinical trials under special protocols and subject safeguards (45). Many pediatric doses are based on body weight or body surface area as noted later in this section.

Elderly persons also present unique therapeutic and dosing problems that require special attention.

Most physiologic functions begin to diminish in adults after the third decade of life. For example, cardiac output declines approximately 1 percent per year from age 20 to age 80. Glomerular filtration rate falls progressively until at age 80, to only about half of what it was at age 20. There is also a decrease in vital capacity, immune capacity and liver microsomal enzyme function (46). The decline in renal and hepatic function in the elderly slows the drug clearance rate and increases the possibil-

Table 2.4. Examples of Therapeutic Indices for Various Drug Substances*

Drug Substances with Therapeutic Indices		
Less than 5	Between 5 and 10	Greater than 10
Amitriptyline	Barbiturates	Acetaminophen
Chlordiazepoxide	Diazepam	Bromide
Diphenhydramine	Digoxin	Chloral hydrate
Ethchlorvynol	Imipramine	Glutethimide
Lidocaine	Meperidine	Meprobamate
Methadone	Paraldehyde	Nortriptyline
Procainamide	Primodone	Pentazocine
Quinidine	Thioridazine	Propoxyphene

*Reprinted with permission from Niazi S. Textbook of Biopharmaceutics and Clinical Pharmacokinetics. New York: Appleton-Century-Crofts, 1979;254.

ity of drug accumulation and toxicity. Elderly persons may also respond differently to drugs than younger patients because of changes in drug-receptor sensitivity or because of age-related alterations in target tissues or organs (47).

Further, the chronic disorders present in the majority of geriatric patients requires concomitant drug therapy, increasing the possibility of drug–drug interactions, and adverse drug effects. In the clinical evaluation of a new drug, consideration is given to other drugs most likely to be taken concomitantly by the intended patient, with studies directed toward determining potential drug-drug effects or interactions.

To assist the pharmacist in pediatric and geriatric patient dosing, the American Pharmaceutical Association publishes the *Pediatric Dosage Handbook* and the *Geriatric Dosage Handbook* (48).

Body Weight

The usual doses for drugs are considered generally suitable for 70 kg (150 pound) individuals. The ratio between the amount of drug administered and the size of the body influences drug concentration in body fluids. Therefore, drug dosage may require adjustment from the usual adult dose for abnormally lean or heavy patients. The doses for certain drugs are determined based on body weight and are expressed on a *milligram* (drug) *per kilogram* (body weight) basis (e.g., 1 mg/kg).

As noted earlier, drug dosage for youngsters based on body weight is considered more dependable than that based strictly on age and for many drugs the dose is determined on a mg/kg basis. In some instances, a pediatric dose may be based on a combination of age and weight (e.g., 6 months to 2 years of age—3 mg/kg/ day).

Body Surface Area

Due to the correlation that exists between a number of physiological processes and body surface area (BSA), some drug doses are determined based on this relationship (e.g., 1 mg/M^2 BSA). The body surface area for a child or an adult may be determined using a nomogram (Fig. 2.10). The BSA is determined at the intersect of a straight line drawn to connect an individual's height and weight. For example, an adult measuring 67 inches in height and weighing 132 pounds would have a BSA of approximately 1.7 square meters.

Sex

Because men and women have different responses to certain drugs and drug dosages due to biochemical and physiologic factors, both sexes should be included in clinical drug trials. Pharmacokinetic differences between women and men may be particularly important for drugs having a narrow therapeutic index (NTI), in which the smaller average size of women might necessitate modified dosing. Drugs with narrow therapeutic indices carry the inherent risk that drug blood levels may increase to toxic levels or decrease to ineffective levels with minimal dosing changes. Other important female gender studies include the effects of the menstrual cycle and menopausal status on a drug's pharmacokinetics and the drug interaction potential of concomitant estrogen or oral contraceptive use (49).

Because virtually all clinical investigations have not included pregnant women in their study protocols, and thus drug effects are undetermined in these circumstances, great caution is advised for most drugs' use during pregnancy and in women of child-bearing age. A similar caution is applicable to drug use in nursing mothers because the transfer of drugs from mother's milk to an infant is well documented for a variety of drugs with drug effects (50–51).

Pathologic State

The effects of certain drugs may be modified by the pathologic condition of the patient. For example, if certain drugs are used in the presence of renal impairment, excessive systemic accumulation of the drug may occur with possible toxicity. Under such conditions, lower than usual doses are indicated, and if therapy is prolonged, blood serum levels of the drug should be taken and the patient monitored at regular intervals to assure the maintenance of non-toxic levels of the drug. In these instances, pharmacokinetic dosing is an integral part of the clinical study protocol and of approved product labeling.

Tolerance

The ability to endure the influence of a drug, particularly when acquired by a continued use of the substance, is referred to as *drug tolerance*. It is usually developed to a specific drug and to its chemical congeners; in the latter instance, it is referred to as *cross-tolerance*. The result is that drug dosage must be increased over time to maintain a desired therapeutic response. Tolerance is common with the use of antihistamines and narcotic analgesics. After the development of tolerance, normal response may be regained by suspending the drug's administration for a period of time.

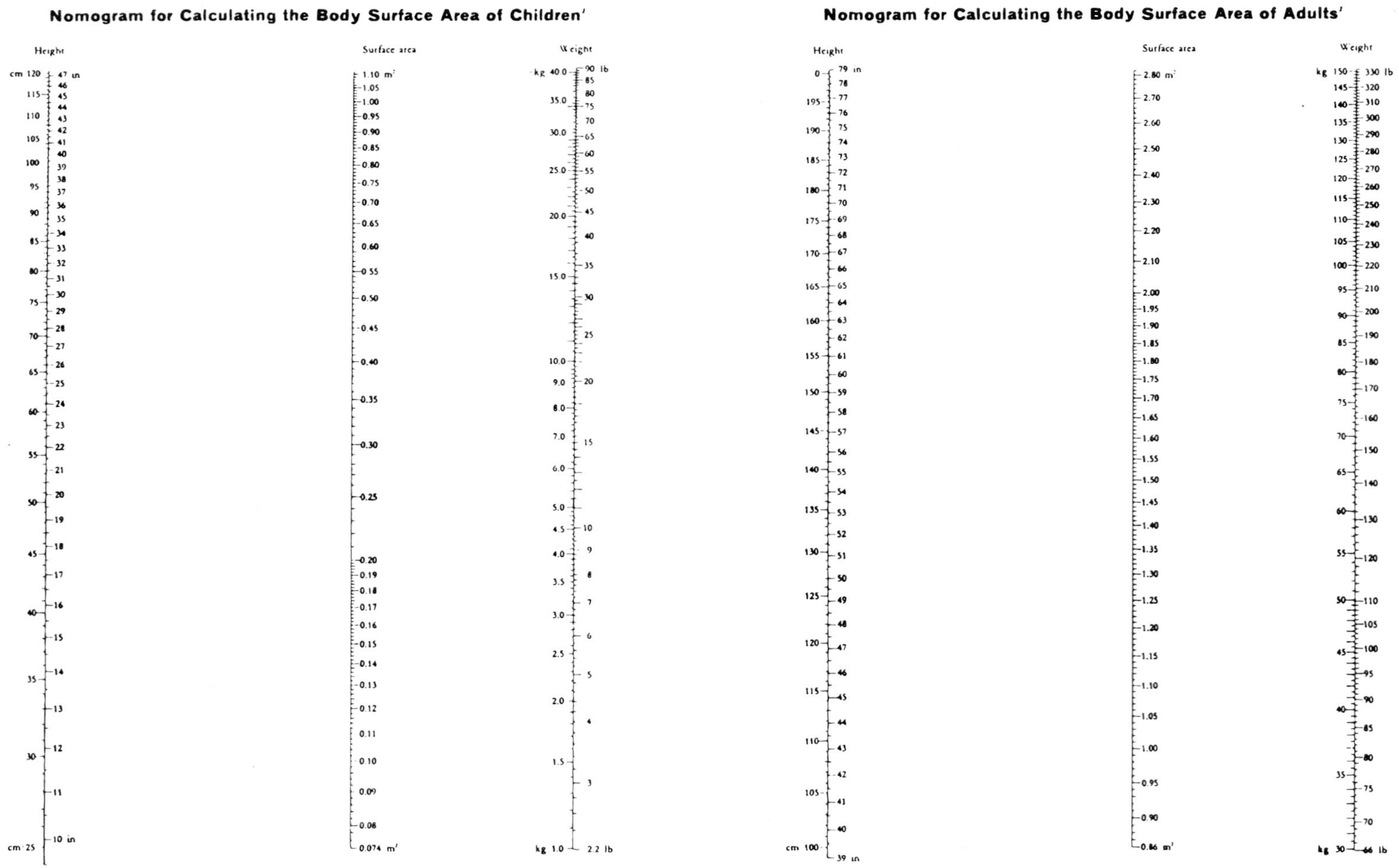

Nomogram for Calculating the Body Surface Area of Children'

Nomogram for Calculating the Body Surface Area of Adults'

'From the formula of DeBois and DeBois, *Arch Intern. Med.*,17, 863 1916 $S = W^{0.425} \times H^{0.725} \times 71.84$ or log $S = 0.425$ log $W + 0.725$ log $H + 1.8564$ where S = body surface area in square centimeters, W = weight in kilograms, H = height in centimeters

Fig. 2.10 *Nomograms for calculating body surface area. (Reprinted with permission from R.J. Geigy S.A. Documenta Geigy Scientific Tables, 6th ed., pp. 632–633.)*

Concomitant Drug Therapy

The effects of a drug may be modified by the prior or concurrent administration of another drug. Such interference between drugs is referred to as a *drug–drug interaction* and may be due to a chemical or physical interaction between the drugs or to an alteration of the absorption, distribution, metabolism, or excretion patterns of one of the drugs. Certain clinical protocols include the evaluation of a new drug in the presence of other drugs most likely to be included in the target patient's therapeutic regimen.

Important drug–drug interactions that are identified during a drug's clinical trials are included in approved product labeling. Additional drug interactions that become known after the drug is marketed are added in labeling revisions. Drug–drug interactions may include "social" agents such as tobacco and alcohol, which affect the pharmacokinetics of a number of drugs and require an alteration in a drug's usual dose.

Time and Conditions of Administration

The time at which a drug is administered may influence dosage. This is especially true for oral therapy in relation to meals. Absorption proceeds more rapidly if the stomach and upper portions of the intestinal tract are empty of food. A dose of a drug that is effective when taken before a meal may be less effective if administered during or after eating. Drug–food interactions can affect a drug's usual absorption pattern. When such interactions are determined, appropriate guidance is provided in the product literature.

Dosage Form and Route of Administration

The effective dose of a drug may vary, depending on the dosage form and the route of administration. Drugs administered intravenously enter the blood stream directly and completely. In contrast, drugs administered orally are rarely, if ever, fully absorbed into the bloodstream due to the various physical, chemical, and biologic barriers to their absorption. Thus, in many instances, a lower parenteral (injectable) dose of a drug is required than the oral dose to achieve the same blood levels or clinical effects. Varying rates and degrees of absorption can occur from drug administration from the rectum, gastrointestinal tract, sublingually, via the skin and from other sites. Therefore for a given drug, different dosage forms and routes of administration are considered "new" by the FDA and must be evaluated individually through clinical studies to determine the effective doses.

"Treatment IND"

A *Treatment IND* or a *treatment protocol* permits the use of an investigational drug in the treatment of patients *not enrolled* in the clinical study but who have a serious or immediately life-threatening disease for which there is no satisfactory alternative therapy. The objective is to make promising new drugs available to desperately ill patients as early as possible in the drug development process. By FDA definition, *"immediately life-threatening"* means "a stage of a disease in which there is a reasonable likelihood that death will occur within a matter of months or in which premature death is likely without early treatment" (1). This would include such conditions as advanced cases of AIDS, herpes simplex encephalitis, advanced metastatic refractory cancers, bacterial endocarditis, Alzheimer's disease, advanced multiple sclerosis, advanced Parkinson's disease, and others.

For products to be considered for a Treatment IND, the drug must be under active investigation in a controlled clinical trial with sufficient evidence of its safety and efficacy demonstrated to support its use in the intended patients. Depending on the sponsor's clinical safety and efficacy data, a drug may be approved for "treatment use" during Phase 2 or Phase 3 of the clinical trials. In applying for a drug's treatment use, a sponsor must submit a *treatment protocol* in addition to the information normally included in an IND application. In making its decision, the FDA renders a risk–benefit judgment after considering the severity of the disease, any alternative therapy, and the potential benefits of the drug against the known and potential risks. In addition to the treatment IND, there is also provision in the law for the *emergency use* of an investigational drug in rare situations before a sponsor's submission of an IND application (1).

IND for an Orphan Drug

Under the Orphan Drug Act of 1983 as amended, an *orphan disease* is defined as a rare disease or condition that affects fewer than 200,000 people in the United States and for which there is no reasonable expectation that costs of research and development for the indication can be recovered by sales of the product in the United States. Examples of such illnesses are chronic lymphocytic leukemia, Gaucher's disease, cystic fibrosis, and conditions related to acquired immune deficiency syndrome (AIDS).

The FDA Office of Orphan Products Development was established to identify and facilitate the development of orphan products, including drugs, biologics, and medical devices. To foster the necessary research and development, the FDA provides support grants to conduct clinical trials on safety and effectiveness. Applicants first request orphan status designation for the disease and file an IND or an investigational device exemption (IDE) with their grant application. In most cases, grants are awarded for Phase 2 and Phase 3 clinical studies based on preliminary clinical research. Regular and Treatment IND protocols may be included in orphan drug clinical trials. An incentive to orphan product development is a provision for a 7-year period of exclusive marketing rights after regulatory approval of a product.

Withdrawal or Termination of an IND

A sponsor may withdraw an IND at any time ending all clinical investigations. All stock of clinical supplies must be returned to the sponsor or otherwise destroyed. If an IND is withdrawn because of safety reasons, the FDA, IRB, and all investigators must be so advised.

If no subjects are entered in an IND for a period of two years or more or if investigations remain on a clinical hold for one year or more, the FDA may place the IND on "inactive status," upon proper notification of the sponsor. An IND may also be placed on inactive status on the initiative of the sponsor.

The FDA may terminate an IND and end related clinical investigations based on safety, efficacy, or regulatory compliance issues.

The New Drug Application (NDA)

If the three phases of clinical testing during the IND period demonstrate sufficient drug safety and therapeutic effectiveness, the sponsor may file a New Drug Application (NDA) with the Food and Drug Administration. This filing may be preceded by a pre-NDA meeting between the sponsor and the FDA to discuss the content and format of the new drug application. The purpose of the NDA is to gain permission to market the drug product in the United States.

General Content of the NDA Submission

An NDA application contains a complete presentation of all of the preclinical and clinical results that the sponsor has obtained during investigation

of the drug. It is a highly organized document that may contain several hundred volumes of information. In recent years, a computer-assisted new drug application (CANDA) process has been implemented whereby the sponsor may interact by computer with the FDA reviewers to facilitate the application review process.

The applicant submits three copies of the NDA: an *archival copy*, maintained by the FDA as the reference document; a *review copy*, used by the FDA review division, and a *field copy*, used by the FDA district office and field inspectors in an on-site *pre-approval inspection* (1). The pre-approval inspection is conducted in the facilities in which the approved product is to be produced. The inspectors assess the sponsor's capability to comply with all control and quality standards contained in the application including the FDA's Current Good Manufacturing Practice (CGMP) standards (discussed in Chapter 5). Final approval of an NDA can be contingent upon this inspection.

In part, an application for a new chemical entity contains the following components:

- Application form (Form FDA 356h) with the name, address, date, and signature of the applicant or of the applicant's authorized representative;
- Chemical, nonproprietary, code and proprietary names of the drug, the dosage form, its strength, and route of administration;
- Statement regarding the applicant's proposal to market the drug product as a prescription-only, or, as an OTC product;
- Detailed summary of all aspects of the application, including the proposed text of the product's intended labeling, chemistry, manufacturing and controls, nonclinical and clinical pharmacology and toxicology, human pharmacokinetics and bioavailability, statistical analysis, clinical trial data, benefit and risk considerations, and proposed additional or planned postmarketing studies;
- Detailed technical sections on the chemistry, manufacturing and controls for the drug substance, including its physical and chemical characteristics, methods of identification, assay, and controls and the drug product, including its composition, specifications, methods of manufacture and equipment used, in-process controls, batch and master production records, container and closure systems, stability, and expiration dating;
- Detailed technical sections for nonclinical pharmacology and toxicology in relation to the pro-

posed therapeutic indication, including acute, subacute, and chronic toxicology, carcinogenicity, reproductive toxicology, and animal studies of absorption, distribution, metabolism, and excretion;

- Detailed technical sections for human pharmacokinetics and bioavailabilty, and microbiology for antibiotic applications;
- Detailed technical sections for clinical data for each controlled and uncontrolled study relating to the proposed indication, a copy of the study protocol, effectiveness and safety data including any updates on safety information, comparison of human and animal pharmacology and toxicology data, support for the dosage and dose intervals and modifications for specific subgroups, as pediatrics, geriatrics, and renally impaired;
- Statement regarding compliance to IRB and informed consent requirements;
- Statistical methods and analysis of the clinical data;
- Samples of the drug substance, drug product proposed for marketing, reference standards, and finished market package, as requested; and
- Clinical case report forms for the archival copy of the application.

The FDA accepts foreign clinical data if they are applicable to the United States population and domestic medical practice; if the studies were conducted by clinical investigatiors of recognized competence; and, if the FDA considers the data to be valid without the need for an on-site inspection. The FDA has entered into certain bilateral agreements with some countries whereby inspections performed by regulatory personnel of those countries are acceptable to the FDA.

Drug Product Labeling

The labeling of all drug products distributed in the United States must meet the specific labeling requirements set forth in *Code of Federal Regulations* and approved for each product by the Food and Drug Administration (52). Specific labeling requirements differ for prescription drugs, nonprescription drugs, and animal drugs. In each instance, however, the objective is the same—to ensure the appropriate and safe use of the approved product.

According to federal regulations, *drug labeling* includes not only the labels placed on an immediate container but also the information on the packaging, in package inserts, and in company literature, advertising, and promotional materials.

For prescription drugs, labeling represents a summary of all of the preclinical and clinical studies conducted over the period of years from drug discovery through product development to FDA approval. The essential prescribing information for a human prescription drug is provided in the package insert, which by law contains a balanced presentation of the usefulness and the risks associated with the product to enable safe and effective use. The package insert is required to contain the following summary information in the order listed.

1. *Description* of the product, including the proprietary and nonproprietary names, dosage form and route of administration, quantitative product composition, pharmacologic or therapeutic class of the drug, chemical name and structural formula of the drug compound, and important chemical and physical information (pH, sterility, etc.).
2. *Clinical Pharmacology,* including a summary of actions of the drug in humans, relevant in-vitro and animal studies essential to the biochemical and/or physiological basis for action, pharmacokinetic information on rate and degree of absorption, biotransformation and metabolite formation, degree of drug binding to plasma proteins, rate or half-time of elimination, uptake by a particular organ or fetus, and any toxic effects.
3. *Indications and Usage,* including the FDA-approved indications in the treatment, prevention, or diagnosis of a disease or condition, evidence of effectiveness demonstrated by results of controlled clinical trials, special conditions to the drug's use for short-term or long-term use.
4. *Contraindications,* stating those situations in which the drug should not be used because the risk of use clearly outweighs any possible beneficial effect. Included are contraindications associated with drug hypersensitivity, concomitant therapy, disease state, and/or factors of age or gender.
5. *Warnings,* including descriptions of serious adverse reactions and potential safety hazards, limitations to use imposed by them, and steps to be taken if they occur.
6. *Precautions,* including special care to be exercised by prescriber and patient in the use of the drug; e.g., drug/drug, drug/food, drug/laboratory test interactions, effects on fertility, use in pregnancy, use in nursing mothers, and in pediatric patients.
7. *Adverse Reactions,* including predictable and potential unpredictable undesired (side) effects, categorized by organ system or severity of reaction and frequency of occurrence.

8. *Drug Abuse and Dependence,* including legal schedule if a controlled substance, types of abuse and resultant adverse reactions, psychological and physical dependence potential, and treatment of withdrawal.
9. *Overdosage,* including signs, symptoms, and laboratory findings of acute overdosage, along with specifics or general principles of treatment.
10. *Dosage and Administration,* stating the recommended usual dose, the usual dosage range, the safe upper limit of dosage, duration of treatment, modification of dosage in special patient populations (children, elders, patients with kidney and/or liver dysfunction), and special rates of administration (as with parenteral medications).
11. *How Supplied,* including information on available dosage forms, strengths, and means of dosage form identification, as color, coating, scoring, and National Drug Code.

FDA Review and "Action Letters"

The completed New Drug Application is carefully reviewed by the Food and Drug Administration, which decides whether to allow the sponsor to market the drug, to disallow marketing, or to require additional data before rendering a judgment. By regulation, the FDA must respond within 180 days of receipt of an application. This 180-day period is called the *review clock* and is often extended by mutual agreement between the applicant and the FDA, as additional information, studies, or clarifications are sought.

The NDA is reviewed by the same FDA division that reviewed the sponsor's original IND. However, for the NDA review, the FDA also obtains the recommendation of an outside Advisory Review Committee, comprised of persons of recognized competence and stature in the clinical area of the proposed drug's use. Although not binding, this committee's recommendation has influence in the FDA's decision to issue one of the following action letters after the entire review of the application is completed.

Approvable Letter. The agency will approve the application if specific additional data or other requested material is submitted, or specified conditions are met. This frequently pertains to development or wording of the final product labeling.

Approval Letter. Approval of the application permitting marketing.

Not Approvable Letter. The application is not considered approvable because of one or more deficiencies.

After an NDA is approved and the product marketed, the FDA requires periodic safety and other reports, schedules plant inspections, and requires continued compliance with control and quality standards and current good manufacturing practices.

Phase 4 Studies and Postmarketing Surveillance

The receipt of marketing status for a new drug product does not necessarily end a sponsor's investigation of the drug. Continued clinical investigations, often referred to as Phase 4 studies, may contribute to the understanding of the drug's mechanism or scope of action; may indicate possible new therapeutic uses for the drug; and/or may demonstrate the need for additional dosage strengths, dosage forms or routes of administration. Postmarketing studies may also reveal additional side effects, serious and unexpected adverse drug effects, and/or drug interactions.

In applying for a new use, strength, dosage form, or route of administration for a previously approved drug, the sponsor must file a new IND, conduct all necessary additional nonclinical and clinical studies, and file a new NDA for FDA review.

Postmarketing Reporting of Adverse Drug Experiences

A drug's sponsor is required to report to the FDA each adverse drug experience that is both serious (life-threatening or fatal) and unexpected (not contained in the approved drug product labeling) regardless of the source of the information within 15 working days of receipt of the information. These "15-day Alert" reports must then be investigated by the sponsor with a follow-up report submitted to the FDA, again within 15 working days. Other adverse experiences, not considered serious and unexpected, are reported on a quarterly basis for three years following the date of approval of the NDA and then annually thereafter. Practicing pharmacists and other health care professionals participate in adverse drug experience reporting through the FDA's "MedWatch" program, using forms provided for this purpose (53).

Depending on the nature, causal relationship, and seriousness of an adverse drug reaction (ADR) report, the FDA may require revised product labeling to reflect the new findings; ask the sponsor to issue special warning notices to health care professionals; undertake or require the sponsor to undertake a review of all available clinical data; restrict the marketing of the product during a review period; issue a product recall notice; or withdraw product approval for marketing.

In the event of information on, or a confirmed incident of, a mislabeled, contaminated, or deteriorated product in distribution, the sponsor is required to file an "NDA-Field Alert Report" to the FDA District office by telephone or other rapid communication within 3 working days of receipt of the information. The FDA follows up with appropriate action.

Annual Reports

Each year the sponsor of an approved drug must file, with the FDA division responsible for the NDA review, a report containing the following information: an annual summary of significant new information that might affect the safety, effectiveness, or labeling of the drug product; data on the quantity of dosage units of the drug product distributed domestically and abroad; a sample of currently used professional labeling, patient brochures, or package inserts, and a summary of any changes since the previous report; reports of experiences, investigations, studies, or tests involving chemical or physical properties of the drug that may affect its safety or effectiveness; a full description of any manufacturing and controls changes (not requiring a Supplemental New Drug Application); copies of unpublished reports and summaries of published reports of new toxicologic findings in vitro and animal studies conducted or obtained by the sponsor; full or abstract reports on published clinical trials of the drug, including studies on safety and effectiveness; new uses; biopharmaceutic, pharmacokinetic, clinical pharmacologic, and epidemiologic reports; pharmacotherapeutic and lay press articles on the drug; summaries of unpublished clinical trials or prepublication manuscripts, as available, conducted or obtained by the sponsor; a statement on the current status of any postmarketing studies performed by, or on behalf of, the sponsor; and specimens of mailing pieces or other forms of promotion of the drug product. Failure to make required reports may lead to FDA withdrawal of approval for marketing.

Supplemental, Abbreviated, and Other Applications

In addition to the IND and NDA the following types of applications are filed with the FDA for the purposes described.

Supplemental New Drug Application (SNDA)

A sponsor of an approved NDA may make changes in that application through the filing of a Supplemental New Drug Application (SNDA). Depending on the changes proposed, some require FDA approval before implementing; others do not.

Among the changes requiring prior approval are: a change in the method of synthesis of the drug substance; use of a different facility to manufacture the drug substance where the facility has not been approved through inspection for Current Good Manufacturing Practice standards within the previous 2 years; change in the formulation, analytical standards, method of manufacture, or in-process controls of the drug product; use of a different facility or contractor to manufacture, process, or package the drug product; change in the container and closure system for a drug product; extension of the expiration date for a drug product based on new stability data; any labeling change that does not add to or strengthen a previously approved label statement.

Examples of changes that may be made without prior approval are: minor editorial or other changes in the labeling that add to or strengthen an approved label section; any analytical changes made to comply with the USP/NF; an extension of the product's expiration date based on full shelf-life data obtained from a protocol in the approved application; and a change in the size (not the type of system) of the container for a solid dosage form.

Abbreviated New Drug Application (ANDA)

An Abbreviated New Drug Application (ANDA) is one in which nonclinical laboratory studies and clinical investigations may be omitted, except those pertaining to the drug's bioavailability. These applications are usually filed for duplicates (generic copies) of drug products previously approved under a full NDA, and for which the FDA has determined that information on the exempted nonclinical and clinical studies is already available at the agency. ANDAs commonly are filed by competing companies following the expiration of patent term protection of the innovator drug/drug product. Bioavailability and product bioequivalency are discussed in Chapter 4.

Biologics License Application (BLA)

Biologics License Applications (BLAs) are submitted to the FDA's Center for Biologics Evaluation and Research (CBER) for the manufacture of biologicals, as blood products, vaccines, and toxins. The applications for biologics approvals follow the regulatory requirements as stated specifically for these products in the relevant parts of the *Code of Federal Regulations* (4).

Animal Drug Applications

The Federal Food, Drug, and Cosmetic Act, as amended, contains specific regulations pertaining to the approval for the marketing and labeling of drugs intended for animal use (6). Regulations apply to Investigational New Animal Drug Applications (INADA), New Animal Drug Applications (NADA), Supplemental New Animal Drug Applications (SNADA) and Abbreviated New Animal Drug Applications (ANADA).

Medical Devices

The Food and Drug Administration has regulatory authority over the manufacture and licensing of all medical devices, from surgeon's gloves and catheters to cardiac pacemakers and cardiopulmonary bypass blood gas monitors (7). Included in the regulations are standards and procedures for manufacturer registration, investigational studies, good manufacturing practices, and premarket approval.

International Conference on Harmonization of Technical Requirements for Registration of Pharmaceuticals for Human Use (ICH)

In recognition of the international marketplace for pharmaceuticals and in an effort to achieve global efficiencies for both regulatory agencies and the pharmaceutical industry, the FDA, counterpart agencies of the European Union and Japan, and geographic representatives of the pharmaceutical industry formed a tripartite organization in 1991 to discuss, identify, and address relevant regulatory issues. This organization, named the International Conference on Harmonization of Technical Requirements for Registration of Pharmaceuticals for Human Use (ICH) has worked toward "harmonizing" or bringing together regulatory requirements with the long range goal of establishing a uniform set of standards for drug registration within these geographic areas.

With ICH success, duplicative technical requirements for registering pharmaceuticals would be

eliminated; new drug approvals would occur more rapidly; patient access to new medicines would be enhanced worldwide; the quality, safety and efficacy of imported products would be improved; and there would be an increase in information transfer between participating countries (54–55).

The ICH's work toward uniform standards is focused in three general areas: drug/drug product quality, safety, and efficacy.

The quality topics include stability, light stability, analytical validation, impurities, and biotechnology. The safety topics include carcinogenicity, genotoxicity, toxicokinetics, reproduction toxicity, and single and repeat dose toxicity. The efficacy topics include population exposure, managing clinical trials, clinical study reports, dose response, ethnic factors, good clinical practices, and geriatrics. For each topic, relevant regulations are identified, addressed, and consensus guidelines developed. The intention is that these guidelines will be incorporated into domestic regulations. In the United States, the resulting guidelines are published in the *Federal Register* as "Notices," with accompanying statements indicating that the guideline should be "useful" or "considered" by applicants conducting required studies or submitting registration applications. Examples of specific ICH-developed guidelines include:

Stability Testing of New Drug Substances and Products
Validation of Analytical Procedures for Pharmaceuticals
Impurities in New Drug Substances
Impurities in New Drug Products
Nonclinical Safety Studies for the Conduct of Human Clinical Trials for Pharmaceuticals
Preclinical Testing of Biotechnology-Derived Pharmaceuticals
General Considerations for Clinical Trials
Studies in Support of Special Populations: Geriatrics
Ethnic Factors in the Acceptability of Foreign Data
Repeated Dose Tissue Distribution Studies
Dose Selection for Carcinogenicity Studies of Pharmaceuticals
Dose Response Information to Support Drug Registration

References

1. *Code of Federal Regulations, Title 21, Parts 300–314.*
2. *Code of Federal Regulations, Title 21, Part 320.*
3. *Code of Federal Regulations, Title 21, Part 430.*

4. *Code of Federal Regulations, Title 21, Parts 600–680.*
5. *Code of Federal Regulations, Title 21, Part 330.*
6. *Code of Federal Regulations, Title 21, Parts 510–555.*
7. *Code of Federal Regulations, Title 21, Parts 800–895.*
8. Federal Register, U.S. Washington, DC: Government Printing Office, Superintendent of Documents.
9. Mathieu M. New Drug Development: A Regulatory Overview. 3rd ed. Cambridge, MA: PAREXEL International Corporation, 1994.
10. Guarino RA, ed. New Drug Approval Process. New York: Marcel Dekker, 1987.
11. Smith CG. The Process of New Drug Discovery and Development. Boca Raton, FL: CRC Press, 1992.
12. Sneader W. Drug Development: From Laboratory to Clinic. New York: John Wiley & Sons, 1986.
13. Spilker B. Multinational Pharmaceutical Companies Principles and Practices. 2nd ed. New York: Raven Press, 1994.
14. Wordell CJ. Biotechnology update. Hosp Pharm 1991;26:897–900.
15. Tami JA, Parr MD, Brown SA, Thompson, JS. Monoclonal antibody technology. Am J Hosp Pharm 1986;43:2816–2826.
16. Brodsky FM. Monoclonal antibodies as magic bullets. Pharm Res 1988;5:1–9.
17. Parasrampuria DA, Hunt CA. Therapeutic delivery issues in gene therapy, part 2: targeting approaches. Pharm Tech 1998;22:34–43.
18. Chew NJ. Cellular and gene therapies, part 1: regulatory health. BioPharmacy 1995;8:22–23.
19. Smith TJ. Gene therapy: opportunities for pharmacy in the 21st century. Am J Pharm Ed 1996;60:213–215.
20. Milestones in gene therapy. BioPharmacy 1997;10:17.
21. Kauvar, LM. Affinity fingerprinting: implications for drug discovery. Pharm News 1996;3:12–15.
22. Harris, AL. High throughput screening and molecular diversity. Pharm News 1995;2:26–30.
23. Silverman RB. Drug discovery, design, and development. In: The organic chemistry of drug design and drug action. New York: Academic Press, 1992; 4–51.
24. Perun TJ, Propst CL, eds. Computer-aided Drug Design: Methods and Applications, New York: Marcel Dekker, Inc., 1989.
25. Benet LZ, Mitchell JR, Sheiner LB. General principles. In: Goodman L, Gilman A, eds. The Pharmacologic Basis of Therapeutics. New York: Pergamon Press, 1990;8:1–2.
26. Katzung BG. Basic and Clinical Pharmacology. Norwalk, CT: Appleton & Lange, 1987;44–51.
27. Spilker B. Extrapolation of preclinical safety data to humans. Drug News Perspect 1991;4:214–216.
28. Guideline for the Format and Content of the Nonclinical/ Pharmacology/Toxicology Section of an Application. Rockville, MD: Food and Drug Administration, 1987.
29. 60 FR 11263–11268. International conference on harmonization; guideline on the assessment of systemic exposure in toxicity studies, 1995.
30. 60 FR 11277–11281. International conference on har-

monization; guidance on dose selection for carcinogenicity study of pharmaceuticals, 1995.
31. 58 FR 21073–21080. International conference on harmonization; draft guideline on detection of toxicity to reproduction for medicinal products, 1993.
32. 59 FR 48734–48737. International conference on harmonization, draft guideline on specific aspects of regulatory genotoxicity tests, 1994.
33. Guideline for the Format and Content of the Chemistry, Manufacturing, and Controls Section of an Application. Rockville, MD: Food and Drug Administration, 1987.
34. Code of Federal Regulations, Title 21, Parts 210–211.
35. 58 Federal Register 39405–39416. Guideline for the study and evaluation of gender differences in the clinical evaluation of drugs, 1993.
36. 59 Federal Register 11145–11151. NIH guidelines on the inclusion of women and minorities as subjects in clinical research, 1994.
37. Richardson ER. Drugs and pregnancy. Wellcome Trends in Pharmacy 1983;7:4.
38. 62 Federal Register 49946–49954. Investigational new drug applications; proposed amendment to clinical hold regulations for products intended for life-threatening diseases, 1997.
39. Wright DT, Chew NJ. Women as subjects in clinical research. Applied Clinical Trials 1996;5:44–52
40. Wick JY. Culture, ethnicity, and medications. JAPhA 1996;NS36:555–563.
41. Code of Federal Regulations, Title 21, Part 56.
42. Code of Federal Regulations, Title 21, Part 50.
43. Hunter JR, Rosen DL, DeChristoforo R. How FDA expedites evaluation of drugs for AIDS and other life-threatening illnesses. Wellcome Programs in Hosp Pharm 1993 (January).
44. Spilker B. Guide to Clinical Trials. New York: Raven Press, 1991.
45. Bush C. When your subject is a child. Appl Clin Trials 1997;6:54–56.
46. Cohen HJ. The elderly patient, a challenge to the art and science of medicine. Drug Ther 1983;13:41.
47. Futerman SS. The geriatric patient—pharmacy care can make a difference. The Apothecary 1982;94:34.
48. American Pharmaceutical Association, Washington, DC
49. Food and Drug Administration. FDA Med Bull 1993;23:2–4.
50. Logsdon BA. Drug use during lactation. JAPhA 1997;NS37:407–418.
51. The transfer of drugs and other chemicals into human breast milk. Washington, DC: American Pharmaceutical Association 1983.
52. Code of Federal Regulations, Title 21, Part 201.
53. MedWatch. Rockville, MD: Food and Drug Administration.
54. Heydorn WE. ICH: background and current status. Pharm News 1994;1:22–24.
55. Report of the FDA task force on international harmonization. Rockville, MD: Food and Drug Administration, 1992.

DOSAGE FORM DESIGN: PHARMACEUTIC AND FORMULATION CONSIDERATIONS

Chapter at a Glance

DRUG SUBSTANCES are seldom administered alone, but rather as part of a formulation in combination with one or more nonmedical agents that serve varied and specialized pharmaceutical functions. Through selective use of these nonmedicinal agents, referred to as *pharmaceutic ingredients,* dosage forms of various types result. The pharmaceutic ingredients solubilize, suspend, thicken, dilute, emulsify, stabilize, preserve, color, flavor, and fashion medicinal agents into efficacious and appealing dosage forms. Each type of dosage form is unique in its physical and pharmaceutical characteristics. These varied preparations provide the manufacturing and compounding pharmacist with the challenges of formulation and the physician with the choice of drug and drug delivery system to prescribe. The general area of study concerned with the formulation, manufacture, stability, and effectiveness of pharmaceutical dosage forms is termed *pharmaceutics.*

The proper design and formulation of a dosage form requires consideration of the physical, chemical and biological characteristics of all of the drug substances and pharmaceutic ingredients to be used in fabricating the product. The drug and pharmaceutic materials utilized must be compatible with one another to produce a drug product that is stable, efficacious, attractive, easy to administer and safe. The product should be manufactured under appropriate measures of quality control and packaged in containers that contribute to product stability. The product should be labeled to promote correct use and be stored under conditions that contribute to maximum shelf life.

Methods for the preparation of specific types of dosage forms and drug delivery systems are described in subsequent chapters. This chapter presents some general considerations regarding physical pharmacy, drug product formulation and pharmaceutic ingredients.

The Need for Dosage Forms

The potent nature and low dosage of most of the drugs in use today precludes any expectation that the general public could safely obtain the appropriate dose of a drug from the bulk material. The vast majority of drug substances are administered in milligram quantities, much too small to be weighed on anything but a sensitive laboratory balance. For instance, how could the layperson accurately obtain the 325 mg of aspirin found in the common aspirin tablet from a bulk supply of aspirin? It couldn't be done. Yet, compared with many other drugs, the dose of aspirin is formidable (Table 3.1). For example, the dose of ethinyl estradiol, 0.05 mg, is 1/6500 the amount of aspirin in an aspirin tablet. To put it another way, 6500 ethinyl estradiol tablets, each containing 0.05 mg of drug, could be made from an amount of ethinyl estradiol equal to the amount of aspirin in just one 325 mg aspirin tablet. When the dose of the drug is minute, as that for ethinyl estradiol, solid dosage forms such as tablets and capsules must be prepared with fillers or diluents so that the size of the resultant dosage unit is large enough to pick up with the fingertips.

Besides providing the mechanism for the safe and convenient delivery of accurate dosage, dosage forms are needed for additional reasons:

1. For the protection of a drug substance from the destructive influences of atmospheric oxygen or humidity (e.g., coated tablets, sealed ampuls)
2. For the protection of a drug substance from the destructive influence of gastric acid after oral administration (e.g., enteric-coated tablets)

Table 3.1. Examples of Some Drugs with Relatively Low Usual Doses

Drug	Usual Dose, mg	Category
Betaxolol HCl	10	Antianginal
Clotrimizole	10	Antifungal
Methylphenidate HCl	10	CNS Stimulant
Medroxyprogesterone acetate	10	Progestin
Mesoridazine besylate	10	Antipsychotic
Morphine Sulfate	10	Narcotic analgesic
Nifedipine	10	Coronary vasodilator
Omeprazole	10	Antiulcer
Quinapril HCl	10	Antihypertensive
Chlorazepate dipotassium	7.5	Tranquilizer
Buspirone HCl	5	Antianxiety
Enalapril maleate	5	Antihypertensive
Hydrocodone	5	Narcotic analgesic
Prednisolone	5	Adrenocortical steroid
Albuterol sulfate	4	Bronchodilator
Chlorpheniramine Maleate	4	Antihistaminic
Felodipine	2.5	Vasodilator
Glyburide	2.5	Antidiabetic
Doxazosin mesylate	2	Antihypertensive
Levorphanol tartrate	2	Narcotic analgesic
Prazosin HCl	2	Antihypertensive
Risperidone	2	Antipsychotic
Estropipate	1.25	Estrogen
Bumetanide	1	Diuretic
Clonazepam	1	Anticonvulsant
Ergoloid mesylates	1	Cognitive adjuvant
Alprazolam	0.5	Antianxiety
Colchicine	0.5	Gout suppressant
Nitroglycerin	0.4	Antianginal
Digoxin	0.25	Cardiotonic (maintenance)
Levothyroxine	0.1	Thyroid
Misoprostol	0.1	Antiulcerative
Ethinyl Estradiol	0.05	Estrogen

3. To conceal the bitter, salty, or offensive taste or odor of a drug substance (e.g., capsules, coated tablets, flavored syrups)
4. To provide liquid preparations of substances that are either insoluble or unstable in the desired vehicle (e.g., suspensions)
5. To provide clear liquid dosage forms of substances (e.g., syrups, solutions)
6. To provide rate-controlled drug action (e.g., various controlled-release tablets, capsules, and suspensions)

7. To provide optimal drug action from topical administration sites (e.g., ointments, creams, transdermal patches, ophthalmic, ear, and nasal preparations)
8. To provide for the insertion of a drug into one of the body's orifices (e.g., rectal or vaginal suppositories)
9. To provide for the placement of drugs directly into the bloodstream or into body tissues (e.g., injections)
10. To provide for optimal drug action through inhalation therapy (e.g., inhalants and inhalation aerosols)

General Considerations in Dosage Form Design

Before formulating a drug substance into a dosage form, the desired product type must be detemined insofar as possible to establish the framework for product development activities. Then, various initial formulations of the product are developed and examined for desired features (e.g., drug release profile, bioavailability, clinical effectiveness) and for pilot plant studies and production scale-up. The formulation that best meets the goals for the product is selected and represents its *master formula.* Each batch of product subsequently prepared must meet the specifications established in the master formula.

There are many different forms into which a medicinal agent may be placed for the convenient and efficacious treatment of disease. Most commonly, a pharmaceutical manufacturer prepares a drug substance in several dosage forms and strengths for the efficacious and convenient treatment of disease (Fig. 3.1). Before a medicinal agent is formulated into one or more dosage forms, among the factors considered are such therapeutic

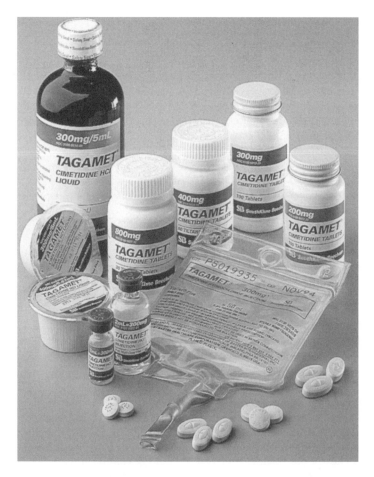

Fig. 3.1 *Examples of varied dosage forms of a drug substance marketed by a pharmaceutical manufacturer to meet the special requirements of the patient. (Courtesy of SmithKline Beecham)*

matters as: the nature of the illness, the manner in which it is treated (locally or through systemic action), and the age and anticipated condition of the patient.

If the medication is intended for systemic use and oral administration is desired, tablets and/or capsules are usually prepared. These dosage units are easily handled by the patient and are most convenient in the self-administration of medication. If a drug substance has application in an emergency situation in which the patient may be comatose or unable to take oral medication, an injectable form of the medication may also be prepared. Many other examples of therapeutic situations affecting dosage form design could be cited, including the preparation of agents for motion sickness, nausea, and vomiting into tablets and skin patches for prevention and suppositories and injections for treatment.

The age of the intended patient also plays a role in dosage form design. For infants and children younger than 5 years of age, pharmaceutical liquids rather than solid dosage forms are preferred for oral administration. These liquids, which are flavored aqueous solutions, syrups or suspensions, are usually administered directly into the infant's or child's mouth by drop, spoon, or oral dispenser (Fig. 3.2) or incorporated into the child's food. A single liquid pediatric preparation may be used for infants and children of all ages, with the dose of the drug varied by the volume administered. When an infant is in the throes of a vomiting crisis, is gagging, has a productive cough, or is simply rebellious, there may be some question as to how much of the medicine administered is actually swallowed and how much is expectorated. In such instances, injections may be required. Infant size rectal suppositories may also be employed although drug absorption from the rectum is often erratic.

During childhood and even in adult years, a person may have difficulty swallowing solid dosage forms, especially uncoated tablets. For this reason, some medications are formulated as chewable tablets that can be broken up in the mouth before swallowing. Many of these tablets are comparable in texture to an after-dinner mint and break down into a pleasant tasting, creamy material. New, rapidly-disintegrating/dissolving tablets are available that dissolve in the mouth in about 10–15 seconds; this allows the patient to take a tablet but actually swallow a liquid. Capsules have been found by many to be more easily swallowed than whole tablets. If a capsule is allowed to become moist in the mouth before swallowing, it becomes slippery and slides down the throat more readily with a glass of water. Also, a teaspoonful of gelatin dessert or syrup placed in the mouth and partially swallowed before placing the solid dosage form in the mouth aids in swallowing them. Also, in instances in which a person has difficulty swallowing a capsule, the contents may be emptied into a spoon, mixed with jam, honey, or other similar food to mask the taste of the medication and swallowed. Medications intended for the elderly are commonly formulated into oral liquids or may be extemporaneously prepared into an oral liquid by the pharmacist. However, certain tablets and capsules that are designed to have controlled release features should not be crushed or chewed to maintain their integrity and intended performance.

Many patients, particularly the elderly, take multiple medications daily. The more distinctive the size, shape, and color of solid dosage forms, the easier is the proper identification of the medications. Frequent errors in taking medications among the elderly occur because of their multiple drug therapy and reduced eyesight. Dosage forms that allow reduced frequency of administration without sacrifice of efficiency are particularly advantageous.

In dealing with the problem of formulating a drug substance into a proper dosage form, research pharmacists employ knowledge that has been gained through experience with other chemically similar drugs and through the proper utilization of the disciplines of the physical, chemical, and biologic and pharmaceutical sciences. The early stages of any new formulation involves studies to collect basic information on the physical and chemical characteristics of the drug substance to be prepared

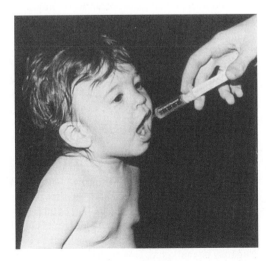

Fig. 3.2 *"Pee Dee Dose" brand of oral liquid dispenser used to administer measured volumes of liquid medication to youngsters. (Courtesy of Baxa Corporation)*

into pharmaceutical dosage forms. These basic studies comprise the *preformulation* work needed before actual product formulation begins.

Preformulation Studies

Before the formulation of a drug substance into a dosage form, it is essential that it be chemically and physically characterized. The following *preformulation studies* (1), and others, provide the type of information needed to define the nature of the drug substance. This information then provides the framework for the drug's combination with pharmaceutic ingredients in the fabrication of a dosage form.

Physical Description

It is important to have an understanding of the physical description of a drug substance prior to dosage form development. The majority of drug substances in use today occur as solid materials. Most of them are pure chemical compounds of either crystalline or amorphous constitution. The purity of the chemical substance is essential for its identification as well as for the evaluation of its chemical, physical, and biologic properties. Chemical properties include structure, form and reactivity. Physical properties include such characteristics as its physical description, particle size, crystalline structure, melting point and solubility. Biologic properties relate to its ability to get to a site of action and elicit a biologic response.

Drugs can be used therapeutically as solids, liquids and gases. Liquid drugs are used to a much lesser extent than solid drugs; gases, even less frequently.

Liquid drugs pose an interesting problem in the design of dosage forms or drug delivery systems. Many of the liquids are volatile substances and as such must be physically sealed from the atmosphere to prevent their loss. Amyl nitrite, for example, is a clear yellowish liquid that is volatile even at low temperatures and is also highly flammable. It is maintained for medicinal purposes in small sealed glass cylinders wrapped with gauze or another suitable material. When amyl nitrite is administered, the glass is broken between the fingertips, and the liquid wets the gauze covering, producing vapors that are inhaled by the patient requiring vasodilation. Propylhexedrine provides another example of a volatile liquid drug that must be contained in a closed system to maintain its presence. This drug is used as a nasal inhalant for its vasoconstrictor action. A cylindrical roll of fibrous material is impregnated with propylhexedrine, and the saturated cylin-

der is placed in a suitable, usually plastic, sealed nasal inhaler. The inhaler's cap must be securely tightened each time it is used. Even then, the inhaler maintains its effectiveness for only a limited period of time due to the volatilization of the drug.

Another problem associated with liquid drugs is that those intended for oral administration cannot generally be formulated into tablet form, the most popular form of oral medication, without undertaking chemical modification of the drug. An exception to this is the liquid drug nitroglycerin, which is formulated into sublingual tablets that disintegrate within seconds after placement under the tongue. However, because the drug is volatile, it has a tendency to escape from the tablets during storage and it is critical that the tablets be stored in tightly sealed glass containers. For the most part, when a liquid drug is to be administered orally and a solid dosage form is desired, two approaches are used. First, the liquid substance may be sealed in a soft gelatin capsule. Clofibrate (Atromid S), vitamins A, D and E, and ethchlorvynol (Placidyl) are examples of liquid drugs commercially available in capsule form. Secondly, the liquid drug may be developed into a solid ester or salt form that will be suitable for tableting or drug encapsulating. For instance, scopolamine hydrobromide is a solid salt of the liquid drug scopolamine and is easily produced into tablets. Another approach to formulate liquids into solids is by mixing the drug with a solid or a melted semisolid material, such as a high molecular weight polyethylene glycol. The melted mixture is poured into hard gelatin capsules where it will harden, and the capsules sealed.

For certain liquid drugs, especially those employed orally in large doses or applied topically, their liquid nature may be of some advantage in therapy. For example, 15-mL doses of mineral oil may be administered conveniently as such. Also, the liquid nature of undecylenic acid certainly does not hinder but rather enhances its use topically in the treatment of fungus infections of the skin. However, for the most part, solid materials are preferred by pharmacists in formulation work because of their ease of preparation into tablets and capsules.

Formulation and stability difficulties arise less frequently with solid dosage forms than with liquid pharmaceutical preparations, and for this reason many new drugs first reach the market as tablets or dry-filled capsules. Later, when the pharmaceutical problems are resolved, a liquid form of the same drug may be marketed. This procedure, when practiced, is doubly advantageous, because for the most part physicians and patients alike prefer small, generally tasteless, accurately dosed tablets or capsules to the analogous liquid forms. Therefore, marketing a drug in solid form first is more practical for the manufacturer and also suits the majority of patients. It is estimated that tablets and capsules comprise the dosage form dispensed 70% of the time by community pharmacists, with tablets dispensed twice as frequently as capsules.

Microscopic Examination

Microscopic examination of the raw drug substance is an important step in preformulation work.

It gives an indication of particle size and particle size range of the raw material as well as the crystal structure. Photomicrographs of the initial and subsequent batch lots of the drug substance can provide important information should problems arise in formulation processing attributable to changes in particle or crystal characteristics of the drug. During some processing procedures, the solid drug powders must flow freely and not become entangled. Spherical and oval-shaped powders flow more easily than needle-shaped powders and make processing easier.

Physical Pharmacy Capsule 3.1   **Melting Point Depression**

The *melting point,* or *freezing point,* of a pure crystalline solid is defined as that temperature where the pure liquid and solid exist in equilibrium. Low melting point drugs may soften during a processing step where heat is generated, such as particle size reduction, compression, sintering, etc. Also, the melting point/range of a drug can be used as an indicator of purity of chemical substances (a pure substance would ordinarily be characterized by a very sharp melting peak). An altered peak or a peak at a different temperature may be indicative of an adulterated or impure drug. This is explained as follows.

The *latent heat of fusion* is the quantity of heat absorbed when 1 g of a solid melts; the molar heat of fusion (ΔH_f) is the quantity of heat absorbed when 1 mole of a solid melts. High-melting-point substances have high heats of fusion and low-melting-point substances have low heats of fusion. These characteristics are related to the types of bonding in the specific substance. For example, ionic materials have high heats of fusion (NaCl melts at 801°C with a heat of fusion of 124 cal/G) and those with weaker van der Waals forces have low heats of fusion (paraffin melts at 52°C with a heat of fusion of 35.1 cal/g). Ice, with weaker hydrogen bonding, has a melting point of 0°C and a heat of fusion of 80 cal/G.

The addition of a second component to a pure compound (A), resulting in a mixture, will result in a melting point that is lower than that of the pure compound. The degree to which the melting point is lowered is proportional to the mole fraction (N_A) of the second component that is added. This can be expressed as:

$$\Delta T = \frac{2.303 \, RTT_0}{\Delta H_f} \log N_A$$

where ΔH_F is the molar heat of fusion,
    T is the absolute equilibrium temperature,
    T_0 is the melting point of pure A, and
    R is the gas constant.

Two things are noteworthy in contributing to the extent of melting-point lowering.

1. Evident from this relationship is the inverse proportion between the melting point and the heat of fusion. When a second ingredient is added to a compound with a low molar heat of fusion, a large lowering of the melting point is observed; substances with a high molar heat of fusion will show little change in melting point with the addition of a second component.
2. The extent of lowering of the melting point is also related to the melting point itself. Compounds with low melting points are affected to a greater extent than compounds with high melting points upon the addition of a second component (i.e., low-melting-point compounds will result in a greater lowering of the melting point than those with high melting points).

Melting Point Depression

A characteristic of a pure substance is a defined melting point or melting range. If not pure, the substance will exhibit a depressed melting point. This phenomenon is commonly used to determine the purity of a drug substnce and, in some cases, the compatibility of various substances before inclusion in the same dosage form. This characteristic is further described in the physical pharmacy capsule entitled "Melting Point Depression."

The Phase Rule

Phase diagrams are often constructed to provide a visual picture of the existence and extent of the presence of solid and liquid phases in binary, ternary and other mixtures. Phase diagrams are normally two-component (binary) representations as shown in the physical pharmacy capsule "The Phase Rule," but multicomponent phase diagrams can also be constructed.

Particle Size

Certain physical and chemical properties of drug substances are affected by the particle size distribution, including drug dissolution rate, bioavailability, content uniformity, taste, texture, color, and stability. In addition, properties such as flow characteristics and sedimentation rates, among others, are also important factors related to particle size. It is essential to establish as early as possible how the particle size of the drug substance may affect formulation and product efficacy. Of special interest is the effect of particle size on the drug's absorption. Particle size significantly influences the oral absorption profiles of certain drugs as griseofulvin, nitrofurantoin, spironolactone, and procaine penicillin. Also, satisfactory content uniformity in solid dosage forms depends to a large degree on particle size and the equal distribution of the active ingredient throughout the formulation. Particle size is discussed further in Chapters 4 and 6.

Polymorphism

An important factor on formulation is the crystal or amorphous form of the drug substance. Polymorphic forms usually exhibit different physical-chemical properties including melting point and solubility. The occurrence of polymorphic forms with drugs is relatively common and it has been estimated that polymorphism is exhibited by at least one-third of all organic compounds.

In addition to the polymorphic forms in which compounds may exist, they also can occur in noncrystalline or amorphous forms. The energy required for a molecule of drug to escape from a crys-

tal is much greater than required to escape from an amorphous powder. Therefore, the amorphous form of a compound is always more soluble than a corresponding crystal form.

Evaluation of crystal structure, polymorphism, and solvate form is an important preformulation activity. The changes in crystal characteristics can influence bioavailability, chemical and physical stability, and have important implications in dosage form process functions. For example, it can be a significant factor relating to the tableting processes due to flow and compaction behaviors, among others. Various techniques are used in determining crystal properties. The most widely used methods are hot stage microscopy, thermal analysis, infrared spectroscopy, and x-ray diffraction.

Solubility

An important physical-chemical property of a drug substance is solubility, especially aqueous system solubility. A drug must possess some aqueous solubility for therapeutic efficacy. For a drug to enter the systemic circulation to exert a therapeutic effect, it must first be in solution. Relatively insoluble compounds often exhibit incomplete or erratic absorption. If the solubility of the drug substance is less than desirable, consideration must be given to improve its solubility. The methods to accomplish this will depend on the chemical nature of the drug and the type of drug product under consideration. The chemical modification of the drug into salt or ester forms is a technique frequently used to obtain more soluble compounds.

A drug's solubility is usually determined by the equilibrium solubility method, by which an excess of the drug is placed in a solvent and shaken at a constant temperature over a prolonged period of time until equilibrium is obtained. Chemical analysis of the drug content in solution is performed to determine degree of solubility.

Solubility and Particle Size

Although solubility is normally considered a physicochemical constant, small increases in solubility can be accomplished by particle size reduction as described in the physical pharmacy capsule, "Solubility and Particle Size."

Solubility and pH

Another technique, if the drug is to be formulated into a liquid product, involves the adjustment of the pH of the solvent in which the drug is to be dissolved to enhance solubility. However, there are many drug substances for which pH adjustment is not an effective means of improving solubility.

Physical Pharmacy Capsule 3.2   **The Phase Rule**

A phase diagram, or temperature-composition diagram, represents the melting point as a function of composition of two or three component systems. The figure is an example of such a representation for a two-component mixture. This phase diagram is of a two-component mixture in which the components are completely miscible in the molten state and no solid solution or addition compound is formed in the solid state. As is evident, starting from the extremes of either pure component A or pure component B, as the second component is added, the melting point of the pure component decreases. There is a point on this phase diagram at which a minimum melting point occurs (i.e., the eutectic point). As is evident, there are four regions, or phases, in this diagram, representing the following:

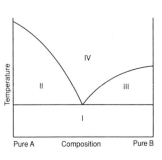

I.   Solid A + Solid B
II. Solid A + Melt
III. Solid B + Melt
IV. Melt

Each phase is a homogenous part of the system, physically separated by distinct boundaries.
A description of the conditions under which these phases can exist is called the *Phase Rule,* which can be presented as:

$$F = C - P + X$$

where F is the number of degrees of freedom,
      C is the number of components,
      P is the number of phases, and

X is a variable dependent upon selected considerations of the phase diagram (1,2 or 3).

"C" describes the minimum number of chemical components that need to be specified to define the phases present. The F is the number of independent variables that must be specified to define the complete system (e.g., temperature, pressure, concentration).

EXAMPLE 1
In a mixture of menthol and thymol, a phase diagram similar to that illustrated can be obtained. To describe the number of degrees of freedom in the part of the graph moving from the curved line starting at pure A, progressing downward to the eutectic point, and then following an increasing melting point to pure B, it is evident from this presentation that either temperature or composition will describe this system, since it is assumed in this instance that pressure is constant. Therefore, the number of degrees of freedom to describe this portion of the phase diagram is given by:

$$F = 2 - 2 + 1 = 1$$

In other words, along this line, either temperature or composition will describe the system.

EXAMPLE 2
When in the area of a single phase of the diagram, such as the melt (IV), the system can be described as:

$$F = 2 - 1 + 1 = 2$$

In this portion of the phase diagram, two factors, temperature and composition, can be varied without a change in the number of phases in the system.

EXAMPLE 3
At the eutectic point,

$$F = 2 - 3 + 1 = 0$$

and any change in the concentration or temperature may cause a disappearance of one of the two solid phases or the liquid phase.

Phase diagrams are valuable in interpreting interactions between two or more components, relating not only to melting point depression and possible liquefaction at room temperature but also the formation of solid solutions, coprecipitates, and other solid-state interactions.

Physical Pharmacy Capsule 3.3   **Solubility and Particle Size**

The particle size and surface area of a drug exposed to a medium can affect actual solubility, within reason. For example, in the following relationship:

$$\log \frac{S}{S_0} = \frac{2\gamma V}{2.303 \ RTr}$$

where S is the solubility of the small particles,
  S_0 is the solubility of the large particles,
  γ is the surface tension
  V is the molar volume
  R is the gas constant
  T is the absolute temperature
  r is the radius of the small particles.

The equation can be used to estimate the decrease in particle size required to result in an increase in solubility. For example, for a desired increase in solubility of 5%, this would require an increase in the S/So ratio to 1.05, that is, the left term in the equation would become "log 1.05." If an example is used for a powder with a surface tension of 125 dynes/cm, the molar volume is 45 cm^3 and the temperature is 27°C, what is the particle size required to obtain the 5% increase in solubility?

$$\log 1.05 = \frac{(2)(125)(45)}{(2.303)(8.314 \times 10^7)(300)r}$$

$$r = 9.238 \times 10^{-6} \ \text{cm or } 0.09238\mu$$

A number of factors are involved in actual solubility enhancement and this is only a basic introduction of the general effects of particle size reduction.

Weak acidic or basic drugs may require extremes in pH that are outside accepted physiologic limits or may cause stability problems with formulation ingredients. Adjustment of pH usually has little effect on the solubility of non-electrolytes. In many cases, it is desirable to utilize co-solvents or other techniques such as complexation, micronization, or solid dispersion to improve aqueous solubility. The effect of pH on solubility is illustrated in the physical pharmacy capsule "Solubility and pH."

In recent years, more and more physicochemical information on drugs is being made available to pharmacists in routinely used reference books. This type of information is important for pharmacists in different types of practice, especially those involved in compounding and pharmacokinetic monitoring.

Dissolution

Variations in the biological activity of a drug substance may be brought about by the rate at which it becomes available to the organism. In many instances, dissolution rate, or the time it takes for the drug to dissolve in the fluids at the absorption site, is the rate-limiting step in the absorption process. This is true for drugs administered orally in solid forms such as tablets, capsules or suspensions, as well as drugs administered intramuscularly in the form of pellets or suspensions. When the dissolution rate is the rate-limiting step, anything which affects it will also affect absorption. Consequently, dissolution rate can affect the onset, intensity, and duration of response, and control the overall bioavailability of the drug from the dosage form, as discussed in the previous chapter.

The dissolution rate of drugs may be increased by decreasing the drug's particle size. It may also be increased by increasing its solubility in the diffusion layer. The most effective means of obtaining higher dissolution rates is to use a highly water soluble salt of the parent substance. Although a soluble salt of a weak acid will subsequently precipitate as the free acid in the bulk phase of an acidic solution, such as gastric fluid, it will do so in the form of fine particles with a large surface area.

The dissolution rates of chemical compounds are determined by two methods: the constant surface

Physical Pharmacy Capsule 3.4   **Solubility and pH**

pH is one of the most important factors involved in the formulation process. Two areas of critical importance are the effects of pH on solubility and stability. The effect of pH on solubility is critical in the formulation of liquid dosage forms, from oral and topical solutions to intravenous solutions and admixtures.

The solubility of a weak acid or base is often pH dependent. The total quantity of a monoprotic weak acid (HA) in solution at a specific pH is the sum of the concentrations of both the free acid and salt (A^-) forms. If excess drug is present, the quantity of free acid in solution is maximized and constant due to its saturation solubility. As the pH of the solution is increased, the quantity of drug in solution increases because the water-soluble ionizable salt is formed. The expression is:

$$HA \underset{}{\overset{K_a}{\rightleftharpoons}} H^+ + A^-$$

where K_a is the dissociation constant.

There may be a certain pH level reached where the total solubility (S_T) of the drug solution is saturated with respect to both the salt and acid forms of the drug, i.e., the pH_{max}. The solution can be saturated with respect to the salt at pH values higher than this, but not with respect to the acid. Also, at pH values less than this, the solution can be saturated with respect to the acid, but not to the salt. This is illustrated in the accompanying figure.

To calculate the total quantity of drug that can be maintained in solution at a selected pH, two different equations can be used, depending on whether the product is to be in a pH region above or below the pH_{max}. The following equation is used when below the pH_{max}:

$$S_T = S_a \left(1 + \frac{K_a}{[H^+]} \right)$$ (Equation 1)

The next equation is used when above the pH_{max}:

$$S_T = S'A \left(1 + \frac{[H^+]}{K_a} \right)$$ (Equation 2)

where S_a is the saturation solubility of the free acid, and

$S'a$ is the saturation solubility of the salt form.

EXAMPLE

A pharmacist prepares a 3.0% solution of an antibiotic as an ophthalmic solution and dispenses it to a patient. A few days later the patient returns the eye drops to the pharmacist because the product contains a precipitate. The pharmacist, checking the pH of the solution and finding it to be 6.0, reasons that the problem might be pH-related. The physicochemical information of interest on the antibiotic includes the following:

Molecular weight	285 (salt) 263 (free acid)
3.0% solution of the drug is a	0.1053 molar solution
Acid form solubility (S_a)	3.1 mg/mL (0.0118 molar)
K_a	5.86×10^{-6}

Using Equation 1, the pharmacist calculates the quantity of the antibiotic that would be in solution at a pH of 6.0 (Note: pH of 6.0 = $[H^+]$ of 1×10^{-6})

$$S_T = 0.0118 \left[1 + \frac{5.86 \times 10^{-6}}{1 \times 10^{-6}} \right] = 0.0809 \text{ molar}$$

Solubility and pH   (Continued)

From this the pharmacist knows that, at a pH of 6.0, a 0.0809 molar solution could be prepared. However, the concentration that was to be prepared was a 0.1053 molar solution; consequently, the drug will not be in solution at that pH. What may have occurred was the pH was all right initially but shifted to a lower pH after a period of time, resulting in precipitation of the drug. The question is then asked, At what pH (hydrogen ion concentration) will the drug remain in solution? This can be calculated using the same equation and the information that is available. The S_T value is 0.1053 molar.

$$0.1053 = 0.0118 \left[1 + \frac{5.86 \times 10^{-6}}{[H^+]}\right]$$

$$[H^+] = 7.333 \times 10^{-7}, \text{ or a pH of } 6.135$$

The pharmacist then prepares a solution of the antibiotic, adjusting the pH to greater than about 6.2 using a suitable buffer system, and dispenses the solution to the patient—with positive results.

An interesting phenomenon can be discussed briefly concerning the close relationship of pH to solubility. At a pH of 6.0, only a 0.0809 molar solution could be prepared, but at a pH of 6.13 a 0.1053 molar solution could be prepared. In other words, a difference of 0.13 pH units resulted in:

$$\frac{0.1053 - 0.0809}{0.0809} = 30.1\% \text{ more drug going into solution at the higher pH}$$
$$\text{compared to the lower pH}$$

In other words, a very small change in pH resulted in about 30% more drug going into solution. According to the figure, the slope of the curve would be very steep for this example drug and a small change in pH (x-axis) results in a large change in solubility (y-axis). From this, it can be reasoned that if one observes the pH:solubility profile of a drug, it is possible to predict the magnitude of the pH change on its solubility.

In recent years, it has been interesting to not that more and more physiochemical information on drugs is being made available to pharmacists in routinely used reference books. This type of information is important for pharmacists in different types of practice, especially those involved in compounding and pharmacokinetic monitoring.

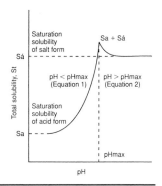

method which provides the intrinsic dissolution rate of the agent, and particulate dissolution in which a suspension of the agent is added to a fixed amount of solvent without exact control of surface area.

The constant surface method utilizes a compressed disc of known area. This method eliminates surface area and surface electrical charges as dissolution variables. The dissolution rate obtained by this method is termed the *intrinsic dissolution rate,* and is characteristic of each solid compound and a given solvent under the fixed experimental conditions. The value is expressed as milligrams dissolved per minute centimeters squared (mg/min/cm²). It has been suggested that this value is useful in predicting probable absorption problems due to dissolution rate. In particulate dissolution, a weighed

amount of powdered sample is added to the dissolution medium in a constant agitation system. This method is frequently used to study the influence of particle size, surface area, and excipients upon the active agent. Occasionally, an inverse relationship of particle size to dissolution is noted due to the surface properties of the drug. In these instances, surface charge and/or agglomeration results in the reduced particle size form of the drug presenting a lower effective surface area to the solvent due to incomplete wetting or agglomeration. Fick's Laws describe the relationship of diffusion and dissolution of the active drug in the dosage form and when administered in the body, as shown in the physical pharmacy capsule entitled Fick's Laws of Diffusion and the Noyes-Whitney Equation.

Early formulation studies should include the

Physical Pharmacy Capsule 3.5   **Fick's Laws of Diffusion and the Noyes-Whitney Equation**

All drugs must diffuse through various barriers when administered to the body. For example, some drugs must diffuse through the skin, gastric mucosa or some other barrier to gain access to the interior of the body. Parenterally administered drugs must diffuse through muscle, connective tissue, etc. to get to the site of action; even intravenous drugs must diffuse from the blood to the site of action. Drugs must also diffuse through various barriers for metabolism and excretion.

Considering all the diffusion processes that occur in the body (passive, active and facilitated), it is not surprising that the laws governing diffusion are very important in designing drug delivery systems. In fact, diffusion is important not only in the body but also in some quality control procedures used to determine batch-to-batch uniformity of products (dissolution test for tablets based on the Noyes-Whitney equation, which can be derived from Fick's law).

When individual molecules move within a substance, diffusion is said to occur. This may occur as the result of a concentration gradient or by random molecular motion.

Probably the most widely used laws of diffusion are known as Fick's laws; the first and second laws. Fick's First Law involving steady-state diffusion (where dc/dx does not change) is derived from the following expression for the quantity of material (M) flowing through a cross-section of a barrier (S) in unit time (t) expressed as the flux (J);

$$J = dM/(S\ dt)$$

Under a concentration gradient (dc/dx), Fick's First Law can be expressed as:

$$J = D[(C_1 - C_2/h]\text{ or }J = -D\ (dC/dx)$$

where J is the flux of a component across a plane of unit area, C_1 and C_2 are the concentrations in the donor and receptor compartments, h is the membrane thickness and D is the diffusion coefficient (or diffusivity). The sign is negative denoting that the flux is in the direction of decreasing concentration. The units of J are $g/(cm^2\ s)$, C is in g/cm^3, M in grams or moles, S in cm^2, x in cm and the units of D would be in cm^2/s.

"D" is appropriately called a diffusion coefficient, not a diffusion constant, as it is subject to change. "D", the diffusion coefficient, may actually change in value with increased concentrations. Also, "D" can be affected by temperature, pressure, solvent properties and the chemical nature of the drug itself. To study the rate of change of the drug in the system, one needs an expression that relates the change in concentration with time at a definite location in place of the mass of drug diffusing across a unit area of barrier in unit time; this expression is known as Fick's Second Law. This law can be summarized as it states that the change in concentration in a particular place with time is proportional to the change in concentration gradient at that particular place in the system.

In summary, Fick's First Law relates to a steady state flow whereas Fick's Second Law relates to a change in concentration of drug with time, at any distance, or a nonsteady state of flow.

The diffusion coefficients $(D \times 10^6)$ of various compounds in water (25°C) and other media have been determined as follows: ethanol, 12.5 cm^2/sec; glycine, 10.6 cm^2/sec; sodium lauryl sulfate, 6.2 cm^2/sec; glucose, 6.8 cm^2/sec.

The concentration of drug in the membrane can be calculated using the partition coefficient (K) and the concentration in the donor and receptor compartments.

$$K = C_1/C_d = C_2/C_r$$

where C_1 and C_d are the concentrations in the donor compartment (g/cm^3) and C_2 and C_r are the concentrations in the receptor compartment (g/cm^3).

K is the partition coefficient of the drug between the solution and the membrane. It can be estimated using the oil solubility of the drug vs. the water solubility of the drug. Usually, the higher the partition coefficient, the more the drug will be soluble in a lipophilic substance. We can now write the expression:

$$dM/dt = [DSK(C_d - C_r)]/h$$

Fick's Laws of Diffusion and the Noyes-Whitney Equation   (Continued)

or, in sink conditions,

$$dM/dt = DSKC_d/h = PSC_d$$

The permeability coefficient (cm/sec) can be obtained by rearranging to:

$$P = DK/h$$

EXAMPLE 1

A drug passing through a 1 mm thick membrane has a diffusion coefficient of 4.23×10^{-7} cm^2/sec, and an o/w partition coefficient of 2.03. The radius of the area exposed to the solution is 2 cm, and the concentration of the drug in the donor compartment is 0.5 mg/mL. Calculate the permeability and the diffusion rate of the drug.

$$h = 1 \text{ mm} = 0.1 \text{ cm}$$
$$D = 4.23 \times 10^{-7} \text{ cm}^2/\text{sec}$$
$$K = 2.03$$
$$r = 2 \text{ cm}, S = \pi(2\text{cm})^2 = 12.57 \text{ cm}^2$$
$$C_d = 0.5 \text{ mg/mL}$$
$$P = [(4.23 \times 10^{-7} \text{ cm}^2/\text{sec}) (2.03)]/0.1 \text{ cm} = 8.59 \times 10^{-6} \text{ cm/sec}$$
$$dM/dt = (8.59 \times 10^{-6} \text{ cm/sec}) (12.57 \text{ cm}^2)(0.5 \text{ mg/mL}) = 5.40 \times 10^{-5} \text{ mg/sec}$$
$$(5.40 \times 10^{-5} \text{ mg/sec})(3600 \text{ sec/hr}) = 0.19 \text{ mg/hr}$$

In the dissolution of particles of drug, the dissolved molecules diffuse away from the individual particle body. An expression to describe this was derived from Fick's equations and is known as the Noyes and Whitney expression, proposed in 1897. It can be written as follows:

$$dC/dt = (DS/Vh)(C_s - C)$$

where C is the concentration of drug dissolved at time t, D is the diffusion coefficient of the solute in solution, S is the surface area of the exposed solid, V is the volume of solution, h is the thickness of the diffusion layer, C_s is the saturation solubility of the drug and C is the concentration of solute in the bulk phase at a specific time, t. It is common practice to utilize sink conditions where C does not exceed about 20% of the solubility of the drug being investigated. Under these conditions, the expression simplifies to:

$$dC/dt = DSC_s/Vh$$

and incorporating the volume of solution (V), the thickness of the diffusion layer (h) and the diffusivity coefficient (D) into a coefficient k (to take into account the various factors in the system), the expression becomes:

$$dC/dt = kSC_s$$

As the factors are held constant, it becomes apparent that the dissolution rate of a drug can be proportional to the surface area exposed to the dissolution media. A number of other expressions have been derived for specific application to various situations and conditions.

It should be obvious to the reader that these relationships expressed as Fick's First and Second Laws and the Noyes-Whitney equation have great importance and relevance in pharmaceutical systems.

EXAMPLE 2

The following data was obtained using the USP 23/NF dissolution apparatus I. The drug is soluble 1 gram in 3 mL of water so sink conditions were maintained, the surface area of the tablet exposed was 1.5 cm^2 (obtained by placing the tablet in a special holder exposing only one side to the dissolution media) and the dosage form studied involved a 16 mg sustained release tablet; the release pattern should be zero order. What is the rate of release of drug?

Fick's Laws of Diffusion and the Noyes-Whitney Equation   (Continued)

Time (hr)	Drug concentration (mg/900 mL of solution)	Graph of Release Profile
0	0	
0.5	1	
1.0	1.9	
2.0	4.1	
4.0	8.0	
6 0	11.8	
8.0	15.9	

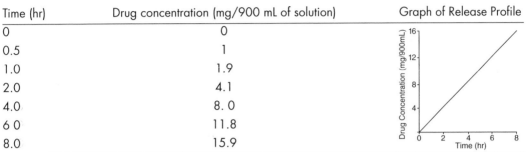

In this problem, since the surface area (S) was maintained constant at 1.5 cm^2 and the solubility (Cs) of the drug is constant at 1 g in 3 mL of water, then the plot of concentration (C) versus time (t) would yield a slope with a value of "kSCs", or "k$_2$", expressing the rate of release of the drug.

$$dC/dt = kSCs$$

the slope of the line would be $= \Delta y/\Delta x = (y_2 - y_1)/(x_2 - x_1)$

$$= (15.9 \text{ mg} - 0 \text{ mg})/(8.0 \text{ h} - 0 \text{ h})$$

$$= 15.9/8 = 1.99 \text{ mg/h}$$

Therefore, the rate of release of the sustained release preparation is 1.99 or approximately 2 mg per hour. From this, the quantity of drug released at any time (t) can be calculated.

effects of pharmaceutic ingredients on the dissolution characteristics of the drug substance.

Membrane Permeability

Modern preformulation studies include an early assessment of passage of drug molecules across biological membranes. To produce a biological response, the drug molecule must first cross a biological membrane. The biological membrane acts as a lipid barrier to most drugs and permits the absorption of lipid soluble substances by passive diffusion while lipid insoluble substances can diffuse across the barrier only with considerable difficulty, if at all. The interrelationship of the dissociation constant, lipid solubility, and pH at the absorption site and absorption characteristics of various drugs are the basis of the pH-partition theory.

Data obtained from the basic physicochemical studies, specifically, pKa, solubility, and dissolution rate provide an indication of absorption expectations. To enhance these data, a technique using the "everted intestinal sac" may be used in evaluating absorption characteristics of drug substances. In this method, a piece of intestine is removed from an intact animal, everted, filled with a solution of the drug substance, and the degree and rate of passage

of the drug through the membrane sac is determined. Through this method, both passive and active transport can be evaluated.

In the latter stages of preformulation testing or early formulation studies, animals and man must be studied to assess the absorption efficiency, pharmacokinetic parameters and to establish possible *in vitro/in vivo* correlation for dissolution and bioavailability.

Partition Coefficient

The use of the partition coefficient is described in some detail in the physical pharmacy capsule entitled "Partition Coefficient."

Inherent in this procedure is the selection of appropriate extraction solvents, drug stability, use of salting-out additives, and environmental concerns.

In formulation development, the octanol-water partition coefficient is commonly used. Following the illustrations provided above, it is defined as:

$$P = \frac{(\text{Conc. of drug in octanol})}{(\text{Conc. of drug in water})}$$

P is dependent on the drug concentration only if the drug molecules have a tendency to associate in

Physical Pharmacy Capsule 3.6   **Partition Coefficient**

The oil/water partition coefficient is a measure of a molecule's lipophilic character; that is, its preference for the hydrophilic or lipophilic phase. If a solute is added to a mixture of two immiscible liquids, it will distribute between the two phases and reach an equilibrium at a constant temperature. The distribution of the solute (unaggregated and undissociated) between the two immiscible layers can be described as:

$$K = C_U/C_L$$

where K is the distribution constant or partition constant,
    C_U is the concentration of the drug in the upper phase, and
    C_L is the concentration of the drug in the lower phase.

This information can be effectively used in the:

1. Extraction of crude drugs,
2. Recovery of antibiotics from fermentation broths,
3. Recovery of biotechnology-derived drugs from bacterial cultures,
4. Extraction of drugs from biologic fluids for therapeutic drug monitoring,
5. Absorption of drugs from dosage forms (ointments, suppositories, transdermal patches),
6. Study of the distribution of flavoring oil between oil and water phases of emulsions, and
7. In other applications.

The basic relationship given above can be used to calculate the quantity of drug extracted from, or remaining behind in, a given layer and to calculate the number of extractions required to remove a drug from a mixture.

The concentration of drug found in the upper layer (U) of two immiscible layers is given by:

$$U = Kr/(Kr + 1)$$

where K is the distribution partition constant, and
    r is V_u/V_l, or the ratio of the volume of upper and lower phases.

The concentration of drug remaining in the lower layer (L) is given by:

$$L = 1/(Kr + 1)$$

If the lower phase is successively re-extracted with *n* equal volumes of the upper layer, each upper (U_n) contains the following fraction of the drug:

$$U_n = Kr/(Kr + 1)^n$$

where U_n is the fraction contained in the *n*th extraction, and
    n is the *n*th successive volume.

The fraction of solute remaining in the lower layer (L_n) is given by:

$$L_n = 1/(kr + 1)^n$$

More efficient extractions are obtained using successive small volumes of the extraction solvent (as compared to single larger volumes). This can be calculated as follows when the same volume of extracting solvent is used, but in divided portions. For example, the fraction L_n remaining after the *n*th extraction is given by:

$$L_n = \frac{1}{\left(\dfrac{Kr}{n} + 1\right)^n}$$

EXAMPLE 1

At 25°C and at pH 6.8, the K for a second generation cephalosporin is 0.7 between equal volumes of butanol and the fermentation broth. Calculate the U, L, and L_n (using the same volume divided into fourths).

Partition Coefficient (Continued)

$U = 0.7/(0.7 + 1) = 0.41$ The fraction of drug extracted into the upper layer
$L = 1/(0.7 + 1) = 0.59$ The fraction of drug remaining in the lower layer
The total of the fractions in the U and L = 0.41 + 0.59 = 1.

If the fermentation broth is extracted with four successive extractions accomplished by dividing the quantity of butanol used into fourths, the quantity of drug remaining after the fourth extraction is

$$L_{4th} = \cfrac{1}{\left(\cfrac{0.7 \times 1}{4} + 1 \right)^4} = 0.525$$

From this, the quantity remaining after a single volume, single extraction is 0.59, but when the single volume is divided into fourths and four successive extractions are done, the quantity remaining is 0.525; therefore, more was extracted using divided portions of the extracting solvent.

Inherent in this procedure is the selection of appropriate extraction solvents, drug stability, use of salting-out additives, and environmental concerns.

---

solution. For an ionizable drug, the following equation is applicable:

$$P = \frac{\text{(Conc. of drug in octanol)}}{[1 - \alpha](\text{Conc. of drug in water})}$$

where α equals the degree of ionization.

pKa/Dissociation Constants

Among the physicochemical characteristics of interest is the extent of dissociation/ionization of drug substances. This is important because the extent of ionization has an important effect on the formulation and pharmacokinetic parameters of the drug. The extent of dissociation/ionization is, in many cases, highly dependent on the pH of the medium containing the drug. In formulation, often the vehicle is adjusted to a certain pH in order to obtain a certain level of ionization of the drug for solubility and stability purposes. In the pharmacokinetic area, the extent of ionization of a drug is an important affector of its extent of absorption, distribution, and elimination. Dissociation constant or pKa is usually determined by potentiometric titration. For the practicing pharmacist, it is important in predicting precipitation in admixtures and in the calculating of the solubility of drugs at certain pH values. The physical pharmacy capsule on "pKa/Dissociation Constants" presents a brief summary of dissociation/ionization concepts.

Drug and Drug Product Stability

One of the most important activities of preformulation work is the evaluation of the physical and chemical stability of the pure drug substance. It is essential that these initial studies be conducted using drug samples of known purity. The presence of impurities can lead to erroneous conclusions in such evaluations. Stability studies conducted in the preformulation phase include solid state stability of the drug alone, solution phase stability, and stability in the presence of expected excipients. Initial investigation begins through knowledge of the drug's chemical structure which allows the preformulation scientist to anticipate the possible degradation reactions.

Drug Stability: Mechanisms of Degradation

Chemical instability of medicinal agents may take many forms, because the drugs in use today are of such diverse chemical constitution. Chemically, drug substances are alcohols, phenols, aldehydes, ketones, esters, ethers, acids, salts, alkaloids, glycosides, and others, each with reactive chemical groups having different susceptibilities toward chemical instability. Chemically, the most frequently encountered destructive processes are hydrolysis and oxidation.

Hydrolysis is a solvolysis process in which (drug) molecules interact with water molecules to yield breakdown products of different chemical constitution. For example, aspirin or acetylsalicylic acid combines with a water molecule and hydrolyzes into one molecule of salicylic acid and one molecule of acetic acid:

The process of hydrolysis is probably the most important single cause of drug decomposition mainly because a great number of medicinal agents are esters or contain such

Physical Pharmacy Capsule 3.7   **pKa/Dissociation Constants**

The dissociation of a weak acid in water is given by the expression:

$$HA \leftrightarrow H^+ + A^-$$

$$K_1[HA] \leftrightarrow K_2[H^+][A^-]$$

At equilibrium, the reaction rate constants K_1 and K_2 are equal. This can be rearranged, and the dissociation constant defined as

$$K_a = \frac{K_1}{K_2} = \frac{[H^+][A^-]}{[HA]}$$

where K_a is the acid dissociation constant.

For the dissociation of a weak base that does not contain a hydroxyl group, the following relationship can be used:

$$BH^+ \leftrightarrow H^+ + B$$

The dissociation constant is described by:

$$K_a = \frac{[H^+][B]}{[BH^+]}$$

The dissociation of a hydroxyl-containing weak base,

$$B + H_2O \leftrightarrow OH^- + BH^+$$

The dissociation constant is described by:

$$K_b = \frac{[OH^-][BH^+]}{[B]}$$

The hydrogen ion concentrations can be calculated for the solution of a weak acid using:

$$[H^+] = \sqrt{K_a c}$$

Similarly, the hydroxyl ion concentration for a solution of a weak base is approximated by:

$$[OH^-] = \sqrt{K_b c}$$

Some practical applications of these equations are as follows.

EXAMPLE 1
The K_a of lactic acid is 1.387×10^{-4} at 25°C. What is the hydrogen ion concentration of a 0.02 M solution?

$$[H^+] = \sqrt{1.387 \times 10^{-4} \times 0.02} = 1.665 \times 10^{-3} \text{ G-ion/L.}$$

EXAMPLE 2
The K_b of morphine is 7.4×10^{-7}. What is the hydroxyl ion concentration of a 0.02 M solution?

$$[OH] = \sqrt{7.4 \times 10^{-7} \times 0.02} = 1.216 \times 10^{-4} \text{ G-ion/L.}$$

other groupings as substituted amides, lactones, and lactams, which are susceptible to the hydrolytic process (2).

Another destructive process is oxidation. The oxidative process is destructive to many drug types, including aldehydes, alcohols, phenols, sugars, alkaloids, and unsaturated fats and oils. Chemically, oxidation involves the loss of electrons from an atom or a molecule. Each electron lost is accepted by some other atom or molecule, thereby accomplishing the reduction of the recipient. In inorganic chemistry, oxidation is accompanied by an increase in the positive valence of an element—for example, ferrous (+2) oxidizing to ferric (+3). In organic chemistry, oxidation is frequently considered synonymous with the loss of hydrogen (dehydrogenation) from a molecule. The oxidative process frequently involves free chemical radicals, which are molecules or atoms containing one or more unpaired electrons, as molecular (atmospheric) oxygen ($\bullet O—O\bullet$) and free hydroxyl ($\bullet OH$). These radicals tend to take electrons from other chemicals, thereby oxidizing the donor.

Many of the oxidative changes in pharmaceutical preparations have the character of autoxidations. Autoxidations occur spontaneously under the initial influence of atmospheric oxygen and proceed slowly at first and then more rapidly as the process continues. The process has been described as a type of chain reaction commencing by the union of oxygen with the drug molecule and continuing with a free radical of this oxidized molecule participating in the destruction of other drug molecules and so forth.

In drug product formulation work, steps are taken to reduce or prevent the occurrence of drug substance deterioration due to hydrolysis, oxidation, and other processes. These techniques are discussed later.

Drug and Drug Product Stability: Kinetics and Shelf-Life

Stability is defined as the extent to which a product retains, within specified limits, and throughout its period of storage and use (i.e., its shelf-life), the same properties and characteristics that it possessed at the time of its manufacture.

There are five types of stability of concern to pharmacists:

1. *Chemical.* Each active ingredient retains its chemical integrity and labeled potency, within the specified limits.
2. *Physical.* The original physical properties, including appearance, palatability, uniformity, dissolution and suspendability are retained.
3. *Microbiologic.* Sterility or resistance to microbial growth is retained according to the specified requirements. Antimicrobial agents that are present retain effectiveness within specified limits.
4. *Therapeutic.* The therapeutic effect remains unchanged.
5. *Toxicologic.* No significant increase in toxicity occurs.

Chemical stability is important for selecting storage conditions (temperature, light, humidity), selecting the proper container for dispensing (glass vs. plastic, clear vs. amber or opaque, cap liners) and for anticipating interactions when mixing drugs and dosage forms. Stability and expiration dating are based on reaction kinetics, i.e., the study of the rate of chemical change and the way this rate is influenced by conditions of concentration of reactants, products, and other chemical species that may be present, and by factors such as solvent, pressure, and temperature.

In considering chemical stability of a pharmaceutical, one must know the reaction order and reaction rate. The reaction order may be the overall order (the sum of the exponents of the concentration terms of the rate expression), or the order with respect to each reactant (the exponent of the individual concentration term in the rate expression).

Rate Reactions

The reaction rate expression is a description of the drug concentration with respect to time. Most commonly, zero-order and first-order reactions are encountered in pharmacy. These are presented in the physical pharmacy capsule "Rate Reactions," along with some appropriate examples.

Q_{10} Method of Shelf-Life Estimation

The Q_{10} method of shelf-life estimation allows the pharmacist quickly to calculate estimates of shelf-life for a product that may have been stored or is going to be stored under a different set of conditions. It is explained in the physical pharmacy capsule "Q_{10} Method of Shelf-Life Estimation."

Enhancing Stability of Drug Products

Many pharmaceutic ingredients may be utilized in preparing the desired dosage form of a drug substance. Some of these agents may be used to achieve the desired physical and chemical characteristics of the product or to enhance its appearance, odor, and taste. Other substances may be used to increase the stability of the drug substance, particularly against the hydrolytic and oxidative processes. In each instance, the added pharmaceutic ingredient must be compatible with and must not detract from the stability of the drug substance in the particular dosage form prepared.

There are several approaches to the stabilization of pharmaceutical preparations containing drugs subject to deterioration by hydrolysis. Perhaps the most obvious is the reduction, or better yet, the elimination of water from the pharmaceutical system. Even solid dosage forms containing water-labile drugs must be protected from the humidity of the atmosphere. This may be accomplished by applying a waterproof protective coating over tablets or by enclosing and maintaining the drug in tightly closed containers. It is not unusual to detect

Physical Pharmacy Capsule 3.8   **Rate Reactions**

ZERO ORDER RATE REACTIONS

If the loss of drug is independent of the concentration of the reactants and constant with respect to time (i.e., 1 mg/mL/hour), the rate is called zero order. The mathematical expression is:

$$\frac{-dC}{dt} = k_0$$

where k_0 is the zero-order rate constant [concentration(C)/time(t)].

The integrated, and more useful form of the equation, is:

$$C = -k_0 t + C_0$$

where C_0 is the initial concentration of the drug.

EXAMPLE 1

A drug suspension (125 mg/mL) decays by zero-order kinetics with a reaction rate constant of 0.5 mg/mL/hour. What is the concentration of intact drug remaining after 3 days (72 hours)?

$$C = -(0.5 \text{ mg/mL/hr}) \ (72 \text{ hr}) + 125 \text{ mg/mL}$$

$$C = 89 \text{ mg/mL}$$

EXAMPLE 2

How long will it take for the suspension to reach 90% of its original concentration?

$$90\% \times 125 \text{ mg/mL} = 112.5 \text{ mg/mL}$$

$$t = \frac{C - C_0}{-k_0} - \frac{112.5 \text{ mg/mL} - 125 \text{ mg/mL}}{-0.5 \text{ mg/mL/hr}} = 25 \text{ hours}$$

Drug suspensions are examples of pharmaceuticals that ordinarily follow zero-order kinetics for degradation.

FIRST ORDER RATE REACTIONS

If the loss of drug is directly proportional to the concentration remaining with respect to time, it is called a first-order reaction and has the units of reciprocal time, i.e., time^{-1}. The mathematical expression is:

$$\frac{-dC}{dt} = kC$$

where C is the concentration of intact drug remaining, t is time, $(-dC/dt)$ is the rate at which the intact drug degrades, and k is the specific reaction rate constant.

The integrated and more useful form of the equation is:

$$\log C = \frac{-kt}{2.303} + \log C_0$$

where C_0 is the initial concentration of the drug.

In natural log form, the equation is:

$$\ln C = -kt + \ln C_0$$

EXAMPLE 3

An ophthalmic solution of a mydriatic drug, present at a 5 mg/mL concentration, exhibits first-order degradation with a rate of 0.0005/day. How much drug will remain after 120 days?

$$\ln C = -(0.0005/\text{day}) \ (120) + \ln \ (5 \text{ mg/mL})$$

$$\ln C = -0.06 + 1.609$$

$$\ln C = 1.549$$

$$C = 4.71 \text{ mg/mL}$$

Rate Reactions (Continued)

EXAMPLE 4

In the above example, how long will it take for the drug to degrade to 90% of its original concentration?

$$90\% \text{ of } 5 \text{ mg/mL} = 4.5 \text{ mg/mL}$$

$$\ln 4.5 \text{ mg/mL} = -(0.0005/\text{day})t + \ln (5 \text{ mg/mL})$$

$$t = \frac{\ln 4.5 \text{ mg/mL} - \ln 5 \text{ mg/mL}}{-0.0005/\text{day}}$$

$$t = 210 \text{ days}$$

Stability projections for shelf-life (t_{90}) (i.e., the time required for 10% of the drug to degrade with 90% of the intact drug remaining, are commonly based on the Arrhenius equation:

$$\log \frac{k_2}{k_1} = \frac{Ea \, (t_2 - T_1)}{2.3 \, RT_1 T_2}$$

which relates the reaction rate constants (k) to temperatures (T) with the gas constant (R) and the energy of activation (Ea).

The relationship of the reaction rate constants at two different temperatures provides the energy of activation for the degradation. By performing the reactions at elevated temperatures, instead of allowing the process to proceed very slowly at room temperature, the Ea can be calculated and a k value for room temperature determined by using the Arrhenius equation.

EXAMPLE 5

The degradation of a new cancer drug follows first-order kinetics and has first-order degradation rate constants of 0.0001/hr at 60°C and 0.0009 at 80°C. What is its Ea?

$$\log \frac{(0.0009)}{(0.0001)} = \frac{EA \, (353 - 333)}{(2.3)(1.987)(353)(333)}$$

$$Ea = 25,651 \text{ kcal/mol}$$

hydrolyzed aspirin by noticing an odor of acetic acid upon opening a bottle of aspirin tablets. In liquid preparations, water can frequently be replaced or reduced in the formulation through the use of substitute liquids such as glycerin, propylene glycol, and alcohol. In certain injectable products, anhydrous vegetable oils may be used as the drug's solvent to reduce the chance of hydrolytic decomposition.

Decomposition by hydrolysis may be prevented for other drugs to be administered in liquid form by suspending them in a non-aqueous vehicle rather than by dissolving them in an aqueous solvent. In still other instances, particularly for certain unstable antibiotic drugs, when an aqueous preparation is desired, the drug may be supplied to the pharmacist in a dry form for *reconstitution* by adding a specified volume of purified water just before dispensing. The dry powder supplied commercially is actually a mixture of the antibiotic, suspending agents, flavorants, and colorants, which, when reconstituted by the pharmacist, remains a stable suspension or solution of the drug for the time period in which the preparation is normally consumed. Storage under refrigeration is advisable for most preparations considered unstable due to hydrolytic causes. Together with temperature, pH is a major determinant in the stability of a drug prone to hydrolytic decomposition. The hydrolysis of most drugs is dependent upon the relative concentrations of the hydroxyl and hydronium ions, and a pH at which each drug is optimally stable can be easily determined. For most hydrolyzable drugs the pH of optimum stability is on the acid side, somewhere between pH 5 and 6. Therefore, through judicious use of buffering agents, the stability of otherwise unstable compounds can be increased.

Physical Pharmacy Capsule 3.9   **Q_{10} Method of Shelf-Life Estimation**

The Q_{10} approach, based on Ea, is independent of reaction order and is described as:

$$Q_{10} = e^{\{(Ea/R)[(1/T+10) - (1/T)]\}}$$

where Ea is the energy of activation,
    R is the gas constant, and
    T is the absolute temperature.
    In usable terms, Q_{10} is the ratio of two different reaction rate constants, and is defined as:

$$Q_{10} = \frac{K_{(T+10)}}{K_T}$$

Q values of 2, 3 and 4 are commonly used and relate to the energies of activations of the reactions for temperatures around room temperature (25°C). For example, a Q value of 2 corresponds to an Ea (kcal/mol) of 12.2, a Q value of 3 corresponds to an Ea of 19.4, and a Q value of 4 corresponds to an Ea of 24.5.

Reasonable estimates can often be made using the value of 3.

The equation to use for Q_{10} shelf-life estimates is:

$$t_{90}(T_2) = \frac{t_{90}(T_1)}{Q_{10}^{(\Delta T/10)}}$$

where $t_{90}T_2$ is the estimated shelf-life,
    $t_{90}T_1$ is the given shelf-life at a given temperature, and
    ΔT is the difference in the temperatures T_1 and T_2.
    As is evident from this relationship, an increase in ΔT will decrease the shelf-life and a decrease in ΔT will increase shelf-life. This is the same as saying that storing at a warmer temperature will shorten the life of the drug and storing at a cooler temperature will increase the life of the drug.

EXAMPLE 1
An antibiotic solution has a shelf-life of 48 hours in the refrigerator (5°C). What is its estimated shelf-life at room temperature (25°C)?

Using a Q value of 3, we set up the relationship as follows.

$$t_{90}(T_2) = \frac{t_{90}(T_1)}{Q_{10}^{(\Delta T/10)}} = \frac{48}{3^{[(25-5)/10]}} = \frac{48}{3^2} = 5.33 \text{ hours}$$

EXAMPLE 2
An ophthalmic solution has a shelf-life of 6 hours at room temperature (25°C). What would be the estimated shelf-life if stored in a refrigerator (5°C)? (*Note:* Since the temperature is decreasing, $\underline{\Delta T}$ will be negative.)

$$t_{90}(T_2) = \frac{6}{3^{[(5-25)/10]}} = \frac{6}{3^{-2}} = 6 \times 3^2 = 54 \text{ hours}$$

Pharmacists should keep in mind that these are estimates, and actual energies of activation can be often be obtained from the literature for more exact calculations.

Buffers are used to maintain a certain pH as described in the physical pharmacy capsule entitled "Buffer Capacity."

Pharmaceutically, the oxidation of a susceptible drug substance is most likely to occur when it is maintained in other than the dry state in the presence of oxygen, exposed to light, or combined in formulation with other chemical agents without proper regard to their influence on the oxidation process. The oxidation of a chemical in a pharmaceutical preparation is usually attendant with an alteration in the color of that preparation. It may also result in precipitation or a change in the usual odor of a preparation.

Physical Pharmacy Capsule 3.10   **Buffer Capacity**

pH, buffers and buffer capacity are especially important in drug product formulation; especially as they are involved in drug solubility, drug activity, drug absorption drug stability and patient comfort.

A buffer is a system, usually an aqueous solution, that can resist changes in pH upon addition of an acid or base. Buffers are composed of a weak acid and its conjugate base, or a weak base and its conjugate acid. Buffers are prepared by:

a. mixing a weak acid and its conjugate base or a weak base and it's conjugate acid, or

b. mixing a weak acid and a strong base to form the conjugate base or a weak base and a strong acid to form the conjugate acid

Using the Henderson-Hasselbach equation:

$$pH = pKa + \log (base/acid)$$
(Remember that the acid is the proton donor and the base is the proton acceptor)

EXAMPLE 1

A buffer is prepared by mixing 100 mL of 0.2 M phosphoric acid with 200 mL of 0.08 M sodium phosphate monobasic. What is the pH of this buffer? (K_a of phosphoric acid = 7.5×10^{-3})

Moles acid = (0.2 mol/1000 mL)(100 mL) = 0.02 mol; (0.02 mol)/(0.3 L) = 0.067 M

Moles base = (0.08 mol/1000 mL)(200 mL) = 0.016 mol; (0.016 mol(/(0.3 L) = 0.053 M

pKa = $-\log 7.5 \times 10^{-3}$ = 2.125

pH = 2.125 + log (0.016 mol/0.02 mol) = 2.028

EXAMPLE 2

Determine the pH of the buffer prepared as shown below.

Sodium acetate 50 g

Conc. HCl 10 mL

Water q.s. 2 L

Helpful numbers:

pK_a acetic acid = 4.76

m.w. sodium acetate = 82.08

m.w. acetic acid = 60.05

m.w. HCl = 36.45

Conc.HCl $\approx$ 44% HCl w/v

NaAc   +   HCl   →   NaCl   +   HAc   +   NaAc
(0.609 mol)   (0.121 mol)   (0.121 mol)   ((0.121 mol)   (0.488 mol)

HCl: {(10 mL) [(44g)/(100 mL)] (l mol)/(36.45g)} = 0.121 mol

NaAc: {(50 g)[(1 mol)/(82.08g)] = 0.609 mol
(0.609 mol) − (0.121 mol) = 0.488 mol

pH = 4.76 + log (0.488 mol)/(0.121 mol) = 5.367

The ability of a buffer solution to resist changes in pH upon the addition of an acid or a base is called buffer capacity (β) and is defined as:

$$\beta = \Delta B/\Delta pH$$

where ΔB = molar concentration of acid or base added
ΔpH = change in pH due to addition of acid or base
ΔpH can be determined experimentally or calculated using the Henderson-Hasselbach equation.

Buffer Capacity (Continued)

EXAMPLE 3

If 0.2 mole of HCl is added to a 0.015 M solution of ammonium hydroxide and the pH falls from 9.5 to 8.9, what is the buffer capacity?

$$\Delta pH = 9.5 - 8.9 = 0.6$$

$$\Delta B = 0.2 \text{ mol/L} = 0.2 \text{ M}$$

$$\beta = 0.2 \text{ M}/0.6 = 0.33 \text{ M}$$

EXAMPLE 4

If 0.002 mole of HCl is added to the buffer in Example No. 1, what is its buffer capacity? After adding 0.002 mole HCl:

$$H_3PO_4: 0.02 \text{ mol} + 0.002 \text{ mol} = 0.022 \text{ mol}$$

$$NaH_2PO_4: 0.016 \text{ mol} - 0.002 \text{ mL} = 0.014 \text{ mol}$$

$$pH = 2.125 + \log (0.014 \text{ mol}/0.022 \text{ mol}) = 1.929$$

$$\Delta pH = 2.028 - 1.929 = 0.099$$

$$\Delta AB = 0.002 \text{ mol}/0.3 \text{ L} = 0.0067 \text{ M}$$

$$\beta = 0.0067 \text{ M}/0.099 = 0.067 \text{ M}$$

Another approach to calculating buffer capacity involves the use of Van-Slyke's equation, given as:

$$\beta = 2.3C \{Ka[H^+]/(Ka[H^+])^2\}$$

where C = sum of the molar concentrations of the acid and base, and

$$[H^+] = 10^{-pH}$$

EXAMPLE 5

What is the Van Slyke's buffer capacity of the buffer prepared in Example No. 1?

$$C = 0.0067 \text{ M} + 0.0053 \text{ M} = 0.12 \text{ M}$$

$$Ka = 7.5 \times 10^{-3}$$

$$[H+] = 10^{-2.028} = 9.38 \times 10^{-3} \text{ M}$$

$$\beta = 2.3(0.12M)\{[(7.5 \times 10^{-3}M)(9.38 \times 10^{-3}M)/[(7.5 \times 10^{-3}M)/(9.38 \times 10^{-3}M)^2]\} = 0.68 \text{ M}$$

The oxidative process is diverted, and the stability of the drug is preserved by agents called *antioxidants*, which react with one or more compounds in the drug to prevent progress of the chain reaction. In general, antioxidants act by providing electrons and easily available hydrogen atoms that are accepted more readily by the free radicals than are those of the drug being protected. Various antioxidants are employed in pharmacy. Among those more frequently used in aqueous preparations are sodium sulfite (Na_2SO_3), sodium bisulfite ($NaHSO_3$), hypophosphorous acid (H_3PO_2), and ascorbic acid. In oleaginous (oily or unctuous) preparations, alpha-tocopherol, butylhydroxyanisole, and ascorbyl palmitate find application.

In June 1987, FDA labeling regulations went into effect requiring a warning about possible allergic-type reactions, including anaphylaxis in the package insert for prescription drugs to which sulfites have been added to the final dosage form. Sulfites are used as preservatives in many injectable drugs, such as antibiotics and local anesthetics. Some inhalants and ophthalmic preparations also contain sulfites, but relatively few oral drugs contain these chemicals. The purpose of the regulation is to protect the estimated 0.2% of the population who suffer allergic reactions from the chemicals. Many of the sulfite-sensitive persons suffer from asthma or other allergic conditions. Previous to the regulations dealing with prescription medication, the FDA issued regulations for the use of sulfites in food. Asthmatics and other patients who may be sulfite-sensitive should be reminded to read the labels of packaged foods and medications to check for the presence of these agents. Sulfiting agents covered by the regulations are potassium bisulfite, potassium metabisulfite, sodium bisulfite, sodium metabisulfite, sodium sulfite and sulfur dioxide. The FDA permits the use of sulfites in prescription products, with the proper labeling, because there are no generally suitable substitutes for sulfites to maintain potency in certain medications. Some, but not all, epinephrine injections contain sulfites.

The proper use of antioxidants involves their specific application only after appropriate biomedical and pharmaceutical studies. In certain instances other pharmaceutical additives can inactivate a given antioxidant when used in the same formulation. In other cases certain antioxidants can react chemically with the drugs they were intended to stabilize, without a noticeable change in the appearance of the preparation.

Because the stability of oxidizable drugs may be adversely affected by oxygen, certain pharmaceuticals may require an oxygen-free atmosphere during their preparation and storage. Oxygen may be present in pharmaceutical liquids in the airspace within the container or may be dissolved in the liquid vehicle. To avoid these exposures, oxygen-sensitive drugs may be prepared in the dry state and they, as well as liquid preparations, may be packaged in sealed containers with the air replaced by an inert gas such as nitrogen. This is common practice in the commercial production of vials and ampuls of easily oxidizable preparations intended for parenteral use.

Trace metals originating in the drug, solvent, container, or stopper are a constant source of difficulty in preparing stable solutions of oxidizable drugs. The rate of formation of color in epinephrine solutions, for instance, is greatly increased by the presence of ferric, ferrous, cupric, and chromic ions. Great care must be taken to eliminate these trace metals from labile preparations by thorough purification of the source of the contaminant or by chemically complexing or binding the metal through the use of specialized agents that make it chemically unavailable for participation in the oxidative process. These agents are referred to as chelating agents and are exemplified by calcium disodium edetate and ethylenediamine tetra-acetic acid (EDTA).

Light can also act as a catalyst to oxidation reactions. As a photocatalyst, light waves transfer their energy (photon) to drug molecules, making the latter more reactive through increased energy capability. As a precaution against the acceleration of the oxidative process, sensitive preparations are packaged in light-resistant or opaque containers.

Because most drug degradations proceed more rapidly with an advanced temperature, it is also advisable to maintain oxidizable drugs in a cool place. Another factor that could affect the stability of an oxidizable drug in solution is the pH of the preparation. Each drug must be maintained in solution at the pH most favorable to its stability. This, in fact, varies from

Table 3.2. Examples of Some Official Drugs and Preparations Especially Subject to Chemical or Physical Deterioration

Preparation	Category	Monograph or Label Warning
Epinephrine Bitartrate Ophthalmic Solution, USP Epinephrine Inhalation Solution, USP Epinephrine Injection, USP Epinephrine Nasal Solution, USP Epinephrine Ophthalmic Solution, USP	Adrenergic	Do not use the inhalation, injection, nasal or ophthalmic solution if it is brown or contains a precipitate.
Isoproterenol Sulfate Inhalation, Solution, USP Isoproterenol Inhalation Solution, USP	Adrenergic (bronchodilator)	Do not use the inhalation or injection if it is pink to brown in color or contains a precipitate.
Nitroglycerin Tablets, USP	Antianginal	To prevent loss of potency, keep these tablets in the original container or in a supplemental nitroglycerin container specifically labeled as being suitable for nitroglycerin tablets.
Paraldehyde, USP	Hypnotic	Paraldehyde is subject to oxidation to form acetic acid.

preparation to preparation and must be determined on an individual basis for the drug in question.

Statements in the USP, as those in Table 3.2, warn of the oxidative decomposition of drugs and preparations. In some instances the specific agent to employ as a stabilizer is mentioned in the monograph, and in others the term "suitable stabilizer" is used. An example in which a particular agent is designated for use is in the monograph for Potassium Iodide Oral Solution, USP. Potassium iodide in solution is prone to photocatalyzed oxidation and the release of free iodine with a resultant yellow to brown discoloration of the solution. The use of light-resistant containers is essential to its stability. As a further precaution against decomposition if the solution is not to be used within a short time, the USP recommends the addition of 0.5 mg of sodium thiosulfate for each gram of potassium iodide in the preparation. In the event free iodine is released during storage, the sodium thiosulfate converts it to colorless and soluble sodium iodide:

$$I_2 + 2Na_2S_2O_3 \longrightarrow 2\,NaI + Na_2S_4O_6$$

In summary, for easily oxidizable drugs, the formulation pharmacist may stabilize the respective preparations by the selective exclusion from the system of oxygen, oxidizing agents, trace metals, light, heat, and other chemical catalysts to the oxidation process. Antioxidants, chelating agents, and buffering agents may be added to create and maintain a favorable pH.

In addition to oxidation and hydrolysis, other destructive processes such as polymerization, chemical decarboxylation, and deamination may occur in pharmaceutical preparations. However, these processes occur less frequently and are peculiar to only small groups of chemical substances. Drug polymerization involves a reaction between two or more identical molecules with resultant formation of a new and generally larger molecule. Formaldehyde is an example of a drug capable of polymerization. In solution it may polymerize to paraformaldehyde $(CH_2O)_n$, a slowly soluble white crystalline substance that may cause the solution to become cloudy. The formation of paraformaldehyde is enhanced by cool storage temperatures, especially in solutions with high concentrations of formaldehyde. The official formaldehyde solution contains approximately 37% formaldehyde and according to the USP should be stored at temperatures not below 15°C (59°F). If the solution becomes cloudy upon standing in a cool place, it usually may be cleared by gentle warming.

Formaldehyde is prepared by the limited oxidation of methanol (methyl alcohol), and the USP permits a residual amount of this material to remain in the final product, since it has the ability to retard the formation of paraformaldehyde. Formaldehyde solution must be maintained in tight containers because oxidation of the formaldehyde yields formic acid.

$$\underset{\text{methanol}}{CH_3OH} \xrightarrow{\text{(O)}} \underset{\text{formaldehyde}}{HCHO} \xrightarrow{\text{(O)}} \underset{\text{formic acid}}{HCOOH}$$

Other organic drug molecules may be degraded through processes in which one or more of their active chemical groups are removed. These processes may involve various catalysts, including light and enzymes. Decarboxylation and deamination are examples of such processes, with the former involving the decomposition of an organic acid (R•COOH) and the consequent release of carbon dioxide gas and the latter involving the removal of the nitrogen-containing group from an organic amine. For example, insulin, a protein, deteriorates rapidly in acid solutions, due to extensive deamination. (3) Thus, most preparations of insulin are neutralized to reduce its rate of decomposition.

Stability Testing

The Food and Drug Administration's Current Good Manufacturing Practice regulations include sections on the stability and stability testing of pharmaceutical components and finished pharmaceutical products. In addition, agency and International Conference on Harmonization (ICH) guidelines and guidances provide working recommendations to support the regulatory requirements. Among these are the following (4):

"Stability Testing of New Drug Substances and Products"
"Quality of Biotechnological Products: Stability Testing of Biotechnology/Biological Drug Products"
"Photostability Testing of New Drug Substances and Products"
"Stability Testing of New Dosage Forms"

Drug and drug product stability testing during every stage of development is critical to the quality of the pharmaceutical product. Drug stability is important during preclinical testing and in clinical (human) trials in order to obtain a true and accurate assessment of the drug/drug product being evaluated. For a marketed drug product, assurance of drug stability is vital to the safety and effectiveness of the product when distributed and during the entire course of its shelf-life and use.

The FDA-required demonstration of drug stability is necessarily different for each stage of drug development, i.e., for a 2-week preclinical study, an early Phase I study, a limited Phase II trial, a pivotal Phase III clinical study, or for a New Drug Application for approval for marketing. As a drug development program progresses, so does the requisite data to demonstrate and document the drug/drug product's stability profile. Before approval for marketing, a product's stability must be assessed with regard to its formulation, the influence of pharmaceutic ingredients present, the influence of the container and closure, the manufacturing and processing conditions (e.g. heat), packaging components and conditions of warehousing/storage, the anticipated conditions of shipping, temperature, light and humidity, and anticipated duration and conditions of pharmacy shelf-life and patient utilization. It is important to recognize, that the"holding"of intermediate product components (as drug granulations for tableting) for undue lengthy periods before processing into finished pharmaceutical products could affect the stability of both the intermediate component and the finished product. Therefore, in-process stability testing including the retesting of intermediate components is important.

Product containers, closures, and other packaging features must be considered in stability testing. For instance, tablets or capsules packaged in glass or plastic bottles, blister packs or strip packaging would require different stability test protocols. Drugs particularly subject to hydrolysis or oxidative decomposition must be evaluated accordingly. And, parenteral and other sterile products must meet sterility test standards to ensure protection 'against microbial contamination. Any preservatives used must be tested for effectiveness in the finished product.

As noted elsewhere in this section, drug products must meet stability standards for long-term storage at room temperatures and under conditions of relative humidity. Products are also subjected to accelerated stability studies as an indication of shelf-life stability. It is an FDA requirement that if not submitted in the approved application, the first three postapproval production batches of a drug substance be placed on long-term stability studies and the first three postapproval production batches of drug product be subject to both long-term and accelerated stability studies (5,6).

Drug instability in pharmaceutical formulations may be detected in some instances by a change in the physical appearance, color, odor, taste or texture of the formulation whereas in other instances chemical changes may occur which are not self-evident and may only be ascertained through chemical analysis. Scientific data pertaining to the stability of a formulation leads to the prediction of the expected shelf-life of the proposed product and, when necessary, to the redesign of the drug (e.g. into more stable salt or ester form) and to the reformulation of the dosage form. Obviously the rate or speed at which drug degradation occurs in a formulation is of prime importance. The study of the rate of chemical change and the way in which it is influenced by such factors as the concentration of the drug or reactant, the solvent employed, the conditions of temperature and pressure, and the presence of other chemical agents in the formulation is termed reaction kinetics.

In general a kinetic study begins by measuring the concentration of the drug being examined at given time intervals under a specific set of conditions including temperature, pH, ionic strength, light intensity, and drug concentration. The measurement of the drug's concentration at the various time intervals reveals the stability or instability of the drug under the specified conditions with the passage of time. From this starting point, each of the original conditions may be varied on an individual basis to determine the influence that such changes make on the drug's stability. For example, the pH of the solution may be changed, whereas the temperature, light intensity, and original drug concentration remain as they were in the original or baseline experiment.

The data collected may be presented graphically, by plotting the drug concentration as a function of time. From the experimental data, the reaction rate may be determined and a rate constant and half-life calculated.

The use of exaggerated conditions of temperature, humidity, light, and others, to test the stability of drug formulations is termed accelerated stability testing. Accelerated temperature stability studies, for example, may be conducted for six months at 40°C with 75% relative humidity. If a significant change occurs in the drug/drug product under these conditions, lesser temperature and humidity may be used, such as 30°C and 60% relative humidity. The use of short-term accelerated studies is for the purpose of determining the most stable of the proposed formulations for a drug product. In stress testing, temperature elevations, in 10°

increments higher than used in accelerated studies, are employed until chemical or physical degradation. Once the most stable formulation is ascertained, its long-term stability is predicted from the data generated from continuing stability studies. Depending on the types and severity of conditions employed, it is not unusual to maintain samples under exaggerated conditions of both temperature and varying humidity for periods of 6 to 12 months. Such studies lead to the prediction of shelf-life for a drug product.

In addition to the accelerated stability studies, drug products are also subjected to long-term stability studies under the usual conditions of transport and storage expected during product distribution. In conducting these studies, the different climatic zones, nationally and internationally, to which the product may be subjected must be borne in mind, and expected variances in conditions of temperature and humidity included in the study design. Geographic regions of the world are defined by climatic zones: zone I, "temperate"; zone II, "subtropical"; zone III, "hot and dry"; and zone IV, "hot and humid." A given drug product may encounter more than a single zone of temperature/humidity variations during its production and shelf-life. Further, it may be warehoused, transported, placed on a pharmacy's shelf, and subsequently in the patient's medicine cabinet, over a varying time course and at a wide range of temperature and humidity. In general, however, the long-term (12 months minimum) testing of new drug entities is conducted at 25° C ± 2° C and at a relative humidity of 60% ± 5%. Samples maintained under these conditions may be retained for periods of 5 years or longer during which time they are observed for physical signs of deterioration and chemically assayed. These studies, considered with the accelerated stability studies previously performed, then lead to a more precise determination of drug product stability, actual shelf-life, and the possible extension of expiration dating.

When chemical degradation products are detected, the FDA requires the manufacturer to report their chemical identities, including structures, mechanism of formation, physical and chemical properties, procedures for isolation and purification, specifications and directions for determination at levels expected to be present in the pharmaceutical product, and the pharmacologic action and biologic significance, if any, to their presence.

In addition, signs of degradation of the specific dosage forms must be observed and reported. For the various dosage forms, this includes the following (1).

Tablets: appearance, friability, hardness, color, odor, moisture content, and dissolution.

Capsules: strength, moisture, color, appearance, shape, brittleness, and dissolution.

Oral solutions and suspensions: appearance, strength, pH, color, odor, redispersibility (suspensions), and clarity (solutions).

Oral powders: appearance, strength, color, odor, moisture.

Metered-dose inhalation aerosols: strength, delivered dose per actuation, number of metered doses, color, particle-size distribution, loss of propellant, pressure, valve corrosion, spray pattern, absence of pathogenic microorganisms.

Topical nonmetered aerosols: appearance, odor, pressure, weight loss, net weight dispensed, delivery rate, and spray pattern.

Topical creams, ointments, lotions, solutions, and gels: appearance, color, homogeneity, odor, pH, resuspendibility (lotions), consistency, particle-size distribution, strength, weight loss.

Ophthalmic preparations: appearance, color, consistency, pH, clarity (solutions), particle size and resuspendibility (suspensions, creams, ointments), strength, and sterility.

Small-volume parenterals: strength, appearance, color, particulate matter, dispersibility (suspensions), pH, sterility, pyrogenicity, and closure integrity.

Large-volume parenterals: strength, appearance, color, clarity, particulate matter, pH, volume and extractables (when plastic containers are used), sterility, pyrogenicity, and closure integrity.

Suppositories: strength, softening range, appearance, and dissolution.

Emulsions: appearance (as phase separation), color, odor, pH, viscosity, and strength.

Controlled-release membrane drug delivery systems: seal strength of the drug reservoir, decomposition products, membrane integrity, drug strength, and drug release rate.

Under usual circumstances, most manufactured products require a shelf-life of 2 or more years to ensure their stability at the time of patient consumption. Commercial products must bear an appropriate expiration date. This date identifies the time during which the product may be expected to maintain its potency and remain stable under the designated storage conditions. The expiration date limits the time during which the product may be dispensed by the pharmacist or used by the patient.

Prescriptions requiring extemporaneous compounding by the pharmacist do not require the extended shelf-life that commercially manufactured and distributed products do because they are intended to be used immediately on their receipt by the patient and used only during the immediate course of the prescribed treatment. However, these compounded prescriptions must remain stable and efficacious during the course of their use and the compounding pharmacist must employ formulative components and techniques which will result in a stable product (7).

In years past pharmacists were confronted primarily with innocuous, topical prescriptions that required extemporaneous formulation. However, in recent years there has been a need to compound other drug delivery systems as well, e.g., progesterone vaginal suppositories, oral suspensions, from existing tablets or capsules. When presented with a prescription that requires extemporaneous compounding, the pharmacist is confronted with a difficult situation because the potency and the stability of these prescriptions is a serious matter. Occasionally, the results of compatibility and stability studies on such prescriptions are published in scientific and professional journals. These are very useful; however, there are also prescriptions for which stability and compatibility information is not readily available. In these instances, it behooves the pharmacist to at least contact the drug manufacturer of the active ingredient(s) to solicit stability information. Also, a compilation of published stability information is included in Trissel's Stability of Compounded Formulations (8). The published stability data are applicable only to products that are prepared identically to the products that are reported.

USP guidelines on stability of extemporaneous compounded formulations state that, in the absence of stability information that is applicable to a specific drug and preparation, the following guidelines can be utilized: nonaqueous liquids and solid formulations where the manufactured drug is the source of the active ingredient-not later than 25% of the time remaining until the product's expiration date or 6 months, whichever is earlier; nonaqueous liquids and solid formulations where a USP or NF substance is the source of active ingredient—a beyond-use date of 6 months; for water-containing formulations prepared from ingredients in solid form—a beyond-use date of not later than 14 days when stored at cold temperatures; for all other formulations—a beyond-use date of the intended du-

ration of therapy or 30 days, whichever is earlier (9). Thus, in the instance where an oral aqueous liquid preparation is made from an existing tablet or capsule formulation, the pharmacist should make up only at most a 14 days supply and it must be stored in a refrigerator. Further, the pharmacist must also dispense the medication in a container conducive to stability and use and must advise the patient of the proper method of use and conditions of storage of the medication.

Finally, when compounding on the basis of extrapolated or less than concrete information it is best for the pharmacist to keep the formulation simple and not to shortcut but use the necessary pharmaceutical adjuvants to prepare the prescription.

Pharmaceutic Ingredients

Definitions and Types

To prepare a drug substance into a final dosage form, pharmaceutic ingredients are required. For example, in the preparation of pharmaceutic solutions, one or more *solvents* are used to dissolve the drug substance, *flavors and sweeteners* are used to make the product more palatable, *colorants* are added to enhance product appeal, *preservatives* may be added to prevent microbial growth and *stabilizers,* such as antioxidants and chelating agents, may be used to prevent drug decomposition, as previously discussed. In the preparation of tablets, *diluents* or *fillers* are commonly added to increase the bulk of the formulation, *binders* to cause the adhesion of the powdered drug and pharmaceutic substances, *antiadherents* or *lubricants* to assist the smooth tableting process, *disintegrating agents* to promote tablet break-up after administration, and coatings to improve stability, control disintegration, or to enhance appearance. Ointments, creams, and suppositories achieve their characteristic features due to the pharmaceutic bases which are utilized. Thus, for each dosage form, the pharmaceutic ingredients establish the primary features of the product, and contribute to the physical form, texture, stability, taste and overall appearance.

Table 3.3 presents the principal categories of pharmaceutic ingredients, with examples of some of the official and commercial agents currently used. Additional discussion of many of the pharmaceutic ingredients may be found in the chapters where they are most relevant; for example, pharmaceutic materials used in tablet and capsule formulations

Table 3.3.   Examples of Pharmaceutic Ingredients

Ingredient Type	Definition	Examples
Acidifying Agent	Used in liquid preparations to provide acidic medium for product stability.	Citric acid Acetic acid Fumaric acid Hydrochloric acid Nitric acid
Alkalinizing Agent	Used in liquid preparations to provide alkaline medium for product stability.	Ammonia solution Ammonium carbonate Diethanolamine Monoethanolamine Potassium hydroxide Sodium borate Sodium carbonate Sodium hydroxide Triethanolamine Trolamine
Adsorbent	An agent capable of holding other molecules onto its surface by physical or chemical (chemisorption) means.	Powdered cellulose Activated charcoal
Aerosol Propellant	Agent responsible for developing the pressure within an aerosol container and expelling the product when the valve is opened.	Carbon dioxide Dichlorodifluoromethane Dichlorotetrafluoroethane Trichloromonofluoromethane
Air Displacement	Agent employed to displace air in a hermetically sealed container to enhance product stability.	Nitrogen Carbon dioxide
Antifungal Preservative	Used in liquid and semi-solid preparations to prevent the growth of fungi. The effectiveness of the parabens is usually enhanced when they are used in combination.	Butylparaben Ethylparaben Methylparaben Benzoic acid Propylparaben Sodium benzoate Sodium propionate
Antimicrobial Preservative	Used in liquid and semi-solid preparations to prevent the growth of microorganisms.	Benzalkonium chloride Benzethonium chloride Benzyl alcohol Cetylpyridinium chloride Chlorobutanol Phenol Phenylethyl alcohol Phenylmercuric nitrate Thimerosal
Antioxidant	Agent that inhibits oxidation and thus is used to prevent the deterioration of preparations by the oxidative process.	Ascorbic acid Ascorbyl palmitate Butylated hydroxyanisole Butylated hydroxytoluene Hypophophorous acid Monothioglycerol Propyl gallate Sodium ascorbate Sodium bisulfite Sodium formaldehyde Sulfoxylate Sodium metabisulfite
Buffering Agent	Used to resist change in pH upon dilution or addition of acid or alkali. potassium metaphosphate	Potassium phosphate, monobasic Sodium acetate Sodium citrate anhydrous and dihydrate

continued

Table 3.3.   Examples of Pharmaceutic Ingredients

Ingredient Type	Definition	Examples
Chelating Agent	Substance that forms stable, water soluble complexes (chelates) with metals. Chelating agents are used in some liquid pharmaceuticals as stabilizers to complex heavy metals which might promote instability. In such use they are also called *sequestering* agents.	Edetic acid Edetate disodium
Colorant	Used to impart color to liquid and solid (e.g., tablets and capsules) pharmaceutical preparations.	FD&C Red No. 3 FD&C Red No. 20 FD&C Yellow No. 6 FD&C Blue No. 2 D&C Green No. 5 D&C Orange No. 5 D&C Red No. 8 Caramel Ferric oxide, red
Clarifying Agent	Used as a filtering aid because of adsorbent qualities.	Bentonite
Emulsifying Agent	Used to promote and maintain the dispersion of finely subdivided particles of a liquid in a vehicle in which it is immiscible. The end product may be a liquid emulsion or semisolid emulsion (e.g., a cream).	Acacia Cetomacrogol Cetyl alcohol Glyceryl monostearate Sorbitan monooleate Polyoxyethylene 50 stearate
Encapsulating Agent	Used to form thin shells for the purpose of enclosing a drug substance or drug formulation for ease of administration.	Gelatin Cellulose acetate phthalate
Flavorant	Used to impart a pleasant flavor and often odor to a pharmaceutical preparation. In addition to the natural flavorants listed, many synthetic flavorants are also used.	Anise oil Cinnamon oil Cocoa Menthol Orange oil Peppermint oil Vanillin
Humectant	Used to prevent the drying out of preparations—particularly ointments and creams—due to the agent's ability to retain moisture.	Glycerin Propylene glycol Sorbitol
Levigating Agent	Liquid used as an intervening agent to reduce the particle size of a drug powder by grinding together, usually in a mortar.	Mineral oil Glycerin
Ointment Base	Semisolid vehicle into which drug substances may be incorporated in preparing medicated ointments.	Lanolin Hydrophilic ointment Polyethylene glycol ointment Petrolatum Hydrophilic petrolatum White ointment Yellow ointment Rose water ointment
Plasticizer	Used as a component of film-coating solutions to enhance the spread of the coat over tablets, beads, and granules.	Diethyl phthalate Glycerin
Solvent	An agent used to dissolve another pharmaceutic substance or a drug in the preparation of a solution. The solvent may be aqueous or nonaqueous (e.g., oleaginous). Cosolvents, such as water and alcohol (hydroalcoholic) and water and glycerin, may be used when needed. Solvents rendered sterile are used in certain preparations (e.g., injections).	Alcohol Corn oil Cottonseed oil Glycerin Isopropyl alcohol Mineral oil Oleic acid Peanut oil Purified water Water for injection Sterile water for injection Sterile water for irrigation

continued

Table 3.3. Examples of Pharmaceutic Ingredients

Ingredient Type	Definition	Examples
Stiffening Agent	Used to increase the thickness or hardness of a pharmaceutical preparation, usually an ointment.	Cetyl alcohol Cetyl esters wax Microcrystalline wax Paraffin Stearyl alcohol White wax Yellow wax
Suppository Base	Used as a vehicle into which drug substances are incorporated in the preparation of suppositories.	Cocoa butter Polyethylene glycols (mixtures)
Surfactant (surface active agent)	Substances that absorb to surfaces or interfaces to reduce surface or interfacial tension. May be used as wetting agents, detergents or emulsifying agents.	Benzalkonium chloride Nonoxynol 10 Oxtoxynol 9 Polysorbate 80 Sodium lauryl sulfate Sorbitan monopalmitate
Suspending Agent	A viscosity increasing agent used to reduce the rate of sedimentation of (drug) particles dispersed throughout a vehicle in which they are not soluble. The resultant suspensions may be formulated for use orally, parenterally, ophthalmically, topically, or by other routes.	Agar Bentonite Carbomer (e.g., Carbopol) Carboxymethylcellulose sodium Hydroxyethyl cellulose Hydroxypropyl cellulose Hydroxypropyl methylcellulose Kaolin Methylcellulose Tragacanth Veegum
Sweetening Agent	Used to impart sweetness to a preparation.	Aspartame Dextrose Glycerin Mannitol Saccharin sodium Sorbitol Sucrose
Tablet Antiadherents	Agents that prevent the sticking of tablet formulation ingredients to punches and dies in a tableting machine during production.	Magnesium stearate Talc
Tablet Binders	Substances used to cause adhesion of powder particles in tablet granulations.	Acacia Alginic acid Carboxymethylcellulose sodium Compressible sugar (e.g., Nu-Tab) Ethylcellulose Gelatin Liquid glucose Methylcellulose Povidone Pregelatinized starch
Tablet and Capsule Diluent	Inert substances used as fillers to create the desired bulk, flow properties, and compression characteristics in the preparation of tablets and capsules.	Dibasic calcium phosphate Kaolin Lactose Mannitol Microcrystalline cellulose Powdered cellulose Precipitated calcium carbonate Sorbitol Starch

continued

Table 3.3.   Examples of Pharmaceutic Ingredients

Ingredient Type	Definition	Examples
Tablet Coating Agent	Used to coat a formed tablet for the purpose of protecting against drug decomposition by atmospheric oxygen or humidity, to provide a desired release pattern for the drug substance after administration, to mask the taste or odor of the drug substance, or for aesthetic purposes. The coating may be of various types, including sugar-coating, film coating, or enteric coating. Sugar coating is water-based and results in a thickened covering around a formed tablet. Sugar-coated tablets generally start to break up in the stomach. A film coat is a thin cover around a formed tablet or bead. Unless it is an enteric coat, the film coat will dissolve in the stomach. An enteric-coated tablet or bead will pass through the stomach and break up in the intestines. Some coatings that are water-insoluble (e.g., ethylcellulose) may be used to coat tablets and beads to slow the release of drug as they pass through the gastrointestinal tract.	
Sugar coating:		Liquid glucose Sucrose
Film coating:		Hydroxyethyl cellulose Hydroxypropyl cellulose Hydroxypropyl methylcellulose Methylcellulose (e.g., Methocel) Ethylcellulose (e.g., Ethocel)
Enteric coating:		Cellulose acetate phthalate Shellac (35% in alcohol, ('pharmaceutical glaze")
Tablet Direct Compression Excipient	Used in direct compression tablet formulations. .	Dibasic calcium phosphate (e.g., Ditab)
Tablet Disintegrant	Used in solid dosage forms to promote the disruption of the solid mass into smaller particles which are more readily dispersed or dissolved.	Alginic acid Carboxymethylcellulose calcium Microcrystalline cellulose (e.g., Avicel) Polacrilin potassium (e.g., Amberlite) Sodium alginate Sodium starch glycollate Starch
Tablet Glidant	Agents used in tablet and capsule formulations to improve the flow properties of the powder mixture.	Colloidal silica Cornstarch Talc
Tablet Lubricant	Substances used in tablet formulations to reduce friction during tablet compression.	Calcium stearate Magnesium stearate Mineral oil Stearic acid Zinc stearate
Tablet/Capsule Opaquant	Used to render a capsule or a tablet coating opaque. May be used alone or in combination with a colorant.	Titanium dioxide
Tablet Polishing Agent	Used to impart an attractive sheen to coated tablets.	Carnauba wax White wax
Tonicity Agent	Used to render a solution similar in osmotic characteristics to physiologic fluids. Ophthalmic, parenteral, and irrigation fluids are examples of preparations in which tonicity is a consideration.	dextrose Sodium chloride

continued

Table 3.3. Examples of Pharmaceutic Ingredients

Ingredient Type	Definition	Examples
Vehicle	A carrying agent for a drug substance. They are used in formulating a variety of liquid dosage for oral and parenteral administration. Generally, oral liquids are aqueous preparations (as syrups) or hydroalcoholic (as elixirs). Parenteral solutions for intravenous use are aqueous, whereas intramuscular injections may be aqueous or oleaginous.	
Flavored/Sweetened		Acacia Syrup Aromatic Syrup Aromatic Elixir Cherry Syrup Cocoa Syrup Orange Syrup Syrup
Oleaginous		Corn Oil Mineral Oil Peanut Oil Sesame Oil
Sterile		Bacteriostatic Sodium chloride injection Bacteriostatic Water for Injection
Viscosity Increasing Agent	Used to change the consistency of a preparation to render it more resistant to flow. Used in suspensions to deter sedimentation, in ophthalmic solutions to enhance contact time (e.g., methylcellulose), to thicken topical creams, etc.	Alginic acid Bentonite Carbomer Carboxymethylcellulose Sodium Methylcellulose Povidone Sodium alginate Tragacanth

are discussed in Chapter 7, Capsules and Tablets and Chapter 8, Modified-Release Dosage Forms and Drug Delivery Systems.

Handbook of Pharmaceutical Excipients

The reader should also be aware of the *Handbook of Pharmaceutical Excipients* (10), which presents monographs on over 200 excipients used in pharmaceutical dosage form preparation. Included in each monograph is such information as: nonproprietary, chemical, and commercial names; empirical and chemical formulas and molecular weight; pharmaceutic specifications and chemical and physical properties; incompatibilities and interactions with other excipients and drug substances; regulatory status; and applications in pharmaceutic formulation or technology.

Harmonization of Standards

There is great interest currently in the international "harmonization" of standards applicable to pharmaceutical excipients. This is due to the fact that the pharmaceutical industry is multinational, with major companies having facilities in more than a single country, with products sold in markets worldwide, and with regulatory approval for these products required in each individual country. Standards for each drug substance and excipient used in pharmaceuticals are contained in pharmacopeias—or, for new agents, in an application for regulatory approval by the FDA or another nation's governing authority. The four pharmacopeias with the largest international use are the *United States Pharmacopeia/National Formulary* (USP/NF), *British Pharmacopeia* (BP), *European Pharmacopeia* (EP), and the *Japanese Pharmacopeia* (JP). Uniform standards for excipients in these and other pharmacopeias would facilitate production efficiency, enable the marketing of a single formulation of a product internationally, and enhance regulatory approval of pharmaceutical products worldwide. The goal of harmonization is an ongoing effort undertaken by corporate representatives and international regulatory authorities.

A few of the more common and widely used pharmaceutical excipients, including sweeteners, flavors, colors and preservatives will be discussed here.

Appearance and Palatability

Although most drug substances in use today are unpalatable and unattractive in their natural state, modern pharmaceutical preparations present them to the patient as colorful, flavorful formulations attractive to the sight, smell, and taste. These qualities, which are the rule rather than the exception, have virtually eliminated the natural reluctance of many patients to take medications because of disagreeable odor or taste. In fact, the inherent attractiveness of today's pharmaceuticals has caused them to acquire the dubious distinction of being a source of accidental poisonings in the home, particularly among children who are lured by their organoleptic appeal.

There is some psychologic basis to drug therapy, and the odor, taste, and color of a pharmaceutical preparation can play a part. An appropriate drug will have its most beneficial effect when it is accepted and taken properly by the patient. The proper combination of flavor, fragrance, and color in a pharmaceutical product contributes to its acceptance.

Flavoring and Sweetening Pharmaceuticals

The flavoring of pharmaceuticals applies primarily to liquid dosage forms intended for oral administration. The 10,000 taste buds, found on the tongue, roof of the mouth, cheeks, and throat, have 60–100 receptor cells each (11). These receptor cells interact with molecules dissolved in the saliva and produce a positive or negative taste sensation. Medication in liquid form obviously comes into immediate and direct contact with these taste buds. By the addition of flavoring agents to liquid medication, the disagreeable taste of drugs may be successfully masked. Drugs placed in capsules or prepared as coated tablets may be easily swallowed with avoidance of contact between the drug and the taste buds. Tablets containing drugs that are not especially distasteful may remain uncoated and unflavored. Swallowing them with water usually is sufficient to avoid undesirable drug taste sensations. However, tablets of the chewable type as certain antacid and vitamin products, which are intended for mastication in the mouth, usually *are* sweetened and flavored to receive better patient acceptance.

The flavor sensation of a food or pharmaceutical is actually a complex blend of taste and smell with lesser influences of texture, temperature, and even sight. In flavor formulating a pharmaceutical product, the pharmacist must give consideration to the color, odor, texture, and taste of the preparation. It would be incongruous, for example, to color a liquid pharmaceutical red, give it a banana taste, and a mint odor. The color of a pharmaceutical must have a psychogenic balance with the taste, and the odor must also enhance that taste. Odor greatly affects the flavor of a preparation or foodstuff. If one's sense of smell is impaired, as during a head cold, the usual flavor sensation of food is similarly diminished.

The medicinal chemist and the formulation pharmacist are well acquainted with the taste characteristic of certain chemical types of drugs and strive to mask effectively the unwanted taste through the appropriate use of flavoring agents. Although there are no dependable rules for unerringly predicting the taste sensation of a drug based on its chemical constitution, experience permits the presentation of several observations. For instance, although we recognize and assume the salty taste of sodium chloride, the formulation pharmacist knows that all salts are not salty, but that their taste is a function of both the cation and anion. Whereas salty tastes are evoked by sodium, potassium, and ammonium chlorides and by sodium bromide, potassium and ammonium bromides elicit simultaneous bitter and salty sensations, and potassium iodide and magnesium sulfate (epsom salt) are predominantly bitter. In general, low molecular weight salts are salty, and higher molecular weight salts are bitter. With organic compounds, an increase in the number of hydroxyl groups (—OH) seems to increase the sweetness of the compound. Sucrose, which has eight hydroxyl groups, is sweeter than glycerin, another pharmaceutical sweetener, which has but three hydroxyl groups. In general, the organic esters, alcohols, and aldehydes are pleasant to the taste, and since many of them are volatile, they also contribute to the odor and thus the flavor of preparations in which they are used. Many nitrogen-containing compounds are extremely bitter, especially the plant alkaloids (as quinine), but certain other nitrogen-containing compounds are extremely sweet (as aspartame). The medicinal chemist recognizes that even the most simple structural change in an organic compound can alter its taste. D-glucose is sweet, but L-glucose has a slightly salty taste; saccharin is very sweet, but N-methyl-saccharin is tasteless (12).

Thus, the predictability of the taste characteristics of a new drug is only speculative. However, it is soon learned, and the formulation pharmacist is then put to the task of increasing the drug's palatability in the environment of other formulative agents. The selection of an appropriate flavoring agent depends upon several factors, but primarily upon the taste of the drug substance itself. Certain flavoring materials are more effective than others in masking or disguising the particular bitter, salty, sour, or otherwise undesirable taste of medicinal agents. Although individuals' tastes and flavor preferences differ, cocoa-flavored vehicles are considered effective for masking the taste of bitter drugs. Fruit or citrus flavors are frequently used to combat sour or acid tasting drugs, and cinnamon, orange, raspberry, and other flavors have been successfully used to make preparations of salty drugs more palatable.

The age of the intended patient should also be considered in the selection of the flavoring agent, because certain age groups seem to prefer certain flavors. Children prefer sweet, candy-like preparations with fruity flavors, but adults seem to prefer less sweet preparations with a tart rather than a fruit flavor.

In addition to sucrose, a number of artificial sweetening agents have been utilized in foods and pharmaceuticals over the years. Some of these, as aspartame, saccharin and cyclamate, have faced challenges over their safety by the FDA and restrictions to their use and sale; in fact, the cyclamates were banned from use in the United States by the FDA in 1969.

The introduction of diet soft drinks in the 1950s provided the spark for the widespread use of artificial sweeteners today. Besides dieters, diabetics are regular users of artificial sweeteners. Over the years, each of the artificial sweeteners has undergone long periods of review and debate. Critical to the evaluation of food additives are issues of metabolism and toxicity. For example, almost none of the saccharin a person consumes is metabolized; it is excreted by the kidneys virtually unchanged. Cyclamate, on the other hand, is metabolized, or processed, in the digestive tract, and its byproducts are excreted by the kidneys. Aspartame breaks down in the body into three basic components: the amino acids phenylalanine and aspartic acid, and methanol. These three components, which also occur naturally in various foods, are in turn metabolized through regular pathways in the body. Be-

cause of its metabolism to phenylalanine, the use of aspartame by phenylketonurics is discouraged and diet foods and drinks must bear an appropriate label warning indicating that the particular foodstuff not be consumed by such individuals. Persons with phenylketonuria (PKU) cannot metabolize phenylalanine adequately, resulting in an increase in the serum levels of the amino acid (hyperphenylalaninemia). This can result in mental retardation, and also can affect the fetus of a pregnant woman who has the disorder.

Passage in 1958 of the Food Additives Amendment to the Food, Drug, and Cosmetic Act produced a major change in how food additives are regulated by the federal government. For one thing, no new food additive may be used if animal feeding studies or other appropriate tests showed that it caused cancer. This is the now-famous Delaney Clause. The *amount* of the substance one would have to consume to induce cancer is not of significance under the Delaney Clause.

Another critical feature of the 1958 amendment, however, was that it did not apply to additives that were generally recognized by experts as safe for their intended uses. Saccharin, cyclamate and a long list of other substances were being used in foods before the amendment's passage and were considered "generally recognized as safe"—or what is known today as GRAS. Aspartame, on the other hand, became the first artificial sweetener to fall under the 1958 amendment's requirement for premarketing proof of safety because the first petition to FDA for its approval was filed in 1973. In 1968, the Committee on Food Protection of the National Academy of Sciences issued an interim report on the safety of non-nutritive sweeteners, including saccharin. In the early 1970s, FDA began a major review of hundreds of food additives on the GRAS list to determine whether more current studies still justified their safe status. In 1972, with new studies under way, FDA decided to take saccharin off the GRAS and establish interim limits that would permit its continued use until additional studies were completed. (Previous studies indicated that male and female rats fed doses of saccharin developed a significant incidence of bladder tumors.) In November 1977, Congress passed the Saccharin Study and Labeling Act, which permitted saccharin's continued availability while mandating that warning labels be used to advise consumers that saccharin caused cancer in animals. The law also directed FDA to arrange further studies of carcinogens and toxic substances in foods.

Cyclamate was introduced into beverages and

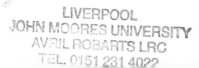

foods in the 1950s and dominated the artificial sweetener market in the 1960s. After much controversy regarding the substance's safety, the FDA issued a final ruling in 1980 stating that the agent's safety has not been demonstrated. Since that date, scientific studies have continued in order to conclusively support or refute the basis for the FDA decision. At question is the agent's possible carcinogenicity and its possible effects in causing genetic damage and testicular atrophy. The student is referred to the indicated references for a review of the recent history of sweeteners including: saccharin, cyclamate, fructose, polyalcohols, sucrose, and aspartame (13–16).

Acesulfame potassium, a nonnutritive sweetener first discovered in 1967, was approved in 1992 by the FDA. It had been used previously in a number of other countries. The substance, structurally similar to saccharin, is 130 times as sweet as sucrose and is excreted unchanged in the urine. Acesulfame is more stable than aspartame at elevated temperatures and was approved by the FDA initially for use in candy, chewing gum, confectionery, and instant coffees and teas.

A relatively new sweetening agent introduced into U.S. commerce is Stevia. Stevia powder is the extract from the leaves of Stevia rebaudiana Bertoni plant. The product is natural, nontoxic, safe and about 30 times sweeter than cane sugar, or sucrose. It can be used in both hot and cold preparations. Table 3.4 compares three of the most used sweeteners in the food and drug industry.

Most large pharmaceutical manufacturers have special laboratories for the taste-testing of proposed formulations of their products. Panels of employees or interested community participants become involved in evaluating the various formulations and their assessments become the basis for the firm's flavoring decisions.

In flavoring liquid pharmaceutical products, the flavoring agent is added to the solvent or vehicle-component of the formulation in which it is most soluble or miscible. That is, water soluble flavorants are added to the aqueous component of a formulation and poorly water-soluble flavorants are added to the alcoholic or other non-aqueous solvent component of the formulation. In a hydroalcoholic or other multi-solvent system, care must be exercised to maintain the flavorant in solution. This is accomplished by maintaining a sufficient level of solvent in which the flavorant is soluble.

Coloring

Coloring agents are used in pharmaceutical preparations for purposes of esthetics. A distinction should be made between agents that have inherent color and those agents which are employed as colorants. Certain agents—sulfur (yellow), cupric sulfate (blue), ferrous sulfate (bluish green), and red mercuric iodide (vivid red)—have inherent color and are not thought of as pharmaceutical colorants in the usual sense of the term.

Although most pharmaceutical colorants in use today are of synthetic origin, a few are obtained from natural mineral and plant sources. For example, red ferric oxide is mixed in small proportions with zinc oxide powder to prepare calamine, giving the latter its characteristic pink color, which is intended to match the skin tone upon application.

The synthetic coloring agents used in pharmaceutical products were first prepared in the middle of the 19th century from principles of coal tar. Coal tar (*pix carbonis*), a thick, black, viscid liquid, is a by-product in the destructive distillation of coal. Its composition is extremely complex, and many of its constituents may be separated by fractional distillation. Among the products obtained are anthracene, benzene, naphtha, creosote, phenol, and pitch. About 90% of

Table 3.4. Comparison of Sweeteners

	Sucrose	*Saccharin*	*Aspartame*
Source:	Sugar cane; sugar beet	Chemical synthesis; phthalic anhydride, a petroleum product	Chemical synthesis; methyl ester dipeptide of phenylalanine and aspartic acid
Relative sweetness:	1	300	180–200
Bitterness:	None	Moderate/strong	None
Aftertaste:	None	Moderate/strong;sometimes metallic or bitter	None
Calories:	4/g	0	4/g
Acid Stability:	Good	Excellent	Fair
Heat Stability:	Good	Excellent	Poor

the total dyes used in the products FDA regulates are synthesized from a single, colorless derivative of benzene, called aniline. These aniline dyes are also known as synthetic organic dyes or as "coal tar" dyes since aniline was originally obtained from bituminous coal. Aniline dyes today come mainly from petroleum.

Many coal-tar dyes were originally used indiscriminately in foods and beverages to enhance their appeal without regard to their toxic potential. It was only after careful scrutiny that some dyes were found to be hazardous to health due to either their own chemical nature or the impurities they carried. As more dyestuffs became available, some expert guidance and regulation was needed to ensure the safety of the public. After passage of the Food and Drug Act in 1906, the United States Department of Agriculture established regulations by which a few colorants were *permitted* or *certified* for use in certain products. Today, the use of color additives in foods, drugs, and cosmetics is regulated by the Food and Drug Administration through the provisions of the Federal Food, Drug, and Cosmetic Act of 1938, as amended in 1960 with the Color Additive Amendments. Lists of color additives *exempt* from certification and those *subject* to certification are codified into law and regulated by the FDA (17). Certified color additives are classified according to their approved use: (a) FD&C color additives, which may be used in foods, drugs, and cosmetics; (b) D&C color additives, some of which are approved for use in drugs, some in cosmetics, and some in medical devices; and (c) external D&C color additives, the use of which is restricted to external parts of the body, not including the lips or any other body surface covered by mucous membrane. Within each certification category there is a variety of basic colors and shades for coloring pharmaceuticals. One may select from a variety of FD&C, D&C, and External D&C reds, yellows, oranges, greens, blues, and violets. By selective combinations of the colorants one can create distinctive colors (Table 3.5).

As a part of the National Toxicology Program of the Department of Health and Human Services, various substances, including color additives, are studied for their toxicology and carcinogenesis. For color additives, the study protocols usually call for a two-year study in which groups of male and female mice and rats are fed diets containing various quantities of the colorant. The nonsurviving and surviving animals are examined for evidence of long-term toxicity and carcinogenesis. Five categories of evidence of carcinogenic activity are used in reporting observations: 1) "clear evidence" of carcinogenic activity; 2) "some evidence"; 3) "equiv-

Table 3.5.   Examples of Color Formulations*

Shade/Color	FD&C Dye	% of Blend
Orange	Yellow #6	100
	or	
	Yellow #5	95
	Red #40	5
Cherry	Red #40	100
	or	
	Red #40	99
	Blue #1	1
Strawberry	Red #40	100
	or	
	Red #40	95
	Red #3	5
Lemon	Yellow #5	100
Lime	Yellow #5	95
	Blue #1	5
Grape	Red #40	80
	Blue #1	20
Raspberry	Red #3	75
	Yellow #6	20
	Blue #1	5
Butterscotch	Yellow #5	74
	Red #40	24
	Blue #1	2
Chocolate	Red #40	52
	Yellow #5	40
	Blue #1	8
Caramel	Yellow #5	64
	Red #3	21
	Yellow #6	9
	Blue #1	6
Cinnamon	Yellow #5	60
	Red #40	35
	Blue #1	5

*From literature of Warner-Jenkinson Co., St. Louis, Mo.

ocal evidence," indicating uncertainty; 4) "no evidence," indicating no observable effect; and 5) "inadequate study," for studies that cannot be evaluated because of major flaws incurred.

The certification status of the colorants is continuously reviewed, and changes are made in the list of certified colors in accordance with toxicologic findings. These changes may involve 1) the withdrawal of certification, 2) the transfer of a colorant from one certification category to another, or 3) the addition of new colors to the list. Before gaining certification, a color additive must be demonstrated to be safe. In the case of pharmaceutical preparations, color additives, like all additives, must not interfere with the therapeutic efficacy of the product in which they are used nor may they interfere with the prescribed assay procedure for that preparation.

In the 1970s, concern and scientific questioning of the safety of some color additives heightened. A color that drew particular attention was FD&C Red No. 2, because of its extensive use in foods, drugs and cosmetics. Researchers in Russia had reported that this color, also known as amaranth, caused cancer in rats. Although the FDA was never able to determine the purity of the amaranth tested in Russia, these reports led to FDA investigations and a series of tests that eventually resulted in withdrawal of FD&C Red No. 2 from the FDA certified list in 1976 because its sponsors were unable to prove safety. That year, the Agency also terminated approval for use of FD&C Red No. 4 in maraschino cherries and ingested drugs because of unresolved safety questions. FD&C Red No. 4 is now permitted only in externally applied drugs and cosmetics.

The dye FD&C Yellow No. 5 (also known as tartrazine) can cause many people to have allergic-type reactions. People who are allergic to aspirin will also likely be allergic to this dye. As a result, the FDA requires the listing of this dye by name on the labels of foods (e.g., butter, cheese, ice cream) and ingested drugs containing the substance.

A colorant becomes an integral part of a pharmaceutical formulation, and its exact quantitative amount must be reproducible each time the formulation is prepared, or else the preparation would have a different appearance from batch to batch. This requires a high degree of pharmaceutical skill, for the amount of colorant generally added to liquid preparations ranges between 0.0005 and 0.001% depending upon the colorant and the depth of color desired. Because of their color potency, dyes generally are added to pharmaceutical preparations in the form of diluted solutions rather than as concentrated dry powders. This permits greater accuracy in measurement and more consistent color production.

In addition to liquid dyes in the coloring of pharmaceuticals, lake pigments may also be used. Whereas a chemical material exhibits coloring power or tinctorial strength when dissolved, pigment is an insoluble material which colors by dispersion. An FD&C lake is a pigment consisting of a substratum of alumina hydrate on which the dye is absorbed or precipitated. Having aluminum hydroxide as the substrate, the lakes are insoluble in nearly all solvents. FD&C lakes are subject to certification and must be made from dyes which have been previously certified. Lakes do not have a specified dye content and range from 10 to 40% pure dye. By their very nature, lakes are suitable for coloring products in which the moisture levels are low. Lakes are commonly used in the form of fine dispersions or suspensions when coloring pharmaceuticals. The pigment particles may range in size from less than 1 μm up to 30 μm. The finer the particle, the less chance there would be for color speckling to occur in the finished product. Blends of various lake pigments may be used to achieve a variety of colors and different vehicles may be employed to disperse the colorants, as glycerin, propylene glycol, and sucrose-based syrup.

In the preparation of capsules, various colored empty gelatin capsule shells may be used to hold the powdered drug mixture. Many commercial capsules are prepared with capsule bodies of one color and a different colored capsule cap, resulting in a two-colored capsule. This makes certain commercial products even more readily identifiable than solid colored capsules. For powdered drugs dispensed as such or compressed into tablets, a generally larger proportion of dye is required (about 0.1%) to achieve the desired hue than with liquid preparations.

Both dyes and lakes have application in the coloring of sugar-coated tablets, film-coated tablets, direct-compression tablets, pharmaceutical suspensions and other dosage forms (18). Traditionally, sugar-coated tablets have been colored with syrup solutions containing varying amounts of the water-soluble dyes, starting with very dilute solutions, working up to concentrated color syrup solutions. As many as 30 to 60 coats are not uncommon. Using the FD&C lakes, fewer color coats are used. Appealing tablets have been made with as few as 8 to 12 coats using lakes dispersed in syrup. Water-soluble dyes in aqueous vehicles or lakes dispersed in organic solvents may be effectively sprayed on tablets to achieve attractive film coatings. There is continued interest today in chewable tablets, due to the availability of many direct-compression materials such as dextrose, sucrose, mannitol, sorbitol, and spray-dried lactose. The direct-compression colored chewable tablets may be prepared utilizing 1 pound of lake per 1000 pounds of tablet mix. For aqueous suspensions, FD&C water-soluble colors or lakes may be satisfactory. In non-aqueous suspensions, FD&C lakes are necessary. The lakes, added either to the aqueous or non-aqueous phase, generally at a level of 1 pound of color per 1000 pounds of suspension, require homogenizing or mechanical blending to achieve uniform coloring.

For the most part, ointments, suppositories, and ophthalmic and parenteral products assume the color of their ingredients and do not contain color additives. Should a dye lose the certification status it held when a product was first formulated, manufactured, and marketed, the manufacturer must, within a reasonable length of time, reformulate, using only color additives certified at the new date of manufacture.

In addition to esthetics and the certification status of a dye, a formulation pharmacist must select the dyes to be used in a particular formula on the basis of the physical and chemical properties of the dyes available. Of prime importance is the solubility of a prospective dye in the vehicle to be used for a liquid formulation or in a solvent to be employed during a pharmaceutical process, as when the dye is sprayed on a batch of tablets. In general, most dyes are broadly grouped into those that are water-soluble and those that are oil-soluble; few, if any, dyes are both. Usually, a water-soluble dye is also adequately soluble in commonly used pharmaceutical liquids like glycerin, alcohol, and glycol ethers. Oil-soluble dyes may also be soluble to some extent in these solvents, as well as in liquid petrolatum (mineral oil), fatty acids, fixed oils, and waxes. It should be remembered that a great deal of solubility is not required, since the concentration of dye in a given preparation is rather minimal.

Another important consideration when selecting a dye for use in a liquid pharmaceutical is the pH and pH stability of the preparation to be colored. Dyes can change color with a change in pH, and a dye must be selected for a product so that any anticipated pH change will not alter the color during the usual shelf-life. The dye also must be chemically stable in the presence of the other formulative ingredients and must not interfere with the stability of the other agents. To maintain their original colors, FD&C dyes must be protected from oxidizing agents, reducing agents (especially metals as iron, aluminum, zinc and tin), strong acids and alkalis, and excessive heating. Dyes must also be reasonably photostable; that is, they must not change color when exposed to light of anticipated intensities and wavelengths under the usual conditions of shelf storage. Certain medicinal agents, particularly those prepared in liquid form, must be protected from light to maintain their chemical stability and their therapeutic effectiveness. These preparations are generally maintained and dispensed in dark amber or opaque containers. For solid dosage forms of photolabile drugs, a colored or opaque capsule shell may actually enhance the drug's stability by shielding out light rays.

Preservatives

In addition to the stabilization of pharmaceutical preparations against chemical and physical degradation due to changed environmental conditions within a formulation, certain liquid and semisolid preparations also must be preserved against microbial contamination.

Sterilization and Preservation

Although some types of pharmaceutical products like ophthalmic and injectable preparations are sterilized by physical methods (autoclaving for 20 minutes at 15 pounds pressure and 120°C, dry heat at 180°C for 1 hour, or by bacterial filtration) during their manufacture, many of them additionally require the presence of an antimicrobial preservative to maintain their aseptic condition throughout the period of their storage and use. Other types of preparations that are not sterilized during their preparation but are particularly susceptible to microbial growth because of the nature of their ingredients, are protected by the addition of an antimicrobial preservative. Preparations that provide excellent growth media for microbes are most aqueous preparations, especially syrups, emulsions, suspensions, and some semisolid preparations, particularly creams. Certain hydroalcoholic and most alcoholic preparations may not require the addition of a chemical preservative when the alcoholic content is sufficient to prevent microbial growth. Generally, 15% alcohol will prevent microbial growth in acid media and 18% in alkaline media. Most alcohol-containing pharmaceuticals such as elixirs, spirits, and tinctures are self-sterilizing and do not require additional preservation. The same would apply to other pharmaceuticals on an individual basis, which by virtue of their vehicles or other formulative agents, may not permit the growth of microorganisms.

Preservative Selection

When experience or shelf-storage experiments indicate that a preservative is required in a pharmaceutical preparation, its selection is based on many cross considerations including some of the following.

1. The preservative prevents the growth of the type of microorganisms considered the most likely contaminants of the preparation being formulated.
2. The preservative is soluble enough in water to achieve adequate concentrations in the aqueous phase of a two or more phase system.
3. The proportion of preservative remaining undissociated at the pH of the preparation makes it capable of penetrating the microorganisms and destroying its integrity.

4. The required concentration of the preservative does not affect the safety or comfort of the patient when the pharmaceutical preparation is administered by the usual or intended route; i.e., nonirritating, nonsensitizing, nontoxic.
5. The preservative has adequate stability and will not be reduced in concentration due to chemical decomposition or volatilization during the desired shelf-life of the preparation.
6. The preservative is completely compatible with all other formulative ingredients and does not interfere with them, nor do they interfere with the effectiveness of the preservative agent.
7. The preservative does not adversely affect the preparation's container or the closure.

General Preservative Considerations

Microorganisms involved include molds, yeasts, and bacteria, with the latter generally favoring a slightly alkaline medium and the others an acid medium. Although few microorganisms can grow below a pH of 3 or above pH 9, most aqueous pharmaceutical preparations are within the favorable pH range and therefore must be protected against microbial growth. To be effective, a preservative agent must be dissolved in sufficient concentration in the aqueous phase of a preparation. Further, only the undissociated fraction or molecular form of a preservative possesses preservative capability, because the ionized portion is incapable of penetrating the microorganism. Thus the preservative selected must be largely undissociated at the pH of the formulation being prepared. Acidic preservatives like benzoic, boric, and sorbic acids are more undissociated and thus more effective as the medium is made more acid. Conversely, alkaline preservatives are less effective in acid or neutral media and more effective in alkaline media. Thus, it is meaningless to suggest preservative effectiveness at specific concentrations unless the pH of the system is mentioned and the undissociated concentration of the agent is calculated or otherwise determined. Also, if formulative materials interfere with the solubility or availability of the preservative agent, its chemical concentration may be misleading, because it may not be a true measure of the effective concentration. Many incompatible combinations of preservative agents and other pharmaceutical adjuncts have been discovered in recent years, and undoubtedly many more will be uncovered in the future as new preservatives, pharmaceutical adjuncts, and therapeutic agents are combined for the first time. Many of the recognized incompatible combinations that result in preservative inactivation involve macromolecules such as various cellulose derivatives, polyethylene glycols, and natural gums such as tragacanth, which can attract and hold preservative agents, such as the parabens and phenolic compounds, rendering them unavailable for their preservative function. It is essential for the research pharmacist to examine all formulative ingredients as one affects the other to assure himself that each agent is free to do the job for which it was included in the formulation. In addition, the preservative must not interact with a container such as a metal ointment tube or a plastic medication bottle or with an enclosure such as a rubber or plastic cap or liner. Such an interaction could result in the decomposition of the preservative or the container closure, or, both, with resultant product decomposition and contamination. Appropriate tests should be devised and conducted to insure against this type of preservative interaction.

Mode of Action

Preservatives interfere with microbial growth, multiplication, and metabolism through one or more of the following mechanisms:

1. Modification of cell membrane permeability and leakage of cell constituents (partial lysis)
2. Lysis and cytoplasmic leakage
3. Irreversible coagulation of cytoplasmic constituents (e.g., protein precipitation)
4. Inhibition of cellular metabolism as through interference with enzyme systems or inhibition of cell wall synthesis
5. Oxidation of cellular constituents
6. Hydrolysis

A few of the commonly used pharmaceutical preservatives and their probable modes of action are presented in Table 3.6.

Preservative Utilization

Suitable substances may be added to a pharmaceutical preparation to enhance its permanency or usefulness. Such additives are suitable only if they are nontoxic and harmless in the amounts administered and do not interfere with the therapeutic efficacy or tests or assays of the preparation. Certain intravenous preparations given in large volumes as blood replenishers or as nutrients are not permitted to contain bacteriostatic additives, because the amounts required to preserve such large volumes would constitute a health hazard when administered to the patient. Thus preparations

Table 3.6.   Probable Modes of Action of Some Preservatives

Preservative	Probable Modes of Action
Benzoic acid, boric acid, and p-hydroxybenzoates	Denaturation of proteins
Phenols and chlorinated phenolic compounds	Lytic and denaturation action on cytoplasmic membranes and for chlorinated preservatives, also by oxidation of enzymes
Alcohols	Lytic and denaturation action on membranes
Quaternary compounds	Lytic action on membranes
Mercurials	Denaturation of enzymes by combining with thiol (-SH) groups)

like Dextrose Injection, USP, and others commonly given as fluid and nutrient replenishers by intravenous injections in amounts of 500 to 1000 mL may not contain antibacterial preservatives. On the other hand, injectable preparations given in small volumes—for example, Morphine Sulfate Injection, USP, which provides a therapeutic amount of morphine sulfate in approximately a 1-mL volume—can be preserved with a suitable preservative without the danger of coadministering an excessive amount of the preservative to the patient.

Examples of the preservatives and their concentrations commonly employed in pharmaceutical preparations are: benzoic acid (0.1 to 0.2%), sodium benzoate (0.1 to 0.2%), alcohol (15 to 20%), phenylmercuric nitrate and acetate (0.002 to 0.01%), phenol (0.1 to 0.5%), cresol (0.1 to 0.5%), chlorobutanol (0.5%), benzalkonium chloride (0.002 to 0.01%), and combinations of methylparaben and propylparaben (0.1 to 0.2%), the latter being especially good against fungus. The required proportion would vary with the factors of pH, dissociation, and others already indicated as well with the presence of other formulative ingredients with inherent preservative capabilities that contribute to the preservation of the preparation and require less additional preservation assistance.

For each type of preparation to be preserved, the research pharmacist must consider the influence of the preservative on the comfort of the patient. For instance, a preservative in an ophthalmic preparation would have to have an extremely low degree of irritant qualities, which is characteristic of chlorobutanol, benzalkonium chloride, and phenylmercuric nitrate, frequently used preservatives in ophthalmic preparations. In all instances, the preserved preparation must be biologically tested to determine its safety and efficacy and shelf-tested to determine its stability for the intended shelf life of the product.

References

1. Poole JW. Preformulation. FMC Corporation, 1982.
2. Brange J, Langkjaer L, Havelund S, Vølund A. Chemical stability of insulin. Hydrolytic degradation during storage of pharmaceutical preparations. Pharm Res 1991;9:715–726.
3. Guideline for Submitting Documentation for the Stability of Human Drugs and Biologics, Rockville, MD: Food and Drug Administration, 1987.
4. FDA/ICH Regulatory Guidance on Stability. In: Federal Register. Washington, DC: Food and Drug Administration, 1998; 63:9795–9843.
5. Sheinin EB. ICH guidlines: History, present status, intent. Athens, GA. International Good Manufacturing Practices Conference, 1998.
6. Rothman B. Stability is the issue. Athens, GA. International Good Manufacturing Practices Conference, 1998.
7. Guidelines on compounding of nonsterile products in pharmacies. Bethesda MD, Am Society Hospital Pharm, 1993.
8. Trissel L. Trissel's Stability of Compounded Formulations. Washington, DC: American Pharmaceutical Association, 1996.
9. U.S. Pharmacopeia 23/National Formulary 18, Supplement 5. Rockville, MD. U.S. Pharmacopeial Convention, Inc., 1996.
10. Handbook of Pharmaceutical Excipients, 3rd Ed. Washington, DC. American Pharmaceutical Association, 1998.
11. Lewis R. When smell and taste go awry. FDA Consumer 1991;25:29–33.
12. Hornstein I, Teranishi R. The chemistry of flavor. Chem Eng News 1967;45:92–108.
13. Murphy DH. A practical compendium on sweetening agents. Am Pharm 1983; NS23:32–37.
14. Jacknowitz AI: Artificial sweeteners: How safe are they? U.S. Pharmacist 1988;13:28–31.
15. Krueger RJ, Topolewski M, Havican S. In search of the ideal sweetener. Pharmacy Times 1991;July:72–77.
16. Lecos CW. Sweetness minus calories = controversy. FDA Consumer 1985;19:18–23.
17. Code of Federal Regulations, Title 21, Parts 70–82.
18. Colorants for drug tablets and capsules. Drug and Cosmetic Industry 1983;133(2):44.

4

DOSAGE FORM DESIGN: BIOPHARMACEUTIC AND PHARMACOKINETIC CONSIDERATIONS

Chapter at a Glance

AS DISCUSSED in the previous chapter, the biologic response to a drug is the result of an interaction between the drug substance and functionally important cell receptors or enzyme systems. The response is due to an alteration in the biologic processes that were present prior to the drug's administration. The magnitude of the response is related to the concentration of the drug achieved at the site of its ac-

tion. This drug concentration depends on the dosage of the drug administered, the extent of its absorption and distribution to the site, and the rate and extent of its elimination from the body. The physical and chemical constitution of the drug substance—particularly its lipid solubility, degree of ionization, and molecular size—determines to a great extent its ability to effect its biological activity. The area of study embracing this relationship between the physical, chemical, and biological sciences as they apply to drugs, dosage forms, and to drug action has been given the descriptive term *biopharmaceutics*.

In general, for a drug to exert its biologic effect, it must be transported by the body fluids, traverse the required biologic membrane barriers, escape widespread distribution to unwanted areas, endure metabolic attack, penetrate in adequate concentration to the sites of action, and interact in a specific fashion, causing an alteration of cellular function. A simplified diagram of this complex series of events between a drug's administration and its elimination is presented in Figure 4.1.

The absorption, distribution, biotransformation (metabolism), and elimination of a drug from the body are dynamic processes that continue from the time a drug is taken until all of the drug has been removed from the body. The *rates* at which these processes occur affect the onset, intensity, and the duration of the drug's activity within the body. The area of study which elucidates the time course of drug concentration in the blood and tissues is termed *pharmacokinetics*. It is the study of the kinetics of absorption, distribution, metabolism and excretion (ADME) of drugs and their corresponding pharmacologic, therapeutic, or toxic response in animals and man. Further, since one drug may alter the absorption, distribution, metabolism or excretion of another drug, pharmacokinetics also may be applied in the study of interactions between drugs.

Once a drug is administered and drug absorption begins, the drug does not remain in a single body location, but rather is distributed throughout the body until its ultimate elimination. For instance, following the oral administration of a drug and its entry into the gastrointestinal tract, a por-

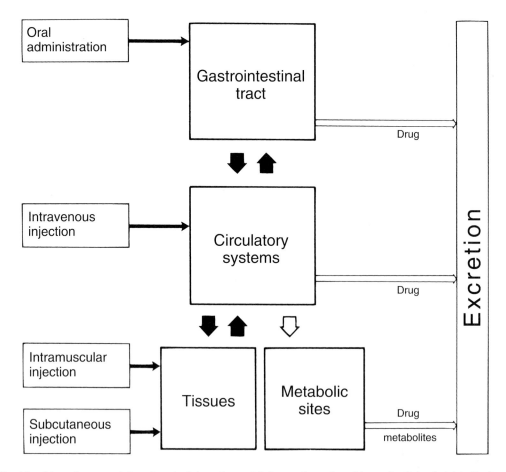

Fig. 4.1   *Schematic representation of events of absorption, metabolism, and excretion of drugs after their administration by various routes.*

tion of the drug is absorbed into the circulatory system from which it is distributed to the various other body fluids, tissues, and organs. From these sites the drug may return to the circulatory system and be excreted through the kidney as such or the drug may be metabolized by the liver or other cellular sites and be excreted as metabolites. As shown in Figure 4.1, drugs administered by intravenous injection are placed directly into the circulatory system, thereby avoiding the absorption process, which is required from all other routes of administration for systemic effects.

The various body locations to which a drug travels may be viewed as separate compartments, each containing some fraction of the administered dose of drug. The transfer of drug from the blood to other body locations is generally a rapid process and is reversible; that is, the drug may diffuse back into the circulation. The drug in the blood therefore exists in equilibrium with the drug in the other compartments. However, in this equilibrium state, the concentration of the drug in the blood may be quite different (greater or lesser) than the concentration of the drug in the other compartments. This is due largely to the physiochemical properties of the drug and its resultant ability to leave the blood and traverse the biological membranes. Certain drugs may leave the circulatory system rapidly and completely, whereas other drugs may do so slowly and with difficulty. A number of drugs become bound to blood proteins, particularly the albumins, and only a small fraction of the drug administered may actually be found at locations outside of the circulatory system at a given time. The transfer of drug from one compartment to another is mathematically associated with a specific rate constant describing that particular transfer. Generally, the rate of transfer of a drug from one compartment to another is proportional to the concentration of the drug in the compartment from which it exits; the greater the concentration, the greater is the amount of drug transfer.

Metabolism is the major process by which foreign substances, including drugs are eliminated from the body. In the process of metabolism a drug substance may be biotransformed into pharmacologically active or inactive metabolites. Often, both the drug substance and its metabolite(s) are active and exert pharmacologic effects. For example, the antianxiety drug prazepam (Centrax) metabolizes, in part, to oxazepam (Serax), which also has antianxiety effects. In some instances a pharmacologically inactive drug (termed a *prodrug*) may be administered for the known effects of its active metabolites. Dipivefrin,

for example, is a prodrug of epinephrine formed by the esterification of epinephrine and pivalic acid. This enhances the lipophilic character of the drug, and as a consequence its penetration into the anterior chamber of the eye is 17 times that of epinephrine. Within the eye, dipivefrin HCl is converted by enzymatic hydrolysis to epinephrine.

The metabolism of a drug to inactive products is usually an irreversible process which culminates in the excretion of the drug from the body, usually via the urine. The pharmacokineticist may calculate an elimination rate constant (termed k_{el}) for a drug to describe its rate of elimination from the body. The term *elimination* refers to both metabolism and excretion. For drugs that are administered intravenously, and therefore involve no absorption process, the task is much less complex than for drugs administered orally or by other routes. In the latter instances, drug absorption and drug elimination are occurring simultaneously but at different rates.

General Principles of Drug Absorption

Before an administered drug can arrive at its site of action in effective concentrations, it must surmount a number of barriers. These barriers are chiefly a succession of biologic membranes such as those of the gastrointestinal epithelium, lungs, blood, and brain. Body membranes are generally classified as three main types: (a) those composed of several layers of cells, as the skin; (b) those composed of a single layer of cells, as the intestinal epithelium; and (c) those of less than one cell in thickness, as the membrane of a single cell. In most instances a drug substance must pass more than one of these membrane types before it reaches its site of action. For instance, a drug taken orally must first traverse the gastrointestinal membranes (stomach, small and large intestine), gain entrance into the general circulation, pass to the organ or tissue with which it has affinity, gain entrance into that tissue, and then enter into its individual cells.

Although the chemistry of body membranes differs one from another, the membranes may be viewed in general as a bimolecular lipoid (fat-containing) layer attached on both sides to a protein layer. Drugs are thought to penetrate these biologic membranes in two general ways: 1) by passive diffusion, and 2) through specialized transport mechanisms. Within each of these main categories, more clearly defined processes have been ascribed to drug transfer.

Passive Diffusion

The term *passive diffusion* is used to describe the passage of (drug) molecules through a membrane which behaves inertly in that it does not actively participate in the process. Drugs absorbed according to this method are said to be *passively absorbed.* The absorption process is driven by the concentration gradient (i.e., the differences in concentration) existing across the membrane, with the passage of drug molecules occurring primarily from the side of high drug concentration. Most drugs pass through biologic membranes by diffusion.

Passive diffusion is described by *Fick's first law,* which states that the rate of diffusion or transport across a membrane (dc/dt) is proportional to the difference in drug concentration on both sides of the membrane:

$$-\frac{dc}{dt} = P(C_1 - C_2)$$

in which C_1 and C_2 refer to the drug concentrations on each side of the membrane and P is a permeability coefficient or constant. The term C_1 is customarily used to represent the compartment with the greater concentration of drug and thus the transport of drug proceeds from compartment one (e.g., absorption site) to compartment two (e.g., blood).

Because the concentration of drug at the site of absorption (C_1) is usually much greater than on the other side of the membrane, due to the rapid dilution of the drug in the blood and its subsequent distribution to the tissues, for practical purposes the value of $C_1 - C_2$ may be taken simply as that of C_1 and the equation written in the standard form for a first order rate equation:

$$-\frac{dc}{dt} = PC_1$$

The gastrointestinal absorption of most drugs from solution occurs in this manner in accordance with *first order kinetics* in which the rate is dependent on drug concentration, i.e., doubling the dose doubles the transfer rate. The magnitude of the permeability constant, depends on the diffusion coefficient of the drug, the thickness and area of the absorbing membrane, and the permeability of the membrane to the particular drug.

Because of the lipoid nature of the cell membrane, it is highly permeable to lipid soluble substances. The rate of diffusion of a drug across the membrane depends not only upon its concentration but also upon the relative extent of its affinity for lipid and rejection of water (a high lipid partition

coefficient). The greater its affinity for lipid and the more hydrophobic it is, the faster will be its rate of penetration into the lipid-rich membrane. Erythromycin base, for example, possesses a higher partition coefficient than other erythromycin compounds, e.g., estolate, gluceptate. Consequently, the base is the preferred agent for the topical treatment of acne where penetration into the skin is desired.

Because biologic cells are also permeated by water and lipid-insoluble substances, it is thought that the membrane also contains water-filled pores or channels that permit the passage of these types of substances. As water passes in bulk across a porous membrane, any dissolved solute molecularly small enough to traverse the pores passes in by *filtration.* Aqueous pores vary in size from membrane to membrane and thus in their individual permeability characteristics for certain drugs and other substances.

The majority of drugs today are weak organic acids or bases. Knowledge of their individual ionization or dissociation characteristics is important, because their absorption is governed to a large extent by their degrees of ionization as they are presented to the membrane barriers. Cell membranes are more permeable to the unionized forms of drugs than to their ionized forms, mainly because of the greater lipid solubility of the unionized forms and to the highly charged nature of the cell membrane which results in the binding or repelling of the ionized drug and thereby decreases cell penetration. Also, ions become hydrated through association with water molecules, resulting in larger particles than the undissociated molecule and again decreased penetrating capability.

The degree of a drug's ionization depends both on the pH of the solution in which it is presented to the biologic membrane and on the pK_a, or dissociation constant, of the drug (whether an acid or base). The concept of pK_a is derived from the Henderson-Hasselbalch equation and is:

For an acid:

$$pH = pK_a + \log \frac{\text{ionized conc. (salt)}}{\text{unionized conc. (acid)}}$$

For a base:

$$pH = pK_a + \log \frac{\text{unionized conc. (base)}}{\text{ionized conc. (salt)}}$$

Since the pH of body fluids varies (stomach, pH 1; lumen of the intestine, pH 6.6; blood plasma, pH 7.4), the absorption of a drug from various body fluids will differ and may dictate to some extent the type of dosage form and the route of administration preferred for a given drug.

By rearranging the equation for an acid:

$$pK_a - pH = \log \frac{\text{unionized concentration (acid)}}{\text{ionized concentration (salt)}}$$

one can theoretically determine the relative extent to which a drug remains unionized under various conditions of pH. This is particularly useful when applied to conditions of body fluids. For instance, if a weak acid having a pK_a of 4 is assumed to be in an environment of gastric juice with a pH of 1, the left side of the equation would yield the number 3, which would mean that the ratio of unionized to ionized drug particles would be about 1000 to 1, and gastric absorption would be excellent. At the pH of plasma the reverse would be true, and in the blood the drug would be largely in the ionized form. Table 4.1 presents the effect of pH on the ionization of weak electrolytes, and Table 4.2 offers some representative pK_a values of common drug substances.

From the equation and from Table 4.1, it may be seen that a drug substance is half ionized at a pH value which is equal to its pK_a. Thus pK_a may be defined as the pH at which a drug is 50% ionized. For example, phenobarbital has a pK_a value of about 7.4, and in plasma (pH 7.4) it is present as ionized and unionized forms in equal amounts. However, a drug substance cannot reach the blood plasma for distribution throughout the body unless it is placed there directly through intravenous injection or is favorably absorbed from a site along its route of entry, as the gastrointestinal tract, and allowed to pass into the general circulation. As shown in Table 4.2, phenobarbital, a weak acid, with a pK_a of 7.4 would

Table 4.2. pK_a Values for Some Acidic and Basic Drugs

		pK_a
Acids:	Acetylsalicylic acid	3.5
	Barbital	7.9
	Benzylpenicillin	2.8
	Boric acid	9.2
	Dicoumarol	5.7
	Phenobarbital	7.4
	Phenytoin	8.3
	Sulfanilamide	10.4
	Theophylline	9.0
	Thiopental	7.6
	Tolbutamide	5.5
	Warfarin	4.8
Bases:	Amphetamine	9.8
	Apomorphine	7.0
	Atropine	9.7
	Caffeine	0.8
	Chlordiazepoxide	4.6
	Cocaine	8.5
	Codeine	7.9
	Guanethidine	11.8
	Morphine	7.9
	Procaine	9.0
	Quinine	8.4
	Reserpine	6.6

be largely undissociated in the gastric environment of pH 1 and would likely be well absorbed. A drug may enter the circulation rapidly and at high concentrations if membrane penetration is easily accomplished or at a low rate and low level if the drug is not readily absorbed from its route of entry. The pH of the drug's current environment influences the rate and the degree of its further distribution because it becomes more or less unionized and therefore more or less lipid-penetrating under some condition of pH than under another. If an unionized molecule is able to diffuse through the lipid barrier and remain unionized in the new environment, it may return to its former location or go on to a new one. However, if in the new environment it is greatly ionized due to the influence of the pH of the second fluid, it likely will be unable to cross the membrane with its former ability. Thus a concentration gradient of a drug usually is reached at equilibrium on each side of a membrane due to different degrees of ionization occurring on each side. A summary of the concepts of dissociation/ionization is found in the physical pharmacy capsule entitled "pKa/Dissociation Constants" in Chapter 3.

It is often desirable for pharmaceutical scientists to make structural modifications in organic drugs

Table 4.1. The Effect of pH on the Ionization of Weak Electrolytes* pK_a-pH % Unionized

	If Weak Acid	If Weak Base
−3.0	0.100	99.9
−2.0	0.990	99.0
−1.0	9.09	90.9
−0.7	16.6	83.4
−0.5	24.0	76.0
−0.2	38.7	61.3
0	50.0	50.0
+0.2	61.3	38.7
+0.5	76.0	24.0
+0.7	83.4	16.6
+1.0	90.9	9.09
+2.0	99.0	0.990
+3.0	99.9	0.100

*Reprinted with permission from Doluisio JT, Swintosky JV. Am J Pharm 1965;137:149.

and thereby favorably alter their lipid solubility, partition coefficients, and dissociation constants while maintaining the same basic pharmacologic activity. These efforts frequently result in increased absorption, better therapeutic response, and lower dosage.

Specialized Transport Mechanisms

In contrast to the passive transfer of drugs and other substances across a biologic membrane, certain substances, including some drugs and biologic metabolites, are conducted across a membrane through one of several postulated *specialized transport* mechanisms. This type of transfer seems to account for those substances, many naturally occurring as amino acids and glucose, that are too lipid-insoluble to dissolve in the boundary and too large to flow or filter through the pores. This type of transport is thought to involve membrane components that may be enzymes or some other type of agent capable of forming a complex with the drug (or other agent) at the surface membrane, after which the complex moves across the membrane where the drug is released, with the carrier returning to the original surface. Figure 4.2 presents the simplified scheme of this process. Specialized transport may be differentiated from passive transfer in that the former process may become "saturated" as the amount of carrier present for a given substance becomes completely bound with that substance resulting in a delay in the "ferrying" or transport process. Other features of specialized transport include the specificity by a carrier for a particular type of chemical

structure so that if two substances are transported by the same mechanism one will competitively inhibit the transport of the other. Further, the transport mechanism is inhibited in general by substances that interfere with cell metabolism. The term *active transport,* as a subclassification of specialized transport, denotes a process with the additional feature of the solute or drug being moved across the membrane against a concentration gradient, that is, from a solution of lower concentration to one of a higher concentration or, if the solute is an ion, against an electrochemical potential gradient. In contrast to active transport, *facilitated diffusion* is a specialized transport mechanism having all of the above characteristics except that the solute is not transferred against a concentration gradient and may attain the same concentration inside the cell as that on the outside.

Many body nutrients, as sugars and amino acids, are transported across the membranes of the gastrointestinal tract by carrier processes. Certain vitamins, as thiamine, niacin, riboflavin and vitamin B_6, and drug substances as methyldopa and 5-fluorouracil, require active transport mechanisms for their absorption.

Investigations of intestinal transport have often utilized *in situ* (at the site) or *in vivo* (in the body) animal models or *ex vivo* (outside the body) transport models; however, recently cell culture models of human small-intestine absorptive cells have become available to investigate transport across intestinal epithelium (1). Both passive and transport-mediated studies have been conducted to investigate mechanisms as well as rates of transport.

Dissolution and Drug Absorption

For a drug to be absorbed, it must first be dissolved in the fluid at the absorption site. For instance, a drug administered orally in tablet or capsule form cannot be absorbed until the drug particles are dissolved by the fluids at some point within the gastrointestinal tract. In instances in which the solubility of a drug is dependent upon either an acidic or basic medium, the drug would be dissolved in the stomach or intestines respectively (Fig. 4.3). The process by which a drug particle dissolves is termed *dissolution.*

As a drug particle undergoes dissolution, the drug molecules on the surface are the first to enter into solution creating a saturated layer of drug-solution which envelops the surface of the solid drug particle. This layer of solution is referred to as the *diffusion layer.* From this diffusion layer, the

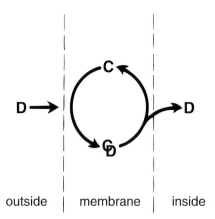

outside | membrane | inside

Fig. 4.2 *Active transport mechanism. D represents a drug molecule; C represents the carrier in the membrane. (Modified from O'Reilly W. Aust J Pharm 1966;47:568.)*

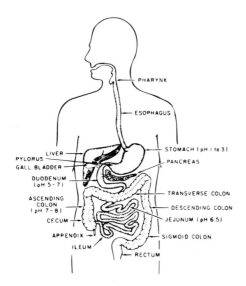

Fig. 4.3 *Anatomical diagram showing the digestive system including the locations involved in drug absorption and their respective pH values.*

for 4 to 10 hours, although there is substantial variation between people, and even in the same person on different occasions. Various techniques have been used to determine gastric emptying time and the gastrointestinal passage of drug from various oral dosage forms, including the tracking of dosage forms labeled with gamma-emitting radionuclides through gamma scintigraphy (2, 3). The gastric emptying time for a drug is most rapid with a fasting stomach, becoming slower as the food content is increased. Changes in gastric emptying time and/or in intestinal motility can affect drug transit time and thus the opportunity for drug dissolution and absorption.

These changes can be affected by drugs the patient may be taking. Certain drugs with anticholinergic properties, e.g., dicyclomine HCl, amitriptyline HCl, have the ability to slow down gastric emptying. This can enhance the rate of absorption of drugs normally absorbed from the stomach, and reduce the rate of absorption of drugs that are primarily absorbed from the small intestine. Alternatively, drugs which enhance gastric motility, e.g., laxatives, may cause some drugs to move so quickly through the gastrointestinal system and past their absorptive site at such a rate to reduce the amount of drug actually absorbed. This effect has been demonstrated with digoxin, whose absorption is significantly decreased by accelerating gastrointestinal motility.

The aging process itself may also influence gastrointestinal absorption. In the elderly, gastric acidity, the number of absorptive cells, intestinal blood flow, the rate of gastric emptying and intestinal motility are all decreased. However, drugs in which absorption depends on passive processes are not affected by these factors as much as those that depend on active transport mechanisms, e.g., calcium, iron, thiamine, and sugars. A decrease in gastric emptying time would be advantageous for those drugs that are absorbed from the stomach but disadvantageous for those drugs which are prone to acid degradation, e.g., penicillins, erythromycin, or inactivated by stomach enzymes, e.g., L-dopa.

The dissolution of a substance may be described by the modified Noyes-Whitney equation:

$$\frac{dc}{dt} = kS(c_s - c_t)$$

in which dc/dt is the rate of dissolution, k is the dissolution rate constant, S is the surface area of the dissolving solid, c_s is the saturation concentration of drug in the diffusion layer (which may be approximated by the maximum solubility of the drug

drug molecules pass throughout the dissolving fluid and make contact with the biologic membranes and absorption ensues. As the molecules of drug continue to leave the diffusion layer, the layer is replenished with dissolved drug from the surface of the drug particle and the process of absorption continues.

If the process of dissolution for a given drug particle is rapid, or if the drug is administered as a solution and remains present in the body as such, the rate at which the drug becomes absorbed would be primarily dependent upon its ability to traverse the membrane barrier. However, if the rate of dissolution for a drug particle is slow, as may be due to the physiochemical characteristics of the drug substance or the dosage form, the dissolution process itself would be a rate-limiting step in the absorption process. Slowly soluble drugs such as digoxin, may not only be absorbed at a slow rate, they may be incompletely absorbed, or, in some cases largely unabsorbed following oral administration, due to the natural limitation of time that they may remain within the stomach or the intestinal tract. Thus, poorly soluble drugs or poorly formulated drug products may result in a drug's incomplete absorption and its passage, unchanged, out of the system via the feces.

Under normal circumstances a drug may be expected to remain in the stomach for 2 to 4 hours (*gastric emptying time*) and in the small intestines in the solvent since the diffusion layer is considered saturated), and c_t is the concentration of the drug in the dissolution medium at time t ($c_s - c_t$ is the concentration gradient). The rate of dissolution is governed by the rate of diffusion of solute molecules through the diffusion layer into the body of the solution. The equation reveals that the dissolution rate of a drug may be increased by increasing the surface area (reducing the particle size) of the drug, by increasing the solubility of the drug in the diffusion layer, and by factors embodied in the dissolution rate constant, k, including the intensity of agitation of the solvent and the diffusion coefficient of the dissolving drug. For a given drug, the diffusion coefficient and usually the concentration of the drug in the diffusion layer will increase with increasing temperature. Also, increasing the rate of agitation of the dissolving medium will increase the rate of dissolution. A reduction in the viscosity of the solvent employed is another means which may be used to enhance the dissolution rate of a drug. Changes in the pH or the nature of the solvent which influence the solubility of the drug may be used to advantage in increasing dissolution rate. Effervescent, buffered aspirin tablet formulations use some of these principles to their advantage. Due to the alkaline adjuvants in the tablet, the solubility of the aspirin is enhanced within the diffusional layer and the evolution of carbon dioxide agitates the solvent system, i.e., gastric juices. Consequently, the rate of aspirin absorbed into the bloodstream is faster than that achieved from a conventional aspirin tablet formulation. If this dosage form is acceptable to the patient, it provides a quicker means for the patient to gain relief from a troublesome headache. Many manufacturers will utilize a particular amorphous, crystalline, salt or ester form of a drug that will exhibit the solubility characteristics needed to achieve the desired dissolution characteristics when administered. Some of these factors that affect drug dissolution briefly are discussed in the following paragraphs, whereas others will be discussed in succeeding chapters in which they are relevant.

The chemical and physical characteristics of a drug substance that can affect drug/drug product safety, efficacy, and stability must be carefully defined by appropriate standards in an application for FDA approval and then sustained and controlled throughout product manufacture.

Surface Area

When a drug particle is reduced to a larger number of smaller particles, the total surface area created is increased. For drug substances that are poorly or slowly soluble, this generally results in an increase in the *rate* of dissolution. This is explained in the Physical Pharmacy Capsule, "Particle Size, Surface Area and Dissolution Rate."

Increased therapeutic response to orally administered drugs due to smaller particle size has been reported for a number of drugs, among them theophylline, a xanthine derivative used to treat bronchial asthma; griseofulvin, an antibiotic with antifungal activity; sulfisoxazole, an anti-infective sulfonamide, and nitrofurantoin, a urinary anti-infective drug. To achieve increased surface area, pharmaceutical manufacturers frequently use *micronized* powders in their solid dosage form products. Micronized powders consist of drug particles reduced in size to about 5 microns and smaller. A slight variation on this is accomplished by blending and melting the poorly water-soluble powders with a water-soluble polymer, such as polyethylene glycol (PEG). In the molten state and if the drug dissolves in this carrier (PEG), a molecular dispersion of the drug in the carrier results. Upon solidification, a solid-dispersion is formed which can be pulverized and tableted or encapsulated. When this powder is placed in water, the water-soluble carrier rapidly dissolves leaving the poorly soluble drug enveloped in water, thus forming a solution.

The use of micronized drugs is not confined to oral preparations. For example, ophthalmic ointments and topical ointments utilize micronized drugs for their preferred release characteristics and nonirritating quality after application.

Due to the different rates and degrees of absorption obtainable from drugs of various particle size, products of the same drug substance prepared by two or more reliable pharmaceutical manufacturers may result in different degrees of therapeutic response in the same individual. A classic example of this occurs with phenytoin sodium capsules where there are two distinct forms. The first is the rapid-release type, i.e., Prompt Phenytoin Sodium Capsules, USP, and the second is the slow-dissolution type, i.e., Extended Phenytoin Sodium Capsules, USP. The former has a dissolution rate of not less than 85% in 30 minutes and is recommended for patient use 3 to 4 times per day. The latter has a slower dissolution rate, e.g., 15 to 35% in 30 minutes, which lends itself for use in patients who could be dosed less frequently. Because of such differences in formulation for a number of drugs and drug products, it is generally advisable for a person to continue taking the same brand of medication, provided it produces the desired therapeutic effect.

Physical Pharmacy Capsule 4.1   **Particle Size, Surface Area and Dissolution Rate**

Particle size has an effect on dissolution rate and solubility. As shown in the Noyes-Whitney equation:

$$\frac{dC}{dT} = kS(C_s - C_t)$$

where dC/dT is the rate of dissolution (concentration with respect to time),
   k is the dissolution rate constant
   S is the surface area of the particles,
   C_s is the concentration of the drug in the immediate proximity of the dissolving particle, i.e., the solubility of the drug,
   C_t is the concentration of the drug in the bulk fluid.

It is evident that the "C_s" cannot be significantly changed, the "C_t" is often under sink conditions (an amount of the drug is used that is less than 20% of its solubility) and "k" comprises many factors such as agitation, temperature. This leaves the "S," surface area, as a factor that can affect the rate of dissolution.

An increase in the surface area of a drug will, within reason, increase the dissolution rate. Circumstances when it may decrease the rate would include a decrease in the "effective surface area," i.e., a condition in which the dissolving fluid would not be able to "wet" the particles. Wetting is the first step in the dissolution process. This can be demonstrated by visualizing a 0.75 inch diameter by 1/4 inch thick tablet. The surface area of the tablet can be increased by drilling a series of 1/16 inch holes in the tablet. However, even though the surface area has been increased, the dissolution fluid, i.e., water, would not necessarily be able to penetrate into the new holes due to surface tension, etc., and displace the air. Adsorbed air and other factors can decrease the effective surface area of a dosage form, including powders. This is the reason that particle size reduction does not always result in an increase in dissolution rate. One can also visualize a powder that has been comminuted to a very fine state of subdivision and when it is placed in a beaker of water, the powder floats due to the entrapped and adsorbed air. The "effective surface area" is not the same as the actual "surface area" of the resulting powder.

Patients who are stabilized on one brand of drug should not be switched to another unless necessary. However, when a change is necessary, appropriate blood or plasma concentrations of the drug should be monitored until the patient is stabilized on the new product.

Occasionally, a rapid rate of drug absorption is not desired in a pharmaceutical preparation. Research pharmacists, in providing sustained rather than rapid action in certain preparations, may employ agents of varying particle size to provide a controlled dissolution and absorption process. Summaries of the physical chemical principles of particle size reduction and the relation of particle size to surface area, dissolution, and solubility may be found in the Physical Pharmacy Capsules in Chapters 3 and 6.

Crystal or Amorphous Drug Form

Solid drug materials may occur as pure crystalline substances of definite identifiable shape or as amorphous particles without definite structure. The amorphous or crystalline character of a drug substance may be of considerable importance to its ease of formulation and handling, its chemical stability, and, as has been recently shown, even its biological activity. Certain medicinal agents may be produced to exist in either a crystalline or an amorphous state. Since the amorphous form of a chemical is usually more soluble than the crystalline form, different extents of drug absorption may result with consequent differences in the degree of pharmacologic activity obtained from each. Experiences with two antibiotic substances, novobiocin and chloramphenicol palmitate, have revealed that these materials are essentially inactive when administered in crystalline form, but when they are administered in the amorphous form, absorption from the gastrointestinal tract proceeds rapidly with good therapeutic response. In other instances, crystalline forms of drugs may be used because of greater stability than the corresponding amorphous forms. For example, the crystalline forms of penicillin G as either the potassium or sodium salt are considerably more stable than the analogous amorphous forms. Thus, in formulation work involving penicillin G, the crystalline forms are preferred and result in excellent therapeutic response.

The hormonal substance insulin presents another striking example of the different degree of activity that may result from the use of different physical forms of the same medicinal agent. Insulin is the active principle of the pancreas gland and is vital to the body's metabolism of glucose. The hormone is produced by two means. The first is by extraction procedures from either beef or pork pancreas. The second process involves a biosynthetic process with strains of *Escherichia coli,* i.e., recombinant DNA. Insulin is used by man as replacement therapy, by injection, when his body's production of the hormone is insufficient. Insulin is a protein, which, when combined with zinc in the presence of acetate buffer, forms an extremely insoluble zinc-insulin complex. Depending on the pH of the acetate buffer solution, the complex may be an amorphous precipitate or a crystalline material. Each type is produced commercially to take advantage of their unique absorption characteristics.

The amorphous form, referred to as *semilente insulin* or Prompt Insulin Zinc Suspension, USP, is rapidly absorbed upon intramuscular or subcutaneous (under the skin) injection. The larger crystalline material, called *ultralente insulin* or Extended Insulin Zinc Suspension, USP, is more slowly absorbed with a resultant longer duration of action. By combining the two types in various proportions, a physician is able to provide his patients with intermediate acting insulin of varying degrees of onset and duration of action. A physical mixture of 70% of the crystalline form and 30% of the amorphous form, called *lente insulin* or Insulin Zinc Suspension, USP, is commercially available and provides an intermediate acting insulin preparation that meets the requirements of many diabetics.

Some medicinal chemicals that exist in crystalline form are capable of forming different types of crystals, depending upon the conditions (temperature, solvent, time) under which crystallization is induced. This property, whereby a single chemical substance may exist in more than one crystalline form, is known as "polymorphism." Only one form of a pure drug substance is stable at a given temperature and pressure with the other forms, called metastable forms, converting in time to the stable crystalline form. It is therefore not unusual for a metastable form of a medicinal agent to change

form even when present in a completed pharmaceutical preparation, although the time required for a complete change may exceed the normal shelf-life of the product itself. However, from a pharmaceutical point of view, any change in the crystal structure of a medicinal agent may critically affect the stability and even the therapeutic efficacy of the product in which the conversion takes place.

The various polymorphic forms of the same chemical generally differ in many physical properties, including their solubility and dissolution characteristics, which are of prime importance to the rate and extent of drug absorption into the body's system. These differences are manifest so long as the drug is in the solid state. Once solution is effected, the different forms are indistinguishable one from another. Therefore, differences in drug action, pharmaceutically and therapeutically, can be expected from polymorphs contained in solid dosage forms as well as in liquid suspension. The use of metastable forms generally results in higher solubility and dissolution rates than the respective stable crystal forms of the same drug. If all other factors remain constant, more rapid and complete drug absorption will likely result from the metastable forms than from the stable form of the same drug. On the other hand, the stable polymorph is more resistant to chemical degradation and because of its lower solubility is frequently preferred in pharmaceutical suspensions of insoluble drugs. If metastable forms are employed in the preparation of suspensions, their gradual conversion to the stable form may be accompanied by an alteration in the consistency of the suspension itself, thereby affecting its permanency. In all instances, the advantages of the metastable crystalline forms in terms of increased physiologic availability of the drug must be balanced against the increased product stability when stable polymorphs are employed. Sulfur and cortisone acetate are two examples of drugs that exist in more than one crystalline form and are frequently prepared in pharmaceutical suspensions. In fact, cortisone acetate is reported to exist in at least five different crystalline forms. It is possible for the commercial products of two manufacturers to differ in stability and in the therapeutic effect, depending upon the crystalline form of the drug used in the formulation.

Salt Forms

The dissolution rate of a salt form of a drug is generally quite different from that of the parent compound. Sodium and potassium salts of weak organic acids and hydrochloride salts of weak organic bases dissolve much more readily than do the respective free acids or bases. The result is a more rapid saturation of the diffusion layer surrounding the dissolving particle and the consequent more rapid diffusion of the drug to the absorption sites.

Numerous examples could be cited to demonstrate the increased rate of drug dissolution due to the use of the salt form of the drug rather than the free acid or base, but the following will suffice: the addition of the ethylenediamine moiety to theophylline increases the water solubility of theophylline 5-fold. The use of the ethylenediamine salt of theophylline has allowed the development of oral aqueous solutions of theophylline and diminished the need to use hydroalcoholic mixtures, e.g., elixirs.

Other Factors

The *state of hydration* of a drug molecule can affect its solubility and pattern of absorption. Usually the anhydrous form of an organic molecule is more readily soluble than the hydrated form. This characteristic was demonstrated with the drug ampicillin, when the anhydrous form was shown to have a greater rate of solubility than the trihydrate form (4). The rate of absorption for the anyhdrous form was greater than that for the trihydrate form of the drug.

Once swallowed, a drug is placed in the gastrointestinal tract where its solubility can be affected not only by the pH of the environment, but by the normal components of the tract and the foodstuffs which may be present. A drug may interact with one of the other agents present to form a chemical complex which may result in reduced drug solubility and decreased drug absorption. The classic example of this complexation phenomenon is that which occurs between tetracycline analogues and certain cations, e.g., calcium, magnesium, aluminum, resulting in a decreased absorption of the tetracycline derivative. Also, if the drug becomes *ad*sorbed onto insoluble material in the tract, its availability for absorption may be correspondingly reduced.

Bioavailability and Bioequivalence

The term *bioavailability* describes the *rate* and *extent* to which an active drug ingredient or therapeutic moiety is absorbed from a drug product and becomes available at the site of drug action. The term *bioequivalence* refers to the *comparison* of bioavail-

abilities of different formulations, drug products, or batches of the same drug product.

The availability to the biologic system of a drug substance formulated into a pharmaceutical product is integral to the goals of dosage form design and paramount to the effectiveness of the medication. The study of a drug's bioavailability depends on the drug's absorption or entry into the systemic circulation, and studying the pharmacokinetic profile of the drug or its metabolite(s) over time in the appropriate biologic system, e.g., blood, plasma, urine. Graphically, bioavailability of a drug is portrayed by a concentration-time curve of the administered drug in an appropriate tissue system, e.g., plasma (Fig. 4.4). Bioavailability data are used to determine: 1) the amount or proportion of drug absorbed from a formulation or dosage form; 2) the rate at which the drug was absorbed; 3) the duration of the drug's presence in the biologic fluid or tissue; and, when correlated with patient response, and 4) the relationship between drug blood levels and clinical efficacy and toxicity.

During the product development stages of a proposed drug product, pharmaceutical manufacturers employ bioavailability studies to compare different formulations of the drug substance to ascertain the one which allows the most desirable absorption pattern. Later, bioavailability studies may be used to compare the availability of the drug substance from different production batches of the product. They may also be used to compare the availability of the drug substance from different dosage forms (as tablets, capsules, elixirs, etc.), or from the same dosage form produced by different (competing) manufacturers.

FDA Bioavailability Submission Requirements

The FDA requires bioavailability data submissions in the following instances (5).

1. *New Drug Applications (NDAs)*. A section of each NDA is required to describe the human pharmacokinetic data and human bioavailability data, or information supporting a waiver of the bioavailability data requirement (see waiver provisions following).
2. *Abbreviated New Drug Applications (ANDAs)*. In vivo bioavailability data are required unless information is provided and accepted supporting a waiver of this requirement (see waiver provisions following).

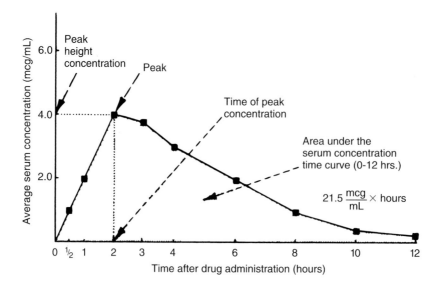

Fig. 4.4 *Serum concentration-time curve showing peak height concentration, time of peak concentration, and area under the curve. (Courtesy of D.J. Chodos and A.R. DiSanto, The Upjohn Company.)*

3. *Supplemental Applications.* In vivo bioavailability data are required if there is a change in the:
   a. Manufacturing process, product formulation or dosage strength, beyond the variations provided for in the approved NDA.
   b. Labeling, to provide for a new indication for use of the drug product and, if clinical studies are required, to support the new indication.
   c. Labeling, to provide for a new or additional dosage regimen for a special patient population (e.g., infants) if clinical studies are required to support the new or additional dosage regimen.

Conditions under which the FDA *may* waive the in-vivo bioavailability requirement include:

1. The product is a solution intended solely for intravenous administration, and contains the same active agent, in the same concentration and solvent, as a product previously approved through a full NDA.
2. The drug product is administered by inhalation as a gas or vapor, and contains the same active agent, in the same dosage form, as a product previously approved through a full NDA.
3. The drug product is an oral solution, elixir, syrup, tincture or similar other solubilized form and contains the same active agent in the same concentration as a previously approved drug product through a full NDA, and contains no inactive

ingredient known to significantly affect absorption of the active drug ingredient.
4. The drug product is a topically applied preparation (e.g., ointment) intended for local therapeutic effect.
5. The drug product is an oral dosage form that is not intended to be absorbed (e.g., antacid or radiopaque medium).
6. The drug product is a solid oral dosage form that has been demonstrated to be identical, or sufficiently similar, to a drug product that has met the in-vivo bioavailability requirement.

Most of the bioavailability studies have been applied to drugs contained in solid dosage forms intended to be administered orally for systemic effects. The emphasis in this direction has been primarily due to the proliferation of competing products on the market in recent years, particularly the nonproprietary (generic) capsules and tablets, and the knowledge that certain drug entities when formulated and manufactured differently into solid dosage forms are particularly prone to variations in biologic availability. Thus, the present discussions will be centered around solid dosage forms. However, this is not to imply that systemic drug absorption is not intended from other routes of administration or other dosage forms, or that bioavailability problems may not exist from these products as well. Indeed, drug absorption from other routes is affected by the physicochemical properties of the drug and the formulative and manufacturing aspects of the dosage form design.

Blood (or Serum or Plasma) Concentration-Time Curve

Following the oral administration of a medication, if blood samples are drawn from the patient at specific time intervals and analyzed for drug content, the resulting data may be plotted on ordinary graph paper to yield the type of drug blood level curve presented in Figure 4.4. The vertical axis of this type of plot characteristically presents the concentration of drug present in the blood (or serum or plasma) and the horizontal axis presents the time the samples were obtained following the administration of the drug. When the drug is first administered (time zero), the blood concentration of the drug should also be zero. As the drug passes into the stomach and/or intestine, it is released from the dosage form, eventually dissolves, and is absorbed. As the sampling and analysis continue, the blood samples reveal increasing concentrations of drug until the maximum (peak) concentration (C_{max}) is reached. Then, the blood level of the drug progres-sively decreases and, if no additional dose is given, eventually falls to zero. The diminished blood level of drug after the peak height is reached indicates that the rate of drug elimination from the blood stream is greater than the rate of drug absorption into the circulatory system. Drug absorption does not terminate after the peak blood level is reached, but may continue for some time. Similarly the process of drug elimination is a continuous one. It begins as soon as the drug first appears in the blood stream and continues until all of the drug has been eliminated. When the drug leaves the blood it may be found in various body tissues and cells for which it has an affinity until ultimately it is excreted as such or as drug metabolites in the urine or via some other route (Fig. 4.5). A urinalysis for the drug or its metabolites may be used to indicate the extent of drug absorption and/or the rate of drug elimination from the body.

Parameters for Assessment and Comparison of Bioavailability

In discussing the important parameters to be considered in the comparative evaluation of the blood

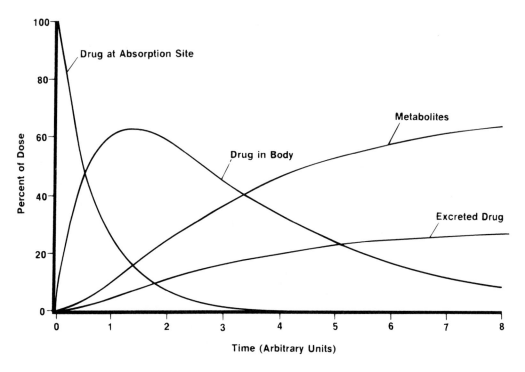

Fig. 4.5 *Time course of drug in the body. (Reprinted with permission from Rowland M, Tozer TN. Clinical Pharmacokinetics. 2nd Ed., Philadelphia: Lea & Febiger, 1989.)*

level curves following the oral administration of single doses of two formulations of the same drug entity, Chodos and DiSanto (6) list the following:

1. The Peak Height Concentration (C_{max})
2. The Time of the Peak Concentration (T_{max})
3. The Area Under the Blood (or serum or plasma) Concentration-Time Curve (AUC)

Using Figure 4.4 as an example, the height of the peak concentration is equivalent to 4.0 μg/mL of drug in the serum; the time of the peak concentration is 2 hours after administration; and the area under the curve from 0 to 12 hours is calculated as 21.5 μg/mL × hours. The meaning and use of these parameters are further explained as follows.

Peak Height

Peak height concentration is the maximum drug concentration (C_{max}) observed in the blood plasma or serum following a dose of the drug. For conventional dosage forms, as tablets and capsules, the C_{max} will usually occur at only a single time point, referred to as T_{max}. The amount of drug is usually expressed in terms of its concentration in relation to a specific volume of blood, serum, or plasma. For example, the concentration may be expressed as g/100 mL, μg/mL or mg% (mg/100 mL). Figure 4.6 depicts concentration-time curves showing different peak height concentrations for *equal* amounts of drug from two different formulations following oral administration. The horizontal line drawn across the figure indicates that the minimum effective concentration (MEC) for the drug substance is

4.0 μg/mL. This means that in order for the patient to exhibit an adequate response to the drug, this concentration in the blood must be achieved. Comparing the blood levels of drug achieved after the oral administration of equal doses of formulations "A" and "B" in Figure 4.6, formulation "A" will achieve the required blood levels of drug to produce the desired pharmacologic effect whereas the administration of formulation "B" will not. On the other hand, if the minimum effective concentration for the drug was 2.0 μg/mL and the mimimum toxic concentration (MTC) was 4.0 μg/mL as depicted in Figure 4.7, equal doses of the two formulations would result in toxic effects produced by formulation "A" but only desired effects by formulation "B." The objective in the individual dosing of a patient is to achieve the MEC but not the MTC.

The *size* of the dose administered influences the blood level concentration and C_{max} for that drug substance. Figure 4.8 depicts the influence of dose on the blood level time curve for a hypothetical drug administered by the same route and in the same dosage form. In this example, it is assumed that all doses are completely absorbed and eliminated at the same rates. As the dose increases, the C_{max} is proportionally higher and the area-under-the-curve (AUC) proportionally greater. The peak time, T_{max}, is the same for each dose.

Time of Peak

The second parameter of importance in assessing the comparative bioavailability of two formulations is the time required to achieve the maximum level of drug in the blood (T_{max}). In Figure 4.6, the

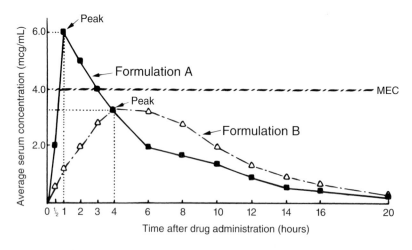

Fig. 4.6   *Serum concentration-time curve showing different peak height concentrations for equal amounts of drug from two different formulations following oral administration. (Courtesy of D.J. Chodos and A.R. DiSanto, The Upjohn Company.)*

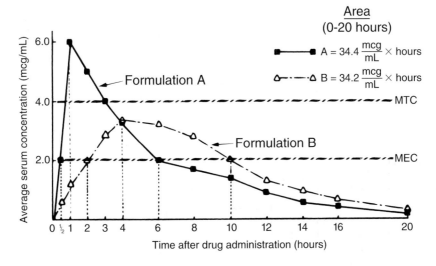

Fig. 4.7 *Serum concentration-time curve showing peak height concentrations, peak height times, times to reach minimum effective concentration (MEC) and areas under the curves for equal amounts of drug from two different formulations following oral administration. (Courtesy of D.I. Chodos and A.R. DiSanto, The Upjohn Company.)*

time required to achieve the peak serum concentration of drug is 1 hour for formulation "A" and 4 hours for formulation "B." This parameter reflects the *rate* of drug absorption from a formulation. It is the rate of drug absorption that determines the time needed for the minimum effective concentration to be reached and thus for the initiation of the desired pharmacologic effect. The rate of drug absorption also influences the period over which the drug enters the blood stream and therefore affects the duration of time that the drug is maintained in the blood. Looking at Figure 4.7, formulation "A" allows the drug to reach the MEC within 30 minutes following administration and a peak concentration in 1 hour. Formulation "B" has a slower rate of drug release. Drug from this formulation reached the MEC 2 hours after administration and its peak concentration 4 hours after administration. Thus formulation "A" permits the greater rate of drug absorption; it allows drug to reach both the MEC and its peak height sooner than drug formulation "B." On the other hand, formulation "B" provides the greater duration of time for drug concentrations maintained above the MEC, 8 hours (from 2 to 10 hours following administration) to 5 1/2 hours (from 30 minutes to 6 hours following administration) for formulation "A." Thus, if a rapid onset of action is desired, a formulation similar to "A" would be preferred, but, if a longer duration of action is desired rather than a rapid onset of action, a formulation similar to "B" would be preferred.

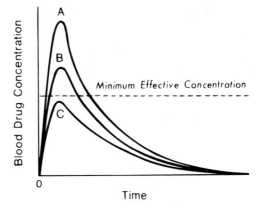

Fig. 4.8 *The influence of dose size on the resultant blood drug concentration-time curves when three different doses of the same drug are administered and the rates of drug absorption and elimination are equal after the three doses. A = 100 mg, B = 80 mg, C = 50 mg. (Reprinted with permission from Ueda CT. Concepts in Clinical Pharmacology. Essentials of Bioavailability and Bioequivalence. The Upjohn Company, 1979).*

In sum, changes in the *rate* of drug absorption will result in changes in the values of both C_{max} and T_{max}. Each product has its own characteristic rate of absorption. When the *rate* of absorption is decreased, the C_{max} is lowered and T_{max} occurs at a later time. If the doses of the drugs are the same and presumed completely absorbed, as in Figure 4.7, the AUC for each is essentially the same.

Area Under the Serum Concentration Time Curve

The area under the curve (AUC) of a concentration-time plot (see Fig. 4.4) is considered representative of the total amount of drug absorbed into the circulation following the administration of a single dose of that drug. Equivalent doses of a drug, when fully absorbed, would produce the same AUC. Thus, two curves dissimilar in terms of peak height and time of peak, as those in Figure 4.7, may be similar in terms of area under the curve, and thus in the amount of drug absorbed. As indicated in Figure 4.7, the area under the curve for formulation "A" is 34.4 µg/mL × hours and for formulation "B" is 34.2 µg/mL × hours, essentially the same. If equivalent doses of drug in different formulation produce *different* AUC values, differences exist in the *extent* of absorption between the formulations. Figure 4.9 depicts concentration-time curves for three different formulations of equal amounts of drug with greatly different areas under the curve. In this example, formulation "A" delivers a much greater amount of drug to the circulatory system than do the other two formulations. In general, the smaller the AUC, the less drug absorbed.

The area under the curve may be measured mathematically, using a technique known as the trapezoidal rule, and is reported in amount of drug/volume of fluid × time (e.g., µg/mL × hours; g/100 × hours; etc.).

According to the trapezoidal rule, the area beneath a drug concentration-time curve can be estimated through the assumption that the AUC can be represented by a series of trapezoids (quadrilateral planes having two parallel and two nonparallel sides). The total AUC would be the sum of the areas of the individual trapezoids. The area of each trapezoid is calculated taking $1/2(C_{n+1} + C_n)(t_n - t_{n-1})$, where C_n and t_n are drug concentrations in the blood plasma, or serum, and time, respectively. The use of the trapezoid is demonstrated by the data reproduced in Table 4.3 and plotted into a plasma drug concentration-time curve as shown in Figure 4.10.

The fraction (F) (or bioavailability) of an orally administered drug may be calculated by comparison of the AUC after oral administration with that obtained after intravenous administration:

$$F = (AUC)_{oral}/(AUC)_{intravenous}$$

In practice, it would be rare for a drug to be completely absorbed into the circulation following oral administration. As noted earlier, many drugs undergo the first-pass effect resulting in some degree of metabolic degradation before entering the general circulation. In addition, factors of drug product formulation, drug dissolution, chemical and physical interactions with the gastrointestinal contents, gastric emptying time, intestinal motility, and others contribute to the incomplete absorption of an administered dose of a drug. The oral dosage strengths of many commerical products are based on considerations of the proportion of the dose administered that is expected to be absorbed and available to its site of action in order to produce the

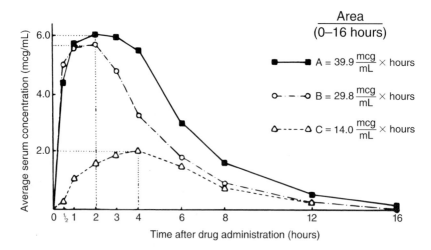

Fig. 4.9   *Serum concentration-time curve showing peak height concentrations, peak height times, and areas under the curves for equal amounts of drugs from three different formulations following oral administration. (Courtesy of Chodos DJ, DiSanto AR, The Upjohn Company.)*

Table 4.3. Determination of AUC Using the Trapezoidal Rule for the Following Plasma Drug Concentration-Time Data*

Sample (n)	Time (hr)	Plasma Concentration (μg/mL)	$AUC/t_n t_{n-1}$ (μg/mL × hr)
1	0	0	½ (0 + 1)(0.5 − 0) = 0.25
2	0.5	1	½ (1 + 11)(1 − 0.5) = 3.00
3	1.0	11	½ (11 + 28)(1.5 − 1) = 9.75
4	1.5	28	½ (28 + 30)(2 − 1.5) = 14.50
5	2	30	½ (30 + 21)(3 − 2) = 25.50
6	3	21	½ (21 + 17)(4 − 3) = 19.00
7	4	17	½ (17 + 9)(6 − 4) = 26.00
8	6	9	½ (9 + 4)(8 − 6) = 13.00
9	8	4	½ (4 + 2)(10 − 8) = 6.00
10	10	2	½ (2 + 1)(12 − 10) = 3.00
11	12	1	½ (1 + 0)(18 − 12) = 3.00
12	18	0	AUC = 123.00

*Reprinted with permission from Ueda CT. Concepts in Clinical Pharmacology. Essentials of Bioavailability and Bioequivalence. The Upjohn Company, 1979.

desired drug blood level and/or therapeutic response. The absolute bioavailability following oral dosing is generally compared to intravenous dosing. As examples, the mean oral absorption of a dose of verapamil (Calan) is reported to be 90%; enalapril (Vasotec) 60%; diltiazem (Cardizem) about 40%, and lisinopril (Zestril) about 25%. However, there is large intersubject variability, and the absorbed doses may vary patient-to-patient.

Bioequivalence of Drug Products

A great deal of discussion and scientific investigation has been devoted recently to the problem of determining the equivalence between drug products of competing manufacturers.

The rate and extent to which a drug in a dosage form becomes available for biologic absorption or utilization depends in great measure upon the materials utilized in the formulation and also on the method of manufacture. Thus, the same drug when formulated in *different* dosage forms may be found to possess different bioavailability characteristics and hence exhibit different clinical effectiveness. Further, two seemingly "identical" or "equivalent" products, of the same drug, in the same dosage strength and in the *same* dosage form type, but differing in formulative materials or method of manufacture, may vary widely in bioavailability and thus in clinical effectiveness.

Dissolution requirements for capsules and tablets are included in the USP and are integral to bioavailability. Experience has shown that where bioinequivalence has been found between two supposedly equivalent products, dissolution testing can help to define the product differences. According to the USP, significant bioavailability and bioinequivalence problems may be revealed through dissolution testing and are generally the result of one or more of the following causal factors: the drug's particle size; excessive amounts of the lubricant magnesium stearate in the formulation; coating materials, especially shellac; and inadequate amounts of tablet or capsule disintegrants.

The following terms are used by the Food and Drug Administration to define the type or level of "equivalency" between drug products (5).

Pharmaceutical equivalents are drug products that contain identical amounts of the identical active

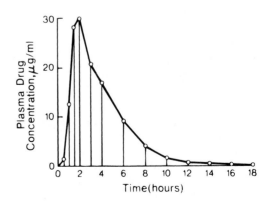

Fig. 4.10 *Estimation of area under the drug concentration-time curve using the trapezoidal rule (see Table 4.3 for raw data). (Reprinted with permission from Ueda CT. Concepts in Clinical Pharmacology. Essentials of Bioavailability and Bioequivalence. The Upjohn Company, 1979).*

drug ingredient, i.e., the same salt or ester of the same therapeutic moiety, in identical dosage forms, but not necessarily containing the same inactive ingredients, and that meet the identical compendial or other applicable standard of identity, strength, quality, and purity, including potency and, where applicable, content uniformity, disintegration times, and/or dissolution rates.

Pharmaceutical alternatives are drug products that contain the identical therapeutic moiety, or its precursor, but not necessarily in the same amount or dosage form or as the same salt or ester. Each such drug product individually meets either the identical or its own respective compendial or other applicable standard of identity, strength, quality, and purity, including potency and, where applicable, content uniformity, disintegration times, and/or dissolution rates.

Bioequivalent drug products are pharmaceutical equivalents or pharmaceutical alternatives whose rate and extent of absorption do not show a significant difference when administered at the same molar dose of the therapeutic moiety under similar experimental conditions, either single dose or multiple dose. Some pharmaceutical equivalents or pharmaceutical alternatives may be equivalent in the extent of their absorption but not in their rate of absorption, and yet may be considered bioequivalent because such differences in the rate of absorption are intentional and are reflected in the labeling, are not essential to the attainment of effective body drug concentrations on chronic use, or are considered medically insignificant for the particular drug product studied.

In addition, the term *therapeutic equivalents* has been used to indicate pharmaceutical equivalents which, when administered to the same individuals in the same dosage regimens, will provide essentially the same therapeutic effect.

Differences in bioavailability have been demonstrated for a number of products involving the following and other drugs: tetracycline, chloramphenicol, digoxin, phenylbutazone, warfarin, diazepam, levodopa, and oxytetracycline. Not only has bio*in*equivalence been shown to exist in products of different manufacturers but there have also been variations in the bioavailability of different batches of drug products from the same manufacturer. Variations in the bioavailability of certain drug products have resulted in some therapeutic failures in patients who have taken two inequivalent drug products in the course of their therapy.

The most common experimental plan to compare the bioavailability of two drug products is the simple *crossover design study*. In this method, each of the 12 to 24 individuals in the group of carefully matched subjects (usually healthy adult males between 18 and 40 years of age of similar height and weight) is administered both products under fasting conditions and essentially serves as his own control. To avoid bias of the test results, each test subject is randomly assigned one of the two products for the first phase of the study. Once the first assigned product is administered, samples of blood or plasma are drawn from the subjects at predetermined times and analyzed for the active drug moiety and its metabolites as a function of time. The same procedure is then repeated (*crossover*) with the second product after an appropriate interval of time, i.e., a washout period to ensure that there is no residual amount of drug from the first administered product that would artificially inflate the test results of the second administered product. Afterward, the patient population data are tabulated and the parameters used to assess and compare bioavailability, i.e., C_{max}, T_{max}, AUC, are then analyzed with statistical procedures. Statistical differences in bioavailability parameters may not always be clinically significant in therapeutic outcome.

Inherent differences in individuals result in different patterns of drug absorption, metabolism and excretion. These differences must be statistically analyzed to separate them from the factors of bioavailability related to the products themselves. The value in the crossover-designed experiment is that each individual serves as his own control by taking each of the products. Thus, inherent differences as mentioned between individuals is minimized.

Absolute bioequivalency between drug products rarely, if ever, occurs. Such absolute equivalency would yield serum concentration-time curves for the products involved that would be exactly superimposable. This simply is not expected of products which are made at different times, in different batches, or indeed by different manufacturers. However, some expectations of bioequivalency are expected of products which are considered to be of equivalent merit for therapy.

In most studies of bioavailability, the originally marketed product (frequently referred to as the "prototype," "pioneer," or "innovator" drug product) is recognized as the established product of the drug and is utilized as the standard for the bioavailability comparative studies.

As a result of the implementation of the Drug Price Competition and Patent Term Restoration Act of 1984, many additional drugs became available in generic form. Prior to the 1984 act, only those drugs marketed before 1962 could be processed by an Abbreviated New Drug Application (ANDA). The ANDA process does not require the sponsor to repeat costly clinical research on active ingredients already found to be safe and effective. The 1984 Act extended the eligibility for ANDA processing to drugs first marketed after 1962, making generic versions immediately possible for many additional off-patent drugs previously available only as brand name (pioneer) products.

According to the FDA, a generic drug is considered bioequivalent if the rate and extent of absorption do not show a significant difference from that of the pioneer drug when administered at the same molar dose of the therapeutic ingredient under the same experimental conditions (7). Because, in the case of a systemically absorbed drug, blood levels even if from an identical product may vary in different subjects, in bioequivalence studies each subject receives both the pioneer and the test drug and thus serves as his own control.

Under the 1984 act, to gain FDA approval a generic drug product must:

- Contain the same active ingredients as the pioneer drug (inert ingredients may vary)
- Be identical in strength, dosage form, and route of administration
- Have the same indications and precautions for use and other labeling instructions
- Be bioequivalent
- Meet the same batch-to-batch requirements for identity, strength, purity, and quality
- Be manufactured under the same strict standards of FDA's Current Good Manufacturing Practice regulations as required for pioneer products

In the design and evaluation of bioequivalence, the FDA employs the "80/20 rule." This rule requires that a study be large enough to provide an 80% probability to detect a 20% difference in average bioavailability. The allowance of a statistical variability of ±20% in bioequivalence applies to both reformulated pioneer drugs and generics. If a pioneer manufacturer reformulates an FDA-approved product, the subsequent formulation must meet the same bioequivalency standards that are required of generic manufacturers of that product (i.e., the approved bioavailability standard for that product).

The FDA recommends generic substitution only among products that it has evaluated to be therapeutically equivalent. Since 1980, the Agency has prepared an annual *Approved Drug Products with*

Therapeutic Equivalence Evaluations (known as the "Orange Book") which is published in the USP-DI, Volume III "Approved Drug Products and Legal Requirements." This publication is regularly updated and contains information on about 10,000 approved prescription drug products. About 7,500 of these are available from more than a single manufacturer, with only about 10% considered therapeutically *in*-equivalent to the pioneer products. For example, the FDA rates all conjugated estrogens and esterified estrogen products as "not therapeutically equivalent," because no manufacturer to date has submitted an acceptable in vivo bioequivalence study. Therefore, the FDA does not recommend that these products be substituted for each other.

The variables that can contribute to the differences between products are many (Table 4.4). For instance in the manufacture of a tablet, different

Table 4.4.   Some Factors Which Can Influence the Bioavailability of Orally Administered Drugs

Drug Substance Physiochemical Properties
 Particle Size
 Crystalline or Amorphous Form
 Salt Form
 Hydration
 Lipid/Water Solubility
 pH and pK_a
Pharmaceutic Ingredients and Dosage Form Characteristics
 Pharmaceutic Ingredients
  Fillers
  Binders
  Coatings
  Disintegrating Agents
  Lubricants
  Suspending Agents
  Surface Active Agents
  Flavoring Agents
  Coloring Agents
  Preservative Agents
  Stabilizing Agents
 Disintegration Rate (Tablets)
 Dissolution Time of Drug in Dosage Form
 Product Age and Storage Conditions
Physiologic Factors and Patient Characteristics
 Gastric Emptying Time
 Intestinal Transit Time
 Gastrointestinal Abnormality or Pathologic Condition
 Gastric Contents
  Other drugs
  Food
  Fluids
 Gastrointestinal pH
 Drug Metabolism (Gut and during first passage
  through liver).

materials or amounts of such formulative components as fillers, disintegrating agents, binders, lubricants, colorants, flavorants and coatings may be used. The particle size or crystalline form of a therapeutic or pharmaceutic component may vary between formulations. The tablet may vary in shape, size, and hardness depending upon the punches and dies selected for use by the manufacturer and the compression forces utilized in the process. During packaging, shipping and storage the integrity of the tablets may be altered by physical impact, or changes in conditions of humidity, temperature, or through interactions with the components of the container. Each of the factors noted may have an effect on the rates of tablet disintegration, drug dissolution, and consequently on the rate and extent of drug absorption. Although the bioequivalency problems are perhaps greater among tablets than for other dosage forms because of the multiplicity of variables, the same types of problems exist for the other dosage forms and must be considered in bioequivalency evaluations.

There are situations in which even therapeutically equivalent drugs may not be equally suitable for a particular patient. For example, a patient may be hypersensitive to an inert ingredient in one product (brand name or generic) that another product does not contain. Or a patient may become confused or upset if dispensed an alternate product that differs in color, flavor, shape, or packaging from that to which he or she has become accustomed. Switching between products can generate concern, and thus pharmacists need to be prudent in both initial product selection and in product interchange.

Routes of Drug Administration

Drugs may be administered by a variety of dosage forms and routes of administration, as presented in Tables 4.5 and 4.6. One of the fundamental considerations in dosage form design is whether the drug is intended for local or systemic effects. *Local* effects are achieved from direct application of the drug to the desired site of action, such as the eye, nose, or skin. *Systemic* effects result from the entrance of the drug into the circulatory system and its subsequent transport to the cellular site of its action. For systemic effects, a drug may be placed directly into the blood stream via intravenous injection or absorbed into the venous circulation following oral, or other routes of administration.

An individual drug substance may be formulated into multiple dosage forms which result in different drug absorption rates and times of onset, peak, and duration of action. This is demonstrated by Figure

Table 4.5.   Routes of Drug Administration

Term	Site
Oral	Mouth
Peroral (per os*)	Gastrointestinal tract via mouth
Sublingual	Under the tongue
Parenteral	Other than the gastrointestinal tract (by injection)
Intravenous	Vein
Intraarterial	Artery
Intracardiac	Heart
Intraspinal or intrathecal	Spine
Intraosseous	Bone
Intraarticular	Joint
Intrasynovial	Joint-fluid area
Intracutaneous or intradermal	Skin
Subcutaneous	Beneath the skin
Intramuscular	Muscle
Epicutaneous (topical)	Skin surface
Transdermal	Skin surface
Conjunctival	Conjunctiva
Intraocular	Eye
Intranasal	Nose
Aural	Ear
Intrarespiratory	Lung
Rectal	Rectum
Vaginal	Vagina

*The abbreviation "po" is commonly used on prescriptions to indicate to be swallowed.

4.11 and Table 4.7, for the drug nitroglycerin in various dosage forms. The sublingual, intravenous, and buccal forms present extremely rapid onsets of action whereas the oral (swallowed), topical ointment and topical disc present slower onsets of action but greater durations of action. The disc provides the longest duration of action, up to 24 hours following application of a single patch to the skin. The transdermal nitroglycerin disc allows a single daily dose, whereas the other forms require multiple dosing to maintain drug levels within the therapeutic window.

The difference in drug absorption between dosage forms is a function of the formulation and the route of administration. For example, a problem associated with the oral administration of a drug is that once absorbed through the lumen of the gastrointestinal tract into the portal vein, the drug may pass directly to the liver and undergo the *first-pass effect*. In essence a portion or all of the drug may be metabolized by the liver. Consequently, as the drug is extracted by the liver, its bioavailability to the body

Table 4.6. Dosage Form/Drug Delivery System Application Route of Administration Primary Dosage Forms

Oral	Tablets
	Capsules
	Solutions
	Syrups
	Elixirs
	Suspensions
	Magmas
	Gels
	Powders
Sublingual	Tablets
	Troches or lozenges
Parenteral	Solutions
	Suspensions
Epicutaneous/	Ointments
transdermal	Creams
	Infusion pumps
	Pastes
	Plasters
	Powders
	Aerosols
	Lotions
	Transdermal patches, discs, solutions
Conjunctival	Contact lens inserts
	Ointments
Intraocular/	Solutions
intraaural	Suspensions
Intranasal	Solutions
	Sprays
	Inhalants
	Ointments
Intrarespiratory	Aerosols
Rectal	Solutions
	Ointments
	Suppositories
Vaginal	Solutions
	Ointments
	Emulsion foams
	Gels
	Tablets
	Inserts, suppositories, sponge
Urethral	Solutions
	Suppositories

The bioavailability is lowest, then, for those drugs that undergo a significant first-pass effect. For these drugs, a hepatic extraction ratio, or the fraction of drug metabolized, E, is calculated. The fraction of drug that enters the system circulation and is ultimately available to exert its effect then is equal to the quantity $(1-E)$. Table 4.8 lists some drugs according to their pharmacologic class that undergo a significant first-pass effect when administered by the oral route.

To compensate for this marked effect, the drug manufacturer may consider other routes of drug administration, e.g., intravenous, intramuscular, sublingual, that avoid the first-pass effect. With these routes there will be a corresponding decrease in the dosage required when compared with oral administration.

Another consideration centers around the metabolites themselves, and whether they are pharmacologically active or inactive. If they are inactive, a larger oral dose will be required to attain the desired therapeutic effect when compared to a lower dosage in a nonfirst-pass effect route. The classic example of drug that exhibits this effect is propranolol. If, on the other hand, the metabolites are the active species, the oral dosage must be carefully tailored to the desired therapeutic effect. First-pass metabolism in this case will result in a quicker therapeutic response than that achieved by a nonfirst-pass effect route.

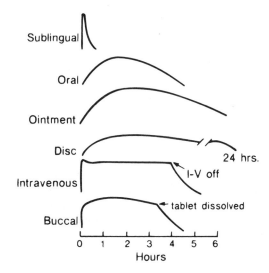

Fig. 4.11 *Blood-level curves of nitroglycerin following administration of dosage forms by various routes. (Reprinted with permission from Abrams J. Nitroglycerin and Long-Acting Nitrates in Clinical Practice. The American Journal of Medicine, Proceedings of a Symposium: First North American Conference on Nitroglycerin Therapy, June 27, 1983).*

is decreased. Thus, the bioavailable fraction is determined by the fraction of drug that is absorbed from the gastrointestinal tract and the fraction that escapes metabolism during its first pass through the liver. The bioavailable fraction (f) is the product of these two fractions as follows:

$$f = \text{Fraction of drug absorbed} \times \text{Fraction escaping first-pass metabolism}$$

Table 4.7. Dosage and Kinetics of Nitroglycerin in Various Dosage Forms

Nitroglycerin, Dosage Form	Usual Dose (mg)	Onset of Action (Minutes)	Peak Action (Minutes)	Duration (Mins/Hours)
Sublingual	0.3–0.8	2–5	4–8	10–30 minutes
Buccal	1–3	2–5	4–10	30–300 minutes[Δ]
Oral	6.5–19.5	20–45	45–120	2–6 hours[Ω]
Ointment (2%)	½–2 inches	15–60	30–120	3–8 hours
Discs	5–10	30–60	60–180	Up to 24 hours

[Δ] Effect persists so long as tablet is intact.
[Ω] Some short-term dosing studies have demonstrated effects to 8 hours.
Reprinted with permission from Abrams J. Nitroglycerin and Long-Acting Nitrates in Clinical Practice. Am J Med. Proceedings of a Symposium: First North American Conference of Nitroglycerin Therapy, June 27, 1983, p. 88.

One must remember also that the flow of blood through the liver can be decreased under certain conditions. Consequently, the bioavailability of those drugs that undergo a first-pass effect then would be expected to increase. For example, during cirrhosis the blood flow to the kidney is dramatically decreased and efficient hepatic extraction by enzymes responsible for a drug's metabolism also falls off. Consequently, in cirrhotic patients the dosage of drug that undergoes a first-pass effect from oral administration will have to be reduced to avoid toxicity.

Oral Route

Drugs are most frequently taken by oral administration. Although a few drugs taken orally are intended to be dissolved within the mouth, the vast majority of drugs taken orally are swallowed. Of these, most are taken for the *systemic* drug effects that result after absorption from the various surfaces along the gastrointestinal tract. A few drugs, such as antacids, are swallowed for their local action within the confines of the gastrointestinal tract.

Compared with alternate routes, the oral route is considered the most natural, uncomplicated, convenient, and safe means of administering drugs. Disadvantages of the oral route include slow drug response (when compared with parenterally administered drugs); chance of irregular absorption of drugs, depending upon such factors as constitutional make-up, the amount or type of food present within the gastrointestinal tract; and the destruction of certain drugs by the acid reaction of the stomach or by gastrointestinal enzymes.

Dosage Forms Applicable

Drugs are administered by the oral route in a variety of pharmaceutical forms. The most popular are tablets, capsules, suspensions, and various pharmaceutical solutions. Briefly, *tablets* are solid dosage forms prepared by compression or molding and contain medicinal substances with or without suitable diluents, disintegrants, coatings, colorants, and other pharmaceutical adjuncts. Diluents are fillers used in preparing tablets of the proper size and consistency. Disintegrants are used for the break-up or separation of the tablet's compressed ingredients. This ensures prompt exposure of drug particles to the dissolution process thereby enhancing drug absorption, as shown in Figure 4.12. Tablet coatings are of several types and for several different purposes. Some called *enteric coatings* are employed to permit safe passage of a tablet through the acid environment of the stomach where certain drugs may be destroyed, to the more suitable juices of the intestines where tablet dissolution safely takes place. Other coatings protect the drug substance from the destructive influences of mois-

Table 4.8. Examples of Drugs that Undergo Significant Liver Metabolism and Exhibit Low Bioavailability when Administered by First-pass Routes

Drug Class	Examples
Analgesics	Aspirin, meperidine, pentazocine, propoxyphene
Antianginal	Nitroglycerin
Antiarrhythmics	Lidocaine
Beta-adrenergic blockers	Labetolol, metoprolol, propranolol
Calcium channel blockers	Verapamil
Sympathomimetic amines	Isoproterenol
Tricyclic antidepressants	Desipramine, imipramine, nortriptyline

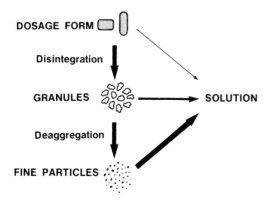

DOSAGE FORM

Disintegration

GRANULES

Deaggregation

FINE PARTICLES

SOLUTION

Fig. 4.12 *Schematic drawing showing disintegration of a tablet dosage form and direct availability of the contents in a capsule dosage form for dissolution and drug absorption after oral administration. (Reprinted with permission from Rowland M, Rozer TN. Clinical Pharmacokinetics. 2nd Ed. Philadelphia: Lea & Febiger, 1989).*

ture, light, and air throughout their period of storage or to conceal a bad or bitter taste from the taste buds of a patient. Commercial tablets, because of their distinctive shapes, colors, and frequently employed monograms of company symbols and code numbers facilitate identification by persons trained in their use and serve as an added protection to public health.

Capsules are solid dosage forms in which the drug substance and appropriate pharmaceutical adjuncts as fillers are enclosed in either a hard or a soft "shell," generally composed of a form of gelatin. Capsules vary in size, depending on the amount of drug to be administered, and are of distinctive shapes and colors when produced commercially. Drug materials are released from capsules faster than from tablets. Capsules of gelatin, a protein, are rapidly disfigured within the gastrointestinal tract, permitting the gastric juices to permeate and reach the contents. Because unsealed capsules have been subject to tampering by unscrupulous individuals, many capsules nowadays are sealed by fusion of the two capsule shells. Also, capsule-shaped and coated tablets, called "caplets," are increasingly utilized. These are easily swallowed but their contents are sealed and protected from tampering like tablets.

Suspensions are preparations of finely divided drugs held in suspension throughout a suitable vehicle. Suspensions taken orally generally employ an aqueous vehicle, whereas those employed for other purposes may utilize a different vehicle. Sus-

pensions of certain drugs to be used for intramuscular injection, for instance, may be maintained in a suitable oil. To be suspended, the drug particles must be insoluble in the vehicle in which they are placed. Nearly all suspensions must be shaken before use because they tend to settle. This ensures not only uniformity of the preparation but more importantly the administration of the proper dosage. Suspensions are a useful means to administer large amounts of solid drugs that would be inconveniently taken in tablet or capsule form. In addition, suspensions have the advantage over solid dosage forms in that they are presented to the body in fine particle size, ready for the dissolution process immediately upon administration. However, not all oral suspensions are intended to be dissolved and absorbed by the body. For instance, kaolin mixture with pectin, an antidiarrheal preparation, contains suspended kaolin, which acts in the intestinal tract by adsorbing excessive intestinal fluid on the large surface area of its particles.

Drugs administered in aqueous *solution* are absorbed much more rapidly than those administered in solid form, because the processes of disintegration and dissolution are not required. Pharmaceutical solutions may differ in the type of solvent employed and therefore in their fluidity characteristics. Among the solutions frequently administered orally are *elixirs*, which are solutions in a sweetened hydroalcoholic vehicle and are more mobile than water; *syrups*, which generally utilize sucrose solutions as the sweet vehicle resulting in a viscous preparation; and *solutions* themselves, which officially are preparations in which the drug substance is dissolved predominantly in an aqueous vehicle and do not for reasons of their method of preparation (e.g., injections, which must be sterilized) fall into another category of pharmaceutical preparations.

Absorption

Absorption of drugs after oral administration may occur at the various body sites between the mouth and rectum. In general, the higher up a drug is absorbed along the length of the alimentary tract, the more rapid will be its action, a desirable feature in most instances. Because of the differences in the chemical and physical nature among drug substances, a given drug may be better absorbed from the environment of one site than from another within the alimentary tract.

The oral cavity is used on certain occasions as the absorption site of certain drugs. Physically, the oral absorption of drugs is managed by allowing the drug substance to be dissolved within the oral cav-

~quent or no swallowing until the taste
~g has dissipated. This process is accom-
~~ated by providing the drug as extremely soluble and rapidly dissolving uncoated tablets. Drugs
capable of being absorbed in the mouth present
themselves to the absorbing surface in a much
more concentrated form than when swallowed,
since drugs become progressively more diluted
with gastrointestinal secretions and contents as
they pass along the alimentary tract.

Currently the oral or *sublingual* (beneath the
tongue) administration of drugs is regularly used for
only a few drugs, with nitroglycerin and certain
steroid sex hormones being the best examples. Nitroglycerin, a coronary vasodilator used in the prophylaxis and treatment of angina pectoris, is available in the form of tiny tablets which are allowed to
dissolve under the tongue, producing therapeutic effects in a few minutes after administration. The dose
of nitroglycerin is so small (usually 400 μg) that if it
were swallowed the resulting dilute gastrointestinal
concentration may not result in reliable and sufficient drug absorption. Even more important, however, is the fact that nitroglycerin is rapidly destroyed
by the liver through the *first-pass effect.* Many sex
hormones have been shown to be absorbed materially better from sublingual administration than
when swallowed. Although the sublingual route is
probably an effective absorption route for many
other drugs, it has not been extensively used, primarily because other routes have proven satisfactory
and more convenient for the patient. Retaining drug
substances in the mouth is unattractive because of
the bitter taste of most drugs.

Drugs may be altered within the gastrointestinal
tract to render them less available for absorption.
This may result from the drug's interaction with or
binding to some normal constituent of the gastrointestinal tract or a foodstuff or even another
drug. For instance, the absorption of the tetracycline group of antibiotics is greatly interfered with
by the simultaneous presence of calcium. Because
of this, tetracycline drugs must not be taken with
milk or other calcium containing foods or drugs.

In some instances it is the intent of the pharmacist to prepare a formulation that releases the drug
slowly over an extended period of time. There are
many methods by which slow release is accomplished, including the complexation of the drug
with another material, the combination of which is
only slowly released from the dosage form. An example of this is the slow-release waxy matrix potassium chloride tablets. These are designed to release
their contents gradually as they are shunted through
the gastrointestinal tract. Because their contents
are leached out gradually there is less incidence of
gastric irritation. The intermingling of food and
drug generally results in delayed drug absorption.
Since most drugs are absorbed more effectively
from the intestines than from the stomach, when
rapid absorption is intended, it is generally desirable to have the drug pass from the stomach into
the intestines as rapidly as possible. Therefore, gastric emptying time is an important factor in effecting drug action dependent upon intestinal absorption. Gastric emptying time may be increased by a
number of factors, including the presence of fatty
foods (more effect than proteins, which in turn
have more effect than carbohydrates), lying on the
back when bedridden (lying on the right side facilitates passage in many instances), and the presence
of drugs (for example, morphine) that have a qui-
eting effect on the movements of the gastrointestinal tract. If a drug is administered in the form of a
solution, it may be expected to pass into the intestines more rapidly than drugs administered in
solid form. As a rule, large volumes of water taken
with medication facilitate gastric emptying and
passage into the intestines.

The pH of the gastrointestinal tract increases
progressively along its length from a pH of about 1
in the stomach to approximately pH 8 at the far end
of the intestines. pH has a definite bearing on the
degree of ionization of most drugs, and this in turn
affects lipid solubility, membrane permeability and
absorption. Because most drugs are absorbed by
passive diffusion through the lipoid barrier, the
lipid/water partition coefficient and the pK_a of the
drugs are of prime importance to both their degree
and site of absorption within the gastrointestinal
tract. As a general rule, weak acids are largely
*un*ionized in the stomach and are absorbed fairly
well from this site, whereas weak bases are highly
ionized in the stomach and are not significantly absorbed from the gastric surface. Alkalinization of
the gastric environment by artificial means (simultaneous administration of alkaline or antacid drugs)
would be expected to decrease the gastric absorption of weak acids and to increase that of weak
bases. Strong acids and bases are generally poorly
absorbed due to their high degrees of ionization.

The small intestine serves as the major absorption pathway for drugs because of its suitable pH
and the great surface area available for drug absorption within its approximate 20-foot length extending from the pylorus at the base of the stomach to the junction with the large intestine at the
cecum. The pH of the lumen of the intestine is

about 6.5 (see Fig. 4.3) and both weakly acidic and weakly basic drugs are well absorbed from the intestinal surface, which behaves in the ionization and distribution of drugs between it and the plasma on the other side of the membrane as though its pH were about 5.3.

Rectal Route

Some drugs are administered rectally for their local effects and others for their systemic effects. Drugs given rectally may be administered as solutions, suppositories, or ointments. *Suppositories* are defined as solid bodies of various weights and shapes intended for introduction into a body orifice (usually rectal, vaginal, or urethral) where they soften, melt, or dissolve, release their medication, and exert their drug effects. These effects simply may be the promotion of laxation (as with glycerin suppositories), the soothing of inflamed tissues (as with various commercial suppositories used to relieve the discomfort of hemorrhoids), or the promotion of systemic effects (as antinausea or antimotion sickness). The composition of the suppository base, or carrier of the medication, can greatly influence the degree and rate of drug release and should be selected on an individual basis for each drug. The use of rectal ointments is generally limited to the treatment of local conditions. Rectal solutions are usually employed as enemas or cleansing solutions.

The rectum and the colon can absorb many soluble drugs. Rectal administration for systemic action may be preferred for those drugs destroyed or inactivated by the environments of the stomach and intestines. The administration of drugs by the rectal route may also be indicated when the oral route is precluded because of vomiting or when the patient is unconscious or incapable of swallowing drugs safely without choking. Approximately 50% of a dose of drug absorbed from rectal administration is likely to bypass the liver, an important factor when considering those orally administered drugs that are rapidly destroyed in the liver by the first-pass effect. On the negative side, compared with oral administration, rectal administration of drugs is inconvenient, and the absorption of drugs from the rectum is frequently irregular and difficult to predict.

Parenteral Route

The term *parenteral* is derived from the Greek words *para,* meaning beside, and *enteron,* meaning intestine, which together indicate something done outside of the intestine and not by way of the alimentary tract. A drug administered parenterally is one injected through the hollow of a fine needle into the body at various sites and to various depths. The three primary routes of parenteral administration are subcutaneous, intramuscular (IM), and intravenous (IV) although there are others such as intracardiac and intraspinal.

Drugs destroyed or inactivated in the gastrointestinal tract or too poorly absorbed to provide satisfactory response may be parenterally administered. The parenteral route is also preferred when rapid absorption is essential, as in emergency situations. Absorption by the parenteral route is not only faster than after oral administration, but the blood levels of drug that result are far more predictable, because little is lost after subcutaneous or intramuscular injection, and virtually none by intravenous injection; this also generally permits the administration of smaller doses. The parenteral route of administration is especially useful in treating patients who are uncooperative, unconscious, or otherwise unable to accept oral medication.

One disadvantage of parenteral administration is that once the drug is injected, there is no retreat. That is, once the substance is within the tissues or is placed directly into the blood stream, removal of the drug warranted by an untoward or toxic effect or an inadvertent overdose is most difficult. By other means of administration, there is more time between drug administration and drug absorption, which becomes a safety factor by allowing for the extraction of unabsorbed drug (as by the induction of vomiting after an orally administered drug). Also, because of the strict sterility requirements for all injections, they are more expensive than other dosage forms and require competent trained personnel for their proper administration.

Dosage Forms Applicable

Pharmaceutically, injectable preparations are usually either sterile suspensions or solutions of a drug substance in water or in a suitable vegetable oil. Drugs in solution act more rapidly than drugs in suspension, with an aqueous vehicle providing faster action in each instance than an oleaginous vehicle. As in other instances of drug absorption, a drug must be in solution to be absorbed, and a suspended drug must first submit to the dissolution process. Also, because body fluids are aqueous, they are more receptive to drugs in an aqueous vehicle than those in an oily one. For these reasons, the rate of drug absorption can be varied in parenteral products by selective combinations of drug state and supporting vehicle. For instance, a suspension of a drug in a vegetable oil likely would be much more slowly absorbed than an aqueous solution of the same drug. Slow absorption means prolonged drug action, and when this is achieved through pharmaceutical means, the resulting preparation is referred to as a *depot* or *repository* injection, because it represents a storage reservoir of the drug substance within the body from which it is slowly removed into the systemic circulation. In this regard, even more sustained drug action may be achieved through the use of subcutaneous implantation of compressed tablets, termed pellets that are only slowly dissolved from their site of implantation, releasing their medication at a rather constant rate over a period of several weeks to many months. The repository type of injection is mainly limited to the subcutaneous or intramscular route. It is obvious that drugs injected intraveously do not encounter absorption barriers and thus produce only rapid drug effects. Preparations for intravenous injection must not interfere with the blood components or with circulation and therefore, with few exceptions, are aqueous solutions.

Subcutaneous Injections

The subcutaneous (hypodermic) administration of drugs involves their injection through the layers of skin into the loose subcutaneous tissue. Subcutaneous injections are prepared as aqueous solutions or as suspensions and are administered in relatively small volumes of 2 mL or less. Insulin is an example of a drug administered by the subcutaneous route. Subcutaneous injections are generally given in the forearm, upper arm, thigh, or buttocks. If the patient is to receive frequent injections, it is best to alterate injection sites to reduce tissue irritation. After injection, the drug comes into the immediate vicinity of blood capillaries and permeates them by diffusion or filtration. The capillary wall is an example of a membrane that behaves as a lipid pore barrier, with lipid-soluble substances penetrating the membrane at rates varying with their oil/water partition coefficients. Lipid-insoluble (generally more water-soluble) drugs penetrate the capillary membrane at rates which appear to be inversely related to their molecular size, with smaller molecules penetrating much more rapidly than larger ones. All substances, whether lipid-soluble or not, cross the capillary membrane at rates that are much more rapid than the rates of their transfer across other body membranes. The blood supply to the site of injection is an important factor in considering the rate of drug absorption, conse-

quently the more proximal capillaries are to the site of injection, the more prompt will be the drug's entrance into the circulation. Also, the more capillaries, the more surface area for absorption, and the faster the rate of absorption. Some substances have the capability of modifying the rate of drug absorption from a subcutaneous site of injection. The addition of a vasconstrictor to the injection formulation (or its prior injection) will generally diminish the rate of drug absorption by causing constriction of the blood vessels in the area of injection and thereby reducing blood flow and the capacity for absorption. This principle is used in the administration of local anesthetics by employing the vasoconstrictor epinephrine. Conversely, vasodilators may be used to enhance subcutaneous absorption by increasing blood flow to the area. Physical exercise can also influence the absorption of drug from an injection site. Diabetic patients who rotate subcutaneous injection sites and then do physical exercise, e.g., jogging, must realize the onset of insulin activity might be influenced by the selected site of administration. Because of the movement of the leg and blood circulation to it during running, the absorption of insulin from a thigh injection site would be expected to be faster than that from an abdominal injection site.

Intramuscular Injections

Intramuscular injections are performed deep into the skeletal muscles, generally the gluteal or lumbar muscles. The site is selected where the danger of hitting a nerve or blood vessel is minimal. Aqueous or oleaginous solutions or suspensions may be used intramuscularly. Certain drugs, because of their inherent low solubilities, provide sustained drug action after an intramuscular injection. For instance, one deep intramuscular injection of a suspension of penicillin G benzathine results in effective blood levels of the drug for seven to ten days.

Drugs that are irritating to subcutaneous tissue are often administered intramuscularly. Also, greater volumes (2 to 5 mL) may be administered intramuscularly than subcutaneously. When a volume greater than 5 mL is to be injected, it is frequently administered in divided doses using two injection sites. Injection sites are best rotated when a patient is receiving repeated injections over a period of time.

Intravenous Injections

In the intravenous administration of drugs, an aqueous solution is injected directly into the vein at a rate commensurate with efficiency, safety, comfort to the patient, and the desired duration of drug response. Drugs may be administered intravenously as a single, small-volume injection or as a large volume, slow intravenous drip infusion (as is common following surgery). Intravenous injection allows the desired blood level of drug to be achieved in an optimal and quantitative manner. Intravenous injections are usually made into the veins of the forearm and are especially useful in emergency situations where immediate drug response is desired. It is essential that the drug be maintained in solution after injection and not be precipitated within the circulatory system, an event that might produce emboli. Because of a fear of the development of pulmonary embolism, oleaginous bases are not usually intravenously administered. However, an intravenous fat emulsion is used therapeutically as a caloric source for patients receiving parenteral nutrition whose caloric requirements cannot be met by glucose. It may be administered either through a peripheral vein or a central venous catheter at a distinct rate to help prevent the occurrence of untoward reactions.

Intradermal Injections

These injections are administered into the corium of the skin, usually in volumes of about a tenth of a milliliter. Common sites for the injection are the arm and the back. The injections are frequently performed as diagnostic measures, as in tuberculin and allergy testing.

Epicutaneous Route

Drugs are administered topically, or applied to the skin, for their action at the site of application or for systemic drug effects.

Drug absorption via the skin is enhanced if the drug substance is in solution, if it has a favorable lipid/water partition coefficient, and if it is a nonelectrolyte. Drugs that are absorbed enter the skin by way of the pores, sweat glands, hair follicles, sebaceous glands, and other anatomic structures of the skin's surface. Because blood capillaries are present just below the epidermal cells, a drug that penetrates the skin and is able to traverse the capillary wall finds ready access to the general circulation.

Among the few drugs currently employed topically to the skin surface for percutaneous absorption and systemic action are nitroglycerin (antianginal), nicotine (smoking cessation), estradiol (estrogenic hormone), clonidine (antihypertensive), and scopolamine (antinausea/antimotion sickness). Each of these drugs is available for use in the form of transdermal delivery systems fabricated as an adhesive disc or patch which slowly releases the medication for percutaneous absorption. Additionally, nitroglycerin is available in an ointment form for application to the skin's surface for systemic absorption. Nitroglycerin is used therapeutically for ischemic heart diease, with the transermal dosage forms becoming increasingly popular because of the benefit in patient compliance through their long-acting (24 hours) characteristics. The nitroglycerin patch is generally applied to the arm or chest, preferably in a hair-free or shaven area. The transdermal scopolamine sytem is also in the form of a patch to be applied to the skin; in this case, behind the ear. The drug system is indicated for the prevention of nausea and vomiting associated with motion sickness. The commercially available product is applied to the postauricular area several hours before need (as prior to an air or sea trip) where it releases its medication over a period of 3 days. The concepts of transdermal therapeutic systems are discussed further in Chapter 10.

For the most part, pharmaceutical preparations applied to the skin are intended to serve some local action and as such are formulated to provide prolonged local contact with minimal absorption. Drugs applied to the skin for their local action include antiseptics, antifungal agents, anti-inflammatory agents, local anesthetic agents, skin emollients, and protectants, against environmental conditions, as the effects of the sun, wind, pests, and chemical irritants. For these purposes, drugs are most commonly administered in the form of ointments and related semisolid preparations such as creams and pastes, as solid dry powders, aerosol sprays or as liquid preparations such as solutions and lotions.

Pharmaceutically, ointments, creams, and pastes are semisolid preparations in which the drug is contained in a suitable base (ointment base), which is itself semisolid and either hydrophilic or hydrophobic in character. These bases play an important role in the proper formulation of semisolid preparations, and there is no single base universally suitable as a carrier of all drug substances or for all therapeutic indications. The proper base for a drug must be determined individually to provide the desired drug release rate, staying qualities after application, and texture. Briefly, *ointments* are simple mixtures of drug substances in an ointment base, whereas *creams* are semisolid emulsions and are less viscid and lighter than ointments. Creams are considered to have greater esthetic appeal due to their nongreasy character and their ability to "vanish" into the skin upon rubbing. *Pastes* contain more solid materials than do ointments and are therefore stiffer and less penetrating. Pastes are usually employed for their protective action and for their ability to absorb serous discharges from skin lesions. Thus when protective rather than therapeutic action is desired, the formulation pharmacist will favor a paste, but when therapeutic action is required, he will prefer ointments and creams. Commerically, many therapeutic agents are prepared in both ointment and cream form and are dispensed and used according to the particular preference of the patient and the prescribing practitioner.

Medicinal powders are intimate mixtures of medicinal substances usually in an inert base as talcum powder. Depending upon the particle size of the resulting blend, the powder will have varying dusting and covering capabilities. In any case, the particle size should be small enough to ensure against grittiness and consequent skin irritation. Powders are most frequently applied topically to relieve such conditions as diaper rash, chafing, and athlete's foot.

When topical application is desired in liquid form other than solution, lotions are most frequently employed. *Lotions* are suspensions of solid materials in an aqueous vehicle, although certain emulsions and even some true solutions have been designated as lotions because of either their appearance or application. Lotions may be preferred over semisolid preparations because of their non-greasy character and their increased spreadability over large areas of skin.

Ocular, Oral, and Nasal Routes

Drugs are frequently applied topically to the eye, ear, and the mucous membranes of the nose. In these instances, ointments, suspensions, and solutions are generally employed. Ophthalmic solutions and suspensions are sterile aqueous preparations with other quantities essential to the safety and comfort of the patient. Ophthalmic ointments must be sterile, and also free of grittiness. Innovative new delivery systems for ophthalmic drugs continue to be investigated. One dosage form, the Ocusert, is an elliptically shaped unit designed for continuous release of pilocarpine following its placement into the cul-de-sac of the eye. Further, case reports of the ability of soft contact lenses to absorb drug from the eye have spawned research in the development of soft contact lenses impregnated with drug for therapeutic application in the eye. Nasal preparations are usually solutions or suspensions administered by drops or as a fine mist from a nasal spray container. Current research is directed toward the feasibility of the nasal administration of insulin for diabetes mellitus. Otic, or ear preparations are usually viscid so that they have prolonged contact with the affected area. They may be employed simply to soften ear wax, to relieve an earache, or to combat an ear infection. Eye, ear, and nose preparations usually are not used for systemic effects, and although ophthalmic and otic preparations are not usually absorbed to any great extent, nasal preparations *may* be absorbed, and systemic effects after the intranasal application of solution are not unusual.

Other Routes

The lungs provide an excellent absorbing surface for the administration of gases and for aerosol mists of very minute particles of liquids or solids. The gases employed are mainly oxygen and the common general anesthetic drugs administered to patients entering surgery. The rich capillary area of the alveoli of the lungs, which in man covers nearly a thousand square feet, provides rapid absorption and drug effects comparable in speed to those following an intravenous injection. In the case of drug particles, their size largely determines the depth to which they penetrate the alveolar regions; their solubility, the extent to which they are absorbed. After contact with the inner surface of the lungs, an insoluble drug particle is caught in the mucus and is moved up the pulmonary tree by ciliary action. Soluble drug particles that are approximately 0.5 to 1.0 μ in size reach the minute alveolar sacs and are most prompt and efficient in providing systemic effects. Particles that are smaller than 0.5 μ are expired to some extent, and thus their absorption is not total but variable. Particles from 1 to 10 μ in size effectively reach the terminal bronchioles and to some extent the alveolar ducts and are favored for local therapy. Therefore, in the pharmaceutical manufacture of aerosol sprays for inhalation therapy, the manufacturers not only must attain the proper drug particle size but also must ensure their uniformity for consistent penetration of the pulmonary tree and uniform effects.

In certain instances and for local effects, drugs are inserted into the vagina and the urethra. Drugs are usually presented to the vagina in tablet form, as suppositories, ointments, emulsion foams, gels or solutions, and to the urethra as suppositories or solutions. Systemic drug effects may result after the vaginal or urethral application of drugs due to absorption of the drug from the mucous membranes of these sites.

Fate of Drug after Absorption

After absorption into the general circulation from any route of administration, a drug may become bound to blood proteins and delayed in its passage into the surrounding tissues. Many drug substances may be highly bound to blood protein and others little-bound. For instance, when in the blood stream, naproxen is 99% bound to plasma proteins, penicillin G is 60% bound, amoxicillin only 20% bound, and minoxidil is unbound.

The degree of drug binding to plasma proteins is usually expressed as a percentage or as a fraction (termed *alpha*, or α) of the bound concentration (C_b) to the total concentration (C_t), bound plus unbound (C_u) drug:

$$\alpha = \frac{C_b}{C_u + C_b} = \frac{C_b}{C_t}$$

Thus, if one knows two of the three terms in the equation, the third may be calculated. Drugs having an alpha value of greater than 0.9 are considered highly bound (90%); those drugs with an alpha value of less than 0.2 are considered to be little (20% or less) protein bound. Table 4.9 presents approximate serum protein binding characteristics for representative drugs present in the blood under conditions associated with usual therapy. The drug-protein complex is reversible and involves albumin, although globulins are also involved in the binding of drugs, particularly some of the hormones. The binding of drugs to biologic materials involves the formation of relatively weak bonds (e.g., van der Waals, hydrogen, and ionic bonds). The binding capacity of blood proteins is limited, and once they are saturated, additional drug absorbed into the blood stream remains unbound unless bound drug is released, creating a vacant site for another drug molecule to attach. Any unbound drug is free to leave the blood stream for tissues or cellular sites within the body.

Bound drug is neither exposed to the body's detoxication (metabolism) processes nor is it filtered through the renal glomeruli. Bound drug is therefore referred to as the *inactive* portion in the blood, and unbound drug, with its ability to penetrate cells, is termed the *active* blood portion. The bound portion of drug serves as a drug reservoir or a depot, from which the drug is released as the free form when the level of free drug in the blood no longer is adequate to ensure protein saturation. The free drug may be only slowly released, thereby increasing the duration of the drug's stay in the body. For this reason a drug that is highly protein bound may remain in the body for longer periods of time

Table 4.9. Examples of Drug Binding to Plasma Proteins

Drug	Percent Bound
Naproxen (Naprosyn)	>99
Chlorambucil (Leukeran)	>99
Etodolac (Lodine)	>99
Warfarin (Coumadin)	>97
Fluoxetine (Prozac)	>95
Cloxacillin (Tegopen)	>95
Ceftriaxone (Rocephin)	85–95
Cefoperazone (Cefobid)	82–93
Cefonicid (Monocid)	>90
Indomethacine (Indocin)	>90
Spironolactone (Aldactone)	>90
Digitoxin (Crystodigin)	>90
Cyclosporine (Sandimmune)	>90
Sulfisoxazole (Gantrisin)	>85
Diltiazem (Cardizem)	70–80
Penicillin V (Veetids)	>75
Nitroglycerin (Nitro-Bid)	>60
Penicillin G Potassium	>60
Methotrexate	>50
Methicillin (Staphcillin)	>40
Ceftizoxime (Cefizox)	>30
Captopril (Capozide)	25–30
Ciprofloxacin (Cipro)	20–40
Digoxin (Lanoxin)	20–25
Ampicillin (Omnipen)	>20
Amoxicillin (Amoxil)	>20
Metronidazole (Flagyl)	<20
Mercaptopurine (Purinethol)	>19
Cephradine (Velosef)	8–17
Ranitidine (Zantac)	>15
Ceftazidime (Tazicef)	<10
Nicotine (Prostep)	<5
Minoxidil (Loniten)	>0

Average literature values, based on conditions usually associated with drug therapy.

and require less frequent dosage administration than another drug that may be only slightly protein bound and may remain in the body for only a short period of time. Evidence suggests that the concentration of serum albumin decreases about 20% in the elderly. This may be clinically significant for drugs that bind strongly to albumin, e.g., phenytoin, because if there is less albumin available to bind the drug there will be a corresponding increase of the free drug in the body. Without a downward dosage adjustment in an elderly patient, there could be an increased incidence of adverse effects.

A drug's binding to blood proteins may be affected by the simultaneous presence of a second (or more) drug(s). The additional drug(s) may result in drug effects or durations of drug action quite dissimilar to that found when each is administered alone. Salicylates, for instance, have the effect of decreasing the binding capacity of thyroxin, the thyroid hormone, to proteins. Phenylbutazone is an example of a drug that competitively displaces several other drugs from serum binding sites, including other antiinflammatory drugs, oral anticoagulants, oral antidiabetics, and sulfonamides. Through this action, the displaced drugs become less protein bound and their activity (and toxicity) may be increased. The intensity of a drug's pharmacologic response is related to the ratio of the bound drug *versus* free, active drug, and the therapeutic index of the drug. Warfarin, an anticoagulant is 97% bound to plasma protein leaving 3% in free form to exert its effect. If a second drug, such as naproxen, which is strongly bound to plasma proteins is administered and results in only 90% of the warfarin being bound, this means that 10% of warfarin is now in the free form. Thus, the blood level of the free warfarin (3 to 10%) has tripled and could result in serious toxicity. The displacement of drugs from plasma protein sites is typical in the elderly who normally are maintained on numerous medicines. Coupled with the aforementioned decrease in serum protein through the aging process the addition of a highly protein-bound drug to an elderly patient's existing treatment regimen could pose significant problems if the patient is not monitored carefully for signs of toxicity.

In the same manner as they are bound to blood proteins, drugs may become bound to specific components of certain cells. Thus drugs are not distributed uniformly among all cells of the body, but rather tend to pass from the blood into the fluid bathing the tissues and may accumulate in certain cells according to their permeability capabilities and chemical and physical affinities. This affinity for certain body sites influences their action, for they may be brought into contact with reactive tissues (their *receptor sites*) or deposited in places where they may be inactive. Many drugs, because of their affinity for and solubility in lipids, are found to be deposited in fatty body tissue, thereby creating a storage place or drug reservoir from which they are slowly released to other tissues.

Drug Metabolism (Biotransformation)

Although some drugs are excreted from the body in their original form, many drugs undergo biotransformation prior to excretion. Biotransformation is a term used to indicate the chemical changes that occur with drugs within the body as they are metabolized and altered by various biochemical mechanisms. The biotransformation of a drug results in its conversion to one or more compounds that are more water soluble, more ionized, less capable of binding to proteins of the plasma and tissues, less capable of being stored in fat tissue, and less able to penetrate cell membranes, and thereby less active pharmacologically. Because of its new characteristics, a drug so transformed is rendered less toxic and is more readily excreted. It is for this reason that the process of biotransformation is also commonly referred to as the "detoxification" or "inactivation" process. (However, sometimes the metabolites are more active than the parent compound; see *prodrugs,* following.)

The exact metabolic processes (pathways) by which drugs are transformed represent an active area of biomedical research. Much work has been done with the processes of animal degradation of drugs and in many instances the biotransformation in the animal is thought to parallel that in man. There are four principal chemical reactions involved in the metabolism of drugs: oxidation, reduction, hydrolysis, and conjugation. Most oxidation reactions are catalyzed by enzymes (oxidases) bound to the endoplasmic reticulum, a tubular system within liver cells; only a small fraction of drugs are metabolized by reduction, through the action of reductases, present in the gut and liver; esterases in the liver participate in the hydrolytic breakdown of drugs containing ester groups as well as amides; glucuronide conjugation is the most common pathway for drug metabolism, through combination of the drug with glucuronic acid, forming ionized compounds that are easily eliminated (2). Other metabolic processes, including methylation and acylation conjugation reactions, occur with certain drugs to foster elimination.

In recent years, much interest has been shown in the metabolites of drug biotransformation. Certain metabolites may be as active or even more active pharmacologically than the original compound. Occasionally an active drug may be converted into an active metabolite, which must be excreted as such or undergo further biotransformation to an inactive metabolite, e.g., amitriptyline to nortriptyline. In other instances of drug therapy, an inactive parent compound, referred to as a *prodrug*, may be converted to an active therapeutic agent by chemical transformation in the body. An example is the prodrug enalapril (Vasotec), which after oral administration is hydrolyzed to enalaprilat, an active angiotensin-converting enzyme (ACE) inhibitor used in the treatment of hypertension. Enalaprilat itself is poorly absorbed when taken orally (and thus the prodrug) but may be administered intravenously in aqueous solution. The use of these active metabolites as "original" drugs represents a new area of drug investigation and a vast reservoir of potential therapeutic agents.

Several examples of biotransformations occurring within the body are as follows:

(1) Acetaminophen $\xrightarrow{\text{conjugation}}$ Acetaminophen glucuronide
      (active)   (inactive)

(2) Amoxapine $\xrightarrow{\text{oxidation}}$ 8-hydroxy-amoxapine
      (active)   (inactive)

(3) Procainamide $\xrightarrow{\text{hydrolysis}}$ p-Aminobenzoic acid
      (active)   (inactive)

(4) Nitroglycerin $\xrightarrow{\text{reduction}}$ 1–2 and 1–3 dinitroglycerol
      (active)   (inactive)

Some parent compounds undergo full, partial, or no biotransformation following administration. Lisinopril (Zestril), for example, does not undergo metabolism and is excreted unchanged in the urine. On the other hand, verapamil (Calan) metabolizes to at least 12 metabolites, the most prevalent of which is norverapamil. Norverapamil has 20% of the cardiovascular activity of the parent compound. Diltiazem (Cardizem) is partially metabolized (about 20%) to desacetyldiltiazem, which has 10–20% the coronary vasodilator activity of the parent compound. Indomethacin (Indocin) is metabolized in part to desmethyl, desbenzoyl, and desmethyldesbenzoyl metabolites. Propoxyphene napsylate (Darvon N) is metabolized to norpropoxyphene, which has less central nervous system depressant action than the parent compound but greater local anesthetic effects. The majority of metabolic transformations takes place in the liver, with some drugs as diltiazem and verapamil undergoing extensive first-pass effects. Other drugs, such as terazosin (Hytrin), undergo minimal first-pass metabolism effects. The excretion of both drug and metabolites takes place primarily, but to varying degrees, via the urine and feces. For example, indomethacin and its metabolites are excreted primarily (60%) in the urine, with the remainder in the feces, whereas terazosin and its metabolites are excreted largely (60%) through the feces, and the remainder in the urine.

It is important to mention that several factors influence drug metabolism. For example, there are marked differences between *species* in pathways of hepatic metabolism of a given drug. Species differences make it extremely difficult to extrapolate from one species to another, e.g., laboratory animals to humans. Furthermore, there are many examples of *interindividual variations* in hepatic metabolism of drugs within one species. Genetic factors are involved in the determination of the basal activity of the drug metabolizing enzyme systems. Thus, there can be marked intersubject variation in the rate at which certain individuals metabolically handle drugs. Because of this variation, a physician must individualize therapy to maximize the chances for a constructive therapeutic outcome with minimal toxicity. Studies in humans have demonstrated that these differences have occurred within the cytochrome P-450 genetic codes for a family of isoenzymes responsible for drug metabolism.

Age of the patient is another significant factor that influences drug metabolism. Although pharmacokinetic calculations have not been able to develop a specific correlative relationship with age, it is known, for example, that the ability to metabolize drugs decreases at the extremes of the age scale, i.e., elderly, neonate. Liver blood flow is reduced by aging at about 1% per year beginning around age 30.[9] This decreased blood flow to the liver reduces the capacity for hepatic drug metabolism and elimination. For example, the half-life of chlordiazepoxide increases from about 6 hours at age 20 to about 36 hours at age 80. Further, an immature hepatic system disallows the effective metabolism of drugs by the newborn or premature infant. As mentioned earlier, the half-life of theophylline ranges between 14 to 58 hours in the premature infant to 2.5 to 5 hours in young children between the ages of 1 to 4 whose liver enzyme systems are mature.

Diet has also been demonstrated to modify the metabolism of some drugs. For example, the conversion of an asthmatic patient from a high to a low protein diet will increase the half-life of theophylline. It has also been demonstrated that the production of polycyclic hydrocarbons by the charcoal broiling of beef enhances the hepatic metabolism and shortens the plasma half-life of theophylline. It is conceivable that this effect could also occur with drugs that are metabolized in similar fashion to theophylline. Diet type, e.g., starvation, certain vegetables (brussels sprouts, cabbage, broccoli), has been shown to influence the metabolism of certain drugs. Lastly, it is important to mention that exposure to other drugs or chemicals, e.g., pesticides, alcohol, nicotine, and the presence of disease states, e.g., hepatitis, have all demonstrated an influence on the drug metabolism and consequently the pharmacokinetic profile of certain drugs.

Excretion of Drugs

The excretion of drugs and their metabolites terminates their activity and presence in the body. They may be eliminated by various routes, with the kidney playing the dominant role by eliminating drugs via the urine. Drug excretion with the feces is also important, especially for drugs that are poorly absorbed and remain in the gastrointestinal tract after oral administration. Exit through the bile is significant only when the drug's reabsorption from the gastrointestinal tract is minimal. The lungs provide the exit for many volatile drugs through the expired breath. The sweat glands, saliva, and milk play only minor roles in drug elimination. However, it should be recognized that if a drug gains access to the milk of a mother during lactation, it could easily exert its drug effects in the nursing infant. Examples of drugs that do enter breast milk and may be passed on to nursing infants include theophylline, penicillin, reserpine, codeine, meperidine, barbiturates, diltiazem, and thiazide diuretics. It is generally good practice for the mother to abstain from taking medication during the period of time she is nursing her infant. If she must take medication, she should abide by a dosage regimen and nursing schedule that permit her own therapy yet ensure the safety of her child. Not all drugs gain entrance into the milk; nevertheless, caution is advisable. Manufacturers' package inserts contain product-specific information (usually in the "Precautions" section) on drug migration into breast milk.

The unnecessary use of medications during the early stages of pregnancy is likewise restricted by physicians, because certain drugs are known to have the ability to cross the placental barrier and gain entrance to the tissues and blood of the fetus. Among the many drugs known to do so after administration to an expectant mother are all of the anesthetic gases, many barbiturates, sulfonamides, salicylates, and a number of other potent agents like quinine, meperidine, and morphine, the latter two drugs being narcotic analgesics with great addiction liabilities. In fact, it is not unusual for a newborn infant to be born an addict due to the narcotic addiction of its mother and the passage of the narcotic drugs across the placental barrier.

The kidney, as the main organ for the elimination of drugs from the body, must be functioning adequately if drugs are to be efficiently eliminated. For instance, elimination of digoxin occurs largely through the kidney according to first-order kinetics; that is, the quantity of digoxin eliminated at any time is proportional to the total body content. Renal excretion of digoxin is proportional to the glomerular filtration rate which when normal results in a digoxin half-life that may range from 1.5 to 2.0 days. When the glomerular filtration rate becomes impaired or disrupted, however, as in an anuric patient, the elimination rate decreases. Consequently, the half-life of digoxin may be between 4 to 6 days. Because of this prolongation of digoxin's half-life, the dosage of the drug must be decreased or the dosage interval prolonged. Otherwise, the patient will experience digoxin toxicity. The degree of impairment can be estimated by measurements of glomerular filtration rates, most often by creatinine clearance determination. Usually, however, this is not feasible and the patient's serum creatinine value is used within appropriate pharmacokinetic equations to help determine a drug's dosage regimen.

Some drugs may be reabsorbed from the renal tubule even after having been sent there for excretion. Because the rate of reabsorption is proportional to the concentration of drug in unionized form, it is possible to modify this rate by adjusting the pH of the urine. By acidifying the urine, as with the oral administration of ammonium chloride, or by alkalinizing it, as with the administration of sodium bicarbonate, one can increase or decrease the ionization of the drug and thereby alter its prospect of being reabsorbed. Alkalinization of the urine has been shown to enhance the urinary excretion of weak acids such as salicylates, sulfonamides, and phenobarbital. The opposite effect can be achieved by acidifying the urine. Thus, the duration of a drug's stay within the body may be markedly altered by changing the pH of the urine. Some foods, such as cranberry juice, can also serve to acidify the urine and may alter drug excretion rates.

The urinary excretion of drugs may also be retarded by the concurrent administration of agents capable of inhibiting their tubular secretion. A well-known example is the use of probenecid to inhibit the tubular secretion of various types of penicillin, thereby reducing the frequency of dosage administrations usually necessary to maintain adequate therapeutic blood levels of the antibiotic drug. In this particular instance, the elevation of penicillin blood levels, by whatever route the antibiotic is administered, to twofold and even fourfold levels has been demonstrated by adjuvant therapy with probenecid. The effects are completely reversible upon withdrawal of the probenecid from concomitant therapy.

The fecal excretion of drugs appears to lag behind the rate of urinary excretion partly because a day or so elapses before the feces reach the rectum. It should be easily seen that drugs administered orally for local activity within the gastrointestinal tract and not absorbed will be eliminated completely via the feces. Unless a drug is particularly irritating to the gastrointestinal tract, there is generally no urgency in removing unabsorbable drugs from the system by means other than the normal defecation process. Some drugs that are only partially absorbed after oral administration will naturally be partly eliminated through the rectum.

Pharmacokinetic Principles

This section introduces the concept of pharmacokinetics and how it interrelates the various processes that take place when one administers a drug to a patient, i.e., absorption, distribution, metabolism, excretion. It is not intended to be comprehensive, and thus for further information about the subject the reader is referred to other appropriate literature sources.

A problem encountered when one needs to determine a more accurate dosage of a drug or a more meaningful interpretation of a biologic response to a dose is the inability to determine the drug concentration at the active site in the body. Consequently, to solve this dilemma, the concept of compartmental analysis is used within the discipline of pharmacokinetics in an attempt to quantitatively define what has become of the drug as a function of time from the moment it is administered until it is no longer in the body. Pharmacokinetic analysis utilizes mathematical models to simplify or simulate the disposition of the drug in the body. The idea is to begin with a simple model and then modify as necessary. The principal assumption is that the human body may be represented by one or more *compartments* or pools in which a drug resides in a dynamic state for a short period of time. A compartment is a hypothetical space bound by an unspecified membrane across which drugs are transferred (Fig. 4.13). The transfer of drugs into and out of this compartment is indicated by arrows that point in the direction of drug movement into or out of the compartment. The rate at which a drug is transferred throughout the system is designated by a symbol that usually represents an exponential rate constant. Typically, the letter K or k with numerical or alpha-numerical subscripts is utilized. There are several assumptions associated with

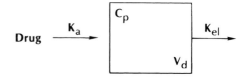

Where:
C_p is the drug concentration in plasma
V_d is the volume of the compartment or volume of distribution

Fig. 4.13 *Schematic of a one-compartment system.*

modeling of drug behavior once in the body. It is assumed that the volume of each compartment remains constant. Thus, an equation that describes the time course of the amount of drug in the compartment can be converted to an equation that depicts the time course of the drug concentration in the compartment by dividing both sides of the equation by the volume of the compartment. Secondly, it is assumed that once a drug enters the compartment it is instantaneously and uniformly distributed throughout the entire compartment. Thus, it is assumed that a sampling of any one portion of the compartment will yield the drug concentration of the entire compartment.

In compartment models it is assumed that drug passes freely into and out of compartments. Thus, these compartmental systems are known as "open" systems. Typically, the process of drug transport between compartments follows first-order kinetics, herein a constant fraction of drug present is eliminated per unit time, and can be described by ordinary differential equations. In these linear systems the time constants that describe the rate at which the plasma or blood concentration curve of a drug decays are independent of the dose of the drug, the volume of distribution of the drug and the route of administration.

The simplest pharmacokinetic model is the single compartment *open-model system* (Figure 4.13). This model depicts the body as one compartment characterized by a certain volume of distribution (V_d) that remains constant. Each drug has its own distinct volume of distribution and this can be influenced by certain patient factors, e.g., age, disease state status. In this scheme a drug can be instantaneously introduced into the compartment, i.e., rapid intravenous administration, or gradually, e.g., oral administration. In the former example it is assumed that the drug distributes immediately to tissues with instantaneous attainment of equilibrium. In the latter example, the drug is absorbed at a certain rate and is characterized by the rate constant K_a. Lastly, the drug is eliminated from the compartment at a certain rate that is characterized by a rate constant K_{el}.

It is relevant at this point to consider the *volume of distribution*, V_d. The volume of distribution is a proportionality constant and is a term that refers to the volume into which the total amount of drug in the body would have to be uniformly distributed to provide the concentration of drug actually measured, e.g., in plasma, in blood. This term can be misleading because it does not represent a specific body fluid or volume. It is influenced by the plasma-protein binding and tissue binding characteristics of a drug. These then influence the distribution of the drug between plasma water, extracellular fluid, intracellular fluid and total body water. Further, because a drug can partition between fat and water according to its unique partition coefficient, this can also influence the volume of distribution. Because of these phenomena, pharmacokineticists find it convenient to describe a drug distribution in terms of compartment models.

To determine the rate of drug transfer into and out of the compartment, plasma, serum, or blood samples are drawn at predetermined times after the drug is administered and analyzed for drug concentration. Once a sufficient number of experimental data points is determined, these are plotted on semi-logarithmic paper and an attempt is made to fit the experimental points with the smoothest curve to fit these points. Figure 4.14 depicts the plasma concentration *versus* time profile for a hypothetical drug following rapid intravenous injection of a bolus dose of the drug with instantaneous distribution. For drugs whose distribution follows first-order, one-compartment pharmacokinetics, a plot of the logarithm of the concentration of drug in the plasma (or blood) versus time will yield a straight line. The equation that describes the plasma decay curve is:

$$C_p = C^0_p \, e^{-K_{el}t} \qquad \text{(Equation 4.1)}$$

where K_{el} is the first-order rate of elimination of the drug from the body, C_p is the concentration of the drug at a time equal to t, and C^0_p is the concentration of drug at time equal to zero, when all the drug administered has been absorbed but none has been removed from the body through elimination mechanisms, e.g., metabolism, renal excretion. The apparent first-order rate of elimination, K_{el}, is usually the sum of the rate constants of a number of individual processes, e.g., metabolic transformation, renal excretion.

For the purpose of pharmacokinetic calculation it is simpler to convert Equation 4–1 to natural logs:

$$\text{Ln } C_p = \text{Ln } C^0_p - K_{el} \, (t) \qquad \text{(Equation 4.2)}$$

and then to log base$_{10}$:

$$\text{Log } C_p = \text{Log } C^0_p - K_{el} \, (t)/2.303 \qquad \text{(Equation 4.3)}$$

Equation 4–3 is then thought of in terms of the Y-intercept form:

$$Y = b + m \times$$
$$\text{Log } C_p = \text{Log } C^0_p - K_{el}/2.303 \, (t)$$

and interpreted as such in the semi-logarithmic plot illustrated in Figure 4.14. Most drugs administered orally can be adequately described using a one-compartment model, whereas drugs administered by rapid intravenous infusion are usually best described by a two-compartment or three-compartment model system.

Assuming that a drug's volume of distribution, V_d, is constant within this system, the total amount of drug in the body (Q_b) can be calculated from the following equation:

$$Q_b = [C^0_p] \, [V_d] \qquad \text{(Equation 4.4)}$$

Usually, C^0_p is determined by extrapolating the drug-concentration time plot back to time zero.

In this simple one-compartment system it is assumed that the administered drug is confined to

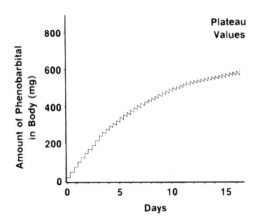

Fig. 4.14 *Plot of the plasma concentration-time data. (Reprinted with permission from Rowland M, Tozer TN. Clinical Pharmacokinetics. 2nd Ed., Philadelphia: Lea & Febiger, 1989).*

the plasma (or blood) and then excreted. Drugs that exhibit this behavior will have small volumes of distribution. For example, a drug such as warfarin which is extensively bound to plasma albumin will have a volume of distribution equivalent to that of plasma water, about 2.8 liters in an average 70 kg adult. Some drugs, however, will initially be distributed at somewhat different rates in various fluids and tissues. Consequently, these drugs' kinetic behavior can best be illustrated by considering an expansion of the one-compartment system to the *two compartment model* (Fig. 4.15).

In the two-compartment system, a drug enters into and is instantaneously distributed throughout the central compartment. Its subsequent distribution into the second or peripheral compartment is slower. For simplicity, on the basis of blood perfusion and tissue-plasma partition coefficients for a given drug, various tissues and organs are considered together and given the designation as central compartment or peripheral compartment. The central compartment is usually considered to include the blood, the extracellular space, and organs with good blood perfusion, e.g., lungs, liver, kidneys, heart. The peripheral compartment is usually constituted by those tissues and organs which are poorly perfused by blood, e.g., skin, bones, fat.

Figure 4.16 depicts the plasma-drug concentration versus time plot for a rapidly administered intravenous dose of a hypothetical drug which exhibits kinetic behavior exemplifying a two-compartment system. Note the initial steep decline of the plasma drug concentration curve. This typifies the distribution of the drug from the central compartment to the peripheral compartment.

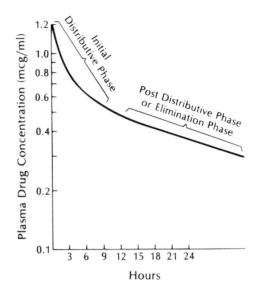

Fig. 4.16 *A semilogarithmic plasma concentration versus time plot of an intravenously administered drug that follows first order, two-compartment pharmacokinetics.*

During this phase the drug concentration in the plasma will decrease more rapidly than in the postdistributive phase, i.e., elimination phase. Whether or not this distributive phase is apparent will depend upon the timing of the plasma samples, particularly in the time immediately following administration. A distributive phase can be very short, a few minutes, or last for hours and even days.

A semi-logarithmic plot of the plasma concentration versus time after rapid intravenous injection of a drug which is best described by a two-compartment model system can often be resolved into two linear components. This procedure can be performed by the method of residuals (or feathering), Figure 4.17. In this procedure, a straight line is fitted through the tail of the original curve and extrapolated back to the Y-axis (the value obtained is B). A plot is then made of the absolute difference values of the original curve and the resultant extrapolated straight line. The slope of the feathered line ($-a/2.303$) and the extrapolated line ($-b/2.303$) and the intercepts, A and B, are determined. Then the following equation is constructed that describes a two-compartment system:
(Equation 4–5)

$$C_p = Ae^{-at} + Be^{-bt}$$

This is a bi-exponential equation which describes the two-compartment system.

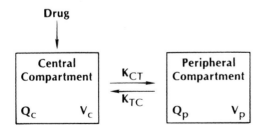

Where:
Q_c = Quantity of drug in central compartment
V_c = Volume of the central compartment
Q_p = Quantity of drug in peripheral compartment
V_p = Volume of the peripheral compartment

Fig. 4.15 *Schematic of a two-compartment system.*

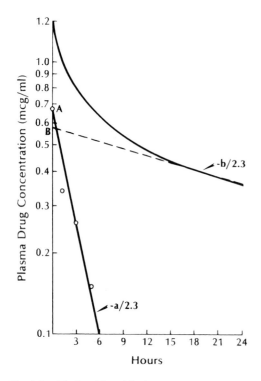

Fig. 4.17 *The logarithm of the drug concentration in plasma plotted versus time (solid line) after intravenous administration of a drug whose disposition can be described by a two-compartment model.*

In this scheme, the slope of the line, i.e., $-a/2.303$, obtained from feathering yields the distributive rate of the drug. The slope of the terminal linear phase or elimination phase, i.e., $-b/2.303$, describes the rate of loss of the drug from the body, and usually is considered to be a reflection of the metabolic processes and renal elimination from the body. Appropriate pharmacokinetic formulas allow the clinician to calculate the various volumes of distribution and rates of distribution and elimination for drugs whose pharmacokinetic behavior is exemplified by the two-compartment system.

Half-Life

The half-life ($T_{1/2}$) of a drug describes the time required for a drug's blood or plasma concentration to decrease by one half. This fall in drug concentration is a reflection of metabolic processes and/or excretion, e.g., renal, fecal. The biological half-life of a drug in the blood may be determined graphically off of a pharmacokinetic plot of a drug's blood-concentration time plot, typically after intra-

venous administration to a sample population. The amount of time required for the concentration of the drug to decrease by one half is considered its half-life. The half-life can also be mathematically determined. Recall Equation 4–3 and rearrange the equation as follows:

$$\frac{K_{el}\,t}{2.303} = \text{Log } C_p^0 - \text{Log } C_p = \text{Log } \frac{C_p^0}{C_p}$$

(Equation 4.6)

Then, if it assumed that C_p is equal to one-half of C_p^0, the equation will become:

$$\frac{K_{el}\,t}{2.303} = \text{Log } \frac{C_p^0}{0.5\,C_p^0} = \text{Log } 2 \qquad \text{(Equation 4.7)}$$

Thus,

$$t_{1/2} = \frac{2.303\,\text{Log } 2}{K_{el}} = \frac{0.693}{K_{el}} \qquad \text{(Equation 4.8)}$$

If this latter equation is rearranged, the half-life finds utility in the determination of drug elimination from the body, provided of course that the drug follows first-order kinetics. Rearranging the prior equation:

$$K_{el} = \frac{0.693}{t_{1/2}} \qquad \text{(Equation 4.9)}$$

Elimination rate constants are reported in time^{-1}, e.g., minutes^{-1}, hours^{-1}. Thus, an elimination constant of a drug is 0.3 hr^{-1} indicates that 30% of the drug is eliminated per hour.

The half-life varies widely between drugs; for some drugs it may be a few minutes, whereas for other drugs it may be hours or even days (Table 4.10). Data on a drug's biologic half-life are useful in determining the most appropriate dosage regimen to achieve and maintain the desired blood level of drug. Such determinations usually result in such recommended dosage schedules for a drug, as the drug to be taken every 4 hours, 6 hours, 8 hours, etc. Although these types of recommendations generally suit the requirements of most patients, they do not suit all patients. The most exceptional patients are those with reduced or impaired ability to metabolize or excrete drugs. These patients, generally suffering from liver dysfunction or kidney disease, retain the administered drug in the blood or tissues for extended periods of time due to their decreased ability to eliminate the drug. The resulting extended biologic half-life of the drug generally ne-

Table 4.10. Some Elimination Half-Life Values

Drug Substance/Product	Elimination Half-Life* ($t_{1/2}$)
Acetaminophen (Tylenol)	1–4 hours
Amoxicillin (Amoxil)	1 hour
Butabarbital Sodium (Butisol Sodium)	100 hours
Cimetidine (Tagamet)	2 hours
Digitoxin (Crystodigin)	7–9 days
Digoxin (Lanoxin)	1.5–2 days
Diltiazem (Cardizem)	2.5 hours
Ibuprofen (Motrin)	1.8–2 hours
Indomethacin (Indocin)	4.5 hours
Lithium Carbonate (Eskalith)	24 hours
Nitroglycerin (Tridil)	3 minutes†
Phenytoin Sodium (Dilantin)	7–29 hours
Pentobarbital Sodium (Nembutal Sodium)	15–50 hours
Propoxyphene (Darvon)	6–12 hours
Propranolol HCl (Inderal)	4 hours
Ranitidine HCl (Zantac)	2.5–3 hours
Theophylline (Theo-Dur)	3–15 hours
Tobramycin Sulfate (Nebcin)	2 hours
Tolbutamide (Orinase)	4.5–6.5 hours

*Mean, average, or value ranges, taken from product information found in *Physicians' Desk Reference*, 52nd ed., 1998, Medical Economics Data, Montvale, New Jersey. Half-life values may vary depending upon patient characteristics (age, liver or renal function, smoking habits, etc.), dose levels administered, and routes of administration.

†After intravenous infusion; nitroglycerin is rapidly metabolized to dinitrates and mononitrates.

cessitates an individualized dosage regimen calling for less frequent drug administration than that called for in patients with normal processes of drug elimination, or a maintenance of the usual dosage schedule, but a decrease in the amount of drug administered.

The drug digoxin presents a good example of a drug having a half-life which is affected by the patient's pathologic condition. Digoxin is eliminated in the urine. Renal excretion of digoxin is proportional to glomerular filtration rate. In subjects with normal renal function, digoxin has a half-life of 1.5 to 2.0 days. In anuric patients (absence of urine formation), the half-life may be prolonged to 4 to 6 days. Theophylline also demonstrates differing half-lives dependent upon certain patient populations. In premature infants with immature liver enzyme systems in the cytochrome P-450 family, the half-life of theophylline ranges from 14 to 58 hours, whereas in young children between the ages of 1 to 4 whose liver enzyme systems are more mature the theophylline half-life ranges between 2 to 5.5 hours.

In adult nonsmokers, the half-life ranges from 6.1 to 12.8 hours, whereas in adult smokers the average half-life of theophylline is 4.3 hours. The increase in theophylline clearance from the body among smokers is believed to be due to an induction of the hepatic metabolism of theophylline. The half-life of theophylline is decreased and total body clearance is enhanced to such a degree in smokers that these individuals may actually require a 50 to 100% increase in theophylline dosage to produce effective therapeutic results. Between 3 months and 2 years may actually be required to normalize the effect of smoking on theophylline metabolism in the body once the patient stops smoking. Because theophylline is metabolized in the liver, the half-life of theophylline will be extended in liver disease. For example, in one study 9 patients with decompensated cirrhosis, the average theophylline half-life was 32 hours.

The half-life of a drug in the blood stream may also be affected by a change in the extent to which it is bound to blood protein or cellular components. Such a change in a drug's binding pattern may be brought about by the administration of a second drug having a greater affinity than the first drug for the same binding sites. The result is the displacement of the first drug from these sites by the second drug and the sudden availability of free (unbound) drug which may pass from the blood stream to other body sites, including those concerned with its elimination. It should be noted that the displacement of one drug from its binding sites by another is generally viewed as an undesired event, since the amount of free drug resulting is greater than the level normally achieved during single drug therapy and may result in untoward drug effects.

Concept of Clearance

The three main mechanisms by which a drug is removed or cleared from the body include (1) the hepatic metabolism, i.e., hepatic clearance, Cl_h, of a drug to either an active or inactive metabolite, (2) the renal excretion, i.e., renal clearance, Cl_r, of a drug unchanged in the urine, and (3) elimination of the drug into the bile and subsequently into the intestines for excretion in feces. An alternate way to express this removal or elimination from the body is to use total body clearance (Cl_B), which is defined as the fraction of the total volume of distribution that can be cleared per unit time. Because most drugs when administered will undergo one or more of these processes, the total body clearance, Cl_B, of a drug is the sum of these clearances, usually hepatic, Cl_h and renal clearances Cl_r. Clearance via the bile and feces is usually not significant for most drugs.

These processes of elimination within the body work together and consequently a drug that is eliminated by renal excretion and hepatic biotransformation will have an overall rate of elimination. K_{el}, that is the sum of the renal excretion, k_u, and hepatic biotransformation, k_m. In the one compartment model described earlier, total body clearance is the product of the volume of distribution, V_d, and the overall rate of elimination, k_{el}:

$$Cl_B = V_d \times k_{el} \qquad \text{(Equation 4.10)}$$

But, recall that k_{el} equals $0.693/t_{1/2}$. If this is substituted into Equation 4–10, and one solves for the half-life, $t_{1/2}$, the following equation is obtained:

$$t_{1/2} = \frac{0.693\,V_d}{Cl_B} \qquad \text{(Equation 4.11)}$$

Recall that total body clearance is a function of one or more processes, thus if a drug were eliminated from the body through hepatic biotransformation and renal clearance, Equation 4–11 becomes:

$$t_{1/2} = \frac{0.693\,V_d}{Cl_h + Cl_r} \qquad \text{(Equation 4.12)}$$

Thus, a drug's half-life is directly proportional to the volume of distribution and inversely proportional to the total body clearance which is comprised of hepatic and renal clearances. Illustratively, if one considers infants and children who exhibit larger volumes of distribution and have lower clearance values, drugs will usually have greater half-lives than that exhibited in adults.

A decrease in the hepatic or renal clearances will prolong the half-life of a drug. This typically occurs for example in renal failure, and consequently, if one can estimate the percentage decrease in excretion due to renal failure one can use Equation 4–12 to calculate the new half-life of the drug in the patient. Thus, an adjusted dosage regimen can then be calculated to decrease the chance of drug toxicity.

Dosage Regimen Considerations

In the previous chapter those factors that can influence the dosage of a drug were mentioned. The question of how much drug and how often to administer it for a desired therapeutic effect is not easily attainable. Basically, there are two approaches to

the development of dosage regimens. The first is the *empirical approach,* which involves the administration of a drug in a certain quantity, noting the therapeutic response and then modifying the dosage of drug and the dosing interval accordingly. Unfortunately, experience with the administration of a drug usually starts with the first patient, and eventually a sufficient number of patients receive the drug so that a fairly accurate prediction can be made. Besides the desired therapeutic effect, consideration must also involve the occurrence and severity of side effects. Empirical therapy is usually employed when the drug concentration in serum or plasma does not reflect the concentration of drug at the receptor site in the body, or the pharmacodynamic effect of the drug is not related (or correlated) with the receptor site drug concentration. Empirical therapy, for example, is utilized for many anticancer drugs that demonstrate effects long after they have been excreted from the body. It is difficult to relate the serum level of these drugs with the desired therapeutic effect.

The second approach to the development of a dosage regimen is through the use of pharmacokinetics or the *kinetic approach.* This approach is based on the assumption that the therapeutic and toxic effects of a drug are related to the amount of drug in the body or to the plasma (or serum) concentration of drug at the receptor site. Through careful pharmacokinetic evaluation of a drug's absorption, distribution, metabolism and excretion in the body from a single dose, the levels of drug attained from multiple dosing can be estimated. One can then determine the appropriateness of a dosage regimen to achieve a desired therapeutic concentration of drug in the body and evaluate the regimen based upon therapeutic response.

When one considers the development of a dosage regimen, pharmacokinetics is but one of a number of factors that should be considered. Table 4.11 illustrates a number of these. Certainly an important factor is the inherent activity, i.e., pharmacodynamics, and toxicity, i.e., toxicology of the drug. A second consideration is the pharmacokinetics of the drug, which are influenced by the dosage form in which the drug is administered to the patient, e.g., biopharmaceutical considerations. The third factor focuses upon the patient to whom the drug will be given and encompasses the clinical state of the patient and how the patient will be managed. Lastly, atypical factors may influence the dosage regimen. Collectively, all of these factors influence the dosage regimen.

Table 4.11. Factors That Determine a Dosage Regimen*

Activity-Toxicity		*Pharmacokinetics*
Minimum therapeutic dose		Absorption
Toxic dose		Distribution
Therapeutic index		Metabolism
Side effects		Excretion
Dose-response relationships		

Dosage Regimen

Clinical Factors		*Other Factors*
Clinical State of Patient	*Management of Therapy*	
Age, weight, urine pH	Multiple drug therapy	Tolerance-dependence
Condition being treated	Convenience of regimen	Pharmacogenetics-idiosyncrasy
Existence of other disease states	Compliance of patient	Drug interactions

*Reprinted with permission from Rowland M, Tozer TN. Clinical Pharmacokinetics. 2nd Ed. Philadelphia: Lea & Febiger, 1989.

The dosage regimen of a drug may simply involve the administration of a drug once for its desired therapeutic effect, e.g., pinworm medication, or encompass the administration of drug for a specific time through multiple doses. In the latter instance, the objective of pharmacokinetic dosing is to design a dosage regimen that will continually maintain a drug's therapeutic serum or plasma concentration within the drug's therapeutic index, i.e., above the minimum effective concentration but below the minimum toxic level.

Frequently drugs are administered between 1 to 4 times per day, most often in a fixed dose, e.g., 75 mg 3 times daily after meals. As mentioned earlier, after a drug is administered its level within the body varies because of the influence of all of the processes, e.g., absorption, distribution, metabolism and excretion. A drug will accumulate in the body when the dosing interval is less than the time needed for the body to eliminate a single dose. For example, Figure 4.18 illustrates the plasma concentration for a drug given by intravenous administration and oral administration. The 50 mg dose of this drug was given at a dosing interval of 8 hours. The drug has an elimination half-life of 12 hours. As one can see with continued dosing the drug concentration reaches a *steady state* or *plateau* concentration. At this limit the amount of drug lost per interval is replenished when the drug is dosed again. Consequently the concentration of drug in the

plasma or serum fluctuates between a minimum concentration and a maximum concentration. Thus for certain patient types it is optimal to target dosing so that the plateau concentration resides within the therapeutic index of a drug to maintain a minimum effective concentration of drug. For example, the asthmatic patient maintained on theophylline must have a serum concentration between 10 and 20 μg/mL. Otherwise the patient may be susceptible to an asthma attack. Thus, when dosing the asthmatic patient it is preferable to give theophylline around the clock 4 times daily to sustain levels at least above the minimum effective concentration. If on the other hand this medicine is only administered every 4 hours during the waking hours, it is possible that the minimum concentration will fall below effective levels between the at-bedtime dose and the next morning dose. Consequently, the patient may awaken in the middle of the night and exhibit an asthma attack.

Patients can be monitored pharmacokinetically through appropriate plasma, serum or blood samples, and some hospital pharmacies have implemented pharmacokinetic dosing services. The intent is to maximize drug efficacy, minimize drug toxicity and keep health care costs at a minimum. Thus, for example, complications associated with overdose are controlled or drug interactions that are known to occur, e.g., smoking-theophylline, can be accommodated. In these services, for exam-

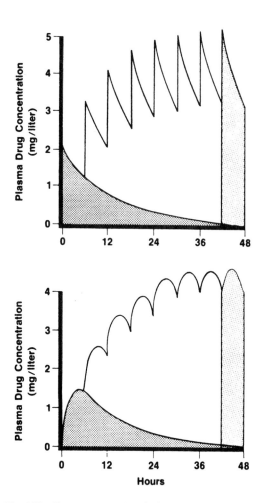

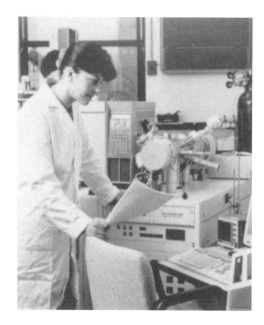

Fig. 4.19 *Computerized gas chromatography mass spectrometry used in bioanalytical studies. Consists of Hewlett Packard Gas Chromatograph (Model 5890 A) and VG Mass Spectrometer (Model UG 12–250). (Courtesy of Elan Corporation, plc.)*

Fig. 4.18 *Plasma concentration of a drug given intravenously (top) and orally (bottom) on a fixed dose of 50 mg and fixed dosing interval of 8 hours. The half-life is 12 hours. Note that the area under the plasma concentration-time curve during a dosing interval at steady state is equal to the total area under the curve for a single dose. The fluctuation of the concentration is diminished when given orally (half-life of absorption is 1.4 hours) but the average steady-state concentration is the same as that after intravenous administration, since F = 1. (Reprinted with permission from Rowland M, Tozer TN. Clinical Pharmacokinetics. Philadelphia: Lea & Febiger, 1989).*

ple, once the physician prescribes a certain amount of drug and monitors the clinical response, it is the pharmacist who coordinates the appropriate sample time to determine drug concentration in the appropriate body fluid. After the level of drug is attained, it is the pharmacist who interprets the result, and consults with the physician regarding subsequent dosages.

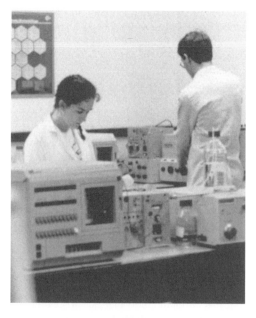

Fig. 4.20 *Assay of biological fluids using Waters HPLC (High Performance Liquid Chromatography) system consisting of (from left to right) Autosampler (Model 712 Wisp), Pump (Model M-45), Shimadzu Fluorescence Detector (Model RF-535). (Courtesy of Elan Corporation, plc.)*

Pharmacokinetic research has demonstrated that the determination of a patient's dosage regimen depends on numerous factors and daily dose formulas exist for a number of drugs that must be administered on a routine maintenance schedule, e.g., digoxin, procainamide, theophylline. For certain drugs such as digoxin, which are not highly lipid soluble, it is preferable to use a patient's lean body weight (LBW) rather than total body weight (TBW) to provide a better estimate of the patient's volume of distribution. Alternatively, even though pharmacokinetic dosing formulas may exist, one must be cognizant that patient factors may be more relevant. For example, with the geriatric patient it is advisable to begin drug therapy with the lowest possible dose and increase the dosage as necessary in small increments to optimize the patient's clinical response. Then the patient should be monitored for drug efficacy and reevaluated periodically. Examples of bioanalytical research laboratories are shown in Figures 4.19 and 4.20.

References

1. Cogburn JN, Donovan MG, Schasteen CS. A model of human small intestinal absorptive cells 1: Transport Barrier. Pharm Res 1991;8:210–216.
2. Christensen FN, et al. The use of gamma scintigraphy to follow the gastrointestinal transit of pharmaceutical formulations. J Pharm Pharmacol 1985; 37:91–95.
3. Coupe AJ, Davis SS, Wilding IR. Variation in gastrointestinal transit of pharmaceutical dosage forms in healthy subjects. Pharm Res 1991;8:360–364.
4. Poole J. Curr Ther Res 1968;10:292–303.
5. Code of Federal Regulations, Title 21, Part 320—Bioavailability and Bioequivalence Requirements.
6. Chodos DJ, DiSanto AR. Basics of Bioavailability. Kalamazoo, MI. The Upjohn Company, 1973.
7. FDA Drug Bulletin, 1986;16, No. 2:1986, pp 14–15.
8. Smith HJ. Process of Drug Handling by the Body. Introduction to the Principles of Drug Design, 2nd ed., London, Butterworth & Co., 1988.
9. Cooper JW. Monitoring of drugs and hepatic status. Clinical Consult 1991;10 (6), 1991.

5

CURRENT GOOD MANUFACTURING PRACTICE AND CURRENT GOOD COMPOUNDING PRACTICE

Chapter at a Glance

Standards for Current Good Manufacturing Practice

CURRENT GOOD Manufacturing Practice (CGMP or GMP) regulations are established by the Food and Drug Administration (FDA) to ensure that minimum standards are met for drug product quality in the United States. The first GMP regulations were promulgated in 1963 under the provisions of the Kefauver-Harris Drug Amendments and since then they have been revised and updated periodically.

The CGMP regulations establish requirements for all aspects of pharmaceutical manufacture. They apply to domestic and to foreign suppliers and manufacturers whose bulk components and finished pharmaceutical products are imported, distributed or sold in this country. To ensure compliance, the FDA inspects the facilities and production records of all firms covered by these regulations.

The Code of Federal Regulations contains requirements for the "Current Good Manufacturing Practice for Finished Pharmaceuticals," (1) and additional CGMP requirements for biologic products (2), medicated articles (3), and medical devices (4). Currency and compliance with CGMP regulations is supported through notices in the Federal Register and through the FDA's Compliance Policy Guide and various other Guidances issued by the FDA.

A topical outline of the CGMP regulations for finished pharmaceuticals is presented in Table 5.1 and summarized in the sections that follow.

CGMP for Finished Pharmaceuticals

General Provisions— Scope and Definitions

The regulations in 21 CFR, Part 211 contain the minimum good manufacturing practice requirements for the preparation of finished pharmaceutical products for administration to humans or animals.

Common terms used in these regulations are defined as follows:

Table 5.1.   Topical Outline of Current Good Manufacturing Practice Regulations*

General Provisions	Calculation of yield
Scope	Equipment identification
Definitions	Sampling and testing of in-process materials and
Organization and Personnel	drug products
Responsibilities of quality control unit	Time limitations on production
Personnel qualifications	Control of microbiological contamination
Personnel responsibilities	Reprocessing
Consultants	Packaging and Labeling Control
Buildings and Facilities	Materials examination and usage criteria
Design and construction features	Labeling issuance
Lighting	Packaging and labeling operations
Ventilation, air filtration, air heating and cooling	Tamper-resistant packaging requirements for
Plumbing	over-the-counter human drug products
Sewage and refuse	Drug product inspection
Washing and toilet facilities	Expiration dating
Sanitation	Holding and Distribution
Maintenance	Warehousing procedures
Equipment	Distribution procedures
Equipment design, size, and location	Laboratory Controls
Equipment construction	General requirements
Equipment cleaning and maintenance	Testing and release for distribution
Automatic, mechanical, and electronic	Stability testing
equipment	Special testing requirements
Filters	Reserve samples
Control of Components and Drug Product Containers	Laboratory animals
and Closures	Penicillin contamination
General requirements	Records and Reports
Receipt and storage of untested components, drug	General requirements
product containers, and closures	Equipment cleaning and use log
Testing and approval or rejection of components, drug	Component, drug product container, closure, and
product containers, and closures	labeling records
Use of approved components, drug product	Master production and control records
containers, and closures	Batch production and control records
Retesting of approved components, drug product	Production record review
containers, and closures	Laboratory records
Rejected components, drug product containers, and	Distribution records
closures	Complaint files
Drug product containers and closures	Returned and Salvaged Drug Products
Production and Process Controls	Returned drug products
Written procedures; deviations	Drug product salvaging
Charge-in of components	

*Code of Federal Regulations, 21, part 211, revised April 1, 1996.

Active Ingredient (AI) or Active Pharmaceutical Ingredient (API)—any component that is intended to furnish pharmacological activity or other direct effect in the diagnosis, cure, mitigation, treatment or prevention of disease or to affect the structure or function of the body of man or other animals.

Batch—a specific quantity of a drug of uniform specified quality produced according to a single manufacturing order during the same cycle of manufacture.

Batchwise Control—the use of validated in-process sampling and testing methods in such a way that results prove the process has done what it purports to do for the specific batch concerned.

Certification—documented testimony by qualified authorities that a system qualification, calibration, validation, or revalidation has been performed appropriately and that the results are acceptable.

Compliance—determination through inspection of the extent to which a manufacturer is complying with prescribed regulations, standards, and practices.

Component—any ingredient used in the manufacture of a drug product, including those which may not be present in the finished product.

Drug Product—a finished dosage form that contains an active drug ingredient in association with inactive ingredients. The term may also include a dosage form that does not contain an active ingredient, as a placebo.

Inactive Ingredient—any component other than the active ingredients in a drug product.

Lot—a batch or any portion of a batch having uniform specified quality and a distinctive identifying "lot number."

Lot Number, Control Number, or Batch Number—any distinctive combination of letters, numbers or symbols from which the complete history of the manufacture, processing, packaging, holding, and distribution of a batch or lot of a drug product may be determined.

Master Record—records containing the formulation, specifications, manufacturing procedures, quality assurance requirements, and labeling of a finished product.

Quality Assurance (QA)—the activity of providing, to all concerned, the evidence needed to establish confidence that the activities relating to quality are being performed adequately.

Quality Audit—a documented activity performed in accordance with established procedures on a planned and periodic basis to verify compliance with the procedures to assure quality.

Quality Control (QC)—the regulatory process through which industry measures actual quality performance, compares it with standards, and acts on the difference.

Quality Control Unit—an organizational element designated by the firm to be responsible for the duties relating to quality control.

Quarantined—an area that is marked, designated, or set aside for the holding of incoming components prior to acceptance testing and qualification for use.

Representative Sample—a sample of a number of units drawn on rational criteria such as random sampling intended to ensure that the sample accurately portrays the entire material being sampled.

Reprocessing—the activity whereby the finished product or any of its components is recycled through all or part of the manufacturing process.

Strength—the concentration of the drug substance per unit dose or volume.

Verified—signed by a second individual or recorded by automated equipment.

Validation—establishing documented evidence that a system does what it purports to do (e.g., equipment, software, controls).

Process Validation—establishing documented evidence that a process does what it purports to do (e.g., sterilization).

Validation Protocol—a prospective experimental plan that, when executed, is intended to produce documented evidence that the system has been validated.

Organization and Personnel

This section of the regulations deals with the responsibilities of the quality control unit, employees, and consultants.

The regulations require that a quality control unit has the authority and responsibility for all functions that may affect product quality. This includes accepting or rejecting product components, product specifications, finished products, packaging, and labeling. Adequate laboratory facilities shall be provided, written procedures followed, and all records maintained.

All personnel engaged in the manufacture, processing, packing, or holding of a drug product, including those in supervisory positions, are required to have the education, training, and/or experience needed to fulfill the assigned responsibility. Appropriate programs of skill development, continuing education and training, and performance evaluations are essential in maintaining quality assurance. Any consultants advising on scientific and technical matters should possess requisite qualifications for the tasks.

Buildings and Facilities

As outlined in Table 5.1, the regulations in this section include the design, structural features, and functional aspects of buildings and facilities. Each building's structure, space, design, and placement of equipment must be such to enable thorough cleaning, inspection, and safe and effective use for the designated operations. Proper considerations must be given to such factors as water quality standards; security; materials used for floors, walls, and ceilings; lighting; segregated quarantine areas for raw materials and product components subject to quality control approval; holding areas for rejected components; storage areas for released components; weighing and measuring rooms; sterile areas for ophthalmic and parenteral products; flammable materials storage areas; finished products storage; control of heat, humidity, temperature, and ventilation; waste handling; employee facilities and safety procedures in compliance with the Occupational Safety and Health Administration (OSHA) regulations; and procedures and practices of personal sanitation.

All work in the manufacture, processing, packing, or holding of a pharmaceutical product must be logged in, supervisor-inspected, and signed off. Similarly, a log of building maintenance must be kept to document this component of the regulations.

Equipment

Each piece of equipment must be of appropriate design and size, and suitably located to facilitate operations for its intended use, cleaning, and maintenance. The equipment's surfaces and parts must not interact with the processes or product's components so as to alter the purity, strength, or quality.

Standard operating procedures (SOPs) must be written and followed for the proper use, mainte-

nance, and cleaning of each piece of equipment, and appropriate logs and records must be kept. Automated equipment and computers used in the processes must be routinely calibrated, maintained, and validated for accuracy.

Filters for liquid filtration in the manufacture or processing of injectable drug products shall not release fibers into such products. If fiber-releasing filters must be used, non–fiber-releasing filters also must be used to reduce any fiber content.

Control of Components, Containers, and Closures

Written procedures are required to be maintained and followed describing the receipt, identification, storage, handling, sampling, testing, and approval or rejection of all drug-product components, product containers, and closures.

Bulk pharmaceutical chemicals, containers, and closures must meet the exact physical and chemical specifications established with the supplier at the time of ordering.

When product components are received from a supplier, each lot must be logged in with the purchase order number, date of receipt, bill of lading, name and vital information on the supplier, supplier's stock or control number, and quantity received. The component is assigned a control number, identifying both the component and the intended product. Raw materials are quarantined until they are verified, through representative sampling and careful qualitative and quantitative analysis. Only those meeting the specifications are approved and released by the quality control unit for use in product manufacture. The assigned control number follows the component throughout production so it can be traced if necessary.

Rejected components, drug product containers, and closures are identified and controlled under a quarantine system to prevent their use in manufacturing and processing operations.

Production and Process Controls

Written procedures are required for production and process controls to ensure that the drug products have the correct identity, strength, quality, and purity. These procedures, which include the charge-in of all components, use of in-process controls, sample-testing, and process and equipment validation must be followed for quality assurance. Any deviation from the written procedures must be recorded and justified. In most instances, a system of time and date recording by the operator and supervisor sign-off is applied to each key operation. When operations are controlled by automated equipment, such equipment must be validated regularly for precision.

All product ingredients, equipment used, and drums or other containers of bulk finished product must be distinctively identified by labeling as to content and/or status.

In-process samples are taken from production batches periodically for product control. In-process controls are of two general types: 1) those performed by production personnel at the time of operation to ensure that the machinery is producing output within preestablished control limits (e.g., tablet size, hardness), and 2) those performed by the quality control laboratory personnel to assure compliance to all product specifications (e.g., tablet content, dissolution) and batch-to-batch consistency. Product found out-of-standard sometimes may be reprocessed for subsequent use. However, in this, as in all instances, procedures must be performed according to established protocol, all materials must be accounted for, all specifications met, and all records meticulously maintained.

Packaging and Labeling Control

Written procedures are required for the receipt, identification, storage, handling, sampling and testing, and issuance of labeling and packaging materials. Labeling for each different drug product, strength, dosage form, or quantity of contents must be stored separately with suitable identification. Obsolete and outdated labels and other packaging materials must be destroyed. Access to the storage area must be limited to authorized personnel.

All materials must be withheld for use in the packaging and labeling of product until approved and released by the quality control unit. Control procedures must be followed and records maintained for the issuance and use of product labeling. Quantities issued, used, and returned must be reconciled and discrepancies investigated. Before labeling operations commence, the labeling facilities must be inspected to assure that all drug products and labels have been removed from the previous operations. During and at the conclusion of an operation, the products are visually or electronically inspected for assurance of correct labeling and packaging. All of these procedures are essential to avoid label mixups and the mislabeling of products. All records of inspections and controls must be documented in the batch production records.

Labels must meet the legal requirements for content, as outlined in Chapter 2 and later in this chapter. Each label must contain expiration dating and the production batch or lot number to facilitate product identification. Special packaging requirements may apply in certain instances, as tamper-evident packaging for OTC products.

Expiration Dating

To ensure that a drug product meets applicable standards of identity, strength, quality and purity at the time of use, it must bear an expiration date determined by appropriate stability testing. Exempt from this requirement are homeopathic drug products, allergenic extracts, and investigational new drugs providing the latter meet the standards established during preclinical and clinical studies.

Tamper-evident Packaging

On November 5, 1982, the Food and Drug Administration published initial regulations on tamper-resistant packaging in the Federal Register. These regulations were promulgated after the criminal tampering with OTC drug products earlier in that year resulting in consumer illness and deaths. In the primary incident, cyanide surreptitiously had been placed in acetaminophen capsules in commercial packages for consumer purchase.

Today, the CGMP regulations require tamper-evident packaging for OTC drug products to improve their security and to ensure their safety and effectiveness. All OTC drug products offered for retail sale are required to have tamper-evident packaging except for some categories as dentifrices, dermatologicals, insulin, and throat lozenge products. For other product categories, a manufacturer may request an exemption for a specific product by filing with the FDA a "Request for Exemption from Tamper Evident Rule." The petition is required to contain specific information on the drug product, the reasons the requirement is unnecessary or cannot be achieved, and alternative steps the petitioner has taken, or may take, to reduce the likelihood of malicious adulteration to the product. Generally exempt from these regulations are products not packaged for retail sale but rather distributed to hospitals, nursing homes, and health care clinics for institutional use.

A tamper-evident package is defined as "one having one or more indicators or barriers to entry which, if breached or missing, can reasonably be expected to provide visible evidence to consumers that tampering has occurred" (1). The indicators or barriers may involve the immediate drug product container and/or an outer container or carton. For two-piece hard gelatin capsule products, a minimum of two tamper-evident packaging features is required unless the capsules are sealed by a tamper-resistant technology.

Even with these safeguards in effect, the possibility of drug product tampering requires the pharmacist and consumer to remain constantly vigilant for signs of product entry. Pharmaceutical manufacturers have the option of determining the type of tamper-resistant packaging to use. Table 5.2 presents some examples of tamper-evident packaging.

Holding and Distribution

Written procedures must be established and followed for the holding and distribution of product. Finished pharmaceuticals must be quarantined in storage until released by the quality control unit. Products must be stored and shipped under conditions that do not affect product quality. Ordinarily, the oldest approved stock is distributed first. A distribution control system must be in place through which the distributed point of each lot of drug product may be readily determined to facilitate its recall if necessary.

Laboratory Controls

This section contains requirements for the establishment of, and conformance to, written specifications, standards, sampling plans, test procedures, and other laboratory control mechanisms. The spec-

ifications apply to each batch of drug product and include provisions for sample size, test intervals, sample storage, stability testing, and special testing requirements for certain dosage forms including parenterals, ophthalmics, controlled-release products and radioactive pharmaceuticals. Reserve samples must be retained for distributed products for specified periods of time depending on their category. Reserve samples must be maintained for 1 to 3 years after the expiration date of the last lot of the drug product.

Records and Reports

Production, control, and distribution records are required to be maintained for at least a year following the expiration date of a product batch. This includes equipment cleaning and maintenance logs, specifications and lot numbers of product components, including raw materials and product containers/closures, and label records. Complete master production and control records for each production batch must be maintained, including the name and strength of the product, dosage form, quantitative amounts of components and dosage units, complete manufacturing and control procedures, specifications, special notations, equipment used, in-process controls, sampling and laboratory methods used and assay results, calibration of instrumentation, distribution records, and dated and employee-identified records documenting that each step in the production, control, packaging, labeling, and distribution of the product was

Table 5.2. Tamper-Evident Packaging Examples

Package Type	Tamper Protection
Film wrappers	Film wrapped and sealed around product and/or product containers; the film must be cut or torn to remove product.
Blister/strip packs	Individually sealed dosage units; removal requires tearing or breaking individual compartment.
Bubble packs	Product and container sealed in plastic, usually mounted on/in display card; plastic must be cut or broken open to remove product.
Shrink seals/bands	Bands or wrappers which are shrunk by heat or drying to conform to cap and containers must be torn to open.
Foil, paper, or Plastic Pouches	Sealed individual packets; must be torn to reach product.
Bottle seals	Paper or foil sealed to mouth of a container under cap; must be torn or broken to reach product.
Tape seals	Paper or foil sealed over carton flap or bottle cap; must be torn or broken to reach product.
Breakable caps	Plastic or metal "tearaway" caps over container; must be broken to remove.
Sealed tubes	Seal over mouth of tube; must be punctured to reach product.
Sealed cartons	Carton flaps are sealed; carton cannot be opened without damage.
Aerosol containers	Tamper-resistant by design.

accomplished and approved by the quality control unit. Depending on the operation, the operator's and/or supervisor's full signatures, initials, or other written or electronic identification codes are required.

Records of written and oral complaints regarding a drug product (e.g., product failure, adverse drug experience) must also be maintained, along with information regarding the internal disposition of each complaint. All records must be made available at the time of inspection by FDA officials.

Returned and Salvaged Drug Products

Returned drug products (as from wholesalers) must be identified by lot number and product quality determined through appropriate testing. Drug products that meet specifications may be salvaged or reprocessed. Those that do not, as well as those that have been subjected to improper storage conditions (e.g., extremes in temperature) shall not be returned to the marketplace. Records for all returned products must be maintained and must include the date and reasons for the return; quantity

and lot number of product returned; procedures employed for holding, testing, and reprocessing the product; and the product's disposition.

Information Technology and Automation

Although not part of the CGMP requirements, the effective deployment of information technologies and automated systems can enhance pharmaceutical process development, production efficiencies, product quality and regulatory compliance (5).

Computers are used extensively in plant operations such as production scheduling, in-process manufacturing, quality control, and packaging and labeling. The networking of computers in the production and quality control areas fully integrates laboratory information and manufacturing operations into sophisticated management systems. These integrated systems support CGMP compliance, process validation, resource management, and cost control. Figure 5.1 presents an example of computer use in the pharmaceutical industry for the management of plant operations.

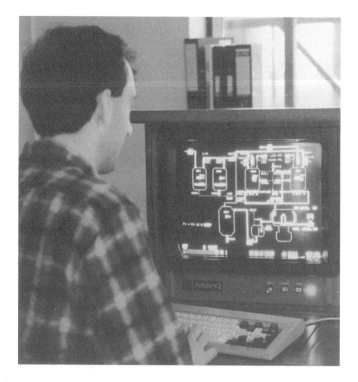

Fig. 5.1 *Example of computer use in the pharmaceutical industry. The machine shown is an Allen Bradley, Advisor 2+ operator interface. This allows the plant operator to communicate with the main programmable logical controller (PLC). The advisor 2+ gives a constant real-time update of the process on a series of screens and allows an operator to perform preprogrammed operations at the push of a button. (Courtesy of Elan Corporation, plc.)*

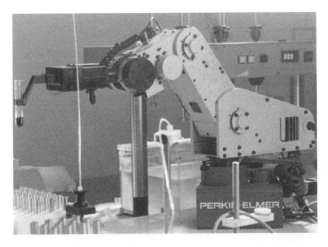

Fig. 5.2 *Robotics in laboratory use. Perkin-Elmer Robotic Arm and Perkin-Elmer Lambda 1a UV/VIS Spectrophotometer. (Courtesy of Elan Corporation, plc.)*

Robotic devices increasingly are being employed to replace manual operations in production lines, analytical sampling, and packaging. Figure 5.2 presents an example of robotic use in the laboratory. Laboratory robotics provides automation in areas as sample preparation and handling, wet chemistry procedures, laboratory process control, and instrumental analysis (6). Pharmaceutical applications of robotics include automated product handling in production lines and in procedures as sampling and analysis, tablet content uniformity, and dissolution testing.

Additional CGMP Regulatory Requirements

Active Pharmaceutical Ingredients (APIs) and Pharmaceutical Excipients

The manufacture of active pharmaceutical ingredients (APIs) come under the aegis of CGMP regulations and requirements. The FDA publication, Guide to the Inspection of Bulk Pharmaceutical Chemicals, (7) identifies the Agency's inspection program for manufactures of chemical components of pharmaceutical products to assure that all required standards for quality are met. Because the quality of any finished pharmaceutical product depends on the quality of the various components, including the active ingredients, compliance with CGMPs is a critical part of the FDA's preapproval inspection program for NDA and ANDA applications.

The broad CGMP areas described previously for finished pharmaceuticals (as facilities, personnel, production and process controls, process validation) apply, but are directed toward the process-specific aspects of bulk pharmaceutical chemicals. The application of the regulations are focused on all of the defining elements of chemical purity and quality, including specifications and analytical methods for all reactive and non-reactive components used in the synthesis, critical chemical reaction steps, handling of chemical intermediates, effect of scale-up of chemical batches on the yield, quality of the water systems, solvent handling and recovery systems, analytical methods to detect impurities or chemical residues and the limits set, and stability studies of the bulk pharmaceutical chemical (8–9).

Pharmaceutical excipients, as they too are components of finished pharmaceutical products, must be produced in accordance with CGMP standards as certified on the application by each sponsor of an NDA or ANDA. Although there is no current FDA approval system specific for pharmaceutical excipients, a comprehensive good manufacturing practices guide has been established by the U.S. affiliate of the International Pharmaceutical Excipients Council (IPEC) and is harmonized with the European counterpart organization (10).

Clinical Trial Materials (CTM)

Clinical trial materials (CTM) must be produced in conformance with CGMP regulations. This applies both to the production of the active pharmaceutical ingredients (API) and investigational drug products.

The API used in a clinical investigation is subject to all of the requirements for the production of bulk pharmaceutical chemicals discussed above. However, the batch size prepared would be different from the commercial-scale used in the production of an FDA-approved pharmaceutical product. In some cases, technology transfer in the production of an API from one production site or laboratory to another may be involved, requiring validation to assure purity and quality standards.

The CTMs used in clinical investigations must be produced in compliance with the CGMP regulatory requirements and standardized as to identity, purity, strength, and quality (11). However, during preclinical testing and the early phases of clinical evaluation, a product's formulation and many of the production processes and analytical controls are under development. Thus, during this period, the regulatory requirements are applied with flexibility. As the clinical trials progress from phase 1 to phase 2, the processes are being characterized and refined, and during phase 3 they are expected to fully meet the regulatory requirements. It is during phase 3 that process optimization is demonstrated to the FDA by the production of at least one-tenth of a commercial-size batch (e.g., 100,000 capsules) of the proposed product. Prior to that, adequate supplies of dosing units from a few hundred to a few thousand or more dosage units may be prepared by hand or in pilot-plant scale operations as is necessary for the conduct of the clinical trials.

In addition to the active drug product, matching placebo and/or comparator products must be prepared. Specific labeling, coding, packaging design, assembly, and distribution protocols are in effect for CTMs to accommodate the clinical trial design and the requirements for investigational drugs as discussed in Chapter 2.

Biologics

As noted previously, current good manufacturing practice standards are defined for biologic products in the Code of Federal Regulations (2). While the basic regulations as described above for finished pharmaceuticals apply to biologic products as well, the nature of blood, bacterial, and viral products requires specific additional mandates. A full discussion of the CGMP requirements and standards for biologics are outside of the scope of this text; however, the following examples of specific areas of activity demonstrates the scope of the additional regulatory content: blood collection procedures; environmental controls; segregation of activities; containment; cell bank and cell line characterization and testing; cell propagation and fermentation; inactivation of infectious agents; aseptic processing validation; use of bioassays; live vaccine work areas; work with spore-bearing organisms; and, evaluation, quantification and validation of risk factors.

Medical Devices

Medical devices follow a path for FDA approval that resembles that for pharmaceuticals. For instance, clinical investigations of devices are conducted on approval of an investigational device exemption (IDE), and approved for marketing when shown to be safe and effective through a Premarket Approval (PMA) application, similar to an IND and NDA respectively for a new drug. Medical devices also are subject to the reporting of adverse events, to recall, and to termination of approval.

The regulations for the "Good Manufacturing Practice for Medical Devices" are similar in organizational structure to those for finished pharmaceuticals and include sections on personnel; buildings; equipment; control of components; production and process controls; packaging and labeling; holding, distribution and installation, device evaluation, and records (4).

There are literally thousands of medical devices that are regulated by the provisions of the Code of Federal Regulations. Each device is of specific design with individual performance features and utility. For many devices, specific standards are stated in the regulations. The range of devices covered by GMP regulations is illustrated by the following: intraocular lenses, hearing aid devices, intrauterine devices, cardiac pacemakers, clinical chemistry analyzers, catheters, cardiopulmonary bypass heart-lung machine console, dental x-ray equipment, surgeon's gloves, condoms, prosthetic hip joint, traction equipment, computed tomography (CT) equipment, and powered wheelchairs.

Noncompliance with CGMP Regulations

Noncompliance with CGMP regulations can lead to a number of regulatory actions by the FDA. Noncompliance determined during a premarket approval inspection of facilities, as part of an NDA or ANDA application, likely would result in a delay of approval of an otherwise approvable application. Noncompliance with CGMP regulations during a regularly scheduled FDA inspection could lead to various actions depending on the severity of the violative offenses. In most instances, time for corrective action is given with the firm required to institute and document corrective measures and undergo reinspection. In a worst case scenario, the FDA is empowered to remove violative products from the market, to withdraw product approvals, and to restrict further applications. All FDA actions are appealable.

CGMP Requirements for Manufacturing in Pharmacies

The FDA's CGMP regulations apply to community or institutional pharmacies engaged in the manufacture, repackaging, or relabeling of drugs and drug products in a supplier function and beyond the usual conduct of professional dispensing. Pharmacies which engage in such activities must register with the FDA as a manufacturer or distributor and be subject to FDA inspection at regular intervals. Included are hospital pharmacies that repackage drug products for their own use as well as the use of other hospitals; chain pharmacy operations that repackage and relabel bulk quantities of products from the manufacturer's original containers for distribution to individual pharmacies within the chain; and similar repackaging and relabeling activities conducted by individual pharmacists or pharmacies for distribution to other pharmacies or retailers.

Recently, professional and legislative attention has been directed toward differentiating between pharmaceutical manufacturing and compounding as practiced by community pharmacists (12). Pharmaceutical manufacturing involves the large-scale production of drugs or drug products for distribution and sale, whereas compounding involves the professional preparation of prescriptions for specific patients as a part of the traditional practice of pharmacy.

Current Good Compounding Practices

In recent years a number of activities have surfaced concerning the ability of pharmacists to compound patient-specific medications. An increase in the incidence of pharmaceutical compounding was noted in the 1970s that continued into the 1980s. By the early and mid 1990s, compounding was making a dramatic comeback in pharmacy practice. A number of reasons have been presented for the increase in preparing patient-specific medications, including the following.

1. Many patients need drug dosages that are not commercially available.

2. Many patients need dosage forms, such as suppositories, oral liquids, topicals, that are not commercially available.
3. Many patients are allergic to excipients in some of the commercially available products.
4. Pediatric medications need to be prepared as liquids, flavored to enhance compliance, and prepared in alternative dosage forms, such as lozenges, gummy-bears, and popsicles.
5. Some medications are not very stable and require preparation and dispensing every few days; they are not really suitable to be manufactured products.
6. Many products are reported in the literature but are not manufactured yet, so pharmacists can compound them for their patients use.
7. Many physicians desire to try products in innovative ways and pharmacists can work with them to solve patient medication problems.
8. Most products are not available for veterinary patients and must be compounded.
9. Home healthcare and the treatment of an increasing number of patients in the home environment has resulted in many community pharmacies and home healthcare pharmacies preparing sterile products for home use; formerly, most sterile products were compounded in hospital pharmacies.

As the extent of compounding increased, many standard-setting agencies and regulatory bodies wanted to ensure quality compounded products; consequently, there was a lot of activity during the mid 1990s to establish guidelines for pharmaceutical compounding.

U.S. Pharmacopeia / National Formulary

In 1990, the U.S. Pharmacopeial Convention approved the appointment of a Pharmacy Compounding Practices Expert Advisory Panel. The activities of the Panel initially were to prepare a chapter for the USP and to begin the process of preparing monographs of compounded products for inclusion in the NF. The prepared chapter, Pharmacy Compounding Practices was published and became official in 1996 (13). The first of the compounding monographs became official in 1998 in the National Formulary section of the USP/NF. For each monograph published, a considerable amount of work is done including a detailed, validated stability study. Some monographs that were previously published in the USP/NF are being reintroduced into the compendia.

The chapter on Pharmacy Compounding Practices includes the following discussions: 1) compounding environment; 2) stability of compounded preparations; 3) ingredient selection and calculations; 4) checklist for acceptable strength, quality and purity; 5) compounded dosage forms; 6) compounding process; 7) compounding records and documents; 8) quality control; and 9) patient counseling.

The introduction to the chapter discusses the difference between manufacturing and compounding. Generally speaking, compounding differs from manufacturing due to the existence of specific practitioner-patient-pharmacist relationships; the quantity of medication prepared in anticipation of receiving a prescription or a prescription order; and the conditions of sale, which are limited to specific prescription orders.

The compounding environment section discusses the design and maintenance of the facilities to be used and the equipment that is selected for compounding. It refers to other specific chapters in the USP, namely the "Weights and Balances and the Prescription Balances" and "Volumetric Apparatus" chapters. Any equipment used for compounding must be of appropriate design and size for compounding and suitable for the intended use.

The discussion on stability includes packaging, sterility, stability criteria and guidelines for assigning beyond-use dates for compounded preparations; the latter detailed as follows:

"In the absence of stability information that is applicable to a specific drug and preparation, the following maximum beyond-use dates are recommended for nonsterile compounded drug preparations that are packaged in tight, light-resistant containers and stored at controlled room temperature unless otherwise indicated."

For nonaqueous liquids and solid formulations, 1) where the manufactured drug product is the source of active ingredient, the beyond-use date is not later than 25% of the time remaining until the product's expiration date or 6 months, whichever is earlier; 2) where a USP or NF substance is the source of active ingredient, the beyond-use date is not later than 6 months.

For water-containing formulations prepared from ingredients in solid form, the beyond-use date is not later than 14 days when stored at cold temperatures.

For all other formulations, the beyond-use date is not later than the intended duration of therapy of 30 days, whichever is earlier.

The chapter goes on to detail that these beyond-use date limits can be exceeded if there is support-

ing valid scientific stability information that is directly applicable to the product being compounded. The product must be of the same drug, in a similar concentration, pH, excipients, vehicle, water content, etc.

The section on ingredient selection describes sources for drugs and excipients as follows:

1. A USP or NF grade substance is the preferred source for compounding.
2. A drug of the highest quality, reasonably available, may be used, preferably one listed as ACS (American Chemical Society) or FCC (Food and Chemicals Codex) grade. Material Safety Data Sheets should be maintained on all materials used for compounding in the pharmacy.
3. A manufactured drug product can be used as a source of a drug, excipient or vehicle. If manufactured drugs are used as the source for the active drugs, then the presence of all excipients must be considered in the overall acceptability of the final product.

Calculations are discussed as they relate to the amount of concentration of drug substances in each unit or dosage portion of a compounded preparation. Special emphasis is placed on calculations involving the purity and potency of drugs, their salt forms, and equivalent potencies.

The chapter also details a checklist that can be used to consider the advisability of preparing a compounded dosage form. It then details many dosage forms and some quality control characteristics that can be checked in the final compounded products. Following is a discussion of the steps involved in a compounding process that can be used as a template for compounding prescriptions. Recordkeeping requirements of various states must be followed and generally include a formulation record and a compounding record.

An emphasis on quality control and the responsibility of the pharmacist in reviewing each procedure and observing the finished preparation is discussed. The chapter ends with the importance of patient counseling in the proper use, storage and observation for instability of the dispensed product. The overall emphasis of the chapter is to support the pharmacist in the compounding of products of acceptable strength, quality and purity.

During the early and mid-1990s, the Food and Drug Administration district offices began investigating a number of pharmacies that were compounding very large quantities of selected drug products. Also during this time period, an unfortunate accident was reported where some ophthalmic products were improperly autoclaved resulting in the loss of sight of a patient. Some other incidences were reported and the Food and Drug Administration became active in investigating individual compounding pharmacies.

At the American Pharmaceutical Association meeting in 1993, FDA Commissioner Kesler stated that it was not the purpose of the FDA to stop the compounding activities of pharmacists but to stop the practice of manufacturing under the guise of compounding. However, over the next few years, the activities of the FDA inspectors and district personnel increased resulting in some pharmacists being threatened with arrest and legal proceedings as their compounded products did not meet the definition of manufactured products as "New Drugs."The FDA was determined to require that all compounded medications meet the requirements set forth as a "New Drug" or else they could not be dispensed to patients. Obviously, this was impossible and seriously threatened pharmaceutical compounding.

The national pharmacy organizations became united in their efforts to protect the rights of pharmacists to compound. The National Association of Boards of Pharmacy promulgated the Good Compounding Practices that have been either adopted or modified and adopted by many states.The U.S. Pharmacopeial Convention became involved in compounding by preparing a chapter for the USP/NF and in establishing monographs for the compendia. In 1997, the efforts of many organizations, politicians and pharmacists resulted in a section of the Food and Drug Administration Modernization Act of 1997 (12) being aimed at supporting pharmacists right to compound, with some guidelines.

Food and Drug Modernization Act of 1997

The purpose of Section 127 of Public Law 105–115 was to ensure patient access to individualized drug therapy and prevent unnecessary FDA regulation of health professional practice. This legislation exempts pharmacy compounding from several regulatory requirements but would not exempt drug manufacturing from the Act's requirements. The legislation also sets forth conditions that must be met in order to qualify for exemption from the Act's requirements.

The Act states that a compounded product is exempt if the drug product is compounded for an individual patient based on the unsolicited receipt of a valid prescription order or a notation, approved by the prescribing practitioner, on the prescription order that a compounded product is necessary for the identified patient, if the product meets certain requirements.

The Act also describes the bulk drug substances and other materials that can be used in compounding and the general requirements for compounding products that are similar to commercially available drugs. Further, a Memorandum of Understanding (MOU) can be established between the Secretary and the individual State Agency in the event a compounding pharmacy needs to compound inordinate amounts of drug products for interstate shipment; generally a 5% limit is set on the amount of compounded products of a pharmacy that can be shipped out of state without this MOU.

A pharmacy cannot advertise or promote the compounding of any particular drug, class of drug, or type of drug but can advertise and promote the compounding service provided by the pharmacy.

This Act removes any doubt that compounding is legal under the FDC Act and Congress has clearly recognized the importance of compounding.

National Association of Boards of Pharmacy

The Good Compounding Practices Applicable to State-Licensed Pharmacies (14) document developed by the National Association of Boards of Pharmacy discuss eight different recommendations. The subparts include (A) general provisions, (B) organization and personnel, (C) drug compounding facilities, (D) equipment, (E) control of components and drug product containers and closures, (F) drug compounding controls, (G) labeling control of excess products and records and reports.

Subpart (A), General Provisions, provides two important definitions, as follows:

> Compounding—the preparation, mixing, assembling, packaging, or labeling of a drug or device (i) as the result of a practitioner's prescription drug order or initiative based on the practitioner/patient/pharmacist relationship in the course of professional practice, or (ii) for the purpose of, or as an incident to, research, teaching, or chemical analysis and not for sale or dispensing. Compounding also includes the preparation of drugs or devices in anticipation of prescription drug orders based on routine, regularly observed prescribing patterns.

Manufacturing—the production, preparation, propagation, conversion, or processing of a drug or device, either directly or indirectly, by extraction from substances of natural origin or independently by means of chemical or biological synthesis, and includes any packaging or repackaging of the substance(s) or labeling or relabeling of its container, and the promotion and marketing of such drugs or devices. Manufacturing also includes the preparation and promotion of commercially available products from bulk compounds for resale by pharmacies, practitioners, or other persons.

Subpart (B), Organization and Personnel, discusses the responsibilities of pharmacists and other personnel engaged in compounding. It also stresses that only personnel authorized by the responsible pharmacist shall be in the immediate vicinity of the drug compounding operation.

Subpart (C), Drug Compounding Facilities, describes the areas that should be set aside for compounding, either nonsterile or sterile compounding. Special attention is required for radiopharmaceuticals and for products requiring special precautions to minimize contamination, such as penicillin, etc.

Subpart (D), Equipment, states that equipment used must be of appropriate design, adequate size and suitably located to facilitate operation for its intended use and for its cleaning and maintenance. If automated, mechanical or electronic equipment is used, controls must be in place to assure proper performance.

Subpart (E), Control of Components and Drug Product Containers and Closures, describes the packaging requirements for compounded products.

Subpart (F), Drug Compounding Controls, discuss the written procedures to ensure that the finished products are of the proper identity, strength, quality and purity, as labeled.

Subpart (G), Labeling Control of Excess Products and Records and Reports, describes the various records and reports that are required under these Guidelines.

Many individual states have used this Model and implemented their own version for their specific states and situations. All pharmacists and pharmacy students should become familiar with the individual state requirements in the state in which they practice.

It will be important as compounding pharmacy increases to ensure reasonable agreement between the national and state agencies so pharmacists will have a set of guidelines within which they can work within the law and provide their patients the needed individualized medications.

Packaging, Labeling, and Storage of Pharmaceuticals

The proper packaging, labeling, and storage of pharmaceutical products all are essential for product stability and efficacious use.

Containers

Standards for the packaging of pharmaceuticals by manufacturers are contained in the Current Good Manufacturing Practice section of Code of Federal Regulations (1), in the United States Pharmacopeia/National Formulary (15), and in the FDA's Guideline for Submitting Documentation for Packaging for Human Drugs and Biologics (16). When submitting a new drug application, the manufacturer must include all relevant specifications for the packaging of the product. During the initial stages of clinical investigations, the packaging must be shown to be effective in providing adequate drug stability for the duration of the clinical trials. As the clinical trials advance to their final stage, information must be developed on the chemical and physical characteristics of the container, closure, and other component parts of the package system for the proposed product to assure drug stability for its anticipated shelf-life.

Different specifications are required for parenteral, nonparenteral, pressurized, and bulk containers, and for those made of glass, plastic, and metal. In each instance, the package and closure system must be shown to be effective for the particular product for which it is intended. Depending on the intended use and type of container, among the tests performed are: physicochemical tests; light-transmission tests for glass or plastic; drug compatibility; leaching and/or migration tests; vapor-transmission test for plastics; moisture barrier tests; toxicity studies for plastics; valve, actuator, metered-dose, particle size, spray characteristics, and leak testing for aerosols; sterility and permeation tests for parenteral containers; and drug stability for all packaging.

Compendial terms applying to types of containers and conditions of storage have defined meanings (15). According to the USP, a container is "that which holds the article and is or may be in direct contact with the article." The immediate container is "that which is in direct contact with the article at all times." The closure is part of the container. The container, including the closure, should be clean and dry prior to its being filled with the drug. The container must not interact physically or chemically with the drug so as to alter its strength, quality, or purity beyond the official requirements.

Containers are classified by the USP according to their ability to protect their contents from external conditions (15). The minimally acceptable container is termed a well-closed container. It "protects the contents from extraneous solids and from loss of the article under ordinary conditions of handling, shipment, storage, and distribution." A tight container "protects the contents from contamination by extraneous liquids, solids, or vapors, from loss of the article, and from efflorescence, deliquescence, or evaporation under the ordinary or customary conditions of handling, shipment, storage, and distribution and is capable of tight re-closure." A hermetic container "is impervious to air or any other gas under the ordinary or customary conditions of handling, shipment, storage, and distribution." Hermetic containers which are sterile are generally used to hold preparations intended for injection or parenteral administration. A single-dose container is one in which the quantity of drug contained is intended as a single dose and when opened cannot be resealed with assurance that sterility has been maintained. These containers include fusion-sealed ampuls, pre-filled syringes and cartridges. A multiple-dose container is a hermetic container that permits withdrawal of successive portions of the contents without changing the strength or endangering the quality or purity of the remaining portion. These containers are commonly referred to as vials. Examples of single-dose and multiple-dose products are shown in Figure 5.3.

Dosage forms, as tablets, capsules, and oral liquids, may be packaged in single-unit or multiple-unit containers. A single-unit container is designed to hold a quantity of drug intended for administration as a single dose promptly after the container is opened. Multiple-unit containers contain more than a single unit or dose of the medication. Examples of single-unit and multiple-unit packages are shown in Figure 5.4. A single-unit package is termed a unit-dose package when dispensed to a patient. The single-unit packaging of drugs may be performed on a large scale by a manufacturer or distributor or on a smaller scale by the pharmacy dispensing the medication. In either instance, the single-unit package must be appropriately labeled with the product identity, quality and/or strength, name of manufac-

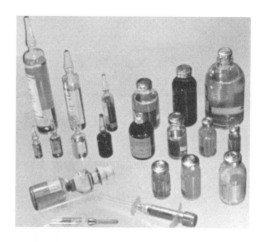

Fig. 5.3 *Examples of injectable products packaged in single-dose (ampuls) and multiple-dose (vials) containers and in unit-dose syringes.*

turer, and lot number of product to ensure the positive identification of the medication.

Although single-unit packaging has particular usefulness in institutional settings as hospitals and extended care facilities it is not limited to such. Many outpatients find single-unit packages a convenient and sanitary means of maintaining and utilizing their medication. Among the advantages cited for single-unit packaging and unit-dose dispensing are: positive identification of each dosage unit and reduction of medication errors; reduced contamination of the drug due to its protective wrapping; reduced dispensing time; greater ease of inventory control in the pharmacy or nursing station; and, elimination of waste through better medication management with less discarded medication.

Many hospitals with unit-dose systems use strip packaging equipment for the packaging of oral solids (Fig. 5.5). Such equipment seals solid dosage forms into four-sided pouches and imprints dose identification on each package at the same time. The equipment can be adjusted to produce individual single-cut packages or perforated strips or rolls of singly packaged dosage units. The packaging materials may be combinations of paper, foil, plastics or cellophane. Some drugs must be packaged in foil-to-foil wrappings to prevent the deteriorating effects of light or the permeation of moisture. The packaging of solid dosage forms in clear plastic or aluminum blister wells is perhaps the most popular method of single-unit packaging (Fig. 5.6).

Oral liquids may be single-unit dispensed in paper, plastic, or foil cups, or pre-packaged and

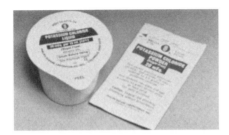
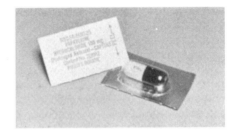
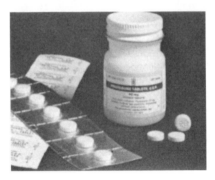

Fig. 5.4 *Examples of multiple-unit and single-unit packaging, including patient cup, unit dose of powder, blister packaging of single capsule, and strip packaging of tablets. (Courtesy of Roxane Laboratories.)*

dispensed in glass containers having threaded caps or crimped aluminum caps. A number of hospital pharmacies package oral liquids for pediatric use in disposable plastic syringes with rubber or plastic tips on the orifice for closure. In these instances, the nursing staff must be fully aware of the novel packaging and special labeling used to indicate "not for injection." Other dosage forms, as suppositories, powders, ointments, creams, and ophthalmic solutions, are also commonly found in single-unit packages provided by their manufacturers. However, the relatively infrequent use of these dosage forms in a given hospital, extended care facility, or community pharmacy does not generally justify the expense of purchasing the specialized packaging machinery necessary for the small-scale packaging of these forms.

Some pharmaceutical manufacturers use unit-of-use packaging; that is, packaging in which the quantity of drug product prescribed is packaged in a container for dispensing. For example, if certain antibiotic capsules are usually prescribed to be taken 4 times a day for 10 days, unit-of-use packaging would contain 40 capsules. Other products may be packaged to contain a month's supply.

Many pharmaceutical products require light-resistant containers to protect them from photochemical deterioration. In most instances a container made of a good quality of amber glass or a light-resistant opaque plastic will reduce light transmission sufficiently to protect a light-sensitive pharma-

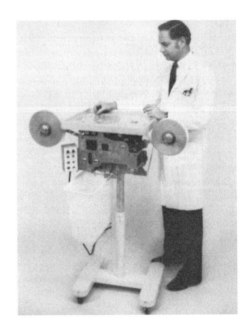

Fig. 5.5 *Strip packaging equipment capable of producing 50 packages per minute. Seals solid dosage units in a variety of wrapping materials and labels each package simultaneously. (Courtesy of Packaging Machinery Associates.)*

ceutical. Agents termed UV-absorbers may be added to plastic to decrease the transmission of short ultraviolet rays. The USP provides tests and standards for

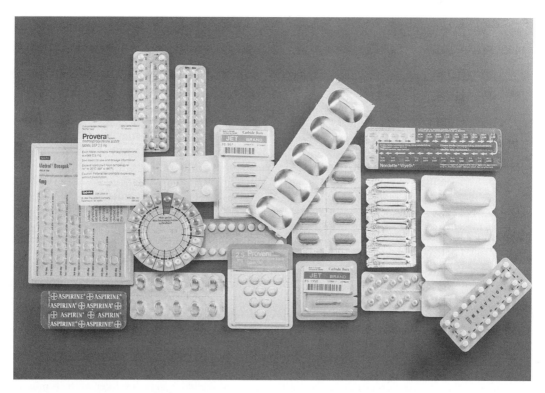

Fig. 5.6 *Examples of the commercial blister packaging of pharmaceuticals. (Courtesy of Hueck Foils L.L.C.)*

glass and plastic containers with respect to their ability to prevent the transmission of light (15). Containers intended to provide protection from light or those offered as "light-resistant" containers must meet the USP standards which define the acceptable limits of light transmission at any wavelength of light between 290 and 450 nm. A recent innovation in plastic packaging is the coextruded two-layer high density polyethylene bottle which has an inner layer of black polyethylene co-extruded with an outer layer of white polyethylene. The container provides both light resistance (exceeding amber glass) and moisture protection. It is increasingly being used in the packaging of tablets and capsules.

The glass used in packaging pharmaceuticals is classified into four categories, depending upon the chemical constitution of the glass and its ability to resist deterioration. Table 5.3 presents the chemical make-up of the various glasses; types I, II, and III are intended for parenteral products and type NP is intended for nonparenteral products. Each type is tested according to its resistance to water attack. The degree of attack is determined by the amount of alkali released from the glass under the test conditions specified. Obviously the leaching of alkali from the glass into a pharmaceutical solution or preparation could alter the pH and thus the stability of the product. Pharmaceutical manufacturers must select and utilize containers which do not adversely affect the composition or stability of their products. Type I is the most resistant glass of the four categories.

Today most pharmaceutical products are packaged in plastic. The modern compact-type container used for oral contraceptives, which contains sufficient tablets for a monthly cycle of administration and permits the scheduled removal of one tablet at a time, is a prime example of contemporary plastic packaging (see Fig. 5.6). Plastic bags for intravenous fluids, plastic ointment tubes, plastic film protected suppositories and plastic tablet and capsule vials are other examples of plastics used in pharmaceutical packaging.

Table 5.3. Constitution of Official Glass Types

Type	General Description
I	Highly resistant, borosilicate glass
II	Treated soda-lime glass
III	Soda-lime glass
NP	General purpose soda-lime glass

The widespread use of plastic containers has been generated by a number of factors including: its advantage over glass in lightness of weight and resistance to impact, thus lowering transportation costs and losses due to container damage; the versatility in container design and in consumer acceptance; consumer preference in utilizing plastic squeeze bottles in the administration of ophthalmics, nasal sprays, and lotions; and, the popularity of blister-packaging and unit-dose dispensing particularly in health care institutions.

The term "plastic" does not apply to a single type of material but rather to a vast number of materials, each developed to have desired features. For example, the addition of methyl groups to every other carbon atom in the polymer chains of polyethylene will give polypropylene a material which can be effectively autoclaved, whereas polyethylene cannot. If a chlorine atom is added to every other carbon in the polyethylene polymer, polyvinyl chloride (PVP) is produced. This material is rigid and has good clarity making it a useful material particularly in the blister packaging of tablets and capsules. However, it has a significant drawback for packaging medical devices (e.g., syringes) since it is unsuitable for gamma sterilization, a method that is being increasingly used. The placement of other functional groups on the main chain of polyethylene or added to other types of polymers can give a variety of alterations to the final plastic material. Among the newer plastic materials used are polyethylene terephthalate (PET), amorphous polyethylene terephthalate glycol (APET) polyethylene terephthalate glycol (PETG). Both APET and PETG have excellent transparency and luster and can be sterilized with gamma radiation (17).

Among the problems encountered in the use of plastics in packaging are 1) permeability of the containers to atmospheric oxygen and to moisture vapor; 2) leaching of the constituents of the container to the internal contents; 3) absorption of drugs from the contents to the container; 4) transmission of light through the container; and 5) alteration of the container upon storage. Added agents are frequently added to alter the properties of plastic, including plasticizers, stabilizers, antioxidants, antistatic agents, antimold agents, colorants, and others.

Permeability is considered a process of solution and diffusion, with the penetrant initially dissolving in the plastic material on one side and diffusing through to the other side. Permeability should be contrasted with porosity, which is a condition in which minute holes or cracks are present in the plastic and through which gas or moisture vapor may move directly. The permeability of a plastic is a function of several factors including the nature of the polymer itself, the amounts and types of plasticizers, fillers, lubricants, pigments and other additives used, the pressure conditions, and the temperature. Generally, increases in temperature, pressure, and the use of additives tend to increase the permeability of the plastic. Glass containers are less permeable than plastic containers.

The movement of moisture vapor or gas, especially oxygen, through a pharmaceutical container can pose a threat to the stability of the product. In the presence of moisture, solid dosage forms may lose their color or physical integrity. A host of pharmaceutical adjuncts, especially those used in tablet formulations, as diluents, binders, and disintegrating agents, are affected by moisture. The majority of these adjuncts are carbohydrates, starches, and natural or synthetic gums, and because of their hygroscopicity they hold moisture and may even serve as nutrient media for the growth of microorganisms. Many of the tablet disintegrating agents act by swelling, and, if exposed to high moisture vapor during storage, can cause tablet deterioration. Many medicinal agents, as aspirin and nitroglycerin, are adversely affected by moisture and require special protection. Sublingual nitroglycerin tablets must be dispensed in their original glass container.

Specially developed "high-barrier" packaging can provide added protection to pharmaceutical products against the effects of humidity. It meets the drug stability requirements for packaging adopted by the International Committee on Harmonization which call for the long-term testing of packaged products for a minimum for 12 months at 25°C ($\pm$ 2 degrees) at 60 percent relative humidity (18). Many capsule and other products are liable under these conditions of humidity unless protected by high barrier packaging. Desiccant protectants, as silica gel in small packets, are commonly included in solid dosage form packaging as added protection against the effects of moisture vapor.

Drug substances that are subject to oxidative degradation may undergo a greater degree of degradation when packaged in plastic as compared to glass. In glass, the container's void space is confined and presents only a limited amount of oxygen to the drug contents. Whereas a drug packaged in a gas-permeable plastic container may be constantly exposed to oxygen due to the replenished air supply entering through the container. Liquid pharmaceuticals packaged in plastic containers that are permeable may lose drug molecules or solvent to the container, altering the concentration of the drug in the product and affecting its potency.

Leaching is a term used to describe the movement of components of a container into the contents. Compounds leached from plastic containers are generally the polymer additives as the plasticizers, stabilizers, or antioxidants. The leaching of these additives occurs predominantly when liquid or semi-solid dosage forms are packaged in plastic. Little leaching occurs when tablets or capsules are packaged in plastic.

Leaching may be influenced by temperature, excessive agitation of the filled container, and by the solubilizing effect of liquid contents on one or more of the polymer additives. The leaching of polymer additives from plastic containers of fluids intended for intravenous administration is a special concern and requires the careful selection of the plastic containers used. Leached material, whether dissolved in an intravenous fluid or present as minute particles would pose a health hazard to the patient. Thus, studies of the leaching characteristics of each plastic material considered for use are undertaken as a part of the drug development process. Soft-walled plastic containers of polyvinyl chloride (PVC) are used to package intravenous solutions and blood for transfusion.

Sorption is a term used to indicate the binding of molecules to polymer materials. Both adsorption and absorption may be considered within this term. Sorption occurs through chemical or physical means due to the chemical structure of the solute molecules and the physical and chemical properties of the polymer. Generally, the unionized species of a solute has a greater tendency to be bound than the ionized species. Because the degree of ionization of a solute may be affected by the pH of a solution, the pH may influence the sorption tendency of a particular solute. Further, the pH of a solution may affect the chemical nature of a plastic container in such a way to either increase or decrease the active bonding sites available to the solute molecules. Plastic materials with polar groups are particularly prone to the sorption process. Because the process of sorption is dependent upon the penetration or diffusion of a solute into the plastic, the pharmaceutical vehicle or solvent used can also play a role in the sorption process by altering the integrity of the plastic.

Sorption may occur with active pharmacologic agents or with pharmaceutical excipients. Thus, each ingredient must be examined in the proposed plastic packaging to determine its tendency. Sorption may be initiated by the adsorption of a solute to the inner surface of a plastic container. After saturation of the surface, the solute may then diffuse into the container and be bound to sites within the plastic. The sorption of an active pharmacologic agent from a pharmaceutical solution would reduce its effective concentration and render the product's potency unreliable. The sorption of pharmaceutical excipients as colorants, preservatives, or stabilizers would likewise alter the quality of the product.

Deformations, softening, hardening, and other physical changes in plastic containers can occur due to the action of the container's contents or to external factors as changes in temperature or the physical stress placed upon the container in handling and shipping.

It is always good practice for the pharmacist to dispense medication to patients in the same type and quality of container as that used by the manufacturer of the product. In some instances the original container may be used to dispense the medication.

Child-Resistant / Adult-Senior Use Packaging

To reduce the occurrence of accidental poisonings through the ingestion of drugs and other household chemicals, the Poison Prevention Packaging Act was passed into law in 1970. The responsibility for the administration and enforcement of the Act, originally with the Food and Drug Administration, was transferred to the Consumer Product Safety Commission in 1973 when this agency was created by passage of the Consumer Product Safety Act. The initial regulations called for the use of "child-proof" closures for aspirin products and certain household chemical products shown to have a significant potential for causing accidental poisoning in youngsters.

As the technical capability to produce effective closures was developed, the regulations were extended to include the use of safety closures in the packaging of both legend and OTC medications. Presently, all legend drugs intended for oral use must be dispensed by the pharmacist to the patient in containers having child-resistant closures unless the prescriber or the patient specifically requests otherwise, or, unless the product is specifically exempt from the requirement.

The Consumer Product Safety Commission may propose the exemption of certain drugs and drug products from the regulations based on toxicologic data or on practical considerations. For instance, certain cardiac drugs, as sublingual tablets of nitroglycerin, are exempt from the regulations because of the importance of a patient's immediate access to the medication. Exemptions are also permitted in the case of OTC products for one package size or specially marked package to be available to consumers for whom safety closures might be unnecessary or too difficult to manipulate. These consumers would include childless persons, arthritic patients, and the debilitated. These packages must be labeled: "This package for households without young children" or "Package not child-resistant."

A child-resistant container is defined as one that is significantly difficult for children under 5 years of age to open or to obtain a harmful amount of its contents within a reasonable time and is not difficult for "normal adults" to use properly (19–20). A testing procedure utilizing children between 42 and 51 months is used by the Consumer Product Safety Commission to evaluate the effectiveness of such containers. The four basic designs commonly used are: align the arrows; press down and turn; squeeze and turn; and latch-top. An example of a child-resistant prescription container is shown in Figure 5.7.

In recognition that many adults, particularly the elderly or those with arthritis or weakened hand-strength, have difficulty opening child-resistant packages, the regulations were amended and (effective in 1998) to require that child-resistant containers be capable of being readily opened by senior adults. The previous requirement which used adults 18 to 45 years of age in the testing evaluation was replaced by protocols using adults in three age groups: 50 to 54, 55 to 59, and 60–70 (20). An example of a specially designed child-resistant and adult-friendly closure for packaging and dispensing medication is shown in Figure 5.8.

Drugs that are used or dispensed within patient-care institutions, as hospitals, nursing homes, and extended care facilities, need not be dispensed with safety closures unless they are intended for patients who are leaving the confines of the institution as outpatients.

Tamper-evident Packaging

This type of packaging borne out of flagrant incidents in which the contents of OTC products were adulterated with toxic substances was presented earlier in this chapter under CGMP "Packaging and Label Control."

Compliance Packaging

Many patients are not compliant with the prescribed schedule for taking their medications. There are many factors associated with noncompliance, as a misunderstanding of the dosing schedule, confusion due to the taking of multiple medications, forgetfulness, or a feeling of well-being leading to premature discontinuance of medication.

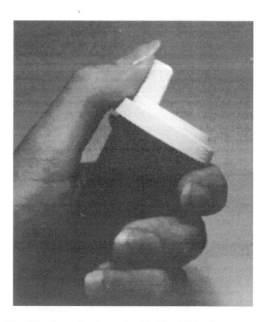

Fig. 5.8 *Example of a senior-friendly child-resistant prescription container. When the arrows on the cap and vial are lined up, leverage on the large tab enables the senior adult patient to push off the cap using a thumb or the side of a hand. The snap cap may also be reversed, with the tab facing in the container, for non-child-resistant use. (Courtesy of Lermer Packaging Corporation)*

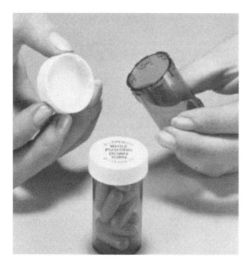

Fig. 5.7 *Example of child-resistant safety closure on a prescription container. (Courtesy of Owens-Brockway Prescription Products).*

To assist patients in taking their medications on schedule, manufacturers and pharmacists have devised numerous educational techniques, reminder aids, compliance packages, and devices. The oral contraceptive compact-type plastic package was among the earliest product packages developed to assist patient adherence to a prescribed dosing schedule. Subsequently, many other packaging innovations were developed including blister-packaging in a calendar pack. For prescriptions dispensed in traditional containers (e.g., capsule vials), pharmacists often provide calendar medication schedules or commercially available compartmentalized devices for the daily or weekly scheduling of solid dosage units. These medication compliance techniques and devices are particularly useful for patients taking multiple medications.

Labeling

The labeling of all drug products distributed in the United States must meet the specific labeling requirements as contained in the Code of Federal Regulations (1–4,21–22). Different labeling requirements apply to investigational drugs, manufacturer's prescription drugs, controlled substances, dispensed prescription medication, OTC products, animal products, medical devices, and to other specific categories and specific products. In every instance, federal labeling requirements may be strengthened by state law.

According to federal regulations, manufacturers' drug product labeling includes not only the labels placed on the immediate container and packaging, but also inserts, company literature, advertising and promotional material including brochures, booklets, mailing pieces, file cards, bulletins, price lists, catalogs, sound recordings, film strips, motion-picture films, slides, exhibits, displays, literature reprints, computer-accessed information, and other materials related to the product.

Important information for a prescription-only drug is provided to health professionals through the manufacturer's product package insert. As discussed in Chapter 2, the package insert must provide full disclosure; that is, a full and balanced presentation of the drug product to enable the prescriber to utilize the drug with sufficient knowledge of important benefit to risk factors.

Manufacturer's Label

Included among the information usually appearing on the manufacturer's or distributor's immediate label affixed to the container of legend drugs is the following:

1. The established or nonproprietary name(s) of the drug(s) present and the proprietary name of the product if one is used.
2. The name of the manufacturer, packer, or distributor of the product.
3. A quantitative statement of the amount of each drug present per unit of weight, volume, or dosage unit, whichever is most appropriate.
4. The pharmaceutical type of dosage form constituting the product.
5. The net amount of drug product contained in the package, in units of weight, volume or number of dosage units, as is appropriate.
6. The logo "Rx-only" or the Federal Legend: "Caution—Federal law prohibits dispensing without prescription," or a similar statement.
7. A label reference to see the accompanying package insert or other product literature for dosage and other information.
8. Special storage instructions, when applicable.
9. The National Drug Code identification number for the product (and often a bar code).
10. An identifying lot or control number.
11. An expiration date.
12. For controlled drug substances, the DEA symbol "C" together with the schedule assigned (e.g. III). The statement: "Warning—May be habit forming" may appear also.

Prescription Label

When filling a prescription, federal law requires the pharmacist to include the following information on the label of the dispensed medication:

1. The name and address of the pharmacy.
2. The serial number of the prescription.
3. The date of the prescription or the date of its filling or refilling (state law often determines which date is to be used).
4. The name of the prescriber.
5. The name of the patient.
6. Directions for use, including precautions, if any, as indicated on the prescription.

In addition to the above, state laws may require additional information as:

7. The address of the patient.
8. The initials or name of the dispensing pharmacist.
9. The telephone number of the pharmacy.
10. The drug name, strength and manufacturer's lot or control number.
11. The expiration date of the drug.
12. The name of the manufacturer or distributor.

OTC Labeling

In 1997, an initiative was taken by the FDA to develop a standardized format for OTC drug product labeling. This initiative was the result of findings that the design and format of labeling information varied considerably among OTC products resulting in difficulty among consumers in reading and understanding the information presented (23). The FDA called for standardized headings and subheadings, a standardized order of presentation, standardized type-face style, and labeling language revised to be simpler to read and more easily understood by the consumer.

The label on the container of OTC products includes the following:

1. Product name.
2. Name and address of the manufacturer, packer or distributor.
3. Statement of the net quantity of the contents.
4. The established names and quantities of all active ingredients per dosage unit. Inactive ingredients are also listed.
5. The name(s) of any habit-forming substance(s) in the preparation.
6. Statement of pharmacologic category or principal intended action (e.g., antacid) and adequate directions for safe and effective use; e.g., dose, frequency of dose, dose-age considerations, route of administration, preparation for use as shaking or dilution.
7. Cautions and warnings needed to protect the consumer; e.g., maximum duration of administration prior to consulting a physician, anticipated side effects, appropriate instructions in the event of accidental overdosage, conditions against which the drug is contraindicated or to be used only with professional supervision, drug interaction precautions, pregnancy-nursing warning if the drug is intended for systemic absorption (unless specifically exempted from this requirement);"Warning: As with any drug, if you are pregnant or nursing a baby, seek the advice of a health professional before using this product."
8. Sodium content for certain oral products intended for ingestion, when the product contains 5 mg of sodium or more per single dose or 140 mg or more in the maximum daily dose.
9. Storage conditions including storage in a safe place out of the reach of children.
10. Description of tamper-evident feature.
11. The product's lot number and expiration date.

As noted, OTC package labeling must include appropriate warning statements whenever the medication is such that indiscriminate use may lead to serious medical complications or mask a condition more serious than that for which the medication was intended. For example, the use of laxatives is a dangerous practice when symptoms of appendicitis are present and can result in an intensification of the problem and even a rupturing of the appendix. For this reason the following statement is required by law to appear on laxative preparations:

Warning: Do not use when abdominal pain, nausea, or vomiting is present. Frequent or prolonged use of this preparation may result in dependence on laxatives.

The seriousness of a cough may be underestimated by a patient if a proprietary cough syrup temporarily relieves the cough; however, coughing is a symptom of many serious conditions requiring specific treatment. Cough remedies sold over-the-counter must therefore bear the following warning statement:

WARNING. A persistent cough may be a sign of a serious condition. If cough persists for more than 1 week, tends to recur, or is accompanied by a fever, rash, or persistent headache, consult a doctor.

These are but two examples of the warning statements required on various types of proprietary products. Serious conditions cannot be diagnosed or successfully treated by the layman with OTC medications.

Storage

To ensure the stability of a pharmaceutical preparation for the period of its intended shelf life, the product must be stored under proper conditions. The labeling of each product includes the desired conditions of storage. The terms generally employed in such labeling have meanings defined by the USP:(15)

Cold—Any temperature not exceeding 8°C (46°F). A refrigerator is a cold place in which the temperature is maintained thermostatically between 2° and 8°C (36° and 46°F). A freezer is a cold place in which the temperature is maintained thermostatically between -20° and -10°C (-4° and 14°F).

Cool—Any temperature between 8° and 15°C (46° and 59°F). An article for which storage in a cool place is directed may, alternatively be stored in a refrigerator unless otherwise specified in the individual monograph.

Room Temperature—The temperature prevailing in a working area. A controlled room temperature encompasses the usual working environment of 20°C to 25°C (68°F to 77°F) but also allows for temperature variations between 15°C and 30°C (59°F and 86°F) that may be experienced in pharmacies, hospitals, and drug warehouses.

Warm—Any temperature between 30° and 40°C (86° and 104°F).

Excessive Heat—Any temperature above 40°C (104°F).

Protection from Freezing—Where in addition to the risk of breakage of the container, freezing subjects a product to loss of strength or potency, or to destructive alteration of the dosage form, the container label bears an appropriate instruction to protect the product from freezing.

Transportation

The stability-protection of a pharmaceutical product during periods of transportation is an important consideration. However, maintenance of satisfactory conditions of temperature and humidity during shipment is not always practiced (24). Temperature and humidity variations to which pharmaceuticals may be exposed may occur during shipment from a manufacturer to a wholesaler or to a pharmacy, from a pharmacy to a patient, during mail-order shipment of prescriptions (and their residence in mailboxes), or when medications are maintained in emergency-care vehicles. Transportation to and within geographic areas of extreme temperatures and humidity requires special consideration.

References

1. Code of Federal Regulations, Title 21, Parts 210–211.
2. Code of Federal Regulations, Title 21, Part 606.
3. Code of Federal Regulations, Title 21, Part 226.
4. Code of Federal Regulations, Title 21, Part 820
5. A strategic view of information technology in the pharmaceutical industry. Philadelphia PA: Deloitte & Touche, 1994.
6. Laboratory robotics handbook. Hopkinton MA: Zymark Corp., 1988.
7. Guide to inspection of bulk pharmaceutical chemicals. Rockville, MD: Food and Drug Administration, 1991.
8. Moore RE. FDA's guideline for bulk pharmaceutical chemicals—a consultant's interpretation. Pharm Tech 1992;16:88–100.
9. Avallone HL. GMP inspections of drug-substance manufacturers. Pharm Tech 1992;16:46–55.
10. Mercill A. A good manufacturing practices guide for bulk pharmaceutical excipients. Pharm Tech 1995;19:34–40.
11. Bernstein DF. Investigational clinical trial material supply operations in new product development. Appl Clin Trials 1993;2:59–69.
12. FDA Modernization Act, Washington DC: Congress of the United States, 1997.
13. Anon. Selections from USP 23-NF 18, Pharmacy compounding practices and sterile drug products for home use. Rockville, MD: United States Pharmacopeial Convention, Inc., 1996.
14. Model State Pharmacy Act and Model Rules of the National Association of Boards of Pharmacy. Park Ridge, IL: National Association of Boards of Pharmacy, 1993.
15. The United States Pharmacopeia 23/National Formulary 18. Rockville MD: The United States Pharmacopeial Convention, Inc., 1995.
16. Guideline for submitting documentation for packaging of human drugs and biologics. Rockville MD: Food and Drug Administration, 1987.
17. Hacker D. Extruder sees future of medical market: rigid PET. Pharmaceut Med Packaging News 1994; 2:22.
18. Wagner J. Pending ICH guidelines and sophisticated drugs add up to the need for higher moisture protection. Pharmaceut Med Packaging News 1996;4:20–24.
19. 60 Federal Register 38671-38674.
20. 60 Federal Register 37709-37744.
21. Code of Federal Regulations, Title 21, Parts 500–599.
22. Code of Federal Regulations, Title 21, Part 1300.
23. 62 Federal Register 9023–9061.
24. Okeke CC, Bailey LC, Medwick T, Grady LT. Temperature fluctuations during mail order shipment of pharmaceutical articles using mean kinetic temperature approach. Pharmaceut Forum 1997;23:4155–4182.

6

POWDERS AND GRANULES

Chapter at a Glance

THE VAST majority of active and non-active pharmaceutical ingredients occur in the solid state as amorphous powders or as crystals of various morphologic structure. The term powder has more than one connotation in pharmacy. The term may be used to describe the physical form of a material, that is, a dry substance composed of finely divided particles. Or, it may be used to describe a type of pharmaceutical preparation, that is, a medicated powder intended for internal (i.e., oral powder) or external (i.e., topical powder) use.

Although the use of medicated powders per se in therapeutics is limited, the use of powdered substances in the preparation of other dosage forms is extensive. For example, powdered drugs may be blended with powdered fillers and other pharmaceutic ingredients to fabricate solid dosage forms as tablets and capsules; or, they may be dissolved or suspended in solvents or liquid vehicles to make various liquid dosage forms; or, they may be incorporated into semisolid bases in the preparation of medicated ointments and creams.

Granules, which are prepared agglomerates of powdered materials, may be used per se for the medicinal value of their content or they may be used for pharmaceutic purposes, as in tableting, as described later in this and in the next chapter.

Powders

Before their use in the preparation of pharmaceutical products, solid materials first are characterized to determine their chemical and physical features including their morphology, purity, solubility, stability, particle size, uniformity, and compatibility with any other formulation components (1). Oftentimes drug and nondrug materials require chemical or pharmaceutical processing to imbue the features desired to enable both the efficient production of a finished dosage form and optimum therapeutic efficacy. This usually includes the adjustment and control of a powder's particle size.

Particle Size and Analysis

The particles of pharmaceutical powders may range from extremely coarse, about 10 mm in diameter, to extremely fine, approaching colloidal dimensions of 1 micron or less. In order to characterize the particle size of a given powder, the USP uses the descriptive terms: Very Coarse, Coarse, Moderately Coarse, Fine, and Very Fine, which are related to the proportion of powder that is capable of passing through the openings of standardized sieves of varying dimensions in a specified time period un-

Table 6.1. Opening of Standard Sieves*

Sieve Number	Sieve Opening
2	9.5 mm
3.5	5.6 mm
4	4.75 mm
8	2.36 mm
10	2.00 mm
20	850 μm
30	600 μm
40	425 μm
50	300 μm
60	250 μm
70	212 μm
80	180 μm
100	150 μm
120	125 μm
200	75 μm
230	63 μm
270	53 μm
325	45 μm
400	38 μm

*Adapted from USP23-NF18.

der shaking, generally in a mechanical sieve shaker (2). Table 6.1 presents the Standard Sieve Numbers and the sieve openings in each, expressed in millimeters and in microns. Sieves for such pharmaceutical testing and measurement are generally made of wire cloth woven from brass, bronze, or other suitable wire. They are not coated or plated.

Powders of vegetable and animal drugs are officially defined as follows:(2)

Very Coarse (or a No. 8) powder—All particles pass through a No. 8 sieve and not more than 20% through a No. 60 sieve.

Coarse (or a No. 20) powder—All particles pass through a No. 20 sieve and not more than 40% through a No. 60 sieve.

Moderately Coarse (or a No. 40) powder—All particles pass through a No. 40 sieve and not more than 40% through a No. 80 sieve.

Fine (or a No. 60) powder—All particles pass through a No. 60 sieve and not more than 40% through a No. 100 sieve.

Very Fine (or a No. 80) powder—All particles pass through a No. 80 sieve. There is no limit as to greater fineness.

The powder fineness for chemicals is defined as follows. There is no "Very Coarse" category.

Coarse (or a No. 20) powder—All particles pass through a No. 20 sieve and not more than 60% through a No. 40 sieve.

Moderately Coarse (or a No. 40) powder—All particles pass through a No. 40 sieve and not more than 60% through a No. 60 sieve.

Fine (or a No. 80) powder—All particles pass through a No. 80 sieve. There is no limit as to greater fineness.

Very Fine (or a No. 120) powder—All particles pass through a No. 120 sieve. There is no limit as to greater fineness.

Granules typically fall within the range of 4- to 12-sieve size, although granulations of powders prepared in the 12- to 20-sieve range are sometimes used in tablet making.

The purpose of particle size analysis in pharmacy is to obtain quantitative data on the size, distribution, and shapes of drug and nondrug components to be used in pharmaceutical formulations. There may be substantial differences in particle size, crystal morphology, and amorphous character within and between substances. Particle size can influence a variety of important factors, including the following:

- Dissolution rate of particles intended to dissolve; drug micronization can increase the rate of drug dissolution and its bioavailablity;
- Suspendability of particles intended to remain undissolved but uniformly dispersed in a liquid vehicle (e.g., fine dispersions have particles from approximately 0.5 to 10 microns);
- Uniform distribution of a drug substance in a powder mixture or solid dosage form to ensure dose-to-dose content uniformity (3);
- Penetrability of particles intended to be inhaled for deposition deep in the respiratory tract (e.g., 1–5 microns) (4); and the
- Nongrittiness of solid particles in dermal ointments, creams, and ophthalmic preparations (e.g., fine powders may be 50–100 microns in size).

A number of methods exist for the determination of particle size, including the following:

- Sieving, in which particles are passed by mechanical shaking through a series of sieves of known and successively smaller size and the determination of the proportion of powder passing through or being withheld on each sieve (range: from about 40 to 9500 microns, depending upon sieve sizes) (2,5)
- Microscopy, in which the particles are sized through the use of a calibrated grid background or other measuring device (range: 0.2 to 100 microns) (6–7)

- Sedimentation rate, in which particle size is determined by measuring the terminal settling velocity of particles through a liquid medium in a gravitational or centrifugal environment (range: 0.8–300 microns)(5). Sedimentation rate may be calculated from Stokes' law.
- Light energy diffraction or light scattering, in which particle size is determined by the reduction in light reaching the sensor as the particle, dispersed in a liquid or gas, passes through the sensing zone (range 0.2–500 microns) (4). Laser scattering, utilizes a He-Ne laser, silicon photo diode detectors and an ultrasonic probe for particle dispersion (range 0.02–2,000 microns) (8).
- Laser Holography, in which a pulsed laser is fired through an aerosolized particle spray and photographed in three dimensions with a holographic camera, allowing the particles to be individually imaged and sized (range: 1.4–100 microns) (9).
- Cascade impaction is based on the principle that a particle, driven by an airstream, will impact on a surface in its path, provided that its inertia is sufficient to overcome the drag force that tends to keep it in the airstream (10). Particles are separated into various size ranges by successively increasing the velocity of the airstream in which they are carried.

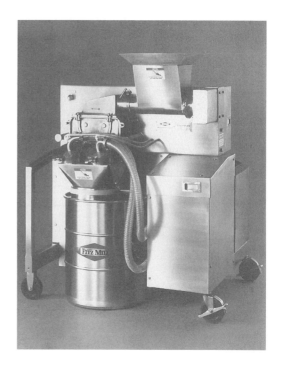

Fig. 6.1 *A FitzMill Comminutor, Model VFS-D6A-PCS, used for particle-reduction with attached containment system for protection of environment and prevention of product contamination. (Courtesy of The Fitzpatrick Company.)*

The above methods and others may be used for the analysis of particle size and shape. For some materials, a single method may be sufficient; however, a combination of methods is frequently preferred to provide greater assurance of size and shape parameters (7). Most of the commercially available particle size analyzers are automated and linked with computers for data processing, distribution analysis, and printout.

The science of small particles is discussed further in the accompanying Physical Pharmacy Capsule, "Micromeritics." The Physical Pharmacy Capsule "Particle Size Reduction" points out that a reduction in a powder's particle size increases the number of particles and the powder's total surface area.

Comminution of Drugs

On a small scale, as in the community pharmacy, the pharmacist reduces the size of chemical substances by grinding with a mortar and pestle. A finer grinding action is accomplished by using a mortar with a rough surface (as a porcelain mortar) than one with a smooth surface (as a glass mortar). The process of grinding a drug in a mortar to reduce

its particle size is termed *trituration*. On a large scale, various types of mills and pulverizers may be used to reduce powder fineness. Figure 6.1 shows one such piece of equipment, a FitzMill comminuting machine with a product containment system. Through the grinding action of rapidly moving blades in the comminuting chamber, particles are reduced in size and passed through a screen of desired dimension to the collection container. The collection/containment system protects the environment from chemical dust, reduces product loss and prevents product contamination.

A process termed *levigation* is commonly used in the small-scale preparation of ointments to reduce the particle size and grittiness of added powders. In the process of levigation, a mortar and pestle or an ointment tile may be used. A paste is formed by combining the powder material and a small amount of liquid (the *levigating agent*) in which the powder is insoluble. The paste is then triturated, effecting a reduction in particle size. The levigated paste may then be added to the ointment base and the mixture made uniform and smooth by rubbing them together using a spatula on the ointment tile. A

Physical Pharmacy Capsule 6.1   **Micromeritics**

Micromeritics is the science of small particles; a particle is any unit of matter having defined physical dimensions. It is important to study particles because the majority of drug dosage forms are solids; solids are not "static" systems—the physical state of particles can be altered by physical manipulation and particle characteristics can alter therapeutic effectiveness.

Micromeritics includes a number of characteristics including particle size, particle size distribution, particle shape, angle of repose, porosity, true volume, bulk volume, apparent density and bulkiness.

PARTICLE SIZE
A number of techniques can be used for determining particle size and particle size distributions. Particle size determinations are complicated by the fact that particles are nonuniform in shape. Only two relatively simple examples will be provided for a detailed calculation of the average particle size of a powder mixture. Other methods will be generally discussed. The techniques used will include the microscopic method and the sieving method.

The microscopic method can include counting not less than 200 particles in a single plane using a calibrated ocular on a microscope. Given the following data, what is the average diameter of the particles?

Size Group of Counted Particles (μ)	Middle Value μ "d"	No. Particles Per Group "n"	"nd"
40–60	50	15	750
60–80	70	25	1750
80–100	90	95	8550
100–120	110	140	15400
120–140	130	80	10400
		$\Sigma n = 355$	$\Sigma nd = 36850$

$$d_{av} = \frac{\Sigma\, nd}{\Sigma n} = \frac{36,850}{355} = 103.8\ \mu$$

The sieving method involves using a set of U.S. Standard sieves in the size range desired. A stack of sieves is arranged in order, the powder placed in the top sieve, the stack shaken, the quantity of powder resting on each sieve weighed, and the following calculation performed.

Sieve No.	Arithmetic Mean Opening (mm)	Weight Retained (G)	% Retained	% Retained × Mean Opening
20/40	0.630	15.5	14.3	9.009
40/60	0.335	25.8	23.7	7.939
60/80	0.214	48.3	44.4	9.502
80/100	0.163	15.6	14.3	2.330
100/120	0.137	3.5	3.3	0.452
		108.7	100.0	29.232

$$d_{av} = \frac{\Sigma\, (\%\ \text{retained}) \times (\text{ave size})}{100} = \frac{29.232}{100} = 0.2923\ mm$$

Another method of particle size determination involves sedimentation using the Andreasen Pipet. The Andreasen Pipet is a special cylindrical container designed such that a sample can be removed from the lower portion at selected time intervals. The powder is dispersed in a nonsolvent in the Andreasen Pipet, agitated, and 20 mL samples removed over a period of time. Each 20 mL sample is dried and weighed. Using the following equation, the particle diameters can be calculated.

Micromeritics (Continued)

$$d = \frac{18\, h\eta}{(\rho_i - \rho_e)\, gt}$$

where

> d is the diameter of the particles
> h is the height of the liquid above the sampling tube orifice,
> η is the viscosity of the suspending liquid,
> $\rho_i - \rho_e$ is the density difference between the suspending liquid and the particles,
> g is the gravitational constant, and
> t is the time in seconds.

Other methods of particle size determinations include the elutriation method, centrifugal method, permeation method, adsorption method, electronic sensing zone (the Coulter Counter), and the light obstruction methods. The latter includes the use of both standard light and laser methods. In general, the resulting average particle sizes by these techniques can provide average particle size by weight (sieve method, light scattering, sedimentation method), and average particle size by volume (light scattering, electronic sensing zone, light obstruction, air permeation and even the optical microscope).

ANGLE OF REPOSE

The angle of repose is a relatively simple technique for estimating the flowability of a powder. It can be easily experimentally determined by allowing a powder to flow through a funnel and fall freely onto a surface. The height and diameter of the resulting cone is measured and, using the following equation, the angle of repose can be calculated.

$$\tan \Theta = h/r$$

where

> h is the height of the powder cone, and
> r is the radius of the powder cone.

EXAMPLE 1

A powder was poured through the funnel and resulted in a cone that was 3.3 cm high and 9 cm in diameter. What is the angle of repose?

$$\tan \Theta = h/r = 3.3/4.5 = 0.73$$

$$\text{arc tan } 0.73 = 36.25°$$

Powders with low angles of repose will flow freely and powders with high angles of repose will flow poorly. A number of factors, including shape and size, determine the flowability of powders. Spherical particles flow better than needles. Very fine particles do not flow as freely as large particles. In general, particles in the size range of 250–2000 μ flow freely if the shape is amenable. Particles in the size range of 75–250 μ may flow freely or cause problems, depending on shape and other factors. With particles less than 100 μ in size, flow is a problem with most substances.

POROSITY, VOID AND BULK VOLUME

If spheres are used as an example, and the different ways they pack together, two possibilities will be considered. First, the closest packing may include the rhombus/triangle packing where angles of 60° and 120° are common. The space between the particles, the void, is about 0.26, resulting in a porosity, as described below, of about 26%. Another packing, called cubical, may be considered where the cubes are packed at 90° angles to each other. This results in a void of about 0.47, or a porosity of about 47%. This is the most open type of packing. It should be noted that if particles are not uniform, the smaller particles will slip into the void spaces between the larger particles and decrease the void areas.

Packing and flow is important, as it will impact the size of container required for packaging, the flow of granulations, the efficiency of the filling apparatus during the tabletting and encapsulating process, and for the ease of working with the powders.

Micromeritics (Continued)

A number of characteristics can be used to describe powders, including porosity, true volume, bulk volume, apparent density, true density, and bulkiness.

Porosity is

$$\text{Void} \times 100$$

This value should be determined experimentally by measuring the volume occupied by a selected weight of a powder. This volume is called the V_{bulk}. The true volume, V, of a powder is the space occupied by the powder exclusive of spaces greater than the intramolecular space.

Void can be defined as

$$\frac{V_{bulk} - V}{V_{bulk}}$$

therefore, porosity is

$$\frac{V_{bulk} - V}{V_{bulk}} \times 100$$

The bulk volume is

$$\text{True volume} + \text{Porosity}$$

APPARENT DENSITY, TRUE DENSITY AND BULKINESS

The apparent density, ρ_a, is

$$\frac{\text{Weight of the sample}}{V_{bulk}}$$

The true density, ρ, is

$$\frac{\text{Weight of the sample}}{V}$$

The bulkiness, B, is the reciprocal of the apparent density,

$$B = 1/\rho a$$

EXAMPLE 2

A selected powder has a true density (ρ) of 3.5 g/cc. Experimentally, 2.5 g of the powder measures 40 mL in a cylindrical graduate. Calculate the true volume, void, porosity, apparent density and bulkiness.

True volume:

$$\text{Density} = \text{Mass (weight)}/\text{Volume}$$
$$\text{Volume} = \text{Mass (weight)}/\text{Density}$$
$$= 2.5 \text{ g}/(3.5 \text{ g/cc}) = 0.715 \text{ cc}$$

Void:

$$\frac{V_{bulk} - V}{V_{bulk}} = \frac{40 \text{ mL} - 0.715 \text{ mL}}{40 \text{ mL}} = 0.982$$

Porosity:

$$\text{Void} \times 100 = 0.982 \times 100 = 98.2\%$$

Apparent density:

$$(\rho a) = \frac{2.5 \text{ g}}{40 \text{ mL}} = 0.0625 \text{ g/mL}$$

Bulkiness:

$$1/\rho a = \frac{1}{0.0625 \text{ (g/mL)}} = 16 \text{ mL/g}$$

Powders with a low apparent density and a large bulk volume are "light" powders, and those with a high apparent density and a small bulk volume are "heavy" powders.

Physical Pharmacy Capsule 6.2   **Particle Size Reduction**

Comminution, the process of reducing the particle size of a solid substance to a finer state of subdivision, is used to facilitate crude drug extraction, increase the dissolution rates of a drug, aid in the formulation of pharmaceutically acceptable dosage forms, and enhance the absorption of drugs. The reduction in the particle size of a solid is accompanied by a great increase in the specific surface area of that substance. An example of the increase in the number of particles formed and the resulting surface area is as follows.

EXAMPLE

Increase in Number of Particles
If a powder consists of cubes 1 mm on edge, and it is reduced to particles 10 μ on edge, what is the number of particles produced?

1. 1 mm equals 1000 μ.
2. 1000 μ/10 μ = 100 pieces produced on each edge, i.e., if the cube is sliced into 100 pieces, each 10 μ long, 100 pieces would result.
3. If this is repeated in each of the other two dimensions, i.e., to include the x, y and z axes, then there would be 100 × 100 × 100 = 1,000,000 particles produced, each 10 μ on edge, for each original particle 1 mm on edge. This can also be written $[(10^2)^3 = 10^6]$.

Increase in Surface Area
What is the increase in the surface area of the powder by decreasing the particle size from 1 mm to 10 μ?

1. The 1 mm cube has 6 surfaces, each 1 mm on edge. Each face has a surface area of 1 mm². Because there are 6 faces, this is 6 mm² surface area for this one particle.
2. Each 10 μ cube has 6 surfaces, each 10 μ on edge. Each face has a surface area of 10 × 10 = 100 μ². Because there are 6 faces, this is 6 × 100 μ², or 600 μ² surface area for this one particle. Since there are 10^6 particles that resulted by comminuting the 1 mm cube into smaller cubes, each 10 μ on edge, there would be 600 μ² × 10^6 or 6 × 10^8 μ² surface area now.
3. To get everything in the same units for ease of comparison, we convert the 6 × 10^8 μ² into mm² as follows.
4. Since there are 1,000 μ/mm, there must be 1,000², or 1,000,000 μ²/mm². This is more appropriately expressed as 10^6 μ²/mm²,

$$\frac{6 \times 10^8 \mu^2}{10^6 \mu^2/mm^2} = 6 \times 10^2 \ mm^2$$

As is evident here, the surface areas have been increased from 6 mm² to 600 mm² by the reduction in particle size of cubes 1 mm on edge to cubes 10 μ on edge (i.e., a hundred-fold increase in surface area). This can have a significant increase in the rate of dissolution of a drug product.

"figure 8" track is commonly used to incorporate the materials. Mineral oil and glycerin are commonly used levigating agents.

Blending Powders

When two or more powdered substances are to be combined to form a uniform mixture, it is best to reduce the particle size of each powder individually before weighing and blending. Depending upon the nature of the ingredients, the amount of pow-

der to prepare, and the equipment available, powders may be blended by spatulation, trituration, sifting, and tumbling.

Spatulation is a method by which small amounts of powders may be blended by the movement of a spatula through the powders on a sheet of paper or an ointment tile. The method is not suitable for large quantities of powders or for powders containing potent substances, because homogeneous blending is not as certain as through other methods. Very little compression or compacting of the

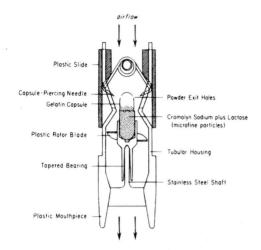

airflow

Plastic Slide

Capsule-Piercing Needle
Gelatin Capsule

Plastic Rotor Blade

Tapered Bearing

Plastic Mouthpiece

Powder Exit Holes

Cromolyn Sodium plus Lactose
(microfine particles)

Tubular Housing

Stainless Steel Shaft

Fig. 6.5 *Cross section of the SPINHALER turbo inhaler, used in the administration of INTAL (cromolyn sodium). (Courtesy of Fisons Corporation).*

containing substances that should be administered in controlled dosage are supplied to the patient in divided amounts in folded papers or packets.

Divided Powders

(Latin, chartulae (pl.); abbrev: charts.) After a powder has been properly blended (using the geometric dilution method for potent substances), it may be divided into individual dosing units based on the amount to be taken or used at a single time. Each divided portion of powder may be placed on a small piece of paper, which is then folded to enclose the medication. A number of commercially prepared pre-measured products are available in folded papers or packets, including headache powders (e.g., BC Powders), powdered laxatives (e.g., Perdiem Packets), and douche powders (e.g., Massengill Powder Packettes).

Divided powders may be prepared as follows by the pharmacist. Depending on the potency of the drug substance, the pharmacist decides whether to weigh each portion of powder separately before enfolding in a paper or to approximate each portion by using the block-and-divide method. By the latter method, used only for nonpotent drugs, the pharmacist places the entire amount of prepared powder on a flat surface such as a porcelain or glass plate, pill tile, or large sheet of paper, and with a large spatula forms a rectangular or square-shaped block of powder having a uniform depth. Then, using the spatula, the pharmacist cuts into the powder vertically and horizontally to delineate the ap-

propriate number of smaller, uniform blocks, each representing a dose or unit of medication. Each of the smaller blocks is then separated from the main block with the spatula and transferred to a powder paper and wrapped.

The powder papers may be of any convenient size to hold the amount of powder required, but the most popular sizes are commercially available and include $2\frac{3}{4} \times 3\frac{3}{4}$ inches, $3 \times 4\frac{1}{2}$ inches, $3\frac{3}{4} \times 5$ inches, and $4\frac{1}{2} \times 6$ inches. The papers may be 1) simple bond paper; 2) vegetable parchment, a thin, semiopaque paper having limited moisture-resistant qualities; 3) glassine, a glazed, transparent paper, also having limited moisture-resistant qualities; and 4) waxed paper, a transparent, waterproof paper. The selection of the type of paper is based primarily on the nature of the powder. If the powder contains hygroscopic or deliquescent materials, a waterproof or a waxed paper should be used. In practice, such powders are double-wrapped in waxed paper, and then for aesthetic appeal they are finally wrapped in bond paper. Glassine and vegetable parchment papers may be used when only a limited barrier against moisture is necessary. Powders containing volatile components should be wrapped in waxed or in glassine papers. Powders containing neither volatile components nor ingredients adversely affected by air or moisture are usually wrapped in white bond paper.

A certain degree of expertise is required in the folding of a powder paper and practice is required for proficiency. The steps are shown in Figure 6.7 and described as follows:

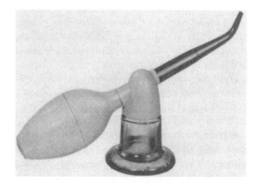

Fig 6.6 *Example of a general purpose powder blower or insufflator. The powder is placed in the device's vessel. When the rubber bulb is depressed, internal turbulence results causing the powder to be dispersed and forced from the orifice. Powders may be delivered to various body locations, as the nose, throat, tooth sockets, or skin. (Courtesy of The DeVilbiss Company.)*

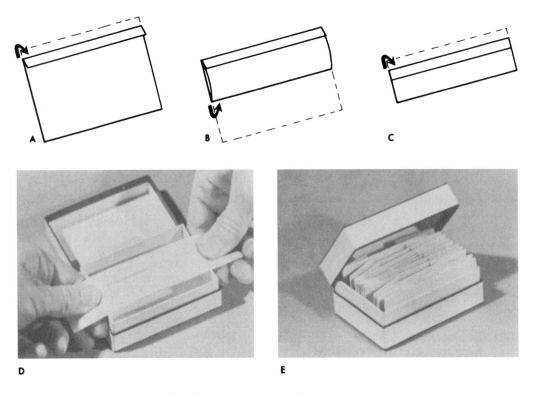

Fig. 6.7 *Steps in the folding of powder papers.*

1. Place the paper flat on a hard surface and fold toward you a uniform flap of about ½ inch of the long side of the paper. To ensure uniformity of all of the papers, this step should be performed on all the required papers concurrently, using the first folded paper as the guide (Fig. 6.7A).
2. With the flap of each paper away and pointing upward, place the weighed or divided amount of powder in the center of each paper.
3. Being careful not to disturb the powder excessively, bring the lower edge of the paper upward, and place it proximate to the crease of the flap (Fig. 6.7B).
4. Grasp the flap, press it down upon the tucked-in bottom edge of the paper and fold again with an amount of paper equal to the size of the original flap (1/2 inch) (Fig. 6.7C).
5. Pick the paper up with the flap upward being careful not to disturb the position of the powder, and place the partially folded paper over the open powder box (to serve as the container) so that the ends of the paper extend equally beyond the sides (lengthwise) of the open container. Then, press the sides of the box slightly inward and the ends of the paper gently downward along the sides of the box to form a crease on each end of the paper. Lift the paper from the box and fold the ends of the paper along each crease sharply so that the powder cannot escape (Fig. 6.7D).
6. The folded papers are then each placed in the box so that the double-folded flaps are at the top, facing the operator, and the ends are folded away from the operator (Fig. 6.7E).

Papers folded properly should fit snugly in the box, have uniform folds, and should be of uniform length and height. There should be no powder in the folds and none should be capable of escape with moderate agitation. Powder boxes, which are generally pasteboard and of the hinged type, should close easily without coming in contact with the tops of the papers. The label for the powders may be placed on the container, but some pharmacists affix a label of directions to each individual paper.

For convenience and uniformity of appearance, pharmacists may use commercially available small cellophane or plastic envelopes to enclose individual doses or units-of-use rather than folding individual powder papers. These envelopes are usually moisture resistant and their use results in uniform packaging.

Granules

As indicated previously, granules are prepared agglomerates of smaller particles of powder. They are irregularly shaped but may be prepared to be spherical. They are usually in the 4- to 12-sieve size range although granules of various mesh sizes may be prepared depending upon their application.

Granules are prepared by wet methods and dry methods. One basic wet method involves moistening the desired powder or powder mixture and then passing the paste-like mass through a screen of the mesh size to produce the desired-size granules. The granules are then placed on drying trays and dried by air or under heat. The granules are periodically moved about on the drying trays to prevent their adhesion into a large mass. Another type of wet method involves the use of fluid-bed processing in which particles are placed in a conical-shaped piece of equipment and then vigorously dispersed and suspended while a liquid excipient is sprayed on them and the fluidized product dried, forming granules or pellets of defined particle size (Fig. 6.8).

The dry granulation method may be performed in a couple of ways. By one method, the dry powder material is passed through a roll compactor and then through a granulating machine (Fig. 6.9). A roll compactor, also called a roll press or roller compactor, processes a fine powder into densified sheets or forms by forcing it through two mechanically rotating metal rolls running counter to each other (12). The surface of the compacting rolls may be smooth or may have pocket indentations or corrugations which allow compactions of different form and texture. The compacted powder is then granulated to

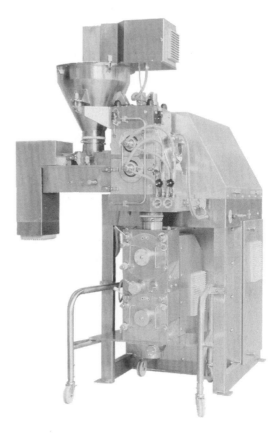

Fig. 6.9 *Roll compactor with granulators, Model WP 170 V, Pharma. The single unit compacts dry powders and crystalline materials with subsequent granulation to reduce compacted material to particles of desired size. (Courtesy of Alexanderwerk, Inc.)*

uniform particle size by passing through a mechanical granulator. Powder compactors are generally combined in sequence in integrated compactor/granulation systems.

An alternative dry method, termed slugging, involves the compression of a powder or powder mixture into large tablets or slugs on a compressing machine under 8,000–12,000 pounds of pressure, depending upon the physical characteristics of the powder. The slugs produced are generally flatface and about 2.5 cm (1 inch) in diameter (12). The slugs are then granulated into the desired particle size, generally for use in the production of tablets. The dry process often results in the production fines, that is, powder which has not agglomerated into granules. These fines are separated, collected and reprocessed. The wet and dry granulation methods are discussed in greater detail in the next chapter as they pertain to tablet making.

Granules flow well compared to powders. For

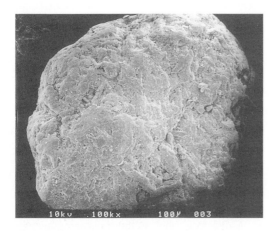

Fig. 6.8 *Granule prepared through fluid-bed technology. (Courtesy of Glatt Air Techniques, Inc.)*

comparison, consider the pouring/flowing characteristics of granulated sugar versus powdered sugar. Because of their flow properties, granulations are commonly used in tablet-making to facilitate the free flow of material from the feeding container (or hopper) into the tableting presses.

In addition to being free-flowing, granules have other important characteristics. Because their surface area is less than a comparable volume of powder, granules are usually more stable to the effects of atmospheric humidity and are less likely to cake or harden upon standing. Granules also are more easily "wetted" by liquids than are certain light and fluffy powders (which tend to float on the surface) and are often preferred for dry products intended to be constituted into solutions or suspensions.

A number of commercial products containing antibiotic drugs that are unstable in aqueous solution are prepared as small granules for constitution by the pharmacist with purified water just prior to dispensing. The granules are prepared to contain not only the medicinal agent, but colorants, flavorants, and other pharmaceutic ingredients. Upon constitution, the resultant liquid has all of the desired medicinal and pharmaceutic features of a liquid pharmaceutical.

Other types of granulated commercial products include the laxative Senokot Granules (Purdue Frederick), which are cocoa-flavored granules containing standardized senna concentrate. The granules are measured and mixed with water or other beverage, sprinkled on food, or eaten plain. Effervescent products as Alka-Seltzer (Bayer) represent another popular type of granulated product. Granulations of effervescent products may be compressed into tablet form, as Zantac EFFERdose Tablets (Glaxo Wellcome). Effervescent granules and tablets are dissolved in water before use. The preparation of effervescent granulated salts is discussed as follows.

Effervescent Granulated Salts

Effervescent salts are granules or coarse to very coarse powders containing a medicinal agent in a dry mixture usually composed of sodium bicarbonate, citric acid, and tartaric acid. When added to water, the acids and base react to liberate carbon dioxide, resulting in effervescence. The resulting carbonated solution masks an undesirable taste of any medicinal agent present. By using granules or coarse particles of the mixed powders rather than small powder particles, the rate of solution is decreased and violent and uncontrollable effervescence is prevented. Sudden and rapid effervescence could overflow the glass and leave little residual carbonation in the solution.

By using a combination of citric and tartaric acids rather than either acid alone, certain difficulties are avoided. When tartaric acid is used as the sole acid, the resulting granules lose their firmness readily and crumble. Citric acid alone results in a sticky mixture difficult to granulate.

A summary of the chemistry of effervescent granules may be found in the accompanying Physical Pharmacy Capsule "Effervescent Granules."

Effervescent granules are prepared by two general methods: 1) the dry or fusion method and 2) the wet method.

Fusion Method

In the fusion method, the one molecule of water present in each molecule of citric acid acts as the binding agent for the powder mixture. Before mixing the powders, the citric acid crystals are powdered and then mixed with the other powders of the same sieve size to ensure uniformity of the mixture. The sieves and the mixing equipment should be made of stainless steel or other material resistant to the effect of the acids. The mixing of the powders is performed as rapidly as is practical, preferably in an environment of low humidity to avoid the absorption of moisture and a premature chemical reaction. After mixing, the powder is placed on a suitable dish in an oven at between 34°C and 40°C. During the heating process, an acid-resistant spatula is used to turn the powder. The heat causes the release of the water of crystallization from the citric acid, which in turn dissolves a portion of the powder mixture, setting of the chemical reaction and the consequent release of some carbon dioxide. This causes the softened mass of powder to become somewhat spongy, and when of the proper consistency (as bread dough), it is removed from the oven and rubbed through a sieve to produce granules of the desired size. A No. 4 sieve produces large granules, a No. 8 sieve prepares medium size granules, and a No. 10 sieve prepares small granules. The granules are dried at a temperature not exceeding 54°C and immediately placed in containers and tightly sealed.

Wet Method

The wet method differs from the fusion method in that the source of binding agent is not the water of crystallization from the citric acid but water added to alcohol as the moistening agent—forming the pliable mass for granulation. In this

Physical Pharmacy Capsule 6.3   **Effervescent Granules**

Granules are dosage forms that consist of particles ranging from about 4 to 10 mesh in size (4.76 mm to 2.00 mm), formed by moistening blended powders and passing through a screen or a special granulator. These moist granules are then either air- or oven-dried. A special form of granules can be used to provide a pleasant vehicle for selected drug products, especially those with either a bitter or salty taste. This special formulation is an "effervescent granule" and may consist of mixtures of citric acid and/or tartaric acid and/or sodium biophosphate combined with sodium bicarbonate.

EXAMPLE

Rx

Active Drug   500 mg/5 g tsp

in effervescent granule qs   120 g

Sig: Dissolve one teaspoonful in one-half glass of cool water and drink. Repeat every 8 hours.

It is desired to dispense this as a granule, where the patient will measure out a teaspoonful (5 g) dose, mix, and administer. Since each dose weighs 5 g and there will be 120 g of the prescription, there will be 24 doses. Each dose contains 0.5 g, which will be 12 g of active drug for the entire prescription. This results in 120 g − 12 g = 108 g of effervescent vehicle that will be required. A good effervescent blend consists of both citric acid and tartaric acid (1:2 ratio), since the former is rather sticky to manipulate and the latter produces a chalky, friable granule. It then becomes necessary to calculate the amount of each ingredient required to prepare 108 g of the granulation.

Citric Acid

$$3\ NaHCO_3 + C_6H_8O_7.H_2O \rightarrow 4\ H_2O + 3CO_2 + Na_3C_6H_5O_7$$
$$3 \times 84 \qquad 210$$

One gram of citric acid (MW = 210) reacts with 1.2 g of sodium bicarbonate (MW = 84) as obtained from the following:

$$\frac{1}{210} = \frac{x}{3 \times 84}$$

$$x = 1.2\ g$$

Tartaric Acid

$$2\ NaHCO_3 + C_4H_6O_6 \rightarrow 2\ H_2O + 2CO_2 + Na_2C_4H_4O_6$$
$$2 \times 84 \qquad 150$$

Since it is desired to use a 1:2 ratio of citric acid to tartaric acid, two grams of tartaric acid (MW = 150) reacts with 2.24 g of sodium bicarbonate according to the following calculation:

$$\frac{2}{150} = \frac{x}{2 \times 84}$$

$$x = 2.24\ g$$

From the above, 1.2g and 2.24 g of sodium bicarbonate is required to react with 1 + 2 g of the citric:tartaric acid combination. Since it is desired to leave a small amount of the acids unreacted to enhance palatability and taste, 2.24 g + 1.2 g = 3.44 g, only 3.4 g of sodium bicarbonate will be utilized. Therefore, the ratio of the effervescent ingredients is 1:2:3.4 for the citric acid:tartaric acid:sodium bicarbonate. Since the prescription requires 108 g of the effervescent mix, the quantity of each ingredient can be calculated as follows:

Effervescent Granules (Continued)

$$1 + 2 + 3.4 = 6.4$$

$$1/6.4 \times 108 \text{ g} = 16.875 \text{ g Citric acid}$$

$$2/6.4 \times 108 \text{ g} = 33.750 \text{ g Tartaric acid}$$

$$3.4/6.4 \times 108 \text{ g} = 57.375 \text{ g Sodium bicarbonate}$$

$$\text{Total} = 108 \text{ g}$$

The prescription will require 12 g of the active drug and 108 g of this effervescent vehicle.

method, all of the powders may be anhydrous as long as water is added to the moistening liquid. Just enough liquid is added (in portions) to prepare a mass of proper consistency; then the granules are prepared and dried in the same manner as described.

References

1. Brittain HG. On the physical characterization of pharmaceutical solids. Pharm Tech 1997;21:100–108.
2. The United States Pharmacopeia 23/National Formulary 18, Rockville, MD: The United States Pharmacopeial Convention, 1995.
3. Yalkowsky SH, Bolton S. Particle size and content uniformity. Pharm Res 1990;7:962–966.
4. Jager PD, DeStefano GA, McNamara DP. Particle-size measurement using right-angle light scattering. Pharm Tech 1993;17:102–110.
5. Carver LD. Particle size analysis. Industrial Res 1971:(August) 39–43.
6. Evans R. Determination of drug particle size and morphology using optical microscopy. Pharm Tech 1993;17:146–152.
7. Houghton ME, Amidon GE. Microscopic characterization of particle size and shape: an inexpensive and versatile method. Pharm Res 1992;9:856–863.
8. Horiba Instruments Inc., Irvine, CA, 1998.
9. Gorman WG, Carroll FA. Aerosol particle-size determination using laser holography. Pharm Tech 1993; 17:34–37.
10. Milosovich SM. Particle-size determination via cascade impaction. Pharm Tech 1992;16:82–86.
11. Hindle M, Byron PR. Size distribution control of raw materials for dry-powder inhalers using aerosizer with aero-dispenser. Pharm Tech 1995:19:64–78.
12. Miller RW. Roller compaction technology. In Parikh DM, ed. Handbook of pharmaceutical granulation technology. New York: Marcel Dekker, 1997;100–150.

7

CAPSULES AND TABLETS

Chapter at a Glance

WHEN MEDICATIONS are to be administered orally to adults, capsules and tablets usually are preferred because they are conveniently carried, readily identified, and easily taken.

Consider the convenience of a patient carrying a day's, week's, or month's supply of capsules or tablets compared with equivalent doses of a liquid medication. With capsules and tablets as dosing units, there is no need for spoons or other measuring devices, which sometimes may be inconvenient and may result in less than accurate dosing. Also, most capsules and tablets are tasteless when swallowed, which is not the case with oral liquid medication.

The characteristic shapes and colors of capsules and tablets and the manufacturer's name and product code number commonly embossed or imprinted on their surface make them readily identified. This enhances communications between the patient and health care providers, assists patient compliance, and fosters safe and effective medication use.

Capsules and tablets are available for many medications in a variety of dosage strengths thereby providing prescribing flexibility to the prescriber and accurate individualized dosage for the patient. Some tablets are *scored*, or grooved, which allows them to be easily broken into two or more parts. This enables the patient to swallow smaller portions as may be desired, or when prescribed, it allows the tablet to be taken in reduced or divided dosage. Tablets that are not scored are not intended to be broken or cut by the patient since they may have special coatings and/or drug-release features that would be compromised by altering the tablet's physical integrity.

From a pharmaceutic standpoint, solid dosage forms are efficiently and productively manufactured; they are packaged and shipped by manufacturers at lower cost and with less breakage than comparable liquid forms; and are more stable and have a longer shelf-life than their liquid counterparts.

As discussed later in this chapter, empty hard gelatin capsules are often used by the pharmacist in the extemporaneous compounding of prescriptions. On occasion, a pharmacist may use commercially available capsules and tablets as the *source* of a medicinal agent when it is not otherwise available. In these instances, the pharmacist must take into account any excipients that are present in the commercial product to ensure compatibility with the other ingredients in the compounded prescription. Capsules and tablets designed to provide modified drug release are discussed in Chapter 8.

Capsules

Capsules are solid dosage forms in which medicinal agents and/or inert substances are enclosed within a small shell of gelatin. Gelatin capsule shells may be *hard* or *soft* depending on their composition.

The vast majority of filled capsules are intended to be swallowed whole by the patient for the benefit of the medication contained therein. However, it is not unusual practice in hospitals and extended care facilities for a caregiver to open capsules or crush tablets to mix with food or drink, especially for children or other patients unable to swallow solid dosage forms. This should be done only with the concurrence of the pharmacist since the drug release characteristics of certain dosage forms could be altered and adversely affect the patient's welfare.

Dosage forms that must be left intact include: enteric coated tablets, designed to pass through the stomach for drug release and absorption in the intestine; extended-release dosage forms, designed to provide prolonged release of the medication; and sublingual or buccal tablets, formulated to dissolve under the tongue or in the oral cavity (1). In instances in which a patient is unable to swallow an intact solid dosage form, an alternative product, such as a chewable tablet, instant dissolving tablet, oral liquid, suppository or injection may be employed.

Hard Gelatin Capsules

Hard gelatin capsule shells are used to manufacture most of the commercially available medicated capsules. They are also commonly employed in clinical drug trials, to compare the effects of an investigational drug to another drug product or placebo. Hard gelatin capsules also are used by the community pharmacist in the extemporaneous compounding of prescriptions. The empty capsule shells are made from a mixture of gelatin, sugar and water. As such, they are clear, colorless, and essentially tasteless. They may be colored with various FD&C and D&C dyes and may be made opaque by adding agents such as titanium dioxide. Most commercially available medicated capsules contain combinations of colorants and opaquants to make them distinctive, many with caps and bodies of different colors.

Gelatin is obtained by the partial hydrolysis of collagen obtained from the skin, white connective tissue, and bones of animals. In commerce, it is available in the form of a fine powder, a coarse powder, shreds, flakes, or sheets (Fig. 7.1).

Gelatin is stable in air when dry but is subject to microbial decomposition when it becomes moist.

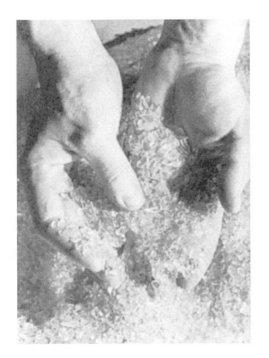

Fig. 7.1 *Pork skin gelatin used as raw material in the manufacture of gelatin capsules. (Courtesy of SmithKline Beecham.)*

Normally, hard gelatin capsules contain between 13 and 16% of moisture (2). However, if stored in an environment of high humidity, additional moisture is absorbed by the capsules, and they may become distorted and lose their rigid shape. In an environment of extreme dryness, some of the moisture normally present in the gelatin capsules is lost and the capsules may become brittle and crumble when handled. Therefore, it is desirable to maintain hard gelatin capsules in an environment free from excess humidity or dryness.

Because moisture may be absorbed by gelatin capsules and affect hygroscopic agents contained within, many capsules are packaged along with a small packet of a desiccant material to protect against the absorption of atmospheric moisture. The desiccant materials most used are dried silica gel, clay, and activated carbon.

Prolonged exposure to high humidity can affect *in vitro* capsule dissolution. Such changes have been observed in capsules containing tetracycline, chloramphenicol, and nitrofurantoin (3). Because such changes could forewarn of possible changes in bioavailability, capsules subjected to such stress conditions must be evaluated on a case by case basis (3).

Although gelatin is insoluble in cold water, it does soften through the absorption of up to ten times its weight of water. Some patients prefer to swallow a capsule wetted with water or saliva because a wetted capsule slides down the throat more readily than a dry capsule. Gelatin is soluble in hot water and in warm gastric fluid a gelatin capsule rapidly dissolves and exposes its contents. Gelatin, being a protein, is digested by proteolytic enzymes and absorbed.

A number of methods have been developed to track the passage of capsules and tablets through the gastrointestinal tract to map their transit time and drug-release patterns. Among these is gamma *scintigraphy,* a noninvasive procedure which involves use of a gamma ray-emitting radiotracer incorporated into the formulation with a gamma camera coupled to a data recording system (4–5). The quantity of material added to allow gamma scintigraphy is small and does not compromise the usual in vivo characteristics of the dosage form being studied. When scintigraphy is combined with pharmacokinetic studies, the resultant *pharmacoscintographic* evaluation provides information of the transit and drug release patterns of the dosage form as well as the rate of drug absorption from the various regions of the gastrointestinal tract (4). This method is particularly useful in: (a) identifying whether a correlation exists between in vitro and in vivo bioavailability for immediate-release products; (b) assessing the integrity and transit time of enteric coated tablets through the stomach enroute to the intestines; and (c) drug/dosage form evaluation in new product development (4–5). A separate technique, using a pH-sensitive, nondigestible, radiotelemetric device termed the Heidelberg capsule, the approximate size of a No. 0 gelatin capsule, has been used as a *non*radioactive means to measure gastric pH, gastric residence time, and gastric emptying time of solid dosage forms in fasting and nonfasting human subjects (6).

As discussed in Chapter 4, drug absorption from the gastrointestinal tract depends on a number of factors, including the solubility characteristics of the drug substance, the type of product formulation (i.e., immediate-release, modified-release, enteric coated), the gastrointestinal contents and intersubject differences in physiologic character and response.

The Manufacture of Hard Gelatin Capsule Shells

Hard gelatin capsule shells are manufactured in two sections, the capsule body and a shorter cap. The two parts overlap when joined, with the cap fitting snugly over the open end of the capsule body.

The shells are produced industrially by the mechanical dipping of pins or pegs of the desired shape and diameter into a temperature-controlled reservoir of melted gelatin mixture (Figs. 7.2, 7.3). The pegs, made of manganese bronze, are affixed to plates, each capable of holding up to about 500 pegs. Each plate is mechanically lowered to the gelatin bath, the pegs submerged to the desired depth and maintained for the desired period to achieve the proper length and thickness of coating. Then the plate and the pegs are slowly lifted from the bath and the gelatin dried by a gentle flow of temperature- and humidity-controlled air. When dried, each capsule part is trimmed mechanically to the proper length, removed from the pegs and the capsule bodies and caps are joined together. It is important that the thickness of the gelatin walls be strictly controlled so that the capsule's body and cap fit snugly to prevent disengagement. The pegs on which the caps are formed are slightly larger in diameter than the pegs on which the bodies are formed, allowing the telescoping of the caps over the bodies. In capsule shell production, there is a continuous dipping, drying, removing and joining of capsules as the peg-containing plates are rotated in and out of the gelatin bath. As noted earlier, capsule shells may be made distinctive by adding colorants and/or opaquants to the gelatin bath.

A manufacturer also may prepare distinctive-looking capsules by altering the usual rounded shape of the capsule-making pegs. By tapering the end of the body-producing peg while leaving the cap-making peg rounded, one manufacturer prepares capsules differentiated from those of other manufacturers (PULVULES, Eli Lilly). Another manufacturer utilizes capsules with the ends of both the bodies and caps highly tapered (SPANSULE Capsules, SmithKline Beecham). Yet another innovation in capsule shell design is the SNAP-FIT, CONI-SNAP, and CONI-SNAP SUPRO hard gelatin capsules depicted in Figures 7.4 and 7.5. The original SNAP-FIT construction enables the two halves of the capsule shells to be positively joined through locking grooves in the shell walls. The two grooves fit into each other and thus ensure reliable closing of the filled capsule. During the closing process, the capsule body is inserted into the cap. With the high-capacity filling rates of the modern capsule filling machines (over 180,000 capsules per hour), capsule splitting ("telescoping") and/or denting of the capsule shell occurs with the slightest contact between the two capsule-part rims when they are joined. This problem, which exists primarily with straight-walled capsule shells, led to the development of the CONI-SNAP capsule, in which the rim of the capsule body is not straight, but tapered slightly (Fig. 7.5). This reduces the risk of the capsule-rims touching on joining, and essentially

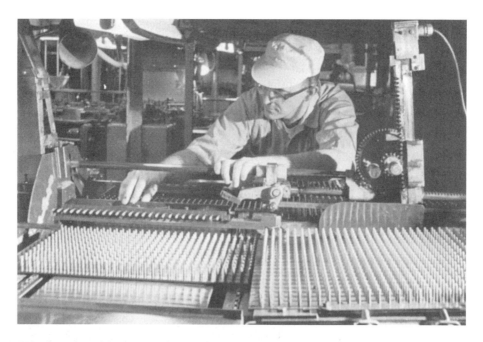

Fig. 7.2 *Body of capsules and their caps are shown as they move through automated capsule-making machine. Each machine is capable of producing 30,000 capsules per hour. It takes a 40-minute cycle to produce a capsule. (Courtesy of SmithKline Beecham.)*

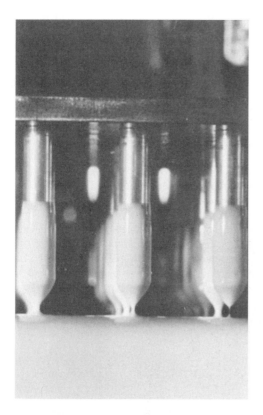

amount of fill material to be encapsulated. The density and compressibility of the fill will largely determine to what extent it may be packed into a capsule shell (7). For estimation, a comparison may be made with powders of well-known features (Table 7.1) and an initial judgment made as to the approximate capsule size needed to hold a specific amount of material. However, the final determination largely may be the result of trial. For human use, empty capsules ranging in size from 000 (the largest) to 5 (the smallest) are commercially available (Fig. 7.7). Larger capsules are available for veterinary use.

For prescriptions requiring extemporaneous compounding, hard gelatin capsules permit a wide prescribing latitude by the physician. The pharmacist may compound capsules of a single medicinal agent or combination of agents at the precise dosage prescribed for the individual patient.

Preparation of Filled Hard Gelatin Capsules

The large-scale or small-scale preparation of filled hard gelatin capsules is divided into the following general steps.

Fig. 7.3 *Capsules being dipped for coloring on automated capsule-making equipment. (Courtesy of SmithKline Beecham.)*

eliminates the problem of splitting during large-scale filling operations. In the CONI-SNAP SUPRO capsules, the upper capsule part extends so far over the lower part that only the rounded edge of the latter is visible (Fig. 7.5). Opening of such a filled capsule is difficult because the lower surface offers less gripping surface to pull the two halves apart. This increases the security of the contents and the integrity of the capsule.

After filling, some manufacturers render their capsules tamper-evident through various capsule sealing techniques. These methods are discussed later in this section. Capsules and tablets also may be imprinted with the names or monograms of the manufacturer, the assigned national drug code (NDC) number and other markings making the product identifiable and distinguishable from other products (Fig. 7.6).

Capsule Sizes

Empty gelatin capsules are manufactured in various sizes, varying in length, in diameter, and capacity. The size selected for use is determined by the

CONI-SNAP™

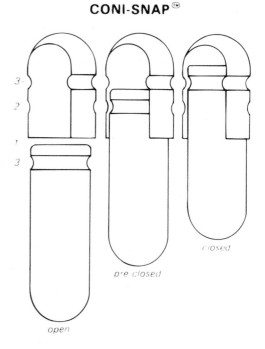

Fig. 7.4 *Line drawings of the CONI-SNAP capsule in open, pre-closed, and closed positions. The tapered rims 1) avoid telescoping; the indentations 2) prevent premature opening, and the grooves 3) lock the two capsule parts together after the capsule has been filled. (Courtesy of Capsugel Division, Warner-Lambert Co.)*

CONI-SNAP ™

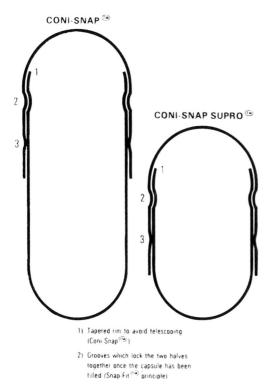

CONI-SNAP SUPRO ™

1) Tapered rim to avoid telescoping
   (Coni Snap ™)

2) Grooves which lock the two halves
   together once the capsule has been
   filled (Snap-Fit ™ principle)

3) Indentations to prevent premature
   opening

Fig. 7.5 *Line drawings of the CONI-SNAP and CONI-SNAP SUPRO (on right) capsules. The latter is designed to be smaller and to have the lower portion of the capsule shell concealed except for the rounded end. This makes separation of the two parts more difficult and contributes to capsule integrity. (Courtesy of Capsugel Division, Warner-Lambert Co.)*

1. Developing and preparing the formulation and selecting the size capsule.
2. Filling the capsule shells.
3. Capsule sealing (optional).
4. Cleaning and polishing the filled capsules.

Developing the Formulation and Selection of Capsule Size

In developing a capsule formulation, the goal is to prepare a capsule with accurate dosage, good bioavailability, ease of filling and production, stability, and elegance.

In dry formulations, the active and inactive components must be blended thoroughly to ensure a uniform powder mix for the capsule fill. Care in blending is especially critical for low-dose drugs since lack of homogeneity could result in significant therapeutic consequences. Preformulation studies

are performed to determine if all of the formulation's bulk powders may be effectively blended together as such or if they require reduction of particle size or other processing to achieve homogeneity.

A diluent or filler may be added to the formulation to produce the proper capsule fill volume. Lactose, microcrystalline cellulose and starch are commonly used for this purpose. In addition to providing bulk, these materials often provide cohesion to the powders, which is beneficial in the transfer of the powder blend into capsule shells (2). Disintegrants are frequently included in a capsule formulation to assist the break-up and distribution of the capsule contents in the stomach. Among the disintegrants used are pregelatinized starch, croscarmellose, and sodium starch glycolate.

To achieve uniform drug distribution, it is advantageous if the density and particle size of the drug and nondrug components are similar. This is par-

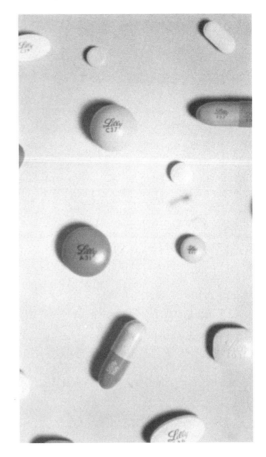

Fig. 7.6 *Examples of tablets and capsules marked with a letter-number code to facilitate identification. (Courtesy of Eli Lilly and Company.)*

Table 7.1. Approximate Capacity of Empty Gelatin Capsules

	Capsule Size							
Volume (mL)	1.40	0.95	0.68	0.50	0.37	0.30	0.21	0.13
*Drug Substance (mg)**								
Quinine Sulfate	650	390	325	227	195	130	97	65
Sodium Bicarbonate	1430	975	715	510	390	325	260	130
Aspirin	1040	650	520	325	260	195	162	97

*Amount may vary according to the degree of pressure used in filling the capsules.

ticularly important when a drug of low dosage is blended with other drugs or nondrug fill (8). When necessary, particle size may be reduced by *milling* to produce particles ranging from about 50 to 1000 microns. Milled powders may be blended effectively for uniform distribution throughout a powder mix when the drug's dosage is 10 mg or greater (8). For drugs of lower dose or when smaller particles are required, *micronization* is employed. Depending on the materials and equipment used, micronization produces particles ranging from about 1 to 20 microns in size.

In preparing capsules on an industrial scale using high-speed automated equipment, the powder mix or granules must be free-flowing to allow steady passage of the capsule fill from the hopper through the encapsulating equipment and into the capsule shells. The addition of a *lubricant or glidant* such as fumed silicon dioxide, magnesium stearate, calcium stearate, stearic acid, or talc (about 0.25–1%) to the powder mix enhances flow properties (2).

When magnesium stearate is used as the lubricant, the water-proofing characteristics of this water-insoluble material can retard penetration by the gastrointestinal fluids and delay drug dissolution and absorption. The addition of surface active agents, as sodium lauryl sulfate, to capsule and tablet formulations is used to facilitate wetting by the gastrointestinal fluids to overcome the problem (9). Even in instances in which a water-insoluble lubricant is not used, after the gelatin capsule shell dissolves, gastrointestinal fluids must displace the air that surrounds the dry powder and penetrate the drug before it can be dispersed and dissolved. Powders of poorly soluble drugs have a tendency to resist such penetration. Disintegration agents included in a capsule formulation facilitate the break up and distribution of the capsule's contents.

Whether it be the presence of a lubricant, surfactant, disintegrating agent, or some other pharmaceutic excipient, formulation can influence the bioavailability of a drug substance and can account for differences in drug effects, which may be encountered between two capsule products of the same medicinal substance. Pharmacists must be aware of this possibility when product-interchange is considered.

Inserting tablets or small capsules within capsules is sometimes a useful technique in the commercial production of capsules and in a pharmacist's extemporaneous preparation of capsules (Fig. 7.8). This may be done to separate chemically incompatible agents or to add premeasured (as tablets) amounts of potent drug substances. Rather

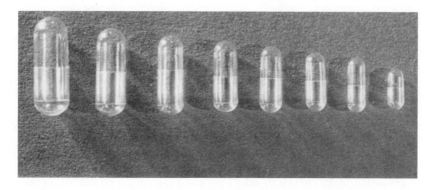

Fig. 7.7　*Actual sizes of hard gelatin capsules. From left to right, sizes 000, 00, 0, 1, 2, 3, 4, and 5.*

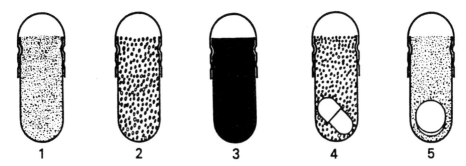

Fig. 7.8 *Examples of fill in hard gelatin capsules. 1, powder or granulate; 2, pellet mixture; 3, paste; 4, capsule; and 5, tablet. (Courtesy of Capsugel, Division of Warner-Lambert)*

than weighing a potent drug, a pharmacist may choose to insert an available prefabricated tablet of the desired strength in each capsule. Other less potent agents and diluents may then we weighed and added. On an industrial scale, coated pellets designed for modified-release drug delivery are also commonly placed in capsule shells.

Gelatin capsules are unsuitable for the encapsulation of aqueous liquids because water softens gelatin and distorts the capsules, resulting in leakage of the contents. However, some liquids such as fixed or volatile oils that do not interfere with the stability of the gelatin shells may be placed in locking gelatin capsules (or the capsules may be sealed with a solution of gelatin thinly coating the interface of the cap and body) to ensure the retention of the liquid. Rather than placing a liquid in a capsule as such, the liquid may be mixed with an inert powder to make a wetted mass or paste, which may then be placed in capsules in the usual manner (Fig. 7.8). *Eutectic mixtures* of drugs, or mixtures of agents that have a propensity to liquefy when admixed, may be mixed with a diluent or absorbent such as magnesium carbonate, kaolin, or light magnesium oxide to separate the interacting agents and to absorb any liquefied material which may form.

In large-scale capsule production, liquids are placed in *soft gelatin* capsules that are sealed during the filling and manufacturing process. Soft capsules are discussed later in this chapter.

In most instances the amount of drug placed in a capsule represents a single dose of the medication. In some instances, when the usual dose of the drug is too large to place in a single capsule, two or more capsules may be required to provide the desired dose. The total amount of formula prepared is that amount necessary to fill the desired number of capsules. On an industrial scale this means hundreds of thousands of capsules. In community practice, an individual prescription may call for the preparation of only six or a dozen capsules. Any slight loss in fill-material during the preparation and capsule-filling process will not materially affect an industrial size batch, but in the community pharmacy, a slight loss of powder would result in an inadequate quantity to fill the last capsule. To ensure enough fill in the compounding of small numbers of capsules, the community pharmacist may calculate for the preparation of one or two more capsules than is required to fill the prescription. However, this procedure may not be followed for capsules containing a controlled substance since the amount of drug used and that called for in the prescription must strictly coincide.

The selection of the capsule size for a commercial product is done during the product development stage. The choice is determined by requirements of the formulation, including the dose of the active ingredient, and the density and compaction characteristics of the drug and nondrug components. If the dose of the drug is inadequate to fill the volume of the capsule body, a diluent is added. Information on the density and compaction characteristics of a capsule's active and inactive components and comparison to other similar materials and prior experiences can serve as a guide in selecting capsule size (7).

Hard gelatin capsules are used to encapsulate between about 65 mg and 1 g of powdered material. As shown in Table 7.1, the smallest capsule (No. 5), may be expected to hold 65 mg of powder or more, depending on the characteristics of the powder substance. Oftentimes, in the extemporaneous compounding of prescriptions, the best capsule size to use is determined by trial. Use of the smallest size capsule, properly filled, is preferred. A properly filled capsule should have its body filled with the drug mixture, not the cap. The cap is intended to fit snugly over the body to retain the contents.

The following examples demonstrate the drug and nondrug contents of a few commercially available capsules.

Tetracycline Capsules

Active ingredient:	Tetracycline hydrochloride, 250 mg
Filler:	Lactose
Lubricant/glidant:	Magnesium stearate
Capsule colorants:	FD&C Yellow No. 6, D&C Yellow No. 10, D&C Red No. 28, FD&C Blue No. 1
Capsule opaquant:	Titanium dioxide

Acetaminophen with Codeine Capsules

Active ingredients:	Acetaminophen, 325 mg Codeine phosphate, 30 mg
Disintegrant:	Sodium starch glycolate
Lubricant/glidants:	Magnesium stearate, stearic acid
Capsule colorants:	D&C Yellow No. 10, Edible Ink, FD&C Blue No. 1 (FD&C Green No. 3 and FD&C Red No. 40)

Diphenhydramine Hydrochloride Capsules

Active ingredient:	Diphenhydramine HCl, 50 mg
Filler:	Confectioner's sugar
Lubricants/glidants:	Talc, colloidal silicon dioxide
Wetting agent:	Sodium lauryl sulfate
Capsule colorants:	FD&C Blue No. 1, FD&C Red No. 3
Capsule opaquant:	Titanium dioxide

Filling Hard Capsule Shells

When filling a small number of capsules in the pharmacy, the pharmacist uses the"punch"method. In this method, the pharmacist takes the precise number of empty capsules to be filled from his stock container. By counting the capsules as the initial step rather than taking a capsule from stock as each one is filled, the pharmacist guards against filling an erroneous number of capsules and avoids contaminating the stock container with drug powder. The powder to be encapsulated is placed on a sheet of clean paper or on a glass or porcelain plate. Using the spatula, the powder mix is formed into a cake having a depth of approximately one-fourth to one-third the length of the capsule body. Then an empty capsule body is held between the thumb

and forefinger and "punched" vertically into the powder cake repeatedly until filled. Some pharmacists wear surgical gloves or latex finger cots to avoid handling the capsules with bare fingers. Because the amount of powder packed into a capsule depends upon the degree of compression, the pharmacist should punch each capsule in the same manner and after capping weigh the product. When nonpotent materials are placed in capsules, the first filled capsule should be weighed (using an empty capsule of the same size on the opposite balance pan to counter the weight of the shell) to determine the capsule size to use and the degree of compaction to be used. After this determination, the other capsules should be prepared and weighed periodically to check the uniformity of the process. When potent drugs are being used, *each capsule* should be weighed after filling to ensure accuracy. Such weighings protect against the uneven filling of capsules and the premature exhaustion or underutilization of the powder. After the body of a capsule has been filled and the cap placed on the body, the body may be squeezed gently to distribute some powder to the cap-end to give the capsule a full appearance.

Granular material that does not lend itself to the "punch" method of filling capsules may be poured into each capsule individually from the powder paper on which it is weighed.

Pharmacists who prepare capsules on a regular or extensive basis may use hand-operated capsule filling machines (Fig. 7.9). The various types of available machines have capacities ranging from 24 to 300 capsules and when efficiently operated are capable of producing from about 200 to 2000 capsules per hour.

Machines developed for industrial use automatically separate the caps from empty capsules, fill the bodies, scrape off the excess powder, replace the caps, seal the capsules as desired, and clean the outside of the filled capsules at a rate of up to 165,000 capsules per hour (Fig. 7.10). The formulation must be such that the filled body contains the accurate drug dosage. This is verified through the use of automated in-process sampling and analysis equipment and processes (Figs. 7.11, 7.12).

As described later, the USP requires adherence to standards for *content uniformity* and *weight variation* for capsules to assure the accuracy of dosage units.

Capsule Sealing

As mentioned previously, some manufacturers make tamper-evident capsules by sealing the joint between the two capsule parts. One manufacturer

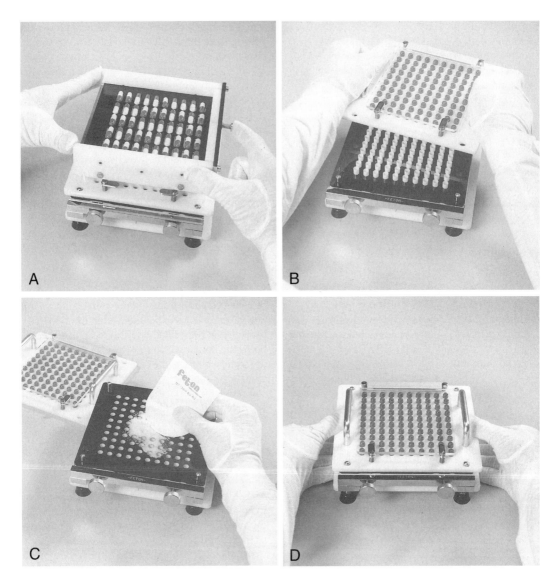

Fig. 7.9 *The Feton capsule filling machine. A, with empty capsules in the loader tray, the tray placed on top of the filler unit; B, the loader inserts the capsules into the filling unit and is removed and the top plate is lifted to separate the caps from the bodies; C, the powder is placed on the unit and the capsule bodies filled; D, the top plate then is returned to the unit and the caps placed on filled capsule bodies. (Courtesy of Chemical and Pharmaceutical Industry Company)*

makes distinctive-looking capsules by sealing them with a colored band of gelatin (KAPSEALS, Parke-Davis). If removed, the band cannot be restored without expert resealing with gelatin. Capsules may also be sealed through a heat welding process that fuses the capsule cap to the body through the double wall thickness at their juncture (10). The process results in a distinctive "ring" around the capsule where heat welded. Still another process utilizes a melting-point-lowering liquid wetting agent in the contact areas of the capsule's cap and body and then thermally bonds the two parts using low temperatures (40–45°C) (11). Industrial capsule sealing machines are capable of producing 60,000 to 150,000 gelatin banded, heat welded, or thermally coupled capsules per hour (12). Figure 7.13 depicts a sealed hard gelatin capsule. Although difficult and tedious, extemporaneously prepared

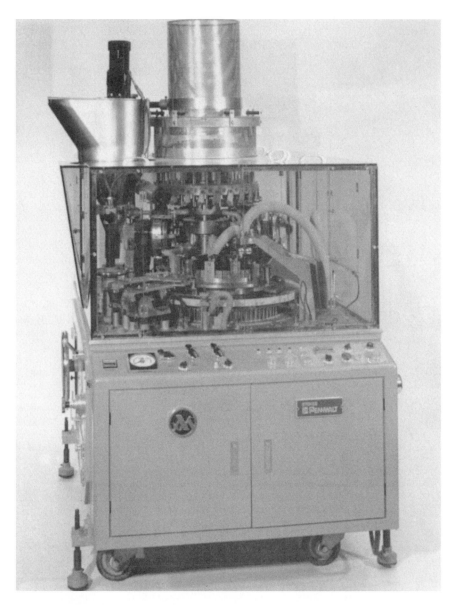

Fig. 7.10   *Osaka Automatic Capsule Filler (Model R-180), capable of filling up to 165,000 capsules per hour. (Courtesy of Sharples-Stokes Div., Stokes-Merrill, Pennwalt Corporation.)*

capsules may be sealed by lightly coating the inner surface of the cap with a warm gelatin solution immediately prior to placement on the filled capsule body.

Cleaning and Polishing Capsules

Small amounts of powder may adhere to the outside of capsules after filling. The powder may be bitter or otherwise unpalatable and should be re-moved before packaging or dispensing. On a small scale, capsules may be cleaned individually or in small numbers by rubbing them with a clean gauze or cloth. On a large scale, many capsule-filling machines are affixed with a cleaning vacuum that removes any extraneous material from the capsules as they exit the equipment. Figure 7.14 shows the industrial cleaning and polishing of hard filled capsules using the Accela-Cota apparatus.

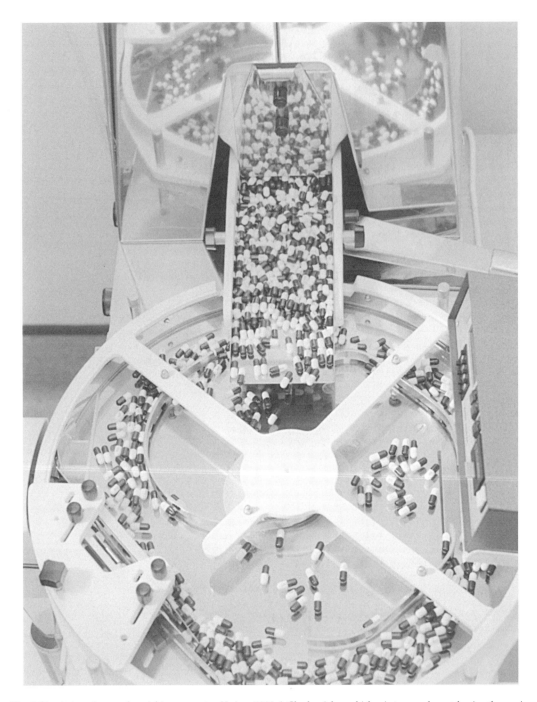

Fig. 7.11 *Automatic capsule weighing apparatus, Vericap 1800 A Checkweigher, which rejects capsules not having the precise weight. (Courtesy of Elan Corporation)*

Soft Gelatin Capsules

Soft gelatin capsules are made of gelatin to which glycerin or a polyhydric alcohol such as sorbitol has been added to render the gelatin elastic or plastic-like. Soft gelatin capsules, which contain more moisture than hard capsules, may have a preservative added as methylparaben and/or propylparaben to retard microbial growth. Soft gelatin capsules may be manufactured to be oblong, oval or round

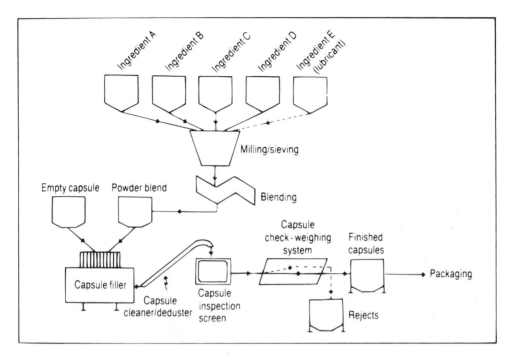

Fig. 7.12 *Process flow diagram for automated capsule filling. (Reprinted with permission from Yelvig M. Principles of process automation for liquid and solid dosage forms. Pharm Technol, 8:47, 1984.)*

in shape. They may be prepared of a single or two-tone color and may be imprinted with identifying markings. As hard gelatin capsules, they may be prepared with opaquants to reduce transparency and render characteristic feature to the capsule shell.

Soft gelatin capsules are used to hermetically seal and encapsulate liquids, suspensions, pasty materials, dry powders and even preformed tablets. Soft gelatin capsules are pharmaceutically elegant and are easily swallowed by the patient.

Preparation of Soft Gelatin Capsules (13)

They may be prepared by the plate process, using a set of molds to form the capsules, or by the more efficient and productive rotary or reciprocating die processes by which they are produced, filled, and sealed in a continuous operation (Fig. 7.15).

By the plate process, a warm sheet of plain or colored gelatin is placed on the bottom plate of the

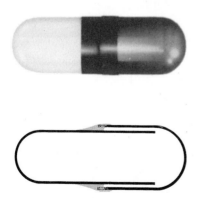

Fig. 7.13 *Z-Weld's gelatin seal fuses the two capsule halves together to create a one-piece capsule that is tamper-evident. (Courtesy of Raymond Automation Co.)*

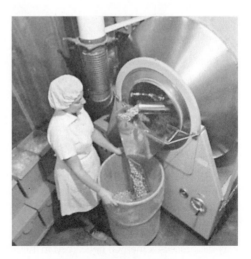

Fig. 7.14 *Cleaning and polishing hard filled capsules using the Accela-Cota apparatus. (Courtesy of Eli Lilly and Company.)*

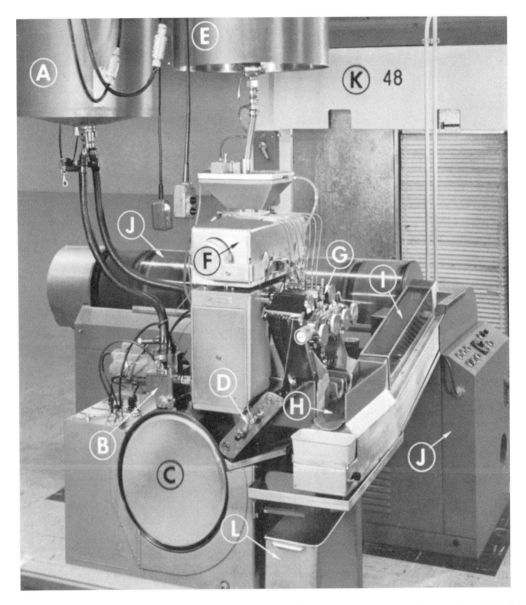

Fig. 7.15 *Rotary die process equipment. A, Gelatin tank; B, spreader box; C, gelatin ribbon casting drum; D, mineral oil lubricant bath; E, medicine tank; F, filling pump; G, encapsulating mechanism; H, capsule conveyor; I, capsule washer; J, infrared dryer; K, capsule drying tunnel; L, gelatin net receiver. (Courtesy of R.P. Scherer Corporation.)*

mold and the liquid-containing medication is evenly poured on it. Then a second sheet of gelatin is carefully placed on top of the medication and the top plate of the mold is put into place. Pressure is then applied to the mold to form, fill, and seal the capsules simultaneously. The capsules are removed and washed with a solvent harmless to the capsules.

Most soft gelatin capsules are prepared by the rotary die process, a method developed in 1933 by Robert P. Scherer. By this method, liquid gelatin flowing from an overhead tank is formed into two continuous ribbons by the rotary die machine and brought together between twin rotating dies (Fig. 7.16). At the same time, metered fill material is injected between the ribbons precisely at the moment that the dies form pockets of the gelatin ribbons. These pockets of fill-containing gelatin are sealed by pressure and heat and then severed from

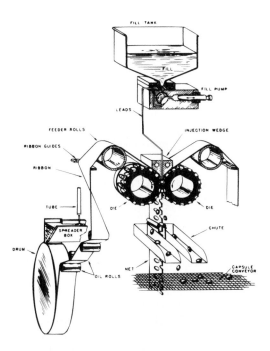

Fig. 7.16 *Schematic drawing of rotary die process. (Courtesy of R.P. Scherer Corporation.)*

the ribbon. Use of ribbons of two different colors results in bicolored capsules.

The reciprocating die process is similar to the rotary process in that ribbons of gelatin are formed and used to encapsulate the fill, but it differs in the actual encapsulating process. The gelatin ribbons are fed between a set of vertical dies that continually open and close to form rows of pockets in the gelatin ribbons. These pockets are filled with the medication and are sealed, shaped, and cut out of the film as they progress through the machinery. As the capsules are cut from the ribbons, they fall into refrigerated tanks which prevent the capsules from adhering to one another.

Utilization of Soft Gelatin Capsules

Soft gelatin capsules are prepared to contain a variety of liquid, pasty, and dry fills. Liquids that may be encapsulated into soft gelatin capsules include the following (13):

1. Water-immiscible volatile and nonvolatile liquids such as vegetable and aromatic oils, aromatic and aliphatic hydrocarbons, chlorinated hydrocarbons, ethers, esters, alcohols and organic acids.

2. Water-miscible, nonvolatile liquids, such as polyethylene glycols, and nonionic surface active agents as polysorbate 80.
3. Water-miscible and relatively nonvolatile compounds, as propylene glycol and isopropyl alcohol, depending on factors as concentration used and packaging conditions.

Liquids that can easily migrate through the capsule shell cannot be encapsulated into soft gelatin capsules. These materials include water above 5%, and low molecular weight water-soluble and volatile organic compounds such as alcohols, ketones, acids, amines, and esters.

Solids may be encapsulated into soft gelatin capsules as solutions in a suitable liquid solvent, suspensions, dry powders, granules, pellets, or small tablets.

Compendial Requirements for Capsules

Added Substances

Substances added to official preparations, including capsules, to enhance their stability, usefulness, elegance, or to facilitate their manufacture, may be used only if they (14):

1. are harmless in the quantities used;
2. do not exceed the minimum amounts required to provide their intended effect;
3. do not impair the product's bioavailability, therapeutic efficacy or safety, and
4. do not interfere with requisite compendial assays and tests.

Containers for Dispensing Capsules

There are specifications listed in the USP prescribing the type of container suitable for the repackaging or dispensing of each official capsule and tablet. Depending on the item, the container might be required to be *tight, well-closed and light resistant.*

Disintegration Test for Capsules

The compendial disintegration test for hard and soft gelatin capsules follows the same procedure and uses the same apparatus described later in this chapter for uncoated tablets. The capsules are placed in the basket-rack assembly, which is repeatedly immersed 30 times per minute into a thermostatically controlled fluid at 37°C and observed over the time described in the individual monograph. To fully satisfy the test, the capsules disintegrate completely into a soft mass having no palpably firm core, and only some fragments of the gelatin shell.

Dissolution Test for Capsules

The compendial dissolution test for capsules uses the same apparatus, dissolution medium and test as that for uncoated and plain coated tablets described later in this chapter. However, in instances in which the capsule shells interfere with the analysis, the contents of a specified number of capsules can be removed and the empty capsule shells dissolved in the dissolution medium before proceeding with the sampling and chemical analysis.

Weight Variation

The uniformity of dosage units may be demonstrated by determining *weight variation* and/or *content uniformity.* The weight variation method is as follows.

HARD CAPSULES. Ten capsules are individually weighed and the contents removed. The emptied shells are individually weighed and the net weight of the contents calculated by subtraction. From the results of an assay performed as directed in the individual monograph, the content of active ingredient in each of the capsules is determined.

SOFT CAPSULES. The gross weight of 10 intact capsules is determined individually. Then each capsule is cut open with a scissors or a sharp open blade, and the contents removed by washing with a suitable solvent. The solvent is allowed to evaporate at room temperature over a period of about 30 minutes, taking precautions to avoid uptake or loss of moisture. The individual shells are weighed and the net contents calculated. From the results of the assay directed in the individual monograph, the content of active ingredient in each of the capsules is determined.

Content Uniformity

Unless otherwise stated in the monograph for an individual capsule, the amount of active ingredient, determined by assay, is within the range of 85% to 115% of the label claim for 9 of 10 dosage units assayed, with no unit outside the range of 70% to 125% of label claim. Additional tests are prescribed when two or three dosage units are outside of the desired range but within the stated extremes.

Content Labeling Requirement

All official capsules must be labeled to express the quantity of each active ingredient in each dosage unit.

Stability Testing

Stability testing of capsules is performed as described in Chapter 3 to determine the intrinsic stability of the active drug molecule and the influence of environmental factors as temperature, humidity, light, formulative components and the container/closure system. The battery of stress testing, long-term stability and accelerated stability tests help determine the appropriate conditions for storage and the product's anticipated shelf-life.

Moisture Permeation Test

The USP requires determination of the moisture-permeation characteristics of single-unit and unit-dose containers to assure their suitability for packaging capsules. The degree and rate of moisture penetration is determined by packaging the dosage unit together with a color-revealing desiccant pellet, exposing the packaged unit to known relative humidity over a specified time, observing the desiccant pellet for color change (indicating absorption of moisture) and comparing the pre- and post-weight of the packaged unit.

Official and Commercially Available Capsules

There are approximately 200 officially recognized medications in capsule form in the USP. However commercially, there are many fold this number of capsule products available from various manufacturers for various drugs and in various dosage strengths.

Examples of official and commercially available medications in hard and soft gelatin capsules are presented in Tables 7.2 and 7.3.

Inspecting, Counting, Packaging, and Storing Capsules

Capsules produced on a small or large scale should be uniform in appearance. Visual or electronic inspection should be undertaken to detect any flaws in the integrity and appearance of the capsules. Defective capsules should be rejected. In commercial manufacture, Current Good Manufacturing Practice regulations require that if the number of production flaws is excessive, the cause must be investigated, documented and steps undertaken to correct the problem.

In the pharmacy, capsules may be counted manually or by automated equipment. For counting small numbers of solid dosage units, specially de-

Table 7.2.   Examples of Some Official Capsules

Official Capsule	Some Representative Commercial Capsules	Capsule Strengths	Category
Amoxicillin	Wymox (Wyeth-Ayerst)	250 and 500 mg	Antibacterial
Ampicillin	Omnipen (Wyeth-Ayerst)	250 and 500 mg	Antibacterial
Cephalexin	Keflex (Dista)	250 and 500 mg	Antibacterial
Diphenhydramine HCl	Benadryl HCl (Parke-Davis)	25 and 50 mg	Antihistaminic
Doxycycline Hyclate	Vibramycin (Pfizer)	50 and 100 mg	Antibacterial
Erythromycin Estolate	Ilosone (Dista)	125 and 250 mg	Antibactetrial
Fluoxitine HCl	Prozac (Dista)	10 and 20 mg	Antidepressant
Flurazepam HCl	Dalmane (Roche)	15 and 30 mg	Hypnotic
Gemfibrozil	Lopid (Parke-Davis)	300 mg	Antihyperlipidemic
Griseofulvin	Grisactin (Wyeth-Ayerst)	125 and 250 mg	Antifungal
Indomethacin	Indocin (Merck)	25 and 50 mg	Antiinflammatory; antipyretic; analgesic
Levodopa	Larodopa (Roche)	100, 250, and 500 mg	Antiparkinsonian
Loperamide HCl	Imodium (Janssen)	2 mg	Antidiarrheal
Oxazepam	Serax (Wyeth-Ayerst)	10, 15 and 30 mg	Antianxiety
Propoxyphene HCl	Darvon (Lilly)	32 and 65 mg	Analgesic
Tetracycline HCl	Achromycin V (Lederle)	250 and 500 mg	Antimicrobial

signed trays are used, as the type depicted in Figure 7.17. In using this tray, the pharmacist pours a supply of capsules or tablets from the bulk source onto the clean tray, and using the spatula counts and sweeps the dosage units into the trough until the desired number is reached. Then the pharmacist closes the trough cover, picks up the tray, returns the uncounted dosage units to the bulk container by means of the lip at the back of the tray, places the prescription container at the opening of the trough, and carefully transfers the capsules or tablets into the container. By this method, the dosage units remain untouched by the pharmacist. To prevent batch-to-batch contamination, the tray must be wiped clean after each use because powder, particularly from counting uncoated tablets, may remain.

In some community and hospital pharmacy settings, small automated counting and filling machines may be used as shown in Figure 7.18.

On the industrial scale, solid dosage forms are counted by large automated pieces of equipment that count and transfer the desired number of dosage units into bulk containers. The containers are then mechanically capped, inspected visually or electronically, labeled, and inspected once more. Some filled containers are then placed into outer packaging cartons. An industrial counting and filling machine is shown in Figure 7.19. Capsules are packaged in glass or in plastic containers, some containing packets of a desiccant to prevent the absorption of excessive moisture.

The unit dose and strip packaging of solid dosage

Table 7.3. Examples of Medications Commercially Prepared into Soft Gelatin Capsules

Drug Substance	Trade Name and Manufacture	Contents and Comments*
Acetazolamide	Diamox Sequels (Lederle)	Acetazolamide is a powder which is very slightly soluble in water. The capsules contain coated pellets of the drug with sustained release features. Acetazolamide is a carbonic anhydrase inhibitor.
Cyclosporine	Sandimmune (Novartis)	Cyclosporine is a slightly water soluble crystalline powder. The capsule also contains corn oil and polyoxyethylated glycolyzed glycerides. Cyclosporine in an immunosuppressive agent.
	Neoral (Novartis)	The capsule contains cyclosporine, dehydrated alcohol, corn oil-mono-ditriglycerides, polyoxyl 40 hydrogenated castor oil. The formulation forms a microemulsion in contact with aqueous fluids for enhanced bioavailability.
Digoxin	Lanoxicaps (Glaxo Wellcome)	Digoxin is a practically water-insoluble powder. The drug is dissolved in a solvent of polyethylene glycol 400, ethyl alcohol, propylene glycol and water. Digoxin is a cardiac glycoside.
Ethchlorvynol	Placidyl (Abbott)	Ethchlorvynol is a liquid immiscible in water. It is a hypnotic. The capsules also contain polyethylene glycol and sorbitol.
Ethosuximide	Zarontin (Parke-Davis)	Ethosuximide is a water soluble powder. The capsule also contains polyethylene glycol 400. Ethosuximide is an anticonvulsant.
Ranitidine HCl	Zantac GELdose (Glaxo Wellcome)	Ranitidine HCl is a water soluble granular powder. The drug is in a nonaqueous matrix of synthetic coconut oil and triglycerides. Ranitidine is a histamine H_2-receptor inhibitor.

*Only a partial listing of the capsule contents is given. The soft capsule shells may also contain colorants, opaquants, preservatives, and other agents.

forms, particularly by pharmacies that service nursing homes and hospitals, provides sanitary handling of the medications, ease of identification, and security in accountability for medications. Typical small scale strip packaging equipment and commercial unit-dose packages of capsules and tablets are presented in Figures 7.20 and 7.21, respectively. Capsules should be stored in tightly capped containers in a cool, dry place.

Tablets

Tablets are solid dosage forms usually prepared with the aid of suitable pharmaceutical excipients. They may vary in size, shape, weight, hardness, thickness, disintegration and dissolution characteristics, and in other aspects, depending upon their intended use and method of manufacture. The ma-

jority of tablets are used in the oral administration of drugs. Many of these are prepared with colorants and coatings of various types. Other tablets, as those administered sublingually, buccally or vaginally are prepared to have features most applicable to their particular route of administration. Advantages of tablets for oral administration were presented at the outset of this chapter.

Tablets are prepared primarily by compression with a limited number prepared by molding. Compressed tablets are manufactured with tablet machines capable of exerting great pressure in compacting the powdered or granulated tableting material (Fig. 7.22). Their shape and dimensions are determined by use of various shaped punches and dies (Fig. 7.23). Molded tablets are prepared on a large-scale by tablet machinery or on a small-scale by manually forcing dampened powder material

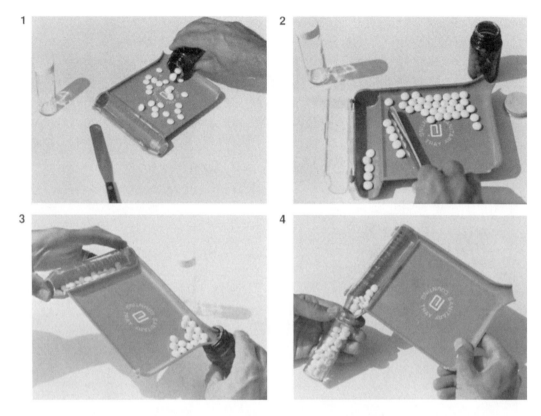

Fig. 7.17   *Steps in the counting of solid dosage units with the Abbott Sanitary Counting Tray: 1) placing units from stock package onto tray, 2) counting and transferring units to trough, 3) returning excess units to stock container, and 4) placing counted units into prescription container.*

into a mold from which the formed tablet is then ejected and allowed to dry.

Types of Tablets

The various types of tablets are described as follows, with their common abbreviations in parentheses.

Compressed Tablets (C.T.)

In addition to the medicinal agent(s), compressed tablets usually contain a number of pharmaceutical adjuncts including (a) *diluents* or *fillers,* which add the necessary bulk to a formulation to prepare tablets of the desired size; (b) *binders* or *adhesives,* which promote the adhesion of the particles of the formulation, enabling a granulation to be prepared and the maintenance of the integrity of the final tablet; (c) *disintegrants* or *disintegrating agents,* which promote the breakup of the tablets after administration to smaller particles for more ready drug availability; (d) *antiadherents, glidants, lubricants* or

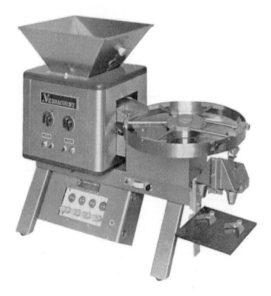

Fig. 7.18   *Versacount Model automatic tablet and capsule counting and filling apparatus. (Courtesy of Production Equipment Co.)*

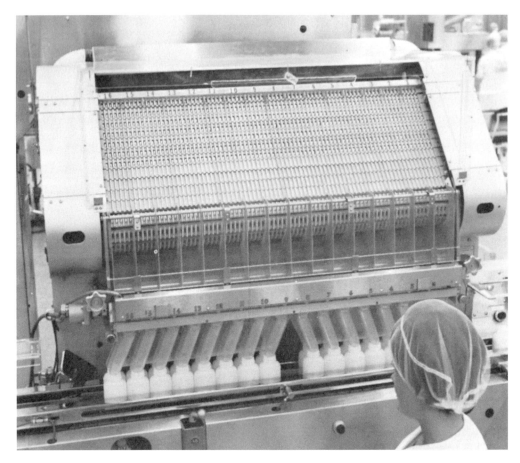

Fig. 7.19 *Large Merrill filling machine that fills 16 bottles with 200 tablets each at one time. A flipper gate in the upper manifold directs the tablets into one row of bottles while the other filled row is evacuated and a new row of bottles moves into place. (Courtesy of The Upjohn Company.)*

lubricating agents, which enhance the flow of the tableting material into the tablet dies, minimize wear of the punches and dies, prevent the sticking of fill material to the punches and dies and produce tablets having a sheen; and (e) *miscellaneous adjuncts* such as colorants and flavorants. After compression, tablets may be coated with various materials as described later. Tablets for oral, buccal, sublingual or vaginal administration may be prepared by compression.

Multiple Compressed Tablets (M.C.T.)

Multiple compressed tablets are prepared by subjecting the fill material to more than a single compression. The result may be a multiple-layered tablet or a tablet-within-a-tablet, the inner tablet being the *core* and the outer portion being the *shell* (Fig. 7.24). Layered tablets are prepared by the initial compaction of a portion of fill material in a die followed by additional fill material and compression to form two- or three-layered tablets, depending upon the number of separate fills. Each layer may contain a different medicinal agent, separated from one another for reasons of chemical or physical incompatibility, staged drug release, or simply for the unique appearance of the multiple-layered tablet. Usually, each portion of fill is colored differently to prepare a distinctive looking tablet. In the preparation of tablets having a compressed tablet as the inner core, special machines are required to place the preformed tablet precisely within the die for the subsequent compression of surrounding fill material.

Sugar-Coated Tablets (S.C.T.)

Compressed tablets may be coated with a colored or an uncolored sugar layer. The coating is water-soluble and is quickly dissolved after swallow-

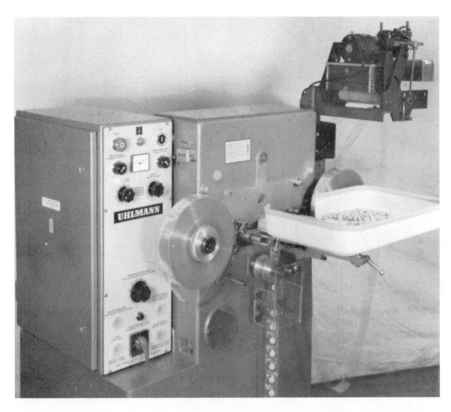

Fig. 7.20   *Strip packager for the unit dose dispensing of solid dosage forms. Drug information is imprinted on each individual package unit. The model shown has a fully automatic cutoff from 1 to 24 dosage units and is especially suited to unit-dose packaging and dispensing in hospitals, dispensaries, nursing homes, and clinics. (Courtesy of Lakso Company, Inc.)*

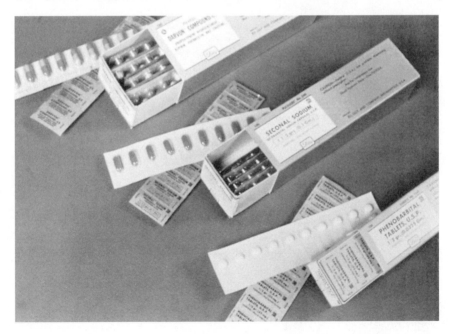

Fig. 7.21   *Example of unit-dose packaging of tablets and capsules. The drug name and other information are imprinted on the backing portion of each unit. (Courtesy of Eli Lilly and Company.)*

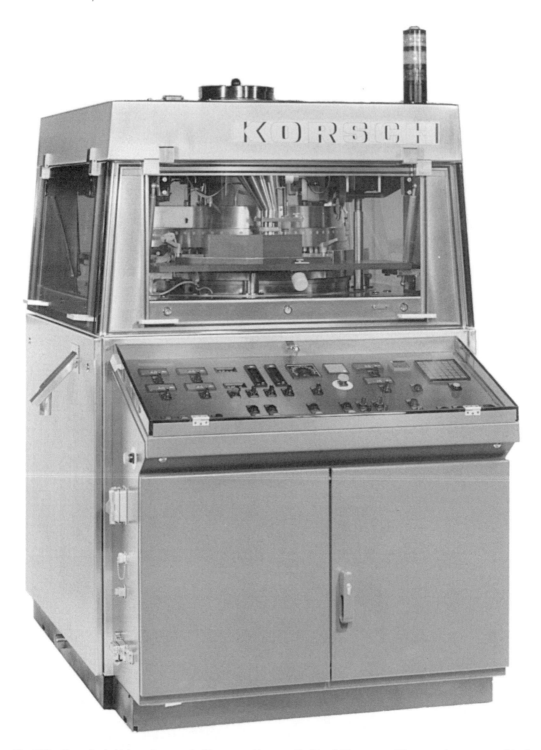

Fig. 7.22 *Example of a high-performance double rotary tablet press. The Korsch PharmapressR has a maximum output of 1 million tablets per hour but for continuous operation it is generally run to produce 600,000 to 800,000 tablets per hour. (Courtesy of Korsch Tableting, Inc.)*

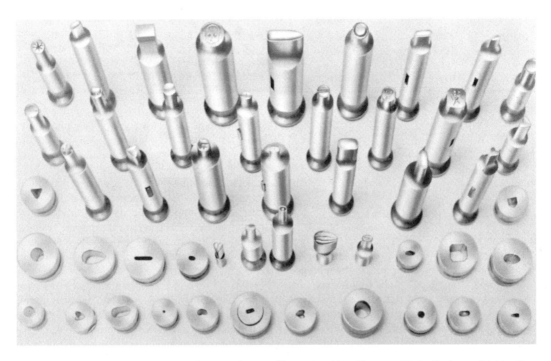

Fig. 7.23 *Various Stokes punches and dies for the production of distinctive tablets. (Courtesy of Stokes Equipment Division, Pennwalt Chemicals Corporation.)*

ing. It serves the purpose of protecting the enclosed drug from the environment and provides a barrier to objectional tasting or smelling drugs. The sugar coating also enhances the appearance of the compressed tablet and permits the imprinting of identifying manufacturer's information. Among the disadvantages to sugar-coating tablets are the time and expertise required in the coating process and the increase in the size, weight, and shipping costs of the tablets. Sugar-coated tablets may be 50% larger and heavier than the original uncoated tablets.

Film-Coated Tablets (F.C.T.)

Film-coated tablets are compressed tablets coated with a thin layer of a polymer capable of forming a skin-like film over the tablet. The film is usually colored and has the advantage over sugar-coatings in that it is more durable, less bulky, and less time-consuming to apply. By its composition, the coating is designed to rupture and expose the core tablet at the desired location within the gastrointestinal tract.

Gelatin-Coated Tablets

A recent innovation in tablet coating is the gelatin-coated tablet. The innovator product, termed GELCAPS, is a capsule-shaped compressed tablet

(Fig. 7.25) that allows the coated product to be about one-third smaller than a capsule filled with an equivalent amount of powder. The gelatin coating facilitates swallowing and compared to unsealed capsules, gelatin-coated tablets are more tamper-evident.

Enteric-Coated Tablets (E.C.T.)

Enteric-coated tablets have delayed-release features. They are designed to pass unchanged through

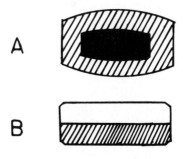

Fig. 7.24 *Diagram of multiple-compressed tablets. A, having a core of one drug and a shell of another, and B, a multiple-layered tablet of two drugs.*

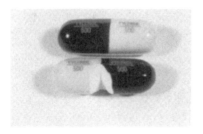

Fig. 7.25 *Cut-away view of "Gelcaps" dosage form. A gelatin-coated capsule-shaped tablet. Dosage form is more easily swallowed than a comparable tablet, smaller than an equivalent capsule, and tamper-evident. (Courtesy of McNeil Consumer Products Co.)*

the stomach with transit to the intestines where the tablets disintegrate and allow drug dissolution and absorption and/or effect. Enteric coatings are employed in instances in which the drug substance is destroyed by gastric acid, is particularly irritating to the gastric mucosa, or when by-pass of the stomach substantially enhances drug absorption.

Buccal or Sublingual Tablets

Buccal or sublingual tablets are flat, oval tablets intended to be dissolved in the buccal pouch (*buccal tablets*) or beneath the tongue (*sublingual tablets*) for absorption through the oral mucosa. They enable the oral absorption of drugs that are destroyed by the gastric juice and/or are poorly absorbed from the gastrointestinal tract. Buccal tablets are designed to erode slowly, whereas those for sublingual use (as nitroglycerin sublingual tablets) dissolve promptly and provide rapid drug effects. *Lozenges* or *troches,* are disc-shaped, solid dosage forms containing a medicinal agent and generally a flavoring substance in a hard candy or sugar base. They are intended to be slowly dissolved in the oral cavity usually for localized effects although some may be formulated for systemic absorption.

Chewable Tablets

Chewable tablets, which have a smooth, rapid disintegration when chewed or allowed to dissolve in the mouth, have a creamy base usually of specially flavored and colored mannitol. Chewable tablets are especially useful for the administration of tablets of large-size to children and adults who have difficulty swallowing solid dosage forms.

Effervescent Tablets

Effervescent tablets are prepared by compressing granular effervescent salts that release gas when in contact with water. These tablets generally contain medicinal substances which dissolve rapidly when added to water.

Molded Tablets (M.T.)

Certain tablets, as tablet triturates, may be prepared by molding rather than by compression. The resultant tablets are very soft, soluble, and are designed for rapid dissolution.

Tablet Triturates (T.T.)

Tablet triturates are small, usually cylindrical, molded (M.T.T.) or compressed tablets (C.T.T.) containing small amounts of usually potent drugs. Today only a few tablet triturate products are available commercially, with most of these produced by tablet compression. Since tablet triturates must be readily and completely soluble in water only a minimal amount of pressure is applied during their manufacture. A combination of sucrose and lactose is usually the diluent. The few tablet triturates which remain are used sublingually, as nitroglycerin tablets.

In the past, pharmacists employed tablet triturates in compounding procedures. For example, they were inserted into capsules or dissolved in liquid preparations to provide accurate amounts of potent drug substances.

Hypodermic Tablets (H.T.)

Hypodermic tablets are no longer available in the United States. They were originally used by physicians in the extemporaneous preparation of parenteral solutions. The required number of tablets was dissolved in a suitable vehicle, sterility attained, and the injection performed. The tablets were a convenience, since they could be easily carried in the physician's medicine bag and injections prepared to meet the needs of the individual patients. However, the difficulty in achieving sterility, the current availability of prefabricated injectable products, some in disposable syringes, have eliminated the need for hypodermic tablets.

Dispensing Tablets (D.T.)

Dispensing tablets are no longer in use. They might better have been termed *compounding tablets* because they were used by the pharmacist in compounding prescriptions and were *not* dispensed as such to the patient. The tablets contained large amounts of highly potent drug substances enabling the pharmacist to rapidly obtain premeasured amounts for compounding multiple dosage units. These tablets had the dangerous potential of being inadvertently dispensed as such to patients.

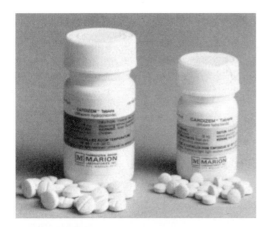

Immediate Release Tablets (I.R.)

Immediate release tablets are designed to disintegrate and release their medication absent of any special rate-controlling features as special coatings and other techniques.

Instant Disintegrating / Dissolving Tablets

Instant-release tablets are characterized by disintegrating/dissolving in the mouth within one minute; some within 10 seconds [e.g., Claritin Reditabs (loratadine), Schering]. Tablets of this type are designed for pediatric and geriatric patients or for any patient who has difficulty in swallowing tablets. After placing them on the tongue they liquefy and the patient swallows the liquid. A number of techniques are used to prepare these tablets involving lyophilization (e.g., Zydis, R.P. Scherer), soft direct compression (e.g., WOW-Tab, Yamanouchi-Shaklee Pharma), and other methods (e.g., Quicksolv, Janssen). These tablets are prepared using very water-soluble excipients designed to "wick" water into the tablet for rapid disintegration/dissolution. They have the stability characteristics of other solid dosage forms.

Extended Release Tablets (E.R.)

Extended-release tablets (sometimes called "controlled release (CR)" tablets) are designed to release their medication in a predetermined manner over an extended period of time. They are discussed in Chapter 8.

Vaginal Tablets

Vaginal tablets, also called *vaginal inserts*, are uncoated and bullet- or ovoid-shaped tablets which are inserted into the vagina for localized effects. They are prepared by compression and shaped to fit snugly on plastic inserter devices which accompany the product. They contain antibacterials for the treatment of vaginitis caused by *Hemophilus vaginalis* or antifungals for the treatment of vulvovaginitis candidiasis caused by *Candida albicans* and related species.

Compressed Tablets

The physical features of compressed tablets are well known. Some are: round, oblong, or unique in shape; thick or thin; large or small in diameter; flat or convex; unscored or *scored* (Fig. 7.26) in halves, thirds, or quadrants; engraved or imprinted with an identifying symbol and/or code number; coated or uncoated; colored or uncolored; single layer, or bi- or tri-layered.

Tablet diameters and shapes are determined by the die and punches used in the compression of the tablet. The less concave the punches, the more flat the resulting tablets; conversely, the more concave the punches, the more convex the resulting tablets (Fig. 7.27). Punches having raised impressions will produce recessed impressions on the tablets; punches having recessed etchings will produce tablets having raised impression or monograms. Monograms may be placed on one or on both sides of a tablet, depending upon whether monogram-producing lower and/or upper punches are used.

Quality Standards and Compendial Requirements

In addition to the apparent features of tablets, pharmacists are aware that tablets must meet other physical specifications and quality standards. These include criteria for tablet weight, weight variation,

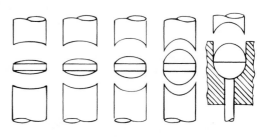

Fig. 7.27   *Contours of the punches determine the shape of the tablets. From left to right, flat face, shallow cup, standard cup, deep cup, and modified ball. (Courtesy of Cherry-Burrell Corporation.)*

content uniformity, tablet thickness, tablet hardness, tablet disintegration, and drug dissolution. These factors must be controlled during production (in-process controls) and verified after the production of each batch to assure that established product quality standards are met (Fig. 7.28).

TABLET WEIGHT AND USP WEIGHT VARIATION TEST. The quantity of fill placed in the die of a tablet press determines the weight of the resulting tablet. The volume of fill is adjusted with the first few tablets produced to yield tablets of the *desired weight and content.* For example, if a tablet is to contain 20 mg of a

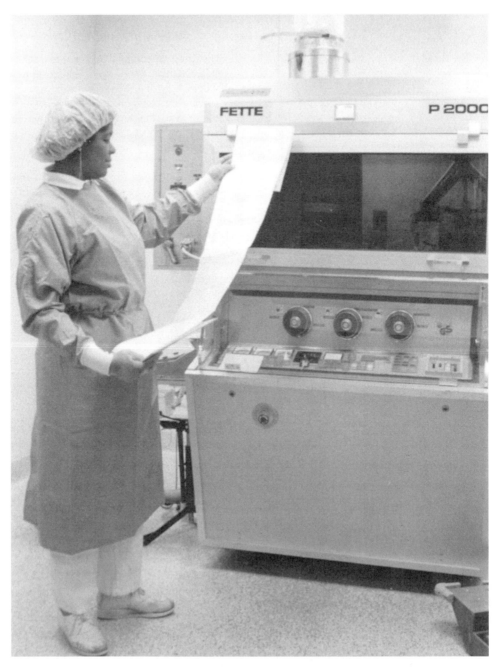

Fig. 7.28   *Quality control in the manufacturing of tablets. (Courtesy of Eli Lilly and Company.)*

drug substance and if 100,000 tablets are to be produced, 2,000 g of drug are included in the formula. After the addition of the pharmaceutical additives such as the diluent, disintegrant, lubricant, and binder, the formulation may weigh 20 kg, which means that each tablet must weigh 200 mg for 20 mg of drug to be present. Thus, the depth of fill in the tablet die must be adjusted to hold a volume of granulation weighing 200 mg. During production, sample tablets are periodically removed for visual inspection and automated physical measurement (Fig. 7.29).

The USP contains a test for the determination of dosage-form uniformity by *weight variation* for uncoated tablets (14). In the test, 10 tablets are weighed individually and the average weight calculated. The tablets are assayed and the content of active ingredient in each of the 10 tablets is calculated assuming homogeneous drug distribution.

CONTENT UNIFORMITY. By the USP method, 10 dosage units are individually assayed for their content according to the assay method described in the individual monograph. Unless otherwise stated in the monograph, the requirements for content uniformity are met if the amount of active ingredient in each dosage unit lies within the range of 85% to 115% of the label claim and the relative standard deviation is less than 6.0%. If one or more dosage units does not meet these criteria, additional tests as prescribed in the USP are required (14).

TABLET THICKNESS. The thickness of a tablet is determined by the diameter of the die, the amount of fill permitted to enter the die, the compactability of the fill material, and the force or pressure applied during compression.

To produce tablets of uniform thickness during batch production and between batch productions for the same formulation, care must be exercised to employ the same factors of fill, die, and pressure. It should be pointed out that the degree of tableting pressure affects not only tablet thickness but also tablet hardness. And, tablet hardness is perhaps the more important criterion since it can affect tablet disintegration and drug dissolution. Thus, for tablets of uniform thickness and hardness, it is doubly important to control tableting pressure. Tablet thickness may be measured by hand gauge during production or by automated equipment.(Figs. 7.30, 7.31).

TABLET HARDNESS AND FRIABILITY. It is not unusual for a tablet press to exert as little as 3000 and as much as 40,000 pounds of force in the production of tablets. Generally, the greater the pressure applied, the harder the tablets, although the characteristics of the granulation also has a bearing on tablet hardness. Certain tablets, such as lozenges and buccal tablets that are intended to dissolve slowly, intentionally are made hard; other tablets, as those for immediate drug release are made soft. In general, tablets should be sufficiently

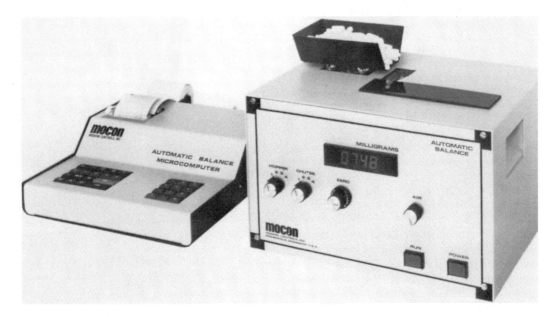

Fig. 7.29 *Automatic balance that weighs product and prints statistics to determine compliance with USP weight variation requirements for tablets. (Courtesy of Mocon Modern Controls, Inc.)*

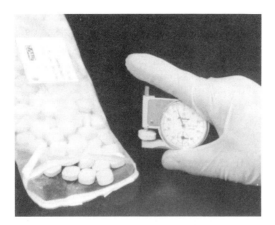

Fig. 7.30   *Tablet thickness gauge. (Courtesy of Eli Lilly and Company.)*

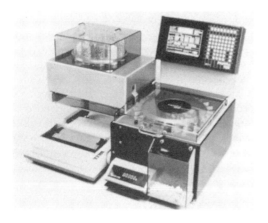

Fig. 7.31   *Automatic weight, hardness, thickness, and tablet diameter test instrument for quality control. Using a microprocessor and monitor for visualization, the instrument can test up to 20 samples at a time. (Courtesy of Scientific Instruments & Technology Corporation.)*

tating apparatus. The tablets are weighed before and after a specified number of rotations and any loss in weight determined. Resistance to loss of weight indicates the tablet's ability to withstand abrasion in handling, packaging, and shipment. A maximum weight loss of not more than 1% of the weight of the tablets being tested generally is considered acceptable for most products.

TABLET DISINTEGRATION. For the medicinal agent in a tablet to become fully available for absorption, the tablet must first disintegrate and discharge the drug to the body fluids for dissolution. Tablet disintegration also is important for those tablets containing medicinal agents (such as antacids and antidiarrheals) that are not intended to be absorbed but rather to act locally within the gastrointestinal tract. In these instances, tablet disintegration provides drug particles with an increased surface area for localized activity within the gastrointestinal tract.

All USP tablets must pass a test for disintegration, which is conducted *in vitro* using a testing apparatus as the one shown in Figure 7.34. The apparatus consists of a basket-rack assembly containing six open-ended transparent tubes of USP-specified dimensions, held vertically upon a 10-mesh stainless steel wire screen. During testing, a tablet is placed in each of the six tubes of the basket and through the use of a mechanical device, the basket is raised and lowered in the immersion fluid at a frequency of between 29 and 32 cycles per minute, the wire screen always being maintained below the level of the fluid. For uncoated tablets, buccal tablets, and sublingual tablets, water maintained at about 37°C serves as the immersion fluid unless another fluid is specified in the individual monograph. For

hard to resist breaking during normal handling and yet soft enough to disintegrate properly after swallowing.

Special dedicated hardness testers (Fig. 7.32) or multifunctional systems (Fig. 7.31) are used to measure the degree of force (in kilograms, pounds, or in arbitrary units) required to break a tablet. A force of about 4 kilograms is considered the minimum requirement for a satisfactory tablet. Multifunctional automated equipment can determine tablet weight, hardness, thickness and diameter.

A tablet's durability may be determined through the use of a *friabilator* (Fig. 7.33). This apparatus determines the tablet's *friability*, or its tendency to crumble by allowing it to roll and fall within the ro-

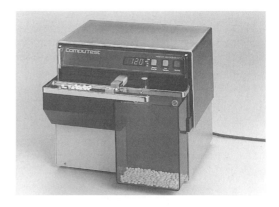

Fig. 7.32   *CompuTest hardness tester, tests in Newtons, Kilopond, and Strong Cobb. Automatic or manually operated. tests up to 100 tablets per run. Integrated software stores product test programs. (Courtesy of Vector Corporation).*

these tests, complete disintegration is defined as "that state in which any residue of the unit, except fragments of insoluble coating or capsule shell, remaining on the screen of the test apparatus is a soft

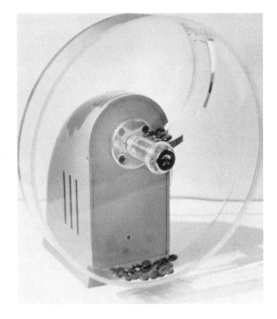

Fig. 7.33   *Erweka tablet testing apparatus for rolling and impact durability. Tablets are weighed and placed in the plexiglass drum in which a curved baffle is mounted. When the motor is activated by setting the timer, the tablets roll and drop. If the free fall within the drum results in the breakage or excessive abrasion of the tablets, they are considered not suited to withstand shipment without being damaged. The motor makes 20 rpm. After the tablets have been tested, they are removed and weighed again. The difference in weight within a given time indicates the rate of abrasion. (Courtesy of Chemical and Pharmaceutical Industry Co.)*

mass having no palpably firm core" (14). Tablets must disintegrate within the times set forth in the individual monograph, usually 30 minutes, but varying from about 2 minutes for Nitroglycerin Tablets to up to 4 hours for buccal tablets. If one or more tablets fail to disintegrate, additional tests prescribed by the USP must be performed.

Enteric-coated tablets are similarly tested, except that the tablets are permitted to be tested in simulated gastric fluid for one hour after which no sign of disintegration, cracking, or softening must be seen. They are then actively immersed in the simulated intestinal fluid for the time stated in the individual monograph during which time the tablets disintegrate completely for a positive test.

TABLET DISSOLUTION. In vitro dissolution testing of solid dosage forms is important for a number of reasons (15).

1. It guides the formulation and product development process toward product optimization. By conducting dissolution studies in the early stages of a product's development, differentiations can be made between formulations and correlations identified with in vivo bioavailability data.
2. The performance of the manufacturing process may be monitored by dissolution testing, as a component of the overall quality assurance program. The conduct of such testing from the early product development through product approval and commercial batch production assures the control of any potential variables of materials and processes which could affect drug dissolution and the product's quality standards.
3. Consistent in vitro dissolution testing results assure bioequivalence from batch-to-batch. In assessing such batch-to-batch bioequivalence, the

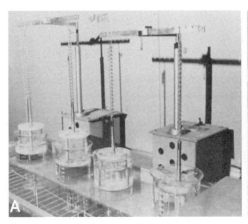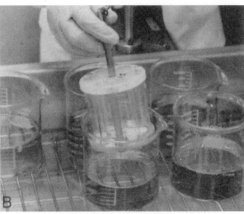

Fig. 7.34   *Tablet disintegration testing apparatus. (Courtesy of Eli Lilly and Company.)*

FDA allows manufacturers to examine scale-up batches of 10% of the proposed size of the actual production batch, or 100,000 dosage units, whichever is greater.

4. As a requirement for regulatory approval for product marketing for products registered with the FDA and regulatory agencies of other countries. New drug applications (NDAs) submitted to the FDA contain in vitro dissolution data generally obtained from batches that have been used in pivotal clinical and/or bioavailability studies and from human studies conducted during product development (16). Once the specifications are established in an approved NDA, they become official (USP) specifications for all subsequent batches and bioequivalent products.

The goal of in vitro dissolution testing is to provide insofar as is possible, a reasonable prediction of, or correlation with, the product's in vivo bioavailability. A system has been developed which relates combinations of a drug's solubility (high or low) and its intestinal permeability (high or low) as a possible basis for predicting the likelihood of achieving a successful in vivo-in vitro correlation (IVIVC) (16–17). Considered are drugs determined to have:

High Solubility and High Permeability
Low Solubility and High Permeability
High Solubility and Low Permeability
Low Solubility and Low Permeability

For a high solubility and high permeability drug, an IVIVC may be expected if the dissolution rate is slower than the rate of gastric emptying (the rate limiting factor) (18). In the case of a low solubility and high permeability drug, drug dissolution may be the rate limiting step for drug absorption and an IVIVC may be expected. In the case of a high solubility and low permeability drug, permeability is the rate-controlling step and only a limited IVIVC may be possible. In the case of a drug with low solubility and low permeability, significant problems would be likely for oral drug delivery (16).

As noted previously, tablet disintegration is the important first step to the dissolution of the drug substance contained in a tablet. A number of formulation and manufacturing factors can affect the disintegration and dissolution of a tablet including: the particle size of the drug substance in the formulation; the solubility and hygroscopicity of the formulation; the type and concentration of the disintegrant, binder, and lubricant used; the manufacturing method, particularly the compactness of the granulation and the compression force used in tableting; and the in-process variables which may occur (19). Together, these factors present a set of complex interrelated conditions which have a bearing on a product's dissolution characteristics. Therefore, it is vitally important for batch-to-batch consistency to establish dissolution test standards and controls for both materials and processes, and to implement them during production and in final testing.

In addition to formulation and manufacturing controls, the method of dissolution testing also must be controlled to minimize important variables, as paddle rotational speed, vibration, and disturbances by sampling probes. Dissolution testing for orally administered dosage forms has been a component of evaluating product quality in the USP since 1970 when only twelve monographs contained such a requirement. Today, the requirement is standard for tablets and capsules.

The USP includes seven apparatus designs for drug release and dissolution testing of immediate release oral dosage forms, extended release products, enteric coated products, and transdermal drug delivery devices. Of primary interest here are USP Apparatus 1 and USP Apparatus 2, used principally for immediate release solid oral dosage forms.

The equipment consist of 1) a variable speed stirrer motor, 2) a cylindrical stainless steel basket on a stirrer shaft (USP Apparatus 1) or a paddle as the stirring element (USP Apparatus 2), 3) a 1000-mL vessel of glass or other inert, transparent material, fitted with a cover having a center port for the shaft of the stirrer, and three additional ports, two for the removal of samples, and one for the placement of a thermometer, and 4) a suitable water bath to maintain the temperature of the dissolution medium in the vessel. In using USP Apparatus 1, the dosage unit is placed inside the basket. In using USP Apparatus 2, the dosage unit is placed in the vessel.

In each test, a volume of the dissolution medium (as stated in the individual monograph) is placed in the vessel and allowed to come to 37°C ± 0.5°C. Then, the stirrer is rotated at the speed specified and at stated intervals, samples of the medium are withdrawn for chemical analysis of the proportion of drug dissolved. The tablet or capsule must meet the stated monograph requirement for rate of dissolution. For example, "not less than 85% of the labeled amount is dissolved in 30 minutes."

There is growing recognition that where problems of inconsistencies in dissolution occur, they occur not between dosage units from the *same* production batch, but rather *between batches* or between products from different manufactures, most likely due to the many factors of formulation, materials, and manufacturing pointed out above. However, since dosage units within a batch are generally not the problem, the concept of "pooled dissolution testing" has emerged. This process recognizes the concept of "batch characteristics" and allows pooled specimens to be tested. The pooled specimens may be sampled from the individual dissolution vessels in the apparatus or from multiple dosage units dissolved in a single vessel (20).

Sophisticated and highly automated equipment is continually being developed to provide high levels of quality assurance and control to the dissolution test process (Figs. 7.35, 7.36).

Compressed Tablet Manufacture

Compressed tablets may be made by three basic methods: *wet granulation, dry granulation,* and *direct compression.* Figure 7.37 presents schematic drawings of each method.

Most powdered medicinal agents require the addition of excipients as diluents, binders, disintegrants, and lubricants to provide the desired characteristics for tablet manufacture and efficacious use. One important requirement in tablet manu-

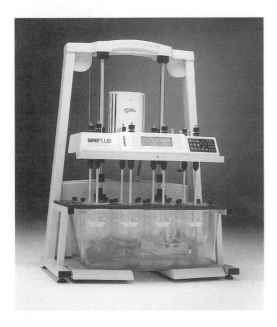

Fig. 7.35 *Hanson SR8-Plus Dissolution Test System. Features microprocessor and templates to create, edit, store, and validate dissolution protocols, graphical displays with menues and icon-based program controls. (Courtesy of Hanson Research Corporation).*

facture is that the drug mixture is free-flowing from the hopper of the tablet press into the dies to enable the high-speed compression of the powder mix into tablets. Granulations of powders provide this free-flowing quality. Granulations also increase material density thereby improving powder compressibility during tableting.

Wet Granulation

Wet granulation is a widely employed method for the production of compressed tablets. The steps required are: 1) weighing and blending the ingredients, 2) preparing a damp mass, 3) screening the damp mass into pellets or granules, 4) drying the granulation, 5) sizing the granulation by dry screening, 6) adding lubricant and blending, and 7) tableting by compression.

WEIGHING AND BLENDING. Specified quantities of active ingredient, diluent or filler, and disintegrating agent are mixed by mechanical powder blender or mixer until uniform.

Among the fillers used are lactose, microcrystalline cellulose, starch, powdered sucrose, and calcium phosphate. The choice of the filler usually is based on the experience of the manufacturer with the material, its relative cost, and its compatibility with the other formulation ingredients. For example, calcium salts must not be used as fillers with tetracycline antibiotics, because of an interaction between the two agents which results in reduced tetracycline absorption from the gastrointestinal tract. Among the fillers most preferred are lactose because of its solubility and compatibility, and microcrystalline cellulose, because of its compactability, compatibility, and the consistent uniformity of supply (21).

Disintegrating agents include croscarmellose, corn and potato starches, sodium starch glycolate, sodium carboxymethylcellulose, polyvinyl polypyrolidone (PVP), crospovidone, cation-exchange resins, alginic acid, and other materials that swell or expand on exposure to moisture and effect the rupture or breakup of the tablet in the gastrointestinal tract. Croscarmellose (2%) and sodium starch glycolate (5%) are often preferred because of their high water uptake and rapid action. One commercial brand of sodium starch glycolate is reported to swell up to 300% of its volume in water (22). When starch is employed, 5% to 10% is usually suitable but up to about 20% may be used to promote more rapid tablet disintegration. The total amount of disintegrant used is not always added in preparing the granulation. Often a portion (sometimes half) is reserved and added to the finished granulation

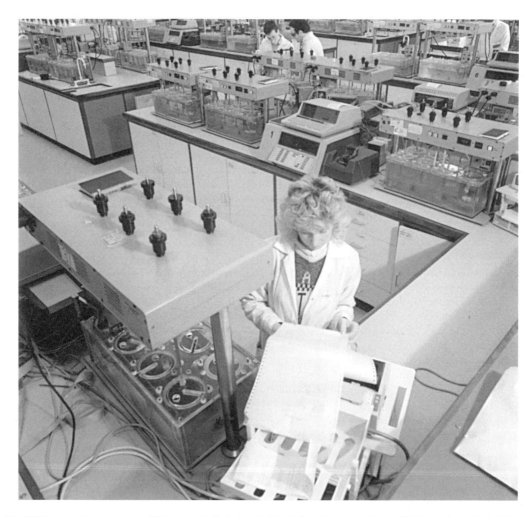

Fig. 7.36 *A modern computerized laboratory dedicated to studies of drug dissolution from solid dosage forms. Included are Erweka dissolution baths, Hewlett-Packard computers, and Hewlett-Packard diode assay spectrophotometers. (Courtesy of Elan Corporation, plc.)*

prior to tableting. This results in a double disintegration of the tablet. One portion assists in the break-up of the tablet into pieces and the other portion assists in the break-up of the pieces into fine particles.

PREPARING THE DAMP MASS. A liquid binder is added to the powder mixture to facilitate the adhesion of the powder particles. A damp mass resembling dough is formed and is used to prepare the granulation. A good binder results in appropriate tablet hardness and does not negatively impact on the release of the drug from the tablet.

Among the binding agents used are povidone, an aqueous preparation of corn starch (10–20%), glucose solution (25–50%), molasses, methylcellu-

lose (3%), carboxymethylcellulose, and microcrystalline cellulose. If the drug substance is adversely affected by an aqueous binder, a nonaqueous solution, or a dry binder may be used. The amount of binding agent used is part of the operator's art; however, the resulting binder-powder mixture should be compactible by squeezing in the hand. The binding agent contributes to the adhesion of the granules to one another and maintains the integrity of the tablet after compression. However, care must be exercised not to over-wet or under-wet the powder. Over-wetting can result in granules that are too hard for proper tableting and under-wetting can result in tablets that are too soft and tend to crumble. When desired, a colorant or

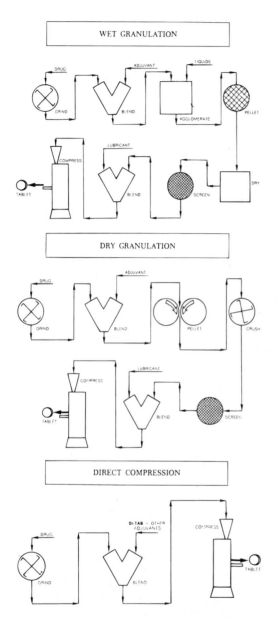

Fig. 7.37 *Schematic drawings of the three main methods for the preparation of tablets: wet granulation (top); dry granulation (center); direct compression (bottom). (Courtesy of Stauffer Chemical Co.)*

flavorant may be added to the binding agent to prepare a granulation having an added feature.

SCREENING THE DAMP MASS INTO PELLETS OR GRANULES. The wet mass is pressed through a screen (usually No. 6- or 8-mesh) to prepare the granules. This may be done by hand or by special equipment which prepares the granules by extru-

sion through perforations in the apparatus. The resultant granules are spread evenly on large pieces of paper in shallow trays and dried.

DRYING THE GRANULATION. Granules may be dried in thermostatically controlled ovens which constantly record the time, temperature, and humidity (Fig. 7.38).

SIZING THE GRANULATION BY DRY SCREENING. After drying, the granules are passed through a screen of a smaller mesh than that used to prepare the original granulation. The degree to which the granules are reduced depends upon the size of the punches to be used. In general, the smaller the tablet to be produced, the smaller are the granules used. Screens from 12- to 20-mesh size are generally used for this purpose. Sizing of the granules is necessary so that the die cavities for tablet compression may be completely and rapidly filled by the free-flowing granulation. Voids or air spaces left by too large a granulation would result in the production of uneven tablets.

ADDING LUBRICATION AND BLENDING. After dry screening, a dry lubricant is dusted over the spread-out granulation through a fine mesh screen. Lubricants contribute to the preparation of compressed tablets in several ways: they improve the flow of the granulation in the hopper to the die cavity; they prevent the adhesion of the tablet formulation to the punches and dies during compression; they reduce friction between the tablet and the die wall during the tablet's ejection from the tablet machine; and, they give a sheen to the finished tablet. Among the more commonly used lubricants are magnesium stearate, calcium stearate, stearic acid, talc, and sodium stearyl fumarate. Magnesium stearate is the most-used (21). The quantity of lubricant used varies from one tableting operation to another, but usually ranges from about 0.1% to 5% of the weight of the granulation.

All-In-One Granulation Methods

Technologic advances now allow the entire process of granulation to be completed in a continuous *fluid-bed process*, using a single piece of equipment, the fluid-bed granulator (Figs. 7.39, 7.40).

The fluid-bed granulator performs the following steps: 1) preblending the formulation powder, including active ingredients, fillers, disintegrants, in a bed by fluidized air, 2) granulating the mixture by spraying onto the fluidized powder bed, a suitable liquid binder, as an aqueous solution of acacia, hydroxypropyl cellulose, or povidone, and 3) drying the granulated product to the desired moisture content.

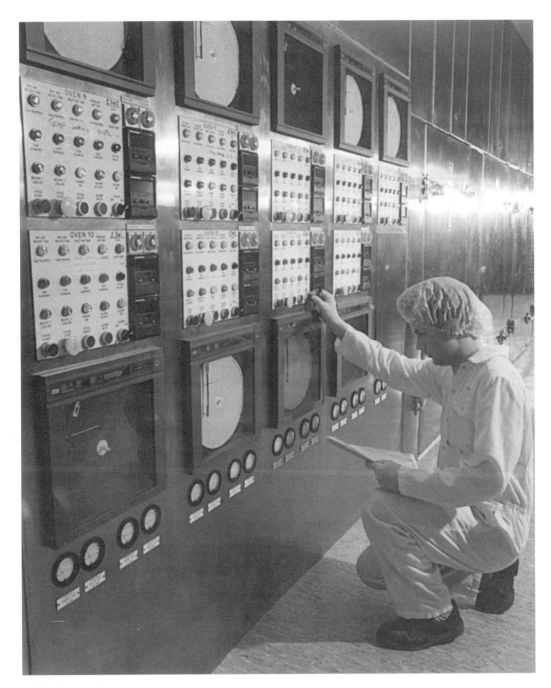

Fig. 7.38 *Temperature controlled Casburt Drying Oven used in the preparation of granules and controlled release beads. (Courtesy of Elan Corporation, plc.)*

Another method, the microwave vacuum processing method, also allows the powders to be tableted to be mixed, wetted, agglomerated, and dried within the confines of a single piece of equipment (Fig. 7.41). The wet mass is dried by gentle mixing, vacuum, and microwave. The use of the microwave for the drying process reduces the drying time considerably, often by one-fourth. The total-batch production time is usually in the range of 90 minutes. After adding lubricants and

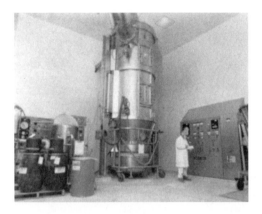

Fig. 7.39 *Example of fluid bed granulator. (Courtesy of Schering Laboratories.)*

screening, the batch is ready for tableting or capsule filling.

Dry Granulation

By the dry granulation method, the powder mixture is compacted in large pieces and subsequently broken down or sized into granules (see Fig. 7.37). By this method, either the active ingredient or the diluent must have cohesive properties. Dry granulation is especially applicable to materials that cannot be prepared by wet granulation due to their degradation by moisture or by the elevated temperatures required for drying the granules.

SLUGGING. In this method, after weighing and mixing the ingredients, the powder mixture is "slugged" or compressed into large flat tablets or pellets of about 1 inch in diameter. The slugs then are broken up by hand or by a mill (Fig. 7.42) and passed through a screen of desired mesh for sizing. Lubricant is added in the usual manner, and tablets are prepared by compression. Aspirin, which is hydrolyzed on exposure to moisture, may be prepared into tablets after slugging.

ROLLER COMPACTION. Instead of slugging, powder compactors may be used to increase the density of a powder by pressing it between high-pressure rollers at 1 ton to 6 tons of pressure. The densified material then is broken up, sized, and lubricated, and tablets are prepared by compression in the usual manner. The *roller compaction* method is often preferred over slugging. Binding agents used in roller compaction formulations include methylcellulose or hydroxymethylcellulose (6 to 12%) and can produce good tablet hardness and friability (23).

Tableting of Granulation

There are a number of types of tablet presses or tableting machines, each varying in productivity but similar in basic function and operation. They all compress a tablet formulation within a steel die cavity by the pressure exerted by the movement of two steel punches, a lower punch and an upper punch (Fig 7.43).

The operation of a single-punch describes the basic mechanical process. As the lower punch drops, the feed shoe filled with granulation from the hopper is positioned over and fills the die cavity. The feed shoe retracts, scrapes away the excessive granulation, and levels the layer of fill in the die cavity. The upper punch lowers and compresses the fill, forming the tablet. The upper punch then retracts as the lower punch rises with the formed tablet to

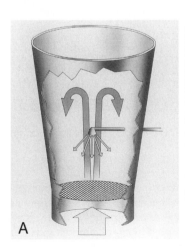
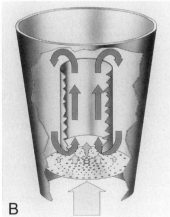
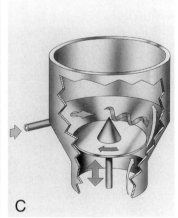

Fig. 7.40 *A, Top-spray; B, bottom-spray (Wurster); and C, tangential-spray methods in the fluid-bed coating of solid particles. (Courtesy of Glatt Air Techniques, Inc.)*

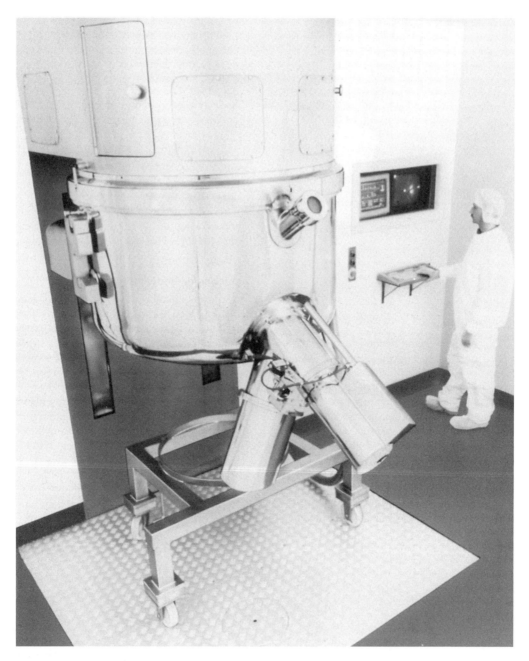

Fig. 7.41 *Microwave vacuum processing in which tableting ingredients are dry mixed, wetted with a binding liquid, and dried by vacuum and microwave within a single piece of equipment. (Courtesy of GEI Processing, Inc.)*

the precise level of the stage. The feed shoe moves over the die cavity, shoves the tablet aside, and once again fills the cavity with granulation to repeat the process. The tablets fall into a collection container. Samples of tablets are assayed/tested for the various quality standards described earlier.

Rotary tablet machines equipped with multiple punches and dies operate through the continuous rotating movement of the punches A single rotary press with 16 stations (16 sets of punches and dies) may produce up to 1150 tablets per minute. Double rotary tablet presses with 27, 33, 37, 41, or 49

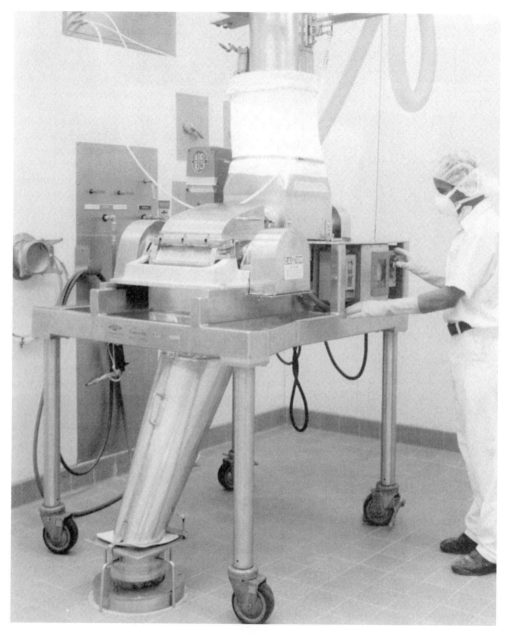

Fig. 7.42   *Frewitt Oscillator or Fitz Mill utilized in the pulverization or granulation process. (Courtesy of Eli Lilly and Company.)*

sets of punches and dies are capable of producing 2 tablets for each die. Some of these machines can produce 10,000 and more tablets per minute of operation (Fig. 7.44). For such high speed production, induced die feeders are required to force fill material into the dies to keep up with the rapidly moving punches (Fig. 7.45). A consequence of high-speed production is the increased occurrence of *lamination* (horizontal striations) and tablet *capping*, in which the top of the tablet separates from the whole because the fill material does not have enough time to bond after compression. Reduced tableting speed remedies the problem (24).

Multiple-layered tablets are produced by the multiple feed and multiple compression of fill material within a single die. Tablets having an inner core

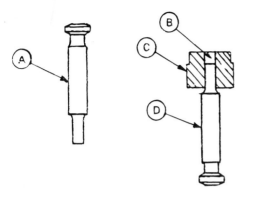

Fig. 7.43 *Punch and die set: A, upper punch; B, die cavity; C, die; and D, lower punch. (Courtesy of Cherry-Burrell Corporation.)*

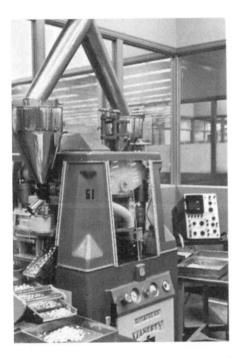

Fig. 7.44 *Manesty Rotapress rotary compression machine making compressed tablets. Tablets leaving the machine run over a tablet duster to screen where they are inspected. Material to be compressed is being fed from overhead hopper through yoke to each of the two compressing machine hoppers. Hardness of tablet is monitored electronically by oscilloscope at the right. (Courtesy of The Upjohn Company.)*

tablet are prepared by machines having a special feed apparatus which strategically places the core tablet within the die for compression with surrounding fill.

Direct Compression Tableting

Some granular chemicals, like potassium chloride, possess free flowing and cohesive properties that enable them to be compressed directly in a tablet machine without need of wet or dry granulation. For chemicals that do not possess this quality, special pharmaceutical excipients may be used which impart the necessary qualities for the production of tablets by direct compression. These tableting excipients include: *fillers,* as spray-dried lactose, microcrystals of alpha-monohydrate lactose, sucrose-invert sugar-corn starch mixtures, microcrystalline cellulose, crystalline maltose, and dicalcium phosphate; *disintegrating agents,* as direct-compression starch, sodium carboxymethyl starch, cross-linked carboxymethylcellulose fibers, and cross-linked polyvinylpyrrolidone; *lubricants,* as magnesium stearate and talc; and *glidants,* as fumed silicon dioxide.

The capping, splitting, or laminating of tablets is sometimes related to air entrapment during direct compression. When air is entrapped, the resulting tablets expand when the pressure of tableting is released, resulting in splits or layers in the tablets. Forced or induced feeders can reduce air entrapment, making the fill powder more dense and amenable to compaction.

Capping also may be caused by punches that are not immaculately clean and perfectly smooth or by a granulation which has too great a proportion of "fines" or fine powder. Fine powder, which results when a dried granulation is sized, is generally 10 to

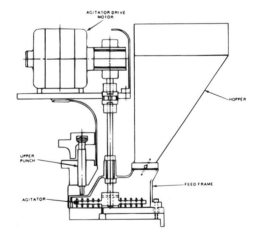

Fig. 7.45 *Induced die feeder. The standard gravity-fed open feed frame can be replaced with an induced die feeder. Using this accessory, granulation is forced into the die by the rotary action of the agitator. (Courtesy of Cherry-Burrell Corporation.)*

20% of the weight of the granulation. Some fine powder is desired to properly fill the die cavity. However, an excess can also lead to tablet softness and capping.

Tablets that have aged or which have been stored improperly also may exhibit splitting or other physical deformations (Fig. 7.46).

Tablet Dedusting

To remove traces of loose powder adhering to tablets following compression, the tablets are conveyed directly from the tableting machine to a tablet deduster. An example of this type of apparatus is shown in Figure 7.47. The compressed tablets may then be coated.

Chewable Tablets

Chewable tablets are pleasant tasting tablets formulated to disintegrate smoothly in the mouth with or without active chewing. They are prepared by wet granulation and compression, using only minimal degrees of tableting pressure in order to produce a soft tablet.

Mannitol, a white crystalline hexahydric alcohol, is used as the excipient in most chewable tablets. Mannitol is about 70% as sweet as sucrose with a cool feel in the mouth resulting from its negative

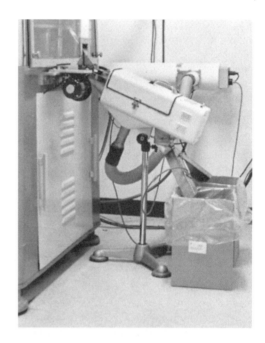

Fig. 7.47 *Model 25 Manesty Tablet Deduster. Tablets leaving tableting machine are dedusted and passed into collection containers. (Courtesy of Eli Lilly and Company.)*

heat of solution. In many chewable tablet formulations, mannitol may account for 50% or more of the weight of the formulation. Sometimes, other sweetening agents, as sorbitol, lactose, dextrose, crystalline maltose, and glucose, may be substituted for part or all of the mannitol. In the preparation of sugar-free chewable tablets, xylitol may be used. Xylitol is sweeter than mannitol and has the desirable negative heat of solution that provides the cool mouth feel upon dissolution.

Lubricants and binders that do not detract from the texture or desired hardness of the tablet may be used. To enhance the appeal of the tablets, colorants and tart or fruity flavorants are commonly employed. Among the types of products prepared as chewable tablets are antacids (e.g., calcium carbonate), antibiotics (e.g., erythromycin), anti-infective agents (e.g., didanosine), anticonvulsants (e.g., carbamazepine), vasodilators (e.g., isosorbide dinitrate), analgesics (e.g., acetaminophen), various vitamins and cold/allergy combination tablets. Chewable tablets are particularly useful for children and adults who have difficulty swallowing other solid dosage forms.

The following is a formula for a typical chewable antacid tablet:(25)

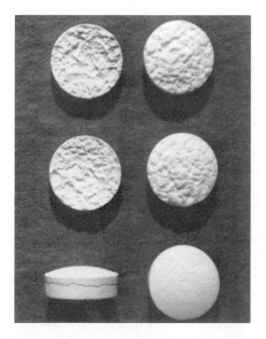

Fig. 7.46 *Tablets that have split on aging, due to conditions of manufacture or storage.*

Per Tablet

Aluminum hydroxide,	325.0 mg
Mannitol,	812.0 mg
Sodium saccharin,	0.4 mg
Sorbitol (10% w/v solution),	32.5 mg
Magnesium stearate,	35.0 mg
Mint flavor concentrate,	4.0 mg

Preparation: Blend the aluminum hydroxide, mannitol, and sodium saccharin. Prepare a wet granulation with the sorbitol solution. Dry at 120°F and screen through a 12-mesh screen. Add the flavor and magnesium stearate, blend, and compress into tablets.

Molded Tablets

The commercial preparation of tablets by molding has been replaced by the tablet compression process. However, molded tablets, or *tablet triturates,* may be prepared on a small laboratory scale as follows.

The mold used in the preparation of molded tablets is made of hard rubber, hard plastic, or metal. It has two parts, the upper part, or *die* portion, and the lower part containing squat, flat *punches.* The die portion is a flat plate the thickness of the tablets to be produced and has 50 to 200 uniformly drilled and evenly spaced circular holes (Fig. 7.48). The lower part of the mold has corresponding punches that fit the holes precisely. When the die is filled with tableting material and placed atop the punches, the punches gently lift the fill material from the holes to rest upon the punches for drying.

The base for molded tablets is generally a mixture of finely powdered lactose with or without a portion of powdered sucrose (5–20%). The addition of sucrose results in less-brittle tablets. In preparing the fill, the drug is mixed uniformly with the base, by geometric dilution when potent drugs are used. The powder mixture is wetted with a 50% mixture of water and alcohol sufficient only to dampen the powder so that is may be compacted. The solvent action of the water on a portion of the lactose/sucrose base effects the binding of the powder mixture upon drying. The alcohol portion hastens the drying process.

The upper mold is placed on a clean flat glass surface and the damp mass added by a rubbing motion. When each opening is filled completely, top and bottom, the mold is fitted on the punch portion of the mold and the tablets raised to dry.

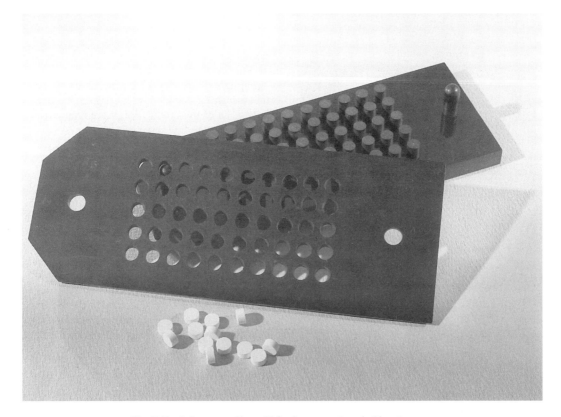

Fig. 7.48   *Laboratory tablet mold for the preparation of tablet triturates.*

Before use, the mold should be "standardized" for the fill material used, since the densities of different formulas result in tablets of different weights. This may be done by preparing a test batch of the formula and weighing and recording the weight of the dry tablets produced. This weight is then used in calculations for production quantities.

Molded tablets are intended to dissolve rapidly in the oral cavity. They do not contain disintegrants, lubricants, or coatings to slow their rate of dissolution.

AUTHORS' NOTE: *A more complete discussion of the preparation of molded tablets and the standardization of laboratory molds may be found in the 5th edition of this textbook.*

Tablet Coating

Tablets are coated for a number of reasons, including to: protect the medicinal agent against destructive exposure to air and/or humidity; mask the taste of the drug; provide special characteristics of drug release (e.g., enteric coatings); and to provide aesthetics or distinction to the product.

In a limited number of instances, tablets are coated to prevent inadvertent contact by nonpatients with the drug substance and the consequent effects of drug absorption. For example, Proscar tablets (finasteride, Merck) are coated for just this reason. The drug is used by men in the treatment of benign prostatic hyperplasia. The labeling instructions warn that women who are pregnant or who could become pregnant should not come into contact with the drug. Drug contact can occur through the handling of broken tablets. If finasteride is absorbed by a woman who is pregnant with a male baby, the drug has the potential capacity to adversely affect the developing male fetus.

The general methods involved in coating tablets are as follows.

Sugarcoating Tablets

The sugarcoating of tablets may be divided into the following steps: 1) waterproofing and sealing (if needed), 2) subcoating, 3) smoothing and final rounding, 4) finishing and coloring (if desired), and 5) polishing. The entire coating process is conducted in a series of mechanically operated acorn-shaped coating pans of galvanized iron, stainless steel, or copper. The pans are partially open in the front, have diameters ranging from about 1 to 4 feet, and are of various capacities (Figs. 7.49, 7.50). The smaller pans are used for experimental, devel-

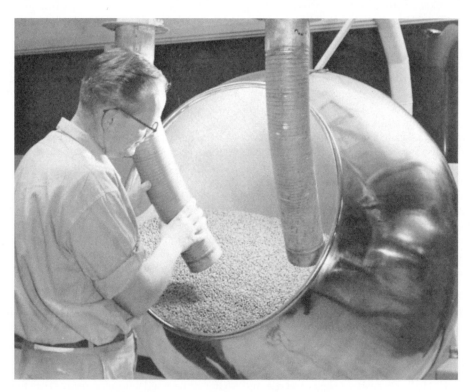

Fig. 7.49 *Tablet coating, an older style coating pan, showing the warm air supply and the exhaust. (Courtesy of Wyeth Laboratories.)*

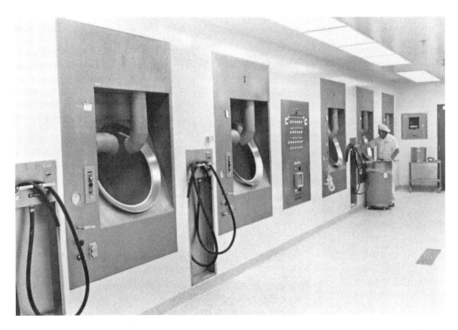

Fig. 7.50   *Modern tablet coating facility. Air and exhaust ducts to assist drying are automatically operated from central board. (Courtesy of Eli Lilly and Company.)*

opmental, and pilot plant operations, the larger pans for industrial production. The pans operate at about a 40° angle to contain the tablets while allowing the operator visual and manual access. During operation, the pan is mechanically rotated at moderate speeds, allowing the tablets to tumble over each other while making contact with the coating solutions which are gently poured or sprayed onto the tablets. To allow gradual build-up of the coatings, the solutions are added in portions, with warm air blown in to hasten drying. Each coat applied only after the previous coat has dried. Tablets intended to be coated are manufactured to be thin-edged and highly convex to allow the coatings to form rounded rather than angular edges.

WATERPROOFING AND SEALING COATS. For tablets containing components that may be adversely affected by moisture, one or more coats of a waterproofing substance, as pharmaceutical shellac or a polymer, is applied to the compressed tablets before the subcoating application. The waterproofing solution (usually alcoholic) is gently poured or sprayed on the compressed tablets rotating in the coating pans. Warm air is blown into the pan during the coating to hasten the drying and to prevent tablets from sticking together.

SUBCOATING. After the tablets are waterproofed (if needed), 3 to 5 subcoats of a sugar-based syrup

are applied. This bonds the sugar coating to the tablet and provides rounding. The sucrose and water syrup also contains gelatin, acacia, or polyvinylpyrrolidone (PVP) to enhance the coating of the tablets. When the tablets are partially dry they are sprinkled with a dusting powder, usually a mixture of powdered sugar and starch but sometimes talc, acacia, or precipitated chalk as well. Warm air is applied to the rolling tablets, and when they are dry, the subcoating process is repeated until the tablets are of the desired shape and size (Fig. 7.51). The subcoated tablets are then scooped out of the coating pan and the excess powder is removed by gently shaking the tablets on a cloth screen.

SMOOTHING AND FINAL ROUNDING. After the tablets have been subcoated, 5 to 10 additional coatings of a thick syrup are applied to complete the rounding and smooth the coatings. This syrup is sucrose-based with or without additional components as starch and calcium carbonate. As the syrup is applied, the operator moves his hand through the rolling tablets to distribute the syrup and to prevent the tablets from sticking to one another. A dusting powder is often used between syrup applications. Warm air is applied to hasten the drying time of each coat.

FINISHING AND COLORING. To attain final smoothness and the appropriate color to the tablets,

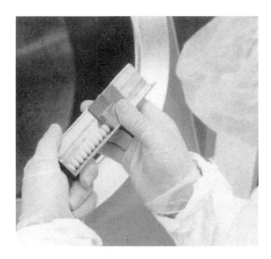

Fig. 7.51 *Tablet gauge used to measure the size of coated tablets. (Courtesy of Eli Lilly and Company.)*

pan and the tablets allowed to tumble over the wax until the desired sheen is attained. A third method involves the light-spraying of the tablets with wax dissolved in a nonaqueous solvent. Two or three coats of wax may be applied depending upon the desired gloss. After each coat has been applied, the addition of a small amount of talc to the tumbling tablets contributes to their high luster (Fig. 7.53).

Film-Coating Tablets

The sugarcoating process, as described, is not only tedious, time-consuming, and specialized, requiring the expertise of highly skilled technicians, but it also results in coated tablets that may be twice the size and weight of the original uncoated tablets. Also, sugar coated tablets may vary slightly in size from batch to batch and within a batch. All of these factors are important considerations for a manufacturer. From a patient's point of view, large

several coats of a thin syrup containing the desired colorant are applied in the usual manner. This step is performed in a clean pan, free from previous coating materials.

IMPRINTING. Solid dosage forms may be passed through special imprinting machines (Fig. 7.52) to impart identification codes and other distinctive symbols. By FDA regulation, effective in 1995, all solid dosage forms for human consumption, including both prescription-only and over-the-counter drug products, must be imprinted with product-specific identification codes. Some exemptions to this requirement are allowed, namely: solid dosage forms used in clinical investigations; solid dosage forms that are extemporaneously compounded in the course of pharmacy practice; radiopharmaceutical drug products; and products that, because of their size, shape, texture or other physical characteristics, make imprinting technologically not feasible.

Technically, the imprint may be *debossed, embossed, engraved,* or printed on the surface with ink. *Debossed* means imprinted with a mark below the dosage form surface; *embossed* means imprinted with a mark raised above the dosage form surface; and *engraved* means imprinted with a code that is cut into the dosage form surface during production.

POLISHING. Coated tablets may be polished in several ways. Special drum-shaped pans or ordinary coating pans lined with fabric or canvas cloth impregnated with carnauba wax and/or beeswax, may be used to polish tablets as they tumble in the pan. Or, pieces of wax may be placed in a polishing

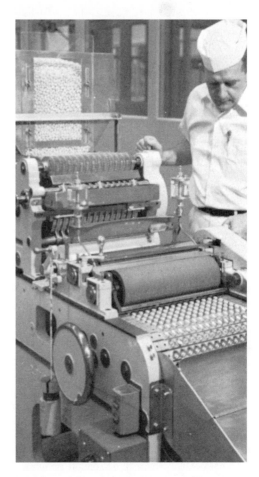

Fig. 7.52 *Branding of coated compression tablets on a Hartnett branding machine. (Courtesy of The Upjohn Company.)*

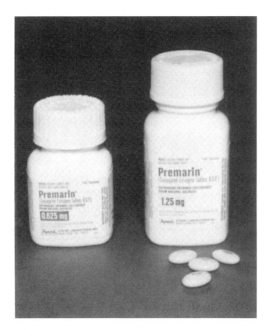

Fig. 7.53 *Example of coated, polished, and monogrammed tablets. (Courtesy of Wyeth-Ayerst Laboratories.)*

tablets are not as easily swallowed as are small tablets.

The film-coating process, which places a thin, skin-tight coating of a plastic-like material over the compressed tablet, was developed to produce coated tablets having essentially the same weight, shape, and size as the originally compressed tablet. And, the coating is thin enough to reveal any identifying monograms embossed in the tablet during its compression by the tablet punches. Film-coated tablets also are far more resistant to destruction by abrasion than are sugar-coated tablets. However, like sugar-coated tablets, the coating may be colored to make the tablets attractive and distinctive.

Film-coating solutions may be nonaqueous or aqueous. The nonaqueous solutions contain the following types of materials to provide the desired coating to the tablets:

1. A *film former* capable of producing smooth, thin films reproducible under conventional coating conditions and applicable to a variety of tablet shapes. Example: cellulose acetate phthalate.
2. An *alloying substance* providing water solubility or permeability to the film to ensure penetration by body fluids and therapeutic availability of the drug. Example: polyethylene glycol.

3. A *plasticizer* to produce flexibility and elasticity of the coating and thus provide durability. Example: castor oil.
4. A *surfactant* to enhance spreadability of the film during application. Example: polyoxyethylene sorbitan derivatives.
5. *Opaquants* and *colorants* to make the appearance of the coated tablets handsome and distinctive. Examples: Opaquant, titanium dioxide; colorant, FD&C or D&C dyes.
6. *Sweeteners, flavors,* and *aromas* to enhance the acceptability of the tablet to the patient. Examples: sweeteners, saccharin; flavors and aromas, vanillin.
7. A *glossant* to provide luster to the tablets without a separate polishing operation. Example: beeswax.
8. A *volatile solvent* to allow the spread of the other components over the tablets while allowing rapid evaporation to permit an effective yet speedy operation. Example: alcohol-acetone mixture.

Tablets are film coated by the application or spraying of the film-coating solution on the tablets in ordinary coating pans. The volatility of the solvent enables the film to adhere quickly to the surface of the tablets.

Due to both the expense of the volatile solvents used in the film-coating process and the environmental problem of the release of solvents, pharmaceutical manufacturers generally favor the use of aqueous-based film-coating solutions. One of the problems attendant to these, however, is the slow evaporation of the water-base compared to the volatile organic solvent-based solutions. One commercially available water-based colloidal coating dispersion is called AQUACOAT (FMC Corporation) and contains a 30% ethyl cellulose pseudolatex. Pseudolatex dispersions have a high solids content for greater coating ability and a relatively low viscosity. The low viscosity allows less water to be used in the coating dispersion, resulting in a lesser requirement for water-evaporation and a reduced likelihood of water interference with the tablet formulation. In addition, the low viscosity permits greater coat penetration into the crevices of monogrammed or scored tablets. A plasticizer may be incorporated into the dispersion to assist in the production of a denser, less-permeable film, with higher gloss and greater mechanical strength. Other aqueous film-coating products use cellulosic materials as methylcellulose, hydroxypropyl cellulose, and hydroxypropyl methylcellulose as the film forming polymer.

A typical aqueous film-coating formulation contains the following:(26)

1. *Film-forming polymer* (7–18%). Examples: cellulose ether polymers as hydroxypropyl methylcellulose, hydroxypropyl cellulose, and methylcellulose.
2. *Plasticizer* (0.5–2.0%). Examples: glycerin, propylene glycol, polyethylene glycol, diethyl phthalate, and dibutyl subacetate.
3. *Colorant and opacifier* (2.5–8%). Examples: FD&C or D&C Lakes and iron oxide pigments.
4. *Vehicle* (water, to make 100%).

There are some problems attendant to aqueous film-coating, including: the appearance of small amounts (*picking*) or larger amounts (*peeling*) of film fragments flaking from the tablet surface; roughness of the tablet surface due to failure of spray droplets to coalesce (*orange peel effect*); an uneven distribution of color on the tablet surface (*mottling*); filling-in of the score-line or indented logo on the tablet by the film (*bridging*); and the disfiguration of the core tablet when subjected for too long a period of time to the coating solution (tablet *erosion*). The cause of each of these problems can be determined and rectified through appropriate changes in formulation, equipment, technique or process (26).

Enteric Coating

Enteric coated solid dosage forms are intended to pass through the stomach intact to disintegrate and release their drug-content for absorption along the intestines. The design of an enteric coating may be based upon the transit time required for the passage of the dosage form from the stomach to the intestines and may be accomplished through coatings of sufficient thickness. However, usually an enteric coating is based upon factors of pH, resisting dissolution in the highly acid environment of the stomach but yielding to the less acid environment of the intestine. Some enteric coatings are designed to dissolve at pH 4.8 and greater.

Enteric coating materials may be applied to either whole compressed tablets or to drug particles or granules used in the subsequent fabrication of tablets or capsules. The coatings may be applied in multiple portions to build a thick coating or they may be applied as a thin film coat. The coating systems may be aqueous-based or organic-solvent-based and are effective so long as the coating material resists breakdown in the gastric fluid. Among the materials used in enteric coatings are pharmaceutical shellac, hydroxypropyl methylcellulose ph-

thalate, polyvinyl acetate phthalate, diethyl phthalate, and cellulose acetate phthalate.

Fluid-Bed or Air Suspension Coating

This process, using equipment of the type shown in Figure 7.54 involves the spray coating of powders, granules, beads, pellets or tablets held in suspension by a column of air. Fluid bed processing equipment is multifunctional and, as described

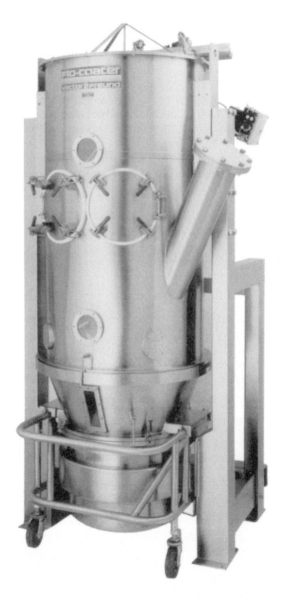

Fig. 7.54 *Vector/Freund Flo-Coater production system. A fluid bed system used in the application of coatings to beads, granules, powders, and tablets. Capacity of models ranges from 5 kg to 700 kg. (Courtesy of Vector Corporation.)*

previously, also may be used in preparing tablet granulations.

In the Wurster process, named after its developer, the items to be coated are fed into a vertical cylinder and are supported by a column of air that enters from the bottom of the cylinder. Within the air stream, the solids rotate both vertically and horizontally. As the coating solution enters the system from the bottom, it is rapidly placed on the suspended, rotating solids, with rounding coats being applied in less than an hour with the assistance of warm air blasts released in the chamber.

In another type of fluidized bed system, the coating solution is sprayed downward onto the particles to be coated as they are suspended by air from below. This method is commonly referred to as the *top-spray* method. This method provided greater capacity, up to 1500 kg, than do the other air suspension coating methods.(27) Both the top-spray and bottom-spray methods may be employed using a modified apparatus used for fluidized bed granulation. A third method, the *tangential-spray technique,* is used in rotary fluid-bed coaters. The bottom-, top-, and tangential-spray methods are depicted in Figure 7.40. Electron microscope images of the results of this process are shown in Fig. 7.55.

The three systems are increasingly used for the application of aqueous- or organic-solvent-based polymers as film coatings. The top-spray coating method is particularly recommended for taste masking, enteric release, and barrier films on particles or tablets. The method is most effective when coatings are applied from aqueous solutions, latexes, or hotmelts (27–28). The bottom-spray coating method is recommended for sustained-release and enteric-release products; and the tangential method for layering coatings, and for sustained-release and enteric-coated products (28).

Among the variables requiring control in order to produce product of desired and consistent quality are: equipment used and the method of spraying (e.g., top, bottom, tangential), spray-nozzle distance from spraying bed, spray (droplet) size, spray rate, spray pressure, volume of fluidization air, batch size, method(s) and time for drying, air temperature and moisture content in processing compartment (28).

Compression Coating

In a manner similar to the preparation of multiple compressed tablets having an inner core and an outer shell of drug material, core tablets may be sugarcoated by compression. The coating material, in the form of a granulation or powder, is compressed onto a tablet core of drug with a special tablet press. Compression coating is an anhydrous operation and thus may be safely employed in the coating of tablets containing a drug that is labile to moisture. Compared to sugarcoating using pans, compression coating is more uniform and uses less coating materials, resulting in tablets that are lighter, smaller, easier to swallow, and less expensive to package and ship.

Irrespective of the method used in coating, all tablets are visually or electronically inspected for physical imperfections (Fig. 7.56).

Impact of Manufacturing Changes on Solid Dosage Forms

The quality and performance of a solid dosage form may be altered by changes in formulation or by changes in the method of manufacture.

The changes in formulation could involve: 1) the

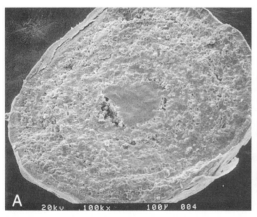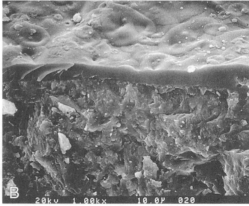

Fig. 7.55 *Scanning electron microscope images of pharmaceutical granules coated through fluid-bed technology: A, layered and coated granule; B, cross-section of top spray enteric coated granule. (Courtesy of Glatt Air Techniques, Inc.)*

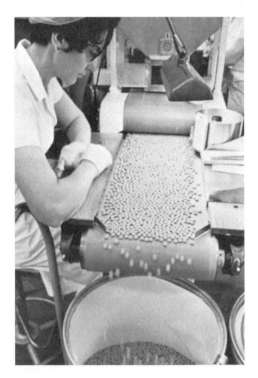

Fig. 7.56 *Checking for physical imperfections in coated tablets. (Courtesy of Smith, Kline & French.)*

use of starting raw materials, including both the active ingredient and pharmaceutical excipients, that have different chemical or physical characteristics (as solubility or particle size) than the standards set for the original components; 2) the use of different pharmaceutical excipients (e.g., magnesium stearate instead of calcium stearate as the lubricant); 3) the use of different quantities of the same excipients in a formulation (e.g., use of a more concentrated wet tablet binder); or 4) the addition of a new excipient to a formulation (as a revised tablet coating formula.

The changes in the method of manufacture could involve: 1) use of processing or manufacturing equipment or a different design; 2) a change in the steps or order in the process or method of manufacture (e.g. different mixing times); 3) different in-process controls, quality tests, or assay methods; 4) production of different batch sizes; 5) employment of different product reprocessing procedures; or 6) employment of a different manufacturing site.

Changes such as these may be proposed or may be implemented during the product development stage, during scale-up of product manufacture before NDA approval, or after NDA approval and product marketing. In all instances, it is critical to assess the impact of the change in meeting the proposed or established standards for product quality (e.g., dissolution rate and bioavailability). It is necessary for a manufacturer to document the change, validate its effect, and provide the necessary information to the FDA. Some changes that are considered minor (as a change in tablet color) and do not affect product quality do not require prior FDA approval for implementation. Other changes that may affect product quality and performance (as use of a substantially different quantity or grade of an excipient, or, use of a piece of manufacturing equipment that changes the basic methodology of manufacture) require prior FDA approval for implementation (29).

Official and Commercially Available Tablets

There are hundreds of tablets recognized by the USP and literally thousands of commercially available tableted products from virtually all pharmaceutical manufacturers, in most therapeutic categories, and in various dosage strengths. Examples of a limited number of these are presented in Table 7.4.

Packaging and Storing Tablets

Tablets are stored in tight containers, in places of low humidity, and protected from extremes in temperature. Products that are prone to decomposition by moisture generally are copackaged with a desiccant packet. Drugs that are adversely affected by light are packaged in light-resistant containers. With a few exceptions, tablets that are properly stored will remain stable for several years or more.

In dispensing tablets, the pharmacist is well advised to use a similar type of container as provided by the manufacturer of the product. The patient is well advised to maintain the drug in the container dispensed. Storage conditions, as recommended for the particular product, should be maintained by the pharmacist and patient alike and expiration dates observed.

The pharmacist should be aware also that the hardness of certain tablets may change upon aging usually resulting in a decrease in the disintegration and dissolution rates of the product. The increase in tablet hardness can frequently be attributed to the increased adhesion of the binding agent and other formulative components within the tablet. Examples of increased tablet hardening with age have been reported for a number of drugs including aluminum hydroxide, sodium salicylate and phenylbutazone (30).

Table 7.4.   Examples of Some Official Tablets

Official Tablet	Some Representative Commercial Products	Tablet Strengths	Category
Acetaminophen	Tylenol (McNeil)	325 and 500 mg	Analgesic and antipyretic
Acyclovir	Zovirax (Glaxo Wellcome)	400 and 800 mg	Antiviral
Allopurinol	Zyloprim (Glaxo Wellcome)	100 and 300 mg	Antigout and antiurolithic
Amitriptyline HCl	Elavil HCl (Zeneca)	10, 25, 50, 100, and 150 mg	Antidepressant
Carbamazepine	Tegretol (Novartis)	200 mg	Anticonvulsant
Chlorambucil	Leukeran (Glaxo Wellcome)	2 mg	Antineoplastic
Chlorpropamide	Diabinese (Pfizer)	100 and 250 mg	Antidiabetic
Cimetidine	Tagamet (SmithKline Beecham)	200 and 300 mg	Histamine H_2 receptor antagonist
Ciprofloxacin	Cipro (Bayer)	150, 500 and 750 mg	Antibacterial
Conjugated Estrogens	Premarin (Wyeth-Ayerst)	0.3, 0.625, 0.9, 1.25, and 2.5 mg	Estrogen
Diazepam	Valium (Roche)	2, 5, and 10 mg	Sedative and skeletal muscle relaxant
Digoxin	Lanoxin (Glaxo Wellcome)	0.125, 0.25, and 0.5 mg	Cardiotonic
Enalapril	Vasotec (Merck)	5, 10, and 20 mg	Antihypertensive
Furosemide	Lasix (Hoechst Marion Roussel)	20, 40, and 80 mg	Diuretic and antihypertensive
Griseofulvin	Fulvicin (Schering)	250 and 500 mg	Antifungal
Haloperidol	Haldol (Ortho McNeil)	0.5, 1, 2, 5, 10 and 20 mg	Traquilizer
Ibuprofen	Motrin (McNeil)	100 mg	Analgesic and antipyretic
Levothyroxine Sodium	Synthroid (Knoll)	0.025, 0.05, 0.075, 0.1, 0.125, 0.15, 0.2, and 0.3 mg	Thyroid hormone
Loratadine	Claritin (Schering)	10 mg	Antihistamine
Lovostatin	Mevacor (Merck)	10, 20 and 40 mg	Antihypercholesteremic
Meperidine HCl	Demerol (Sanofi Winthrop)	50 and 100 mg	Narcotic analgesic
Methyldopa	Aldomet (Merck)	125, 250, and 500 mg	Antihypertensive
Nitroglycerin	Nitrostat (Parke-Davis)	0.150, 0.3, 0.4, and 0.6 mg	Antianginal
Penicillin V	Pen Vee K (Wyeth-Ayerst)	250 and 500 mg	Antiinfective
Pergolide Mesylate	Permax (Athena)	0.05, 0.25, and 1 mg	Dopamine receptor agonist
Propanolol	Inderal (Wyeth-Ayerst)	10, 20, 40, 60, and 80 mg	Antianginal, antiarrhythmic, and antihypertensive
Terbutaline Sulfate	Brethine (Novartis)	2.5 and 5 mg	Antiasthmatic
Verapamil HCl	Calan (Searle)	40, 80, and 120 mg	Antihypertensive
Warfarin Sodium	Coumadin (DuPont)	2, 2.5, 7.5, and 10 mg	Anticoagulant

Certain tablets containing volatile drugs, as nitroglycerin, may experience the migration of the drug between tablets in the container resulting in a lack of uniformity among the tablets (31). Further, packing materials, as cotton and rayon, in contact with nitroglycerin tablets may absorb varying amounts of nitroglycerin rendering the tablets subpotent (32). The USP directs that nitrogen tablets be preserved in tight containers, preferably of glass, at controlled room temperature.

The USP further directs that nitroglycerin tablets must be dispensed in the original, unopened container, labeled with the following statement directed to the patient. "Warning: to prevent loss of potency, keep these tablets in the original container or in a supplemental Nitroglycerin container specifically labeled as being suitable for Nitroglycerin Tablets. Close tightly immediately after use" (14).

The pharmacist also should caution patients about the handling of medication when it poses a potential risk. For example and as noted earlier, finasteride tablets are taken by men to treat benign prostatic hyperplasia. Finasteride has the potential to adversely affect a male fetus if absorbed by a pregnant woman through either direct contact with finasteride or possibly through semen. Therefore, a woman who is pregnant or who may become pregnant should not handle finasteride tablets or come into contact with finasteride powder. In addition, when the male patient's sexual partner is pregnant or may become pregnant, the patient should avoid exposure of his partner to semen or he should discontinue use of the drug.

Oral Administration of Solid Dosage Forms

Solid dosage forms for oral administration are best taken by placing the dosage form upon the tongue and swallowing it with a glassful of water or beverage. Taking solid dosage forms with adequate amounts of water is important. Some patients attempt to swallow a tablet or capsule without water, but this can be dangerous because of the possibility that the dry dosage form will lodge in the esophagus. Esophageal ulceration can occur with the dry ingestion of solid dosage forms, particularly when taken just before bedtime. Among the drugs of greatest concern in this regard are: alendronate sodium, aspirin, ferrous sulfate, any nonsteroidal antiinflammatory drug (NSAID), potassium chloride and tetracycline antibiotics.

The proper administration of alendronate sodium tablets (i.e., Fosamax, Merck), for example, calls for the tablets to be taken with a full 6- or 8-ounce glass of plain water upon rising in the morning and at least one-half hour before taking any food, beverage or other medication to prevent local irritation of the esophagus and other upper gastrointestinal mucosa. Further, the patient is instructed to not recline for at least 30 minutes and until after the first food of the day is eaten due to the possibility of refluxing the drug back up into the esophagus.

In general, patients who suffer from gastroesophageal reflux disease must take their medications with adequate amounts of water and avoid reclining for at least an hour to avoid reflux.

The administration of oral medication in relation to meals is very important since the bioavailability and efficacy of certain drugs may be severely affected by food and certain drink. The pharmacist should be knowledgeable of such instances and advise patients accordingly.

As mentioned earlier in this chapter, oral dosage forms that have special coatings (e.g., enteric) or are designed to provide controlled drug release must not be chewed, broken, or crushed to preserve their drug release features.

When an ordinary tablet is crushed or a capsule opened to facilitate ease of administration, any unpleasant drug taste may be partially masked by mixing with custards, yogurt, rice pudding, other soft food, or fruit juice. The patient should be advised to consume the entire drug-food mixture to obtain the full drug dose and the drug should not be pre-mixed and allowed to set, due to stability considerations.

If a patient cannot swallow a solid dosage form, the pharmacist can suggest using an available chewable or liquid form of the drug. If these are not available, an extemporaneously compounded liquid form may be prepared.

Other Solid Dosage Forms for Oral Administration

Lozenges

Lozenges can be made by compression or molding. When compressed, they are made using a tablet machine and large, flat punches. The machine is operated at a high degree of compression to produce lozenges that are harder than ordinary tablets so that they dissolve or disintegrate slowly in the mouth. Medicinal substances that are heat stable may be molded into a hard, sugar candy lozenge by candy-making machines that process a warm, highly concentrated, flavored syrup as the base and form the lozenges by molding and drying.

Lozenges have a special place in the delivery of medication. For example, a lozenge dosage form containing clotrimazole (MycelexTroche, Bayer), an antifungal agent, is used in the treatment of oropharyngeal candidiasis by the patient allowing the lozenge to slowly dissolve in the mouth, providing salivary levels of the antifungal drug for up to 3 hours. A number of other lozenge dosage forms are available for self-care drugs, e.g., benzocaine, dextromethorphan, phenylpropanolamine, and zinc, to treat self-limiting cough/cold symptoms and minor sore throat.

Pills

By definition, pills are small, round, solid dosage forms containing a medicinal agent and intended to be administered orally. Although the manufacture and administration of pills was at one time quite prevalent, today pills have been replaced by compressed tablets and capsules. A procedure for the extemporaneous preparation of pills on a small-scale may be found in the first edition of this text.

References

1. Mitchell JF. Oral solid dosage forms that should not be crushed: 1996 revision. Hospital Pharmacy 1996; 31:27–37.
2. Jones BE. Hard gelatin capsules and the pharmaceutical formulator. Pharm Tech 1985;9:106–112.
3. Digenis A, Gold TB, Shah VP. Crosslinking of gelatin capsules and its relevance to their in vitro/in vivo performance. Dissolution Technologies 1995;2:1.
4. Gardner D, Casper R, Leith F, Wilding, I. Noninvasive methodology for assessing regional drug absorption from the gastrointestinal tract. Pharm Tech 1997; 21:82–89.
5. Wilding IR. Pharmacoscintigraphic evaluation of oral delivery systems, part I. Pharm Tech 1995; 54–60.
6. Mojaverian P, Reynolds JC, Ouyang A, Wirth F, Kellner PE, Vlasses PH. Mechanism of gastric emptying of a nondisintegrating radiotelemetry capsule in man. Pharm Res 1991;8:97–100.
7. Nash RA. The "rule of sixes" for filling hard-shell gelatin capsules. International Journal of Pharmaceutical Compounding 1997;1:40–41.
8. Yalkowsky SH, Bolton S. Particle size and content uniformity. Pharm Res 1990;7:962–966.
9. Caldwell HC. Dissolution of lithium and magnesium from lithium carbonate capsules containing magnesium stearate. J Pharm Sci 1974;63:770–773.
10. "Etaseal." Windsor, Ontario, Canada: Capsule Technology International, Ltd.
11. "Licaps." Greenwood, SC: Capsugel Division of Warner-Lambert Co.
12. "Quali-seal." Indianapolis, IN: Elanco Qualicaps Division of Ely Lilly and Company.
13. Stanley JP. Soft gelatin capsules. In: Lachman L, Lieberman HA, Kanig JL eds. The theory and practice of industrial pharmacy, 3rd ed. Philadelphia: Lea & Febiger, 1986, 398–429.
14. The United States Pharmacopeia 23/National Formulary 18. Rockville MD: The United States Pharmacopeial Convention, 1995.
15. Skoug JW, Halstead GW, Theis DL, Freeman JE, Fagan DT, Rohrs BR. Strategy for the development and validation of dissolution tests for solid oral dosage forms. Pharm Tech 1996;20:58–71.
16. Guidance for industry: dissolution testing of immediate release solid oral dosage forms. Rockville MD: FDA/CDER, 1997.
17. Amidon GL, Lennernas, Shah VP, Crison JR. A theoretical basis for a biopharmaceutic drug classification: the correlation of in vitro drug product dissolution and in vivo bioavailability. Pharm Res 1995;12: 413–420.
18. Swarbrick J. In vitro dissolution, drug bioavailability, and the spiral of science. Pharm Tech 1997;21:68–72.
19. Chowhan ZT. Factors affecting dissolution of drugs and their stability upon aging in solid dosage forms. PharmTech 1994;18:60–73.
20. Hanson R, Swartz ME, Jarnutowski RJ. Pooled dissolution testing: a primer. Dissolution Technologies 1998;5:15–17.
21. Shangraw RF, Demarest DA. A survey of current industrial practices in the formulation and manufacture of tablets and capsules. Pharm Tech 1993;17:32–44.
22. Explotab. Patterson NY. Mendell, Penmwest Company. 1992.
23. METHOCEL as a granulation binding agent for immediate-release tablet and capsule products. Wilmington DE: Dow Chemical Company, 1996.
24. Rubinstein MH. Lubricant behaviour of magnesium stearate. Acta Pharmaceutica Suecica 1987;24:43.
25. Atlas mannitol, USP tablet excipient. Wilmington, DE: ICI Americas Inc., 1973.
26. Mathur LK, Forbes SJ, Yelvigi M. Characterization techniques for the aqueous film coating process. Pharm Tech 1984;8:42.
27. Jones DM. Factors to consider in fluid-bed processing. Pharm Tech 1985;9:50–62.
28. Mehta AM. Scale-up considerations in the fluid-bed process for controlled-release products. Pharm Tech 1988;12
29. Lucisano LJ, Franz RM. FDA proposed guidance for chemistry, manufacturing, and control changes for immediate-release solid dosage forms: a review and industrial perspective. Pharm Tech 1995;19:30–44.
30. Barrett D, Fell JT. Effect of aging on physical properties of phenylbutazone tablets. J Pharm Sci 1975;64: 335.
31. Page DP, et al. Stability study of nitroglycerin sublingual tablets. J Pharm Sci 1975;64:140.
32. Fusari SA. Nitroglycerin sublingual tablets I: Stability of conventional tablets. J Pharm Sci 1973;62:122.

8

MODIFIED-RELEASE DOSAGE FORMS AND DRUG DELIVERY SYSTEMS

Chapter at a Glance

THIS CHAPTER describes dosage forms and drug delivery systems which, by virtue of formulation and product design, have modified drug release features. In contrast to conventional (immediate release) forms, modified-release products provide either delayed-release or extended-release of drug. *Delayed-release* products usually are enteric-coated tablets or capsules designed to pass through the stomach unaltered, later to release their medication within the intestinal tract. As noted in the previous chapter, enteric coatings are used to either protect a gastric-labile drug substance from destruction by gastric fluids or to reduce stomach distress caused by gastric-irritating drugs. *Extended-release* products are designed to release their medication in a *controlled* manner, at a predetermined rate, duration and location to achieve and maintain optimum therapeutic blood levels of drug.

The vast majority of modified-release products are orally administered tablets and capsules and therefore these dosage forms are emphasized in this chapter. However, examples of some non-oral modified-release dosage forms and drug delivery systems are also described, including ocular, parenteral, subdermal and vaginal products. Transdermal patches, which provide rate-controlled drug delivery are also noted, but are discussed at length in Chapter 10.

The Rationale for Extended-Release Pharmaceuticals

Some drugs are inherently long-lasting and require only once-a-day oral dosing to sustain adequate drug blood levels and the desired therapeutic effect. These drugs are formulated in the conventional manner in immediate-release dosage forms. However, many other drugs are not inherently long-lasting and require multiple daily dosing to achieve the desired therapeutic results.

Multiple daily dosing often is inconvenient for the patient and can result in missed doses, made-up doses and patient noncompliance with the therapeutic regimen. When conventional immediate-release dosage forms are taken on schedule and more than once daily, there are sequential therapeutic blood level peaks and valleys (troughs) associated with the taking of each dose (Fig. 8.1). However, when doses are *not* administered on schedule, the resulting peaks and valleys reflect less than optimum drug therapy. For example, if doses are administered too frequently, minimum toxic concentrations (MTC) of drug may be reached with toxic side effects resulting. If doses are missed, periods of subtherapeutic drug blood levels or those below the minimum effective concentration (MEC) may result, with no patient benefit.

Extended-release tablets and capsules are commonly taken only once or twice daily compared with counterpart conventional forms that may need to be taken three to four times daily to achieve the same therapeutic effect. Typically, extended-release products provide an immediate release of drug which promptly produces the desired therapeutic effect which then is followed by the gradual and continual release of additional amounts of drug to maintain this effect over a predetermined period of time (Fig. 8.2). The sustained plasma drug levels provided by extended-release drug products often-times eliminates the need for night dosing, which provides benefit not only to the patient but to the caregiver as well (1–3). For nonoral rate-controlled drug delivery systems, their drug-release pattern ranges in duration from 24 hours for most transdermal patches, to 3 months for the estradiol vaginal ring insert (Estring, Pharmacia & Upjohn), to 5 years for levonorgestrel subdermal implants (Norplant System, Wyeth-Ayerst).

Some advantages of extended-release systems are given in Table 8.1. Some disadvantages are the loss of flexibility in adjusting the drug dose and/or dosage regimen, and an increased risk of sudden and total drug release or "dose dumping" due to failure of the technology of the dosage unit.

Terminology

Drug products that provide "extended" or "sustained" drug release first appeared as a major new class of dosage form in the late 1940s and early 1950s (4). Over the years, many terms (and abbreviations) as *sustained-release (SR), sustained-action (SA), prolonged-action (PA), controlled-release (CR), extended-release (ER), timed-release (TR), and long-acting (LA)*, have been used by manufacturers to describe product types and features. Although these terms often have been used interchangeably, individual products bearing these descriptions may

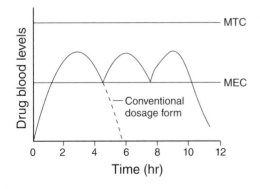

Fig. 8.1 *Hypothetical drug blood level-time curves for a conventional solid dosage form and a multiple-action product.*

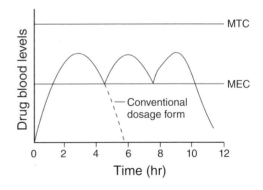

Fig. 8.2 *Hypothetical drug blood level-time curves for a conventional solid dosage form and a controlled release product.*

Table 8.1. Advantages of Extended-Release Dosage Forms Over Conventional Forms

Advantage	Explanation
Reduction in drug blood level fluctuations	By controlling the rate of drug release,"peaks and valleys"of drug-blood levels are eliminated.
Frequency reduction in dosing	Extended-release products deliver frequently more than a single dose of medication and thus they may be taken less often than conventional forms.
Enhanced patient convenience and compliance	With less frequency of dose administration, a patient is less apt to neglect taking a dose. There is also greater patient and/or caregiver convenience with daytime and nighttime medication administration.
Reduction in adverse side effects	Because there are fewer drug blood level peaks outside of the drug's therapeutic range and into the toxic range, adverse side effects occur less frequently.
Reduction in overall health care costs	Although the initial cost of extended-release dosage forms may be greater than that for conventional dosage forms, the overall cost of treatment may be less due to enhanced therapeutic benefit, fewer side-effects, and reduced time required of health care personnel to dispense and administer drugs and monitor patients.

differ in design and performance and must be examined individually to ascertain their respective features. For the most part, these terms are used to describe orally administered dosage forms, whereas the term *rate-controlled delivery* is applied to certain types of drug delivery systems in which the rate of drug delivery is controlled by features of the device rather than by physiological or environmental conditions as gastrointestinal pH or drug transit time through the gastrointestinal tract.

Modified-release

In recent years, this term has come into general use to describe dosage forms having drug release features based on time, course, and/or location which are designed to accomplish therapeutic or convenience objectives not offered by conventional or immediate-release forms (2, 5). The USP differentiates modified-release forms as *extended-release* and *delayed-release* (6).

Extended-release

The FDA defines an extended-release dosage form as one that allows a reduction in dosing frequency to that presented by a conventional dosage form, e.g., a solution or an immediate-release dosage form (2,7).

Delayed-release

A delayed-release dosage form is designed to release the drug from the dosage form at a time other than promptly after administration. The delay may be time-based or based on the influence of environmental conditions, as gastrointestinal pH.

Repeat Action

These forms usually contain two single doses of medication, one for immediate release and the second for delayed release. Bilayered tablets, for example, may be prepared with one layer of drug for immediate release with the second layer designed to release drug later as either a second dose or in an extended-release manner.

Targeted Release

Targeted release describes drug release directed toward isolating or concentrating a drug in a body region, tissue, or site for absorption or for drug action.

Extended-Release Oral Dosage Forms

Not all drugs are suited for formulation into extended-release products and not all medical conditions require treatment with such a product. The drug and the therapeutic indication must be considered jointly in determining whether or not to develop an extended-release dosage form.

Drug-Candidates for Extended-Release Products

For a successful extended-release product, the drug must be released from the dosage form at a predetermined rate, dissolve in the gastrointestinal fluids, maintain sufficient gastrointestinal residence time, and be absorbed at a rate that will replace the amount of drug being metabolized and excreted.

In general, the drugs best suited for incorporation into an extended-release product have the following characteristics.

1. *They exhibit neither very slow nor very fast rates of absorption and excretion.* Drugs with slow rates of absorption and excretion are usually inherently long-acting and their preparation into extended-release dosage forms is not necessary. Drugs with very short half-lives, i.e., <2 hours, are poor candidates for extended-release dosage forms because of the large quantities of drug required for such a formulation. It should also be noted that drugs which act by affecting enzyme systems may be longer acting than indicated by their quantitative half-lives due to residual effects and recovery of the diminished biosystem (8).
2. *They are uniformly absorbed from the gastrointestinal tract.* Drugs prepared in extended-release forms, must have good aqueous solubility and maintain adequate residence time in the gastrointestinal tract. Drugs absorbed poorly or at varying and unpredictable rates are not good candidates for extended-release products.
3. *They are administered in relatively small doses.* Drugs with large single doses frequently are not suitable for the preparation of an extended-release product because the oral dosage unit (tablet or capsule) needed to maintain a sustained therapeutic blood level of the drug would have to be too large for the patient to easily swallow.
4. *They possess a good margin of safety.* The most widely used measure of the margin of a drug's safety is its therapeutic index, i.e., the median toxic dose divided by the median effective dose. For very "potent" drugs the therapeutic index may be "narrow" or very small. The larger the therapeutic index, the safer the drug. Drugs which are administered in very small doses or possess very narrow therapeutic indices are poor candidates for formulation into extended-release formulations because of technologic limitations of precise control over release rates and the risk of dose "dumping" due to a product defect. Patient misuse (e.g., chewing dosage unit) also could result in toxic drug levels.
5. *They are used in the treatment of chronic rather than acute conditions.* Drugs for acute conditions require greater physician adjustment of the dosage than that provided by extended-release products.

Extended-Release Technology for Oral Dosage Forms

For orally administered dosage forms, extended drug action is achieved by affecting the rate at which the drug is released from the dosage form and/or by slowing the transit time of the dosage form through the gastrointestinal tract (2).

The rate of drug release from solid dosage forms may be modified by the technologies described below which, in general, are based on 1) modifying drug dissolution by controlling access of biologic fluids to the drug through the use of barrier coatings; 2) controlling drug diffusion rates from dosage forms; and 3) chemically reacting or interacting between the drug substance or its pharmaceutical barrier and site-specific biologic fluids.

Coated Beads, Granules, or Microspheres

In these systems, the drug is distributed onto beads, pellets, granules or other particulate systems. Using conventional pan-coating or air-suspension coating techniques, a solution of the drug substance is placed onto small inert nonpareil seeds or beads made of sugar and starch or onto microcrystalline cellulose spheres. The nonpareil seeds are most often in the 425 to 850 μm range whereas the microcrystalline cellulose spheres are available ranging from 170 to 600 μm. The microcrystalline spheres are considered more durable during production than sugar-based cores (9).

In instances in which the dose of the drug is large, the starting granules of material may be composed of the drug itself. Some of these granules may remain uncoated to provide immediate drug release. Other granules (about two-thirds to three-fourths) receive varying coats of a lipid material like beeswax, carnauba wax, glycerylmonostearate, cetyl alcohol, or a cellulosic material like ethylcellulose. Then granules of different coating thicknesses are blended to achieve a mix having the desired drug release characteristics. The coating material may be colored with one or more dyes to distinguish granules or beads of different coating thicknesses (by depth of color) and to provide distinctiveness to the product. When properly blended, the granules may be placed in capsules or tableted. Various coating systems are commercially available which are aqueous-based and which utilize ethyl cellulose and plasticizer as the coating material [e.g., Aquacoat (FMC Corporation) and Surelease (Colorcon)]

(10–11). Aqueous-based coating systems eliminate the hazards and environmental concerns associated with organic solvent-based systems.

The variation in the thickness of the coats and in the type of coating material used affects the rate at which the body fluids are capable of penetrating the coating to dissolve the drug. Naturally, the thicker the coat, the more resistant to penetration and the more delayed will be drug release and dissolution. Typically the coated beads are about 1 mm in diameter. They are combined to have three or four release groups among the more than 100 beads contained in the dosing unit (8). This provides the different desired sustained or extended release rates and the targeting of the coated beads to the desired segments of the gastrointestinal tract. An example of this type of dosage form is the Spansule (SmithKline Beecham) capsule shown in Figure 8.3.

Multitablet System

Small spheroid-shaped compressed minitablets 3- to 4 mm in diameter may be prepared to have varying drug release characteristics. They then may be placed in gelatin capsule shells to provide the desired pattern of drug release (12). Each capsule may contain 8–10 minitablets, some uncoated for immediate release and others coated for extended drug release.

Microencapsulated Drug

Microencapsulation is a process by which solids, liquids, or even gases may be encapsulated into microscopic size particles through the formation of thin coatings of "wall" material around the substance being encapsulated. The process had its early origin in the late 1930s as a "clean" substitute for carbon paper and carbon ribbons as sought by the business machines industry. The ultimate development in the 1950s of reproduction paper and ribbons which contained dyes in tiny gelatin capsules released upon impact by a typewriter key or the pressure of a pen or pencil was the stimulus for the development of a host of microencapsulated materials, including drugs. Gelatin is a common wall-forming material but synthetic polymers as polyvinyl alcohol, ethylcellulose, polyvinyl chloride, and other materials also may be used.

The typical encapsulation process usually begins with the dissolving of the prospective wall material, say gelatin, in water. The material to be encapsulated is added and the two-phase mixture thoroughly stirred. With the material to be encapsulated broken up to the desired particle size, a solution of a second material is added, usually acacia. This additive material is chosen to have the ability to concentrate the gelatin (polymer) into tiny liquid droplets. These droplets (the *coacervate*) then form a film or coat around the particles of the substance to be encapsulated as a consequence of the extremely low interfacial tension of the residual water or solvent in the wall material so that a continuous, tight, film coating remains on the particle (Fig. 8.4). The final dry microcapsules are free-flowing, discrete particles of coated material. Of the total particle weight, the wall material usually represents between 2 and 20%. Different rates of drug release may be obtained by changing the core:wall ratio, the polymer used for the coating, and the method of microencapsulation (13).

One of the advantages of microencapsulation is that the administered dose of a drug is subdivided into small units that are spread over a large area of the gastrointestinal tract, which may enhance absorption by diminishing localized drug concentration (13). An example of a drug commercially

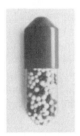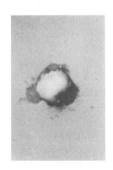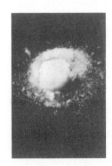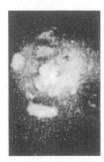

Fig. 8.3 *The Spansule capsule showing the hard gelatin capsule containing hundreds of tiny pellets for sustained drug release and the rupturing of one of the pellets as occurs in the gastric fluid. (Courtesy of SmithKline Beecham.)*

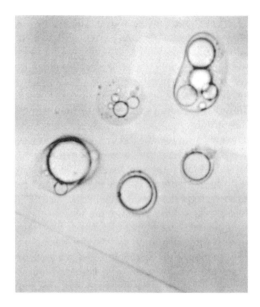

Fig. 8.4 *Microcapsules of mineral oil in a gelatin-acacia coacervate. (Photo courtesy of James C. Price, PhD, College of Pharmacy, The University of Georgia.)*

available in a microencapsulated extended-release dosage form is potassium chloride (Micro-K Exten-caps, A. H. Robins).

Embedding Drug in Slowly Eroding or Hydrophilic Matrix System

By this process, the drug substance is combined and made into granules with an excipient material that slowly erodes in body fluids, progressively releasing the drug for absorption. When these granules are mixed with granules of drug prepared without the excipient, the uncombined granules provide the immediate drug effect whereas the drug-excipient granules provide extended drug action. The granule-mix may be tableted or placed into gelatin capsule shells for oral delivery.

Hydrophilic cellulose polymers are commonly used as the excipient base in tableted matrix systems. The effectiveness of these hydrophilic matrix systems is based on the successive processes of: hydration of the cellulosic polymer; gel formation on the polymer's surface; tablet erosion; and, the subsequent and continuous release of drug. Hydroxypropyl methylcellulose (HPMC), a free-flowing powder, is commonly used to provide the hydrophilic matrix. Tablets are prepared by thoroughly distributing HPMC in the formulation, preparing the granules by wet granulation or roller compaction, and manufacturing the tablets by compression (14).

After ingestion, the tablet is wetted by gastric fluid and the polymer begins to hydrate. A gel layer forms around surface of the tablet and an initial quantity of drug is exposed and released. As water permeates further into the tablet the thickness of the gel layer is increased and soluble drug diffuses through the gel layer. As the outer layer becomes fully hydrated it erodes from the tablet core. If the drug is insoluble, it is released as such with the eroding gel layer. Thus, the rate of drug release is controlled by the processes of diffusion and tablet erosion (15).

If the bulk density of the tablet is less than one, it is buoyant in the gastric fluids, extending its residence time as it slowly erodes and releases its medication contents (16). An example of this type of product is Valrelease (Roche), a 15-mg slow-release dosage form of diazepam (Valium, Roche). The product is formulated using a unique *Hydro-dynamically Balanced Drug-delivery System* (HBS), which achieves, in one administration, plasma concentrations of diazepam equivalent to those obtained with conventional Valium 5 mg tablets taken 3 times daily. On contact with gastric fluid, the dosage form demonstrates a bulk density of less than one and thus remains buoyant and remains in the stomach for a variable period of time, depending on individual patient's physiologic characteristics. When Valrelease passes into the intestine, gradual release of the active drug and absorption continue. Solid dosage forms that have this buoyant characteristic are sometimes referred to as "floating" capsules or tablets.

In formulating a successful hydrophilic matrix system, the polymer selected for use must form a gelatinous layer rapidly enough to protect the inner core of the tablet from disintegrating too rapidly after ingestion. As the proportion of polymer is increased in a formulation so is the viscosity of the gel formed with a resultant decrease in the rate of drug diffusion and drug release (15). In general 20% of HPMC results in satisfactory rates of drug release for an extended-release tablet formulation. However, as with all formulations, consideration must be given to the possible effects of other formulation ingredients as fillers, tablet binders, and disintegrants. An example of a proprietary product using a hydrophilic matrix base of HPMC for extended drug release is Oramorph SR Tablets (Roxane), which contains morphine sulfate.

When hydrophilic matrix formulations are used in the preparation of extended-release capsules, the same concept applies. When ingested, water penetrates the capsule shell, comes in contact with the capsule fill, hydrates the outer layer of powder, and forms a gelatinous plug from which the drug content diffuses gradually over time as hydration continues and the gelatinous plug dissolves.

Manufacturers may prepare two-layered tablets, with one layer containing the uncombined drug for immediate release and the other layer having the drug imbedded in a hydrophilic matrix for extended-release. Three-layered tablets may be similarly prepared, with both outer layers containing the drug for immediate release. Some commercial tablets are prepared with an inner core containing the extended-release portion of drug and an outer shell enclosing the core and containing drug for immediate release.

Embedding Drug in Inert Plastic Matrix

By this method, the drug is granulated with an inert plastic material such as polyethylene, polyvinyl acetate, or polymethacrylate, and the granulation is compressed into tablets. The drug is slowly released from the inert plastic matrix by diffusion. The compression of the tablet creates the matrix or plastic form that retains its shape during the leaching of the drug and through its passage through the alimentary tract. An immediate-release portion of drug may be compressed onto the surface of the tablet. The inert tablet matrix, expended of drug, is excreted with the feces. The primary example of a dosage form of this type is the Gradumet (Abbott).

Complex Formation

Certain drug substances when chemically combined with certain other chemical agents form chemical complexes that may be only slowly soluble in body fluids, depending upon the pH of the environment. This slow dissolution rate provides the extended release of the drug. Salts of tannic acid, tannates, provide this quality in a variety of proprietary products by the tradename Rynatan (Wallace) (8).

Ion-exchange Resins

A solution of a cationic drug may be passed through a column containing an ion-exchange resin, forming a complex by the replacement of hydrogen atoms. The resin-drug complex is then washed and may be tableted, encapsulated, or suspended in an aqueous vehicle. The release of the drug is dependent upon the pH and the electrolyte concentration in the gastrointestinal tract. Release is greater in the acidity of the stomach than in the less acidic environment of the small intestine. Examples of drug products of this type include hy-

drocodone polistirex and chlorpheniramine polistirex suspension [Tussionex Pennkinetic Extended Release Suspension (Medeva)] and phentermine resin capsules [Ionamin Capsules (Pharmanex)].

The mechanism of action of drug release from ion exchange resins may be depicted as follows.

In the stomach:

1. Drug resinate + HCl $\rightleftharpoons$ acidic resin + drug hydrochloride
2. Resin salt + HCl $\rightleftharpoons$ resin chloride + acidic drug

In the intestine:

1. Drug resinate + NaCl $\rightleftharpoons$ sodium resinate + drug hydrochloride
2. Resin salt + NaCl $\rightleftharpoons$ resin chloride + sodium salt of drug.

This system incorporates a polymer barrier coating and bead technology in addition to the ion-exchange mechanism. The initial dose comes from an uncoated portion, and the remainder from the coated beads. The coating does not dissolve, and release is extended over a 12-hour period by ionic exchange. The drug-containing polymer particles are minute, and may be suspended to produce a liquid with extended-release characteristics as well as solid dosage forms.

Osmotic Pump

The pioneer *oral osmotic* pump drug delivery system is the *Oros* system, developed by Alza. The system is composed of a core tablet surrounded by a semipermeable membrane coating having a 0.4 mm diameter hole produced by laser beam. (Fig. 8.5). The core tablet has two layers, one containing the drug (the "active" layer) and the other containing a polymeric osmotic agent (the "push" layer). The system operates on the principle of osmotic pressure.

When the tablet is swallowed, the semipermeable membrane permits water to enter from the patient's stomach into the core tablet, dissolving or suspending the drug. As pressure increases in the osmotic layer it forces or pumps the drug solution out of the delivery orifice on the side of the tablet (Fig. 8.6). Only the drug solution (not the undissolved drug) is capable of passing through the hole in the tablet. The system is designed such that only a few drops of water are drawn into the tablet each hour. The rate of inflow of water and the function of the tablet depends upon the existence of an osmotic gradient between the contents of the bi-layer

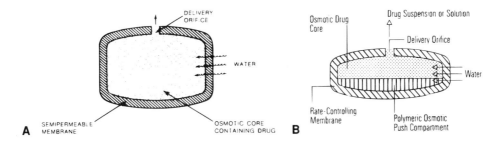

Fig. 8.5   *A, Depiction of the elementary OROS osmotic pump drug delivery system; B, the OROS Push-Pull Osmotic System. (Courtesy of Alza Corporation.)*

core and the fluid in the GI tract. Drug delivery is essentially constant as long as the osmotic gradient remains constant. The drug release rate may be altered by changing the surface area, the thickness or composition of the membrane, and/or by changing the diameter of the drug release orifice. The drug-release rate is not affected by gastrointestinal acidity, alkalinity, fed conditions, or GI motility. The biologically inert components of the tablet remain intact during GI transit and are eliminated in the feces as an insoluble shell.

This type of osmotic system, termed the "gastrointestinal therapeutic system ["GITS"(Pfizer)] is employed in the manufacture of Glucotrol XL Extended Release Tablets and Procardia XL Extended Release Tablets. Another example of the osmotic system is the controlled-onset extended release ["COER" (Searle)] system used in Covera-HS Tablets, in which initial drug is released 4–5 hours after tablet ingestion. The delay in drug release is effected by a slowly solubilized coated layer between the active drug core and the outer semipermeable membrane.

Repeat Action Tablets

Repeat action tablets are prepared so that an initial dose of drug is released immediately followed later by a second dose. The tablets may be prepared with the immediate-release dose in the tablet's outer shell or coating with the second dose in the tablet's inner core, separated by a slowly permeable barrier coating. In general, the drug from the inner core is exposed to body fluids and released 4 to 6 hours after administration. An example of this type of product is Repetabs (Schering). Repeat action dosage forms are best suited for the treatment of chronic conditions requiring repeated dosing. The drugs utilized should have low dosage and fairly rapid rates of absorption and excretion.

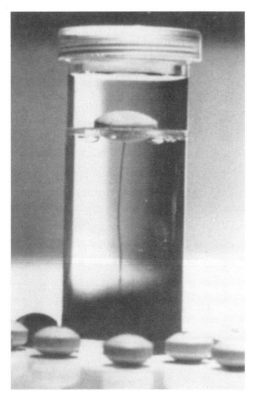

Fig. 8.6   *The OROS (Oral Osmotic) drug delivery system. A tablet core of drug is surrounded by a semipermeable membrane that is pierced by a small laser-drilled hole. After ingestion, water is drawn into the tablet from the digestive tract by osmosis. As water enters the tablet core, the drug gradually goes into solution. The solution is pushed out through the small hole at a controlled rate of about 1 to 2 drops per hour. (Courtesy of ALZA Corporation.)*

Delayed-Release Oral Dosage Forms

The release of a drug from an oral dosage form may be intentionally delayed until it reaches the intestines for several reasons. The purpose may be to protect a drug destroyed by gastric fluids, to reduce gastric distress caused by drugs particularly irritating to the stomach, or to facilitate GI transit for drugs which are better absorbed from the intestines. As stated previously, capsules and tablets specially coated to remain intact in the stomach later to yield their ingredients in the intestines are termed *enteric coated.* The enteric coating may be pH-dependent breaking down in the less acidic environment of the intestine, time-dependent and eroding by moisture over time during GI transit, or enzyme-dependent and deteriorating due to the hydrolysis-catalyzing action of intestinal enzymes. Among the many agents used to enteric coat tablets and capsules are fats, fatty acids, waxes, shellac, and cellulose acetate phthalate.

Examples of modified-release tablets and capsules official in the USP are presented in Table 8.2 and examples of proprietary modified-release oral dosage forms are presented in Table 8.3.

USP Requirements and FDA Guidance for Modified-Release Dosage Forms

The USP contains general chapters and specific tests to determine the drug release capabilities of extended-release and delayed-release tablets and capsules (6).

Table 8.2. Examples of Modified-Release Tablets and Capsules Official in the USP

Delayed-Release
  Aspirin Delayed-release Tablets
  Doxycycline Hyclate Delayed-release Capsules
  Erythromycin Delayed-release Capsules
  Oxtriphylline Delayed-release Tablets
Extended-Release
  Aspirin Extended-release Tablets
  Diazepam Extended-release Capsules
  Diltiazem Extended-release Capsules
  Disopyramide Phosphate Extended-release Capsules
  Ferrous Fumarate and Docusate Sodium
    Extended-release Tablets
  Indomethacin Extended-release Capsules
  Isosorbide Dinitrate Extended-release Tablets and
    Capsules
  Lithium Carbonate Extended-release Tablets
  Oxtriphylline Extended-release Tablets
  Phenylpropanolamine Hydrochloride
    Extended-release Capsules
  Potassium Chloride Extended-release Tablets
  Procainamide Hydrochloride Extended-release Tablets
  Propranolol Hydrochloride Extended-release Capsules
  Quinidine Gluconate Extended-release Tablets
  Theophylline Extended-release Capsules

Drug Release

The USP test for drug release for extended-release and delayed-release articles is based on drug dissolution from the dosage unit against elapsed test time. Descriptions of the various test apparatus and procedures may be found in the USP, Chapter <724> (6). The individual monographs contain specific criteria for compliance with the test and the apparatus and test procedures to be used. For example, for Aspirin Extended-release Tablets, the USP requires the following aspirin dissolution rate to meet the stated drug release test:

Time (hr)	Amount Dissolved
1.0	between 15% and 40%
2.0	between 25% and 60%
4.0	between 35% and 75%
8.0	not less than 70%

Uniformity of Dosage Units

Modified-release tablets and capsules must meet the USP standard for uniformity as described in the previous chapter for conventional dosage units. Uniformity of dosage units may be demonstrated by either of two methods, weight variation or content uniformity, as described in USP Chapter <905> (6).

In Vitro/In Vivo Correlations (IVIVCs)

In vitro/in vivo relationships (IVIVRs) or *in vitro/in vivo* correlations (IVIVCs) are critical to the development of oral extended-release products. Assessing IVICRs are important throughout the periods of product development, clinical evaluation, submission of an application for FDA-approval for marketing, and during postapproval for any formulation or manufacturing changes which are proposed (17).

In 1997, the Food and Drug Administration (FDA) published a guidance document entitled "Extended Release Oral Dosage Forms: Development, Evaluation, and Application of In Vitro/In Vivo Correlations" (7). The document provides guidance to sponsors of New Drug Applications (NDAs) and Abbreviated New Drug Applications (ANDAs) for extended-release oral products. The guidance provides methods of: 1) developing an IVIVC and evaluating its predictability; 2) using an IVIVC to establish dissolution specifications; and 3) applying an IVIVC as a surrogate for in vivo bioequivalence when it is necessary to document bioequivalence during the approval process or during postapproval for certain formulation or manufacturing changes.

Table 8.3. Examples of Proprietary Modified-Release Oral Dosage Forms

Drug Product and Manufacturer	*Dosage Form Characteristics*
Delayed-Release	
E-Mycin (erythromycin) Delayed-Release Tablets (Knoll)	Tablets enteric coated with cellulose acetate phthalate, carnauba wax, and cellulose polymers. Use: antibiotic.
Asacol (mesalamine) Delayed-Release Tablets (Procter & Gamble)	Tablets coated with Eudragit S (methylacrylic acid copolymer B), a resin that bypasses the stomach dissolves in the ileum and beyond. Use: treat ulcerative colitis
Prilosec (omeprazole) Delayed-Release Capsules (Astra-Merck)	Enteric coated granules of omeprazole placed in capsules. Omeprazole is acid-labile and is degraded by gastric acid. Use: treatment of duodenal ulcer.
Extended-Release Coated Particles/Beads	
Toprol-XL (metoprolol succinate) Tablets (Astra)	Drug pellets coated with cellulose polymers compressed into tablets. Use: treatment of hypertension.
Indocin SR (indomethacin) Capsules (Merck)	Coated pellets for sustained release. The formulation includes polyvinyl acetate-crotonic acid copolymer and hydroxypropyl methylcellulose. Use: analgesic/antiinflammatory.
Compazine (prochlorperazine) Spansule Capsules (SmithKline Beecham)	Coated pellets in capsule formulated to release initial dose promptly with additional drug for prolonged-release. Use: antinausea/antivomiting.
Extended-Release Inert Matrix	
Desoxyn (methamphetamine HCl) Gradumet Tablets (Abbott)	Drug impregnated in an inert, porous, plastic matrix. Drug leaches out as it passes slowly through the GI tract. Expended matrix is excreted in stool. Use: attention deficit disorder.
Procanbid (procainamide HCl) Tablets (Parke-Davis)	Extended-release tablets with a core tablet of a non-erodible wax matrix coated with cellulose polymers. Use: an antiarrhythmic.
Extended-Release Hydrophilic/Eroding Matrix	
Quinidex (quinidine sulfate) Tablets (Robins)	Extended-release is provided by a hydrophilic matrix which swells and slowly erodes. Use: an antiarrhythmic.
Oramorph SR (morphine sulfate) Tablets (Roxane)	Sustained-release hydrophilic matrix system, based on the polymer hydroxypropyl methylcellulose. Use: analgesic for severe pain.
Extended-Release Microencapsulated	
K-Dur Microburst Release System (potassium chloride) Tablets (Key)	Immediately dispersing drug microencapsulated with ethylcellulose and hydroxypropyl cellulose. Use: treat potassium depletion.
Extended-Release Osmotic	
Glucotrol XL (glipizide) Tablets (Pfizer)	Controlled-release "Gastrointestinal Therapeutic System (GITS)" osmotic system (described in the text). Ingredients include polyethylene oxide, hydroxypropyl cellulose, and cellulose acetate. Use: antihyperglycemic.
Covera-HS (verapamil HCl) Tablets (Searle)	A controlled-onset extended-release ("COER") osmotic system (described in the text). Use: antihypertensive/antianginal.

Three categories of IVIVCs are included in the document:

Level A—A predictive mathematical model for the relationship between the entire in vitro dissolution/release time course and the entire in vivo response time course; e.g., the time course of plasma drug concentration or amount of drug absorbed.

This is the most common type of correlation submitted.

Level B—A predictive mathematical model of the relationship between summary parameters that characterize the in vitro and in vivo time courses; e.g., models that relate the mean in vitro dissolution time to the mean in vivo dissolution time; the mean in vitro dissolution time to the mean residence time in vivo; or the in vitro dissolution rate constant to the absorption rate constant.

Level C —A predictive mathematical model of the relationship between the amount dissolved in vitro at a particular time (or the time required for in vitro dissolution of a fixed percent of the dose; e.g., T_{50}%) and a summary parameter that characterizes the in vivo time course (e.g., C_{max} or AUC). The level of IVIVCs may be useful in the early stages of formulation development when pilot formulations are being selected.

The most common process for developing an IVIVC model (Level A) is to: 1) develop formulations with different release rates (e.g., slow, fast, and intermediate) or a single release rate if dissolution is condition-independent; 2) obtain in vitro dissolution profiles and in vivo plasma concentration profiles for these formulations; and 3) estimate the in vivo absorption or dissolution time course for each formulation and subject using appropriate mathematical approaches.

Among the criteria applicable to the development of IVIVCs are the following (7):

- In determining in vitro dissolution, USP dissolution apparatus, type I (basket) or type II (paddle) is preferred although type III (reciprocating cylinder) or type IV (flow through cell) may be applicable in some instances.
- An aqueous medium with a pH not exceeding pH 6.8 is preferred as the medium for dissolution studies. For poorly soluble drugs, the addition of a surfactant (e.g. 1% sodium lauryl sulfate) may be employed.
- The dissolution profiles of at least 12 individual dosage units from each lot should be determined.
- For in vivo studies, human subjects are used in the fasted state unless the drug is not well tolerated, in which case the studies may be conducted in the fed state. Six to 36 human subjects have been shown to produce acceptable data sets.
- Crossover studies are preferred, but parallel studies or cross-study analysis may be acceptable using a common reference treatment product as an IV solution, an aqueous oral solution, or an immediate release product.

Labeling

The USP indicates labeling requirements for modified-release dosage form articles in addition to general labeling requirements. The requirements are specific to the monograph article.

For example, the label of Aspirin Delayed-release Tablets must state that *the tablets are enteric coated* whereas the labeling for Theophylline Extended-release Capsules must indicate *whether the product is intended for dosing every 12 or 24 hours, and states with which in-vitro Drug Release Test the product complies* (seven tests are described in the monograph, each with different drug-release times and tolerances).

Clinical Considerations in the Use of Oral Modified-Release Dosage Forms

Patients should be advised of the dose and dosing frequency of modified drug release products and instructed to not use them interchangeably or concomitantly with immediate-release forms of the same drug. Patients stabilized on a modified-release product should not be changed to an immediate-release product without consideration of any existing blood level concentrations of the drug. Also, once stabilized, patients should not be changed to another extended-release product unless there is assurance of equivalent bioavailability. A different product could result in a marked shift in the patient's drug blood level due to differences in drug release characteristics.

Patients should be advised that modified-release tablets and capsules should not be crushed or chewed since such action would compromise their drug release features (18). Patients being fed by enteral nutrition through a nasogastric feeding tube may receive conventional or modified-release medication. For example, coated pellets from inside capsules simply may be mixed with water and poured down the feeding tube (19).

Patients and caregivers should be advised that nonerodible plastic matrix shells and osmotic tablets remain intact throughout gastrointestinal transit and the empty shells or "ghosts" from osmotic tablets may be seen in the stool. The patient should be assured of the normalcy of this event and that drug absorption has taken place (2).

Packaging and Storing Modified-Release Tablets and Capsules

Modified-release tablets and capsules are packaged and stored in the same manner as conventional products as discussed in Chapter 7.

Nonoral Modified-Release Systems

Dosage forms delivered by nonoral routes of administration may be designed to provide extended

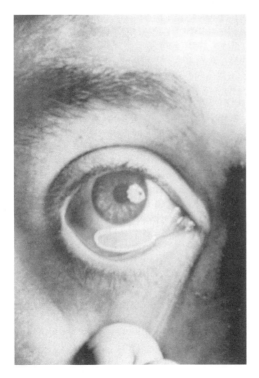

Fig. 8.7   *Ocusert Ocular Therapeutic Systems are thin, flexible wafers placed under the eyelid to provide a week's dosage of pilocarpine in the treatment of glaucoma. Ocusert systems cause less blurring of vision than conventional pilocarpine eye drops, which must be administered 4 times daily. (Courtesy of Alza Corporation.)*

drug action. As indicated below, extended drug action may be achieved through a modification of the physical or chemical characteristics of the drug substance, a change in the characteristics of the drug carrier or vehicle, or by the fabrication of rate-controlled drug delivery systems.

Ocular

One of the problems associated with the use of ophthalmic solutions is the rapid loss of administered drug due to the blinking of the eye and the flushing effect of lacrimal fluids. Up to 80% of an administered dose may be lost through tears and the action of nasolacrimal drainage within 5 minutes of installation (20). Extended periods of therapy may be achieved by formulations which increase the contact time between the medication and the corneal surface. This may be accomplished through use of agents that increase the viscosity of solutions; by ophthalmic suspensions in which the drug particles slowly dissolve; by slowly dissipating

ophthalmic ointments; or by the use of ophthalmic inserts.

Although ophthalmic dosage forms are discussed at length in Chapter 16, it is useful within the context of the present chapter to note certain preparations designed to extend drug action. The following are but two examples of proprietary products which utilize viscosity-increasing agents to increase corneal contact time are: Pilopine HS Gel (pilocarpine, Alcon), which employs Carbopol 940, a synthetic high molecular weight cross-linked polymer of acrylic acid; and, Timoptic-XE (timolol maleate, Merck), which employs Gelrite (gellan gum) which forms a gel upon contact with the precorneal tear film.

The development and use of ophthalmic inserts represents an innovative achievement in the delivery of medication to the eye. One such insert, the OCUSERT system (Alza) is shown in Figures 8.7 and 8.8. The insert is elliptical with the dimensions of one of the pilocarpine-containing systems being 13.4 by 5.7 mm by 0.3 mm (thickness). The insert is flexible and has a drug-containing core surrounded on each side by a layer of hydrophobic ethylene/vinyl acetate copolymer membranes through which the drug diffuses at a constant rate. The white margin around the system contains titanium dioxide for visibility. The rate of drug diffusion is controlled by the polymer composition, the membrane thickness, and the solubility of the drug. During the first few hours after insertion, the drug release rate is greater than that which occurs thereafter in order to achieve initially adequate drug levels. The pilocarpine-containing inserts are placed in the conjunctival sac from which they release their medication over a 7-day period in the treatment of glaucoma.

Another ophthalmic insert is Lacrisert (Merck) which is a rod-shaped, water soluble form of hydroxypropyl cellulose. The insert is placed into the inferior cul-de-sac of the eye once or twice daily in

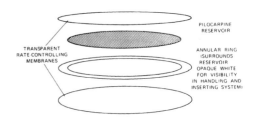

Fig. 8.8   *Construction of the Ocusert Ocular Therapeutic System containing pilocarpine between transparent rate-controlling membranes. (Courtesy of Alza Corporation.)*

the treatment of dry eyes. The inserts soften and slowly dissolve, thickening the precorneal tear film and prolonging the tear film breakup.

Parenteral Systems

Extended rates of drug action following injection may be achieved in a number of ways, including the use of: crystal or amorphous drug forms having prolonged dissolution characteristics; slowly dissolving chemical complexes of the drug entity; solutions or suspensions of drug in slowly absorbed carriers or vehicles (as oleaginous); increased particle size of drug in suspension; or, by injection of slowly eroding microspheres of drug (22). The duration of action of the various forms of insulin for example is based in part on its physical form (amorphous or crystalline), complex formation with added agents, and its dosage form (solution or suspension) (23).

Matrix carrier systems based on biodegradable materials for parenteral application have been examined as a potential means of delivering peptides and proteins (22). In such systems, a material as purified insoluble collagen is used as a matrix from which its drug contents are released through controlled diffusion and enzymatic matrix degradation.

In addition to the above means of achieving extended drug action, the rate and duration of drug delivery may be controlled by slow intravenous infusion, using mechanically-controlled drug infusion pumps.

Examples of proprietary parenteral products having long-acting features are presented in Table 8.4. Conventional parenteral products and methods of their administration are discussed in Chapter 14.

Vaginal Insert

Cervidil Vaginal Insert (Forest Pharmaceuticals) is an example of a vaginal product having extended drug action. The insert is a rectangular polymeric pouch containing the drug dinoprostone (prostaglandin E_2) in a cross-linked polyethylene oxide/urethane polymer which releases the drug at a predetermined controlled release rate for the induction of labor. The insert, administered by trained obstetrical hospital personnel, is designed to release drug over a 12 hour period, after which time (or upon onset of active labor) it is removed.

Another type of vaginal product with extended drug action is the bioadhesive vaginal gel, Crinone Gel (Wyeth-Ayerst), which contains micronized progesterone and the polymer polycarbophil in an oil-in-water emulsion system. The polymer, which is insoluble in water, swells within the vagina and forms a bioadhesive gel coating on the walls of the vagina. This allows the absorption of progesterone through the vaginal tissue over a 25–50 hour period. The product is used to assist in reproduction.

A unique method of administering estradiol is through the use of the estradiol vaginal ring [Estring (Pharmacia & Upjohn)] shown in Figure 8.9. The core of the ring contains a reservoir of estradiol, which is released immediately and then at a continuous rate of 75 μg/24 hours over 90 days. The ring, composed of silicone polymers and barium sulfate, has an outer diameter of 55 mm and a core diameter of 2 mm. The ring is inserted into the upper one-third of the vaginal vault and is worn continuously for the treatment of urogenital symptoms associated with postmenopausal atrophy of the vagina.

Table 8.4. Examples of Proprietary Extended Action Parenteral Products

Product	Contents and Comments
Bicillin C-R Injection (Wyeth-Ayerst)	Contains penicillin G benzathine and penicillin G procaine which have a low solubility and thus are slowly released from intramuscular injection sites. The drugs are hydrolyzed to penicillin G. The combination of hydrolysis and slow absorption results in prolonged blood serum levels. Usual dose intervals, 2–3 days.
Decadron-LA Sterile Suspension (Merck)	Contains dexamethasone acetate, a very insoluble ester of dexamethasone. The repository intramuscular injection may be repeated as needed at intervals of 1–3 weeks.
Depo-Provera Contraceptive Injection (Pharmacia & Upjohn)	Medroxyprogesterone acetate, a water-insoluble drug, in aqueous suspension. The single intramuscular dose is repeated every 3 months.
Abelcet Amphotericin B Lipid Complex Injection (Liposome Company)	An intravenous suspension of amphtericin B complexed with two phospholipids administered by IV infusion once a day.
Lupron Depot for Suspension (TAP Pharmaceuticals)	Sterile lyophilized microspheres which when mixed with diluent form a suspension administered by IM injection once every 3 to 4 months.

Subdermal Implant

Solid dosage forms designed to be inserted under the skin by special injectors or by surgical incision are termed *implants*. They are designed to provide continuous long-term drug therapy through the slow release of medication. Examples of drugs administered as subdermal implants are goserelin acetate (Zoladex Implant, Zeneca) and levonorgestrel (Norplant System, Wyeth-Ayerst).

Zoladex Implant is a sterile, biodegradable product for subcutaneous injection with continuous medication release over a 4- to 12-week period, depending on the product strength administered. The

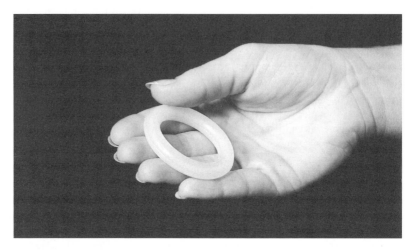

Fig. 8.9 *Estring vaginal ring which provides continuous release of estradiol over a 90-day period. (Courtesy of Pharmacia & Upjohn)*

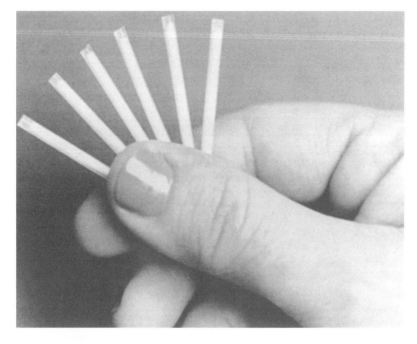

Fig. 8.10 *Norplant System of levonorgestrel implants for the long-term (up to 5 years) prevention of pregnancy. Six implants are inserted subdermally in the midportion of the inner upper arm about 8 to 10 cm above the elbow crease. The implants are inserted in a fanlike pattern about 15 degrees apart. (Courtesy of Wyeth-Ayerst Laboratories.)*

drug is used in the treatment of advanced prostatic cancer. The active agent is dispersed in a matrix of a completely biodegradable D,L-lactic and glycolic acids copolymer. The 1-mm diameter cylinder pre-loaded in a special use syringe is implanted subcutaneously in the upper abdomen.

The Norplant System of levonorgestrel implants (Fig. 8.10) provides up to 5 years of protection from pregnancy after subcutaneous insertion (23). The implants are sterile flexible closed capsules made of silicone rubber tubing (Silastic), a dimethylsiloxane/methylvinylsiloxane copolymer, containing the synthetic progestin levonorgestrel. Each capsule is 2.4 mm in diameter and 34 mm in length. Six capsules are inserted in a fan-like pattern in a superficial plane beneath the skin of the upper arm by small 2 mm incision and special injector. The insertion pattern facilitates removal of the expended capsules. Following their term of use, the capsules are surgically removed and may be replaced with fresh capsules.

Transdermal Systems

A number of drugs are delivered to the systemic circulation through intact skin in a controlled manner by transdermal drug delivery systems. These systems, which are discussed in Chapter 10, allow once-a-day dosing.

References

1. Rogers JD, Kwan KC. Pharmacokinetic requirements for controlled-release dosage forms. In: John Urquhart, ed. Controlled-release pharmaceuticals. Washington DC: Academy of Pharmaceutical Sciences, American Pharmaceutical Association, 1979; 95–119.
2. Bogner RH. Bioavailability and bioequivalence of extended-release oral dosage forms. US Pharmacist 1997;22(Suppl):3–12.
3. Madan PL. Sustained-release drug delivery systems: part II, preformulation considerations. Pharmaceutical Manufacturing 1985;2:41–45.
4. Madan PL. Sustained-release drug delivery systems: part I, an overview. Pharmaceutical Manufacturing 1985;2:23–27.
5. Scale-up of oral extended-release dosage forms. AAPS/FDA Workshop Committee. Pharm Tech 1995; 19:46–54.
6. The United States Pharmacopeia 23/National Formulary 18, The United States Pharmacopeial Convention, Inc., Rockville, MD, 1995.
7. Guidance for industry. Extended release oral dosage forms: development, evaluation, and application of in vitro/in vivo correlations. Rockville, MD: Center for Drug Evaluation and Research, Food and Drug Administration, 1997.
8. Madan PL. Sustained release dosage forms. US Pharmacist 1990;15:39–50.
9. Celphere microcrystalline cellulose spheres. Philadelphia: FMC Corporation, 1996.
10. Aquacoat aqueous polymeric dispersion. Philadelphia: FMC Corporation, 1991.
11. Surelease aqueous controlled release coating system. West Point, PA: Colorcon, 1990.
12. Butler J, Cumming I, Brown J, et al. A novel multiunit controlled-release system. Pharm Tech 1998;22: 122–138.
13. Yazici E, Oner L, Kas HS, Hincal AA. Phenytoin sodium microcapsules: bench scale formulation, process characterization and release kinetics. Pharmaceut Dev Technol 1996;1:175–183.
14. Sheskey PJ, Cabelka TD, Robb RT, Boyce BM. Use of roller compaction in the preparation of controlled-release hydrophilic matrix tablets containing methylcellulose and hydroxypropyl methylcellulose polymers. Pharm Tech 1994;18:132–150.
15. Formulating for controlled release with Methocel Premium cellulose ethers. Midland, MI: Dow Chemical Company, 1995.
16. Banakar UV. Drug delivery systems of the 90s. Innovations in controlled release. Am Pharm 1987;NS27: 39–48.
17. Devane J, Butler J. The impact of in vitro-in vivo relationships on product development. Pharm Tech 1997; 21:146–159.
18. Mitchell JF. Oral dosage forms that should not be crushed: 1998 update. Hosp Pharm 1998;33:399–415.
19. Beckwith MC, Barton RG, Graves C. A guide to drug therapy in patients with enteral feeding tubes: dosage form selection and administration methods. Hosp Pharm 1997;32:57–64.
20. Madan PL. Sustained-release drug delivery systems: part VI, special devices. Pharmaceutical Manufacturing 1985;2:33–40.
21. Madan PL. Sustained-release drug delivery systems: part V, parenteral products. Pharmaceutical Manufacturing 1985;2:51.
22. Friess W, Lee G, Groves MJ. Insoluble collagen matrices for prolonged delivery of proteins. Pharmaceutical Development and Technology 1996;1:185–193.
23. Norplant System, Product Information. Philadelphia, PA: Wyeth-Ayerst Laboratories, 1998.

9

OINTMENTS, CREAMS AND GELS

Chapter at a Glance

OINTMENTS, CREAMS, and gels are semisolid dosage forms intended for topical application. They may be applied to the skin, placed onto the surface of the eye, or used nasally, vaginally or rectally. The majority of these preparations are used for the effects of the therapeutic agents they contain. Those which are nonmedicated are used for their physical effects as protectants or lubricants.

For the most part, topical preparations are used for the localized effects produced at the site of their application by virtue of drug penetration into the underlying layers of skin or mucous membranes.

Although some unintended systemic drug absorption may occur, it is usually in subtherapeutic quantities and generally only of minor concern. However, systemic drug absorption can be an important consideration in certain instances, as when the patient is pregnant or nursing because drugs can enter the fetal blood supply and breast milk and be transferred to the fetus or nursing infant.

Some topical applications, most notably transdermal drug delivery systems, *are* designed for the systemic absorption of drug substances in therapeutic quantities. The following distinction is an important one with regard to dermatologic applications. A *topical dermatological* product is designed to deliver drug *into* the skin in treating dermal disorders, *with the skin as the target organ*. A *transdermal* drug delivery system is designed to deliver drugs *through* the skin (*percutaneous absorption*) to the general circulation for systemic effects, *with the skin not being the target organ* (1). Transdermal drug delivery systems are discussed in the next chapter.

Ointments

Ointments are semisolid preparations intended for external application to the skin or mucous membranes. Ointments may be medicated or nonmedicated. Nonmedicated ointments are used for the physical effects that they provide as protectants, emollients or lubricants. *Ointment bases,* as described, may by used for their physical effects or as vehicles in the preparation of medicated ointments.

Ointment Bases

Ointment bases are classified by the USP (2) into four general groups: 1) hydrocarbon bases, 2) absorption bases, 3) water-removable bases, and 4) water-soluble bases.

Hydrocarbon Bases

Hydrocarbon bases are also termed *oleaginous bases.* On application to the skin, they have an emollient effect, protect against the escape of moisture, are effective as occlusive dressings, can remain on the skin for prolonged periods of time without "drying out," and because of their immiscibility with water are difficult to wash off. Water and aqueous preparations may be incorporated into them, but only in small amounts and with some difficulty. Petrolatum, White Petrolatum, White Ointment, and Yellow Ointment are examples of hydrocarbon ointment bases.

When powdered substances are to be incorporated into hydrocarbon bases, liquid petrolatum (mineral oil) may be used as the levigating agent.

Petrolatum, USP

Petrolatum, USP, is a purified mixture of semisolid hydrocarbons obtained from petroleum. It is an unctuous mass, varying in color from yellowish to light amber. It melts at temperatures between 38° and 60°C and may be used alone or in combination with other agents as an ointment base. Petrolatum is also known as "Yellow Petrolatum" and "Petroleum Jelly." A commercial product is Vaseline (Chesebrough-Ponds)

White Petrolatum, USP

White Petrolatum, USP, is a purified mixture of semisolid hydrocarbons from petroleum that has been wholly or nearly decolorized. It is used for the same purpose as Petrolatum, but due to its lighter color it is considered more esthetic by some pharmacists and patients. White Petrolatum is also known as "White Petroleum Jelly." A commercial product is White Vaseline (Chesebrough-Ponds)

Yellow Ointment, USP

This ointment has the following formula for the preparation of 1000 g:

Yellow Wax	50 g
Petrolatum	950 g

Yellow wax is the purified wax obtained from the honeycomb of the bee (*Apis mellifera*). The ointment is prepared by melting the yellow wax on a water bath, adding the petrolatum until the mixture is uniform, then cooling with stirring until congealed. The ointment also has been called "Simple Ointment."

White Ointment, USP

This ointment differs from Yellow Ointment by substituting White Wax (bleached and purified Yellow Wax) and White Petrolatum in the formula.

Absorption Bases

Absorption bases are of two types: 1) those that *permit* the incorporation of aqueous solutions resulting in the formation of water-in-oil emulsions (e.g., *Hydrophilic Petrolatum*), and (2) those that *are* water-in-oil emulsions (syn: *emulsion bases*) and permit the incorporation of additional quantities of aqueous solutions (e.g., Lanolin). These bases may be used as emollients although they do not provide the degree of occlusion afforded by the hydrocarbon bases. Absorption bases are not easily removed from the skin with water washing since the external phase of the emulsion is oleaginous. Absorption bases are useful as pharmaceutical adjuncts to incorporate small volumes of aqueous solutions into hydrocarbon bases. This is accomplished by incorporating the aqueous solution into the absorption base and then incorporating this mixture into the hydrocarbon base.

Hydrophilic Petrolatum, USP

Hydrophilic Petrolatum, USP has the following formula for the preparation of 1000 g:

Cholesterol	30 g
Stearyl Alcohol	30 g
White Wax	80 g
White Petrolatum	860 g

It is prepared by melting the stearyl alcohol and the white wax on a steam bath, adding the cholesterol with stirring until dissolved, adding the white petrolatum and allowing the mixture to cool while being stirred until congealed.

A commercial product, Aquaphor, is a variation of Hydrophilic Petrolatum and has the capacity to absorb up to three times its weight in water.

Lanolin, USP

Lanolin, USP, obtained from the wool of sheep (*Ovis aries*), is a purified, wax-like substance that has been cleaned, deodorized, and decolorized. It contains not more than 0.25% water. Additional water may be incorporated into lanolin by mixing. *Modified Lanolin, USP* is Lanolin that has been processed to reduce the contents of free lanolin alcohols and any detergent and pesticide residues.

Water-removable Bases

Water-removable bases are oil-in-water emulsions resembling creams in appearance. Because the external phase of the emulsion is aqueous, they are easily washed from skin and are often called "water-washable" bases. They may be diluted with water or aqueous solutions. They have the ability to absorb serous discharges. Hydrophilic Ointment, USP is an example of this type of base.

Hydrophilic Ointment, USP

Hydrophilic Ointment has the following formula for the preparation of about 1000 g:

Methylparaben	0.25 g
Propylparaben	0.15 g
Sodium Lauryl Sulfate	10 g
Propylene Glycol	120 g
Stearyl Alcohol	250 g
White Petrolatum	250 g
Purified Water	370 g

In preparing the ointment, the stearyl alcohol and white petrolatum are melted together at about 75°C. The other agents, dissolved in the purified water, are added with stirring until the mixture congeals. Sodium lauryl sulfate is the emulsifying agent with the stearyl alcohol and white petrolatum comprising the oleaginous phase of the emulsion and the other ingredients the aqueous phase. Methylparaben and propylparaben are antimicrobial preservatives.

Water-soluble Bases

Water-soluble bases do not contain oleaginous components. They are completely water-washable and often referred to as "greaseless." Because they soften greatly with the addition of water, large amounts of aqueous solutions are not effectively incorporated into these bases. They mostly are used for the incorporation of solid substances. Polyethylene Glycol Ointment, NF is the prototype example of a water-soluble base.

Polyethylene Glycol Ointment, NF

Polyethylene glycol (PEG) is a polymer of ethylene oxide and water represented by the formula: $H(OCH_2CH_2)_nOH$ in which n represents the average number of oxyethylene groups. The numerical designations associated with PEGs refer to the average molecular weight of the polymer. PEGs having average molecular weights below 600 are clear, colorless liquids; those with molecular weights above 1000 are wax-like white materials; and those with molecular weights in between are semisolids. The greater the molecular weight the greater the viscosity. The NF lists the viscosities of PEGs ranging from average molecular weights of 200 to 8000.

The general formula for the preparation of 1000 g of Polyethylene Glycol Ointment is:

Polyethylene Glycol 3350	400 g
Polyethylene Glycol 400	600 g

The combining of PEG 3350, a solid, with PEG 400, a liquid, results in a very pliable semisolid ointment. If a firmer ointment is desired, the formula may be altered to contain up to equal parts of the two ingredients. When aqueous solutions are to be incorporated into the base, the substitution of 50 g of the polyethylene glycol 3350 with an equal amount of stearyl alcohol is advantageous in rendering the final product more firm.

Selection of the Appropriate Base

The selection of the base to use in the formulation of an ointment depends upon the careful assessment of a number of factors, including the: (a) desired release rate of the drug substance from the ointment base, (b) desirability for topical or percutaneous drug absorption, (c) desirability of occlusion of moisture from the skin, (d) stability of the drug in the ointment base, (e) effect, if any, of the drug on the consistency or other features of the ointment base, and (f) the desire for a base that is easily removed by washing with water. The base that provides the majority of the most desired attributes should be selected.

Preparation of Ointments

Ointments are prepared by two general methods: 1) incorporation, and 2) fusion. The method used depends primarily on the nature of the ingredients.

Incorporation

By the incorporation method, the components are mixed until a uniform preparation is attained (Fig. 9.1). On a small scale, as in extemporaneous compounding, the pharmacist may mix the components using a mortar and pestle, or a spatula may

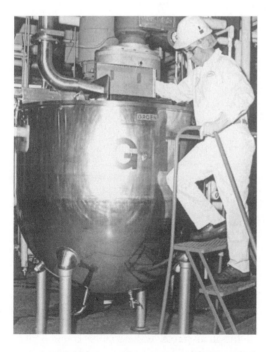

Fig. 9.1 *Creams and ointments in batch sizes up to 1,500 kilos are manufactured in this stainless steel tank, which has counter sweep agitation and a built-in homogenizer. (Courtesy of Lederle Laboratories.)*

be used to rub the ingredients together on an ointment slab (a large glass or porcelain plate). Some pharmacists use nonabsorbent parchment paper to cover the working surface; being disposable, the paper eliminates the time required to clean the ointment slab.

INCORPORATION OF SOLIDS. When preparing an ointment by spatulation, the pharmacist works the ointment with a stainless steel spatula having a long, broad blade and periodically removes the accumulation of ointment on the large spatula with a smaller one. If the components of an ointment are reactive with the metal of the spatula (as is phenol, for example), hard rubber spatulas may be used. The ointment is prepared by thoroughly rubbing and working the components together on the hard surface until the product is smooth and uniform. The ointment base is placed on one side of the working surface and the powdered components, previously reduced to fine powders and thoroughly blended in a mortar, on the other side. A small portion of the powder is mixed with a portion of the base until uniform. The process is continued until all portions of the powder and base are combined and thoroughly and uniformly blended.

It often is desirable to reduce the particle size of a powder or crystalline material before incorporation into the ointment base so that the final product will not be gritty. This may be done by *levigating* or mixing the solid material in a vehicle in which it is insoluble to make a smooth dispersion. The levigating agent used (e.g., mineral oil for oleaginous or bases where oils are the external phase or glycerin for bases where water is the external phase) should be physically and chemically compatible with the drug and base. The amount of levigating agent used should be about equal in volume to the solid material. A mortar and pestle is used for levigation. This allows both reduction of particle size and the dispersion of the substance in the vehicle. After levigation, the dispersion is incorporated into the ointment base by spatulation or with the mortar and pestle until the product is uniform.

Solids that are soluble in a common solvent that will affect neither the stability of the drug nor the efficacy of the product may first be dissolved in that solvent (e.g., water or alcohol) and the solution added to the ointment base by spatulation or by using a mortar and pestle. The mortar and pestle method is preferred when large volumes of liquid are added since the liquid is more captive than when on an ointment slab.

INCORPORATION OF LIQUIDS. Liquid substances or solutions of drugs, as described above, are added to an ointment only after due consideration of an ointment base's capacity to accept the volume required. For example, as noted previously, only very small amounts of an aqueous solution may be incorporated into an oleaginous ointment whereas hydrophilic ointment bases readily accept aqueous solutions. When it is necessary to add an aqueous preparation to a hydro*phobic* base, the solution first may be incorporated into a minimum amount of a hydro*philic* base and then that mixture added to the hydrophobic base. However, all bases, even if hydrophilic, have their limits to retain liquids, beyond which they become too soft or semiliquid.

Alcoholic solutions of small volume may be added quite well to oleaginous vehicles or emulsion bases. Natural balsams, as Peru balsam, are usually mixed with an equal portion of castor oil before incorporation into a base. This reduces the surface tension of the balsam and allows an even distribution of the balsam throughout the base.

On a large scale, roller mills force coarsely formed ointments through stainless steel rollers to produce ointments that are uniform in composition and smooth in texture (Fig. 9.2). Small ointment mills

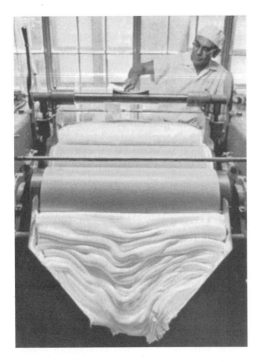

Fig. 9.2 *Day ointment roller mill. Standards of fineness and smoothness require that no grains of material be visible under a ten-power microscope after passage through this machine. (Courtesy of Eli Lilly and Company.)*

also are available and find use in product development laboratories and in small-batch manufacture.

Fusion

By the fusion method, all or some of the components of an ointment are combined by being melted together and cooled with constant stirring until congealed. Components not melted are added to the congealing mixture as it is being cooled and stirred. Naturally, heat-labile substances and any volatile components are added last when the temperature of the mixture is low enough not to cause decomposition or volatilization of the components. Substances may be added to the congealing mixture as solutions or as insoluble powders levigated with a portion of the base. On a small scale, the fusion process may be conducted in a porcelain dish or glass beaker. On a large scale, it is carried out in large steam-jacketed kettles. Once congealed, the ointment may be passed through an ointment mill (in large-scale manufacture) or rubbed with a spatula or in a mortar (in small-scale preparation) to ensure a uniform texture.

Medicated ointments and ointment bases containing components as beeswax, paraffin, stearyl alcohol, and high molecular weight polyethylene glycols, which do not lend themselves well to mixture by incorporation, are prepared by fusion. By this general process, the materials with the highest melting points are heated to the lowest required temperature to produce a melt. The additional materials then are added with constant stirring during cooling of the melt until the mixture is congealed. In this way, not all of the components are subjected to the highest temperature. Alternative methods involve melting the component having the lowest melting point first and adding the remaining components in order of their melting points or simply melting all of the components together under slowly increasing temperature. By these alternative methods, a lower temperature is usually sufficient to achieve fusion due to the solvent action exerted by the first melted components on the others.

In the preparation of ointments having an emulsion base, the method of manufacture often involves both a melting and an emulsification process. The water-immiscible components such as the oil and waxes are melted together in a steam bath to about 70 to 75°C. Meantime, an aqueous solution of the heat-stable, water-soluble components is prepared and heated to the same temperature as the oleaginous components. Then the aqueous solution is slowly added, with mechanical stirring, to the melted oleaginous mixture. The temperature is maintained for 5 to 10 minutes and the mixture is slowly cooled with the stirring continued until congealed. If the aqueous solution were not the same temperature as the oleaginous melt, there would be solidification of some of the waxes upon the addition of the colder aqueous solution to the melted mixture.

Compendial Requirements for Ointments (2)

Ointments and other semisolid dosage forms must meet USP tests for *microbial content, minimum fill, packaging, storage and labeling.* As discussed later in this chapter, ophthalmic ointments must also meet tests for *sterility* and *metal particles* content.

Microbial Content

With the exception of ophthalmic preparations, topical applications are not required to be sterile. They must, however, meet acceptable standards for microbial content and preparations which are prone to microbial growth must be preserved with antimicrobial preservatives. Preparations that contain water tend to support microbial growth to a greater extent than preparations which are water-free. Among the antimicrobial preservatives used to inhibit microbial growth in topical preparations are: methylparaben, propylparaben, phenols, benzoic acid, sorbic acid, and quaternary ammonium salts.

Microbial limits are stated for certain articles in the USP. For example, Betamethasone Valerate Ointment, USP, must *meet the requirements of the tests for absence of Staphylococcus aureus and Pseudomonas aeruginosa.* These particular microbes are of special importance in dermatological preparations because of their capacity to infect the skin which, for patients being treated for a skin condition, is already compromised.

In the USP chapter titled "Microbiological Attributes of Nonsterile Pharmaceutical Products," emphasis is placed on strict adherence to environmental control and application of good manufacturing practices to minimize both the type and the number of microorganisms present in nonsterilized pharmaceutical products (2). This involves the testing of raw materials, use of acceptable water, in-process controls and final product testing. The USP states that certain products should be routinely tested for microorganisms based on their use. Thus, dermatologic products should be examined for *P. aeruginosa* and *S. aureus* and those intended for rectal, urethral, or vaginal use should be tested for the

presence of yeasts and molds, common offenders at these sites of application.

Minimum Fill

The USP's *minimum fill* test involves the determination of the net weight or volume of the contents of filled containers to assure proper contents compared with the labeled amount.

Packaging, Storage, and Labeling

Ointments and other semisolid preparations are packaged either in large-mouth ointment jars or in metal or plastic tubes. Semisolid preparations must be stored in well-closed containers to protect against contamination and in a cool place to protect against product separation due to heat. When required, light-sensitive preparations are packaged in opaque or light-resistant containers.

In addition to the usual labeling requirements for pharmaceutical products, the USP directs that the labeling for certain ointments and creams include the type of base used (e.g., water-soluble or water-insoluble).

Additional Standards

In addition to the USP requirements, manufacturers often examine semisolid preparations for viscosity and for in vitro drug release to ensure intralot and lot-to-lot uniformity (3–4). In vitro drug-release tests involve diffusion cell studies to determine the drug's release profile from the semisolid product.

Creams

Pharmaceutical *creams* are semisolid preparations containing one or more medicinal agents dissolved or dispersed in either an oil-in-water emulsion or in another type of water-washable base. So-called "vanishing creams" are oil-in-water emulsions containing large percentages of water and stearic acid. After application of the cream, the water evaporates leaving behind a thin residue film of the stearic acid. The reader is referred to Chapter 13 for discussion of the types of emulsions, their physical characteristics, and method of manufacture.

Creams find primary application in topical skin products and in products used rectally and vaginally. Many patients and physicians prefer creams to ointments because they are easier to spread and remove than many ointments. Pharmaceutical manufacturers frequently manufacture topical preparations of a drug in both cream and ointment bases to satisfy the preference of the patient and physician.

Gels

Gels are semisolid systems consisting of dispersions of small or large molecules in an aqueous liquid vehicle rendered jelly-like through the addition of a *gelling agent.* Among the gelling agents used are: synthetic macromolecules as carbomer 934, cellulose derivatives as carboxymethylcellulose or hydroxypropylmethyl-cellulose, and natural gums as tragacanth. Carbomers are high molecular weight water-soluble polymers of acrylic acid cross-linked with allyl ethers of sucrose and/or pentaerythritol. Depending on their polymeric composition, different viscosities result. The NF contains monographs for six such polymers: Carbomers 910, 934, 934P, 940, 941, and 1342. They are used as gelling agents at concentrations of 0.5 to 2.0% in water. Carbomer 940 yields the highest viscosity, between 40,000 and 60,000 centipoises as a 0.5% aqueous dispersion. Gels are sometimes called *jellies.*

Single-phase gels are gels in which the macromolecules are uniformly distributed throughout a liquid with no apparent boundaries between the dispersed macromolecules and the liquid. In instances in which the gel mass consists of floccules of small distinct particles, the gel is termed a *two-phase* system often referred to as a *magma.* Milk of magnesia (or magnesia magma), which is comprised of a gelatinous precipitate of magnesium hydroxide, is an example of such a system. Gels may thicken on standing, forming a thixotrope, and must be shaken before use to liquefy the gel and enable pouring.

In addition to the gelling agent and water, gels may be formulated to contain a drug substance, cosolvents as alcohol and/or propylene glycol, antimicrobial preservatives as methylparaben and propylparaben or chlorhexidine gluconate, and stabilizers as edetate disodium. Medicated gels may be prepared for administration by various routes including topically to the skin, to the eye, nasally, vaginally, and rectally.

Miscellaneous Semisolid Preparations: Pastes, Plasters and Glycerogelatins

Pastes

Pastes are semisolid preparations intended for application to the skin. They generally contain a larger proportion of solid material than ointments and therefore are stiffer. When prepared with an oleaginous base they are less greasy than their counterpart ointments due to the reduced amount of base used.

Pastes are prepared in the same manner as ointments. However, when a levigating agent is to be used to render the powdered component smooth, a portion of the base is often used rather than a liquid, which would soften the paste.

Because of the stiffness of pastes, they remain in place after application and are effectively employed to absorb serous secretions. Because of their stiffness and impenetrability, pastes are not suited for application to hairy parts of the body.

Among the few pastes in use today is Zinc Oxide Paste (syn: Lassar's Plain Zinc Paste), which is prepared by levigating and then mixing 25% each of zinc oxide and starch with white petrolatum. The product is very firm and is better able to protect the skin and absorb secretions than is zinc oxide ointment.

Plasters

Plasters are solid or semisolid adhesive masses spread upon a backing material of paper, fabric, moleskin or plastic. The adhesive material used is a rubber base or a synthetic resin. Plasters are applied to the skin to provide prolonged contact at the site. Nonmedicated plasters provide protection or mechanical support at the site of application. Adhesive tape was formerly official under the title "Adhesive Plaster," the use of this material being well known.

Medicated plasters provide effects at the site of application. They may be cut to size to conform to the surface to be covered. Among the few plasters in use today is Salicylic Acid Plaster used on the toes for the removal of corns. The horny layers of skin are removed by the keratolytic action of salicylic acid. The concentration of salicylic acid used in commercial corn plasters ranges from 10 to 40%.

Glycerogelatins

Glycerogelatins are plastic masses containing gelatin (15%), glycerin (40%), water (35%), and an added medicinal substance (10%) as zinc oxide. They are prepared by first softening the gelatin in the water for about 10 minutes, heating on a steam bath until the gelatin is dissolved, adding the medicinal substance mixed with the glycerin, and allowing the mixture to cool with stirring until congealed.

Glycerogelatins are applied to the skin for long-term residence. They are melted before application, cooled to slightly above body temperature, and applied to the affected area with a fine brush. Following application, the glycerogelatin hardens, is usually covered with a bandage and is allowed to remain in place for a period of weeks. The most recently official glycerogelatin was Zinc Gelatin, used in the treatment of varicose ulcers. It was also known as "zinc gelatin boot" due to its ability to form a pressure bandage.

Packaging Semisolid Preparations

Topical dermatologic products are packaged in either jars or tubes whereas ophthalmic, nasal, vaginal and rectal semisolid products are almost always packaged in tubes.

So-called "ointment jars" are made of clear or opaque glass or plastic. Some are colored green, amber or blue. Opaque jars, used for light-sensitive products, are porcelain-white or dark green or amber in color. Commercially available empty ointment jars vary in size from about one-half ounce to one pound.

In the commercial manufacture and packaging of topical products, the jars and tubes are first tested for compatibility and stability for the intended product. This includes stability testing of filled containers at room temperatures (e.g., 70°F) as well as under accelerated stability testing conditions (e.g., 105 and 120°F).

Tubes used to package topical pharmaceutical products are gaining in popularity. They are light in weight, relatively inexpensive, convenient for use by the patient, compatible with most formulative components and provide greater protection against external contamination and environmental conditions than jars (5).

Ointment tubes are made of aluminum or plastic. When the ointment is to be used for ophthalmic, rectal, vaginal, aural, or nasal application they are co-packaged with special applicator tips. Tubes of aluminum generally are coated with an epoxy resin, vinyl or lacquers to eliminate any interactions between the contents and the tube. Plastic tubes are made of high- or low-density polyethylene (HDPE or LDPE) or a blend of each, polypropylene (PP), polyethylene terephthalate (PET) and various plastic/foil/paper laminates sometimes 10 layers thick.

Each type of plastic offers special features and advantages. For example, LDPE is soft, resilient and provides a good moisture barrier. HDPE provides a superior moisture barrier but is less resilient. PP has a high level of heat resistance and PET offers transparency and a high degree of product chemical compatibility. Laminates provide an excellent moisture barrier due to the foil content, high durability and product compatibility (5). These qualities and flexibility make plastic and plastic laminate tubes preferred over metal tubes for the packaging of pharmaceuticals.

The cylindrical bodies of plastic tubes are made by extrusion and then joined to the shoulder-neck-tip piece which is made by molding. Most multiple-dose tubes used for pharmaceuticals have conventional continuous-thread closures. Single-dose tubes may be prepared with a tear-away tip. Metered-dose, tamper-evident, and child-resistant closures are available (5). Empty tubes are available which hold 1.5, 2, 3.5, 5, 15, 30, 45, 60, and 120 grams of contents (6). Topical dermatologicals most frequently are packaged in 5, 15, and 30 g tubes.

Ophthalmic ointments typically are packaged in small aluminum or collapsible plastic tubes holding 3.5 g (about 1/8 oz) of ointment as shown in Chapter 16, Figure 16.4). The tubes are sterilized before being aseptically filled. The tubes are fitted with narrow gauge tips which permit the extrusion and placement of narrow bands of ointment onto the inner margin of the eyelid, the usual site of application.

Filling Ointment Jars

Ointment jars are filled on a small scale in the pharmacy by carefully transferring the weighed amount of ointment into the jar with a spatula. The ointment is packed toward the bottom and along the sides of the jar avoiding the entrapment of air. The size of ointment jar selected should allow the ointment to reach near the top of the jar but not so high as to touch the lid when closed. Through the adept use of the spatula, some pharmacists place a "curl" in the center of the surface of the ointment. Ointments prepared by fusion may be poured directly into the ointment jars for congealing within the jar. This must be done cautiously to prevent stratification of the components. In the large-scale manufacture of ointments, pressure fillers force the specified amount of ointment into the jars.

Filling Ointment Tubes

Tubes are filled from the open back end of the tube, opposite from the cap end (Fig. 9.3). Ointments prepared by fusion may be poured directly into the tubes being cautious to prevent stratification of the components. On a small scale, as in the extemporaneous filling of an ointment in the pharmacy, the tube may be filled manually (Fig. 9.4) or with a small scale filling machine (Fig. 9.5). After filling, the tube

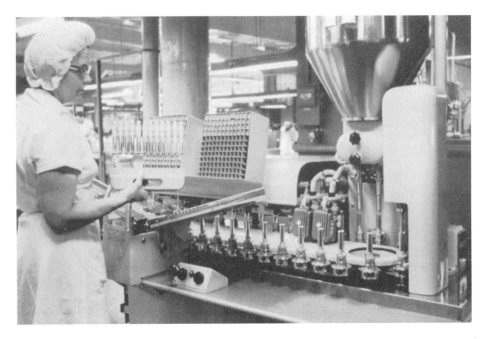

Fig. 9.3   *Arenco tube-filling machine automatically fills 125 tubes a minute with proper amount, tightens cap, orients each tube by electric eye so that label faces forward, then closes and crimps the end. (Courtesy of Eli Lilly and Company.)*

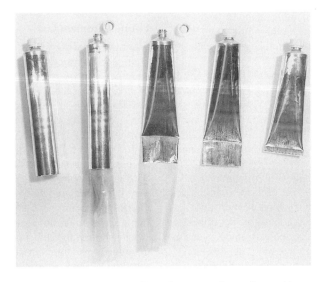

Fig. 9.4   *Steps in the manual filling of ointment tubes as discussed in text.*

is closed and sealed. As depicted in Figure 9.4, the manual filling of an ointment tube requires a number of steps: 1) the prepared ointment, placed on waxed or parchment paper and rolled into a cylindrical shape, is inserted into the open end of the tube and pushed forward as far as allowed; 2) with a spatula pressing against the lower portion of the tube making a crease below the ointment fill, the paper is slowly removed leaving the ointment in the tube; and 3) the bottom of the tube is flattened, folded, and sealed with a crimping tool or clip.

Industrially, automatic tube-filling, closing, crimp-

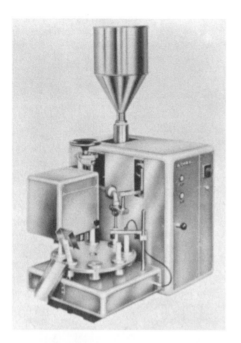

Fig. 9.5 *Example of a small-scale fully automatic filling and crimping machine for collapsible metal tubes. The capacity of the machine is up to 60 units per minute. (Courtesy of Chemical and Pharmaceutical Industry Co.)*

ing, and labeling machines are used for the large-scale packaging of semisolid pharmaceuticals (Fig. 9.3). Depending on the model, machines are available which have the capacity to fill from about 1000 to up to 6000 tubes per hour (5,7). Rotary machines have four stations for tube feeding, cleaning, filling, and closing. Plastic and laminate tubes are closed and sealed by heat and crimping. Metal tubes are sealed by folding and crimping with or without the additional use of a vinyl, latex, or lacquer sealant (5).

Features and Use of Dermatologic Preparations

Among the dosage forms used in the topical treatment of conditions and diseases of the skin are ointments, creams, gels, pastes and plasters. Other dosage forms used include solutions, powders and transdermal drug delivery systems, discussed elsewhere in this text. Oral therapy also may be used, as in the treatment of poison ivy with prednisone.

In treating skin diseases, the drug in a medicated application should *penetrate* and be *retained* in the skin for a period of time. Drug penetration into the skin depends on a number of factors including the physicochemical properties of the medicinal sub-

stance, the characteristics of the pharmaceutical vehicle and the condition of skin itself. Normal unbroken skin acts as a natural barrier limiting both the rate and degree of drug penetration.

The skin is divided histologically into the stratum corneum (the outer layer), the living epidermis, and the dermis, collectively comprising a laminate of barriers protecting against permeation by external agents and loss of water from the body. Blood capillaries and nerve fibers rise from the subcutaneous fat tissue into the dermis and up to the epidermis. Sebaceous glands, sweat glands, and hair follicles originating in the dermis and subcutaneous layers rise to the skin's surface (Fig. 9.6). The stratum corneum is the desquamating "horny layer," a 10 to 15 μm thick layer of flat, partially desiccated, dead epidermal cells (8–9). The stratum corneum is composed of approximately 40% protein (mainly keratin) and 40% water, with the balance being lipid, principally as triglycerides, free fatty acids, cholesterol, and phospholipids. On the surface is a film of emulsified material composed of a complex mixture of sebum, sweat, and desquamating epidermal cells.

The film covering the stratum corneum varies in composition, thickness, and continuity due to differences in the proportion of sebum and sweat produced and the extent of their removal through washing and sweat evaporation. It offers little resistance to drug penetration. Hair follicles and gland ducts can provide entry for drug molecules, but because their relative surface area is so minute compared to the total epidermis they are minor factors in drug absorption.

The stratum corneum, being keratinized tissue, behaves as a semipermeable artificial membrane, and drug molecules can penetrate by passive diffusion. The rate of drug movement across this skin layer depends on the drug concentration in the vehicle, its aqueous solubility, and the oil/water partition coefficient between the stratum corneum and the product's vehicle (10). Substances that possess both aqueous and lipid solubility characteristics are good candidates for diffusion through the stratum corneum. Once through the stratum corneum, drug molecules may then pass through the deeper epidermal tissues and into the dermis. If the drug reaches the vascularized dermal layer, it becomes available for absorption into the general circulation.

Whereas drug blood levels achieved by transdermal drug delivery systems may be measured and equated against desired therapeutic effects, the same is not true for topical *non*systemic dermatologic products. For topical products, the therapeutically effective drug concentration in the skin is not

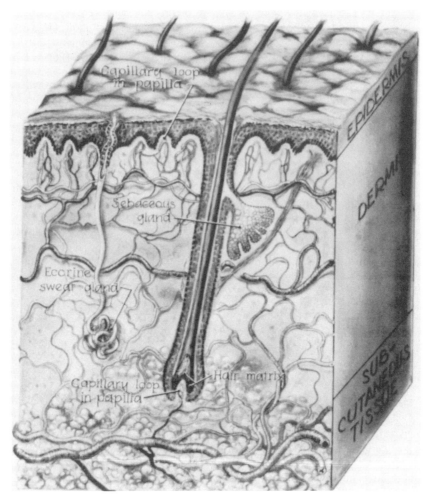

Fig. 9.6   *Stratified organization of the skin. (Pillsbury DM, Heston CL. A Manual of Dermatology. 2nd Ed., Courtesy of W.B. Saunders Co., 1979.)*

known, and thus, treatment is based on qualitative measures with clinical efficacy often varying between patients and products.

Differences in emollient and occlusive effects and ease of application and removal between products is a factor of the base used and product type. As noted earlier, oleaginous bases provide greater occlusion and emollient effects than do hydrophilic or water-washable bases. Pastes offer even greater occlusion and are more effective than ointments at absorbing serous discharge. Creams, usually oil-in-water emulsions, spread more easily than ointments and are easier for the patient to remove. Water-soluble bases are nongreasy and are applied and removed easily.

Unless otherwise directed, before applying a der-

matologic product, the patient should thoroughly clean the affected area with soap and water and dry by patting with a soft cloth. In most instances, a thin layer of medication should be applied to the affected area and spread evenly using gentle pressure with the fingertips. Typically about 1–3 mg of ointment or cream are applied per square centimeter of skin (1). Unless there is a specified need for an occlusive dressing to protect the area from excessive contact or contaminants, a bandage should not be used. After application, the hands should be thoroughly washed.

Upon dispensing a prescription or OTC product, the pharmacist should be certain that the patient understands the proper method of administration, frequency and duration of use, special warnings (as those related to pregnancy or nursing due to possible systemic drug absorption), therapeutic goals and anticipated outcomes, signs of adverse response, allergic sensitivity reactions or treatment failure, and reasons to discontinue treatment and seek further professional guidance.

The patient should be advised that if symptoms persist or if irritation develops, use of the product should be discontinued and their physician or pharmacist advised. It is not uncommon for patients to have an allergic response, as a skin rash, to a topical product due to sensitivity to the medicinal agent or pharmaceutic ingredient. An alternative product that does not contain the suspected offending agent may be substituted to solve the problem.

Examples of dermatologic ointments, creams and gels are presented in Tables 9.1 and 9.2.

Features and Use of Ophthalmic Ointments and Gels

Among the dosage forms used in the topical treatment of conditions and diseases of the eye are ophthalmic ointments and gels. Other dosage forms used topically include ophthalmic solutions, suspensions and inserts, discussed elsewhere in this text. Systemic therapy also may be undertaken, as in the use of diuretics in the adjunctive treatment of glaucoma.

The application of medication to the eye or conjunctival sac results in effects on the surface of the eye and in underlying tissues due to drug penetration. The major route by which drugs enter the eye is by simple diffusion via the cornea. For drugs that are poorly absorbed by the cornea, the conjunctive and sclera provide an alternate route (11). The cornea is a trilaminate structure with a lipophilic epithelial layer, a hydrophilic stromal layer, and an less lipophilic endothelial layer on the inside (11). Drug penetration is dependent on a drug's ability to traverse these three layers. Lipophilic drugs are more capable of penetration than hydrophilic compounds (11).

In general, ocular drug penetration is limited due to the short residence time that ophthalmic preparations have on the surface of the eye because of: their rapid removal by tearing and other natural mechanisms; the small surface area of the cornea for drug absorption; and, the cornea's natural resistance to drug penetration (11). Compared with ophthalmic solutions, ophthalmic ointments, and gels provide extended residence time on the surface of the eye increasing the duration of their surface effects and bioavailability for absorption

into the ocular tissues. Ophthalmic ointments are cleared from the eye as slowly as 0.5% per minute compared with ophthalmic solutions, which can lose up to 16% of their volume per minute (12–13).

The ointment base selected for an ophthalmic ointment must be non-irritating to the eye and must permit the diffusion of the medicinal substance throughout the secretions bathing the eye. Ointment bases used for ophthalmics should have a softening point close to body temperature both for patient comfort and for drug release. Most often, mixtures of white petrolatum and liquid petrolatum (mineral oil) are utilized as the base in medicated and nonmedicated (lubricating) ophthalmic ointments. Sometimes a water-miscible agent as lanolin is added. A gel-base of polyethylene glycol and mineral oil is also used; this form permits water and water-insoluble drugs to be retained within the base.

Medicinal agents are added to an ointment base either as a solution or as a finely micronized powder. The ointment is made uniform and smooth by fine milling.

In addition to the previously stated quality standards for ointments, ophthalmic ointments also must meet the USP *Sterility Tests* and the test *Metal Particles in Ophthalmic Ointments.* Rendering an ophthalmic ointment sterile requires special technique and processing. For a number of reasons, the terminal sterilization of a finished ointment by standard methods is problematic. Steam sterilization or ethylene oxide methods are ineffective because neither is capable of penetrating the ointment base. Although dry heat sterilization can penetrate the ointment base, the high heat required poses a threat to the stability of many drug substances and introduces the possibility of separating the ointment base from the other components (14). Because of these difficulties, terminal sterilization generally is not undertaken. Rather, strict methods of aseptic processing are employed as each drug and nondrug component is rendered sterile and then aseptically weighed and incorporated in preparing a final product which meets the sterility requirement (14). When an antimicrobial preservative is needed, among those used are: methylparaben (0.05%) and propylparaben (0.01%) combinations, phenylmercuric acetate (0.0008%), chlorobutanol (0.5%), and benzalkonium chloride (0.008%).

The USP test for metal particles involves the microscopic examination of a heat-melted ophthalmic ointment. Detected metal particles are counted and measured by a calibrated eye piece micrometer disk. The requirements are met if the total number of particles 50 μm or larger from 10 product tubes

Table 9.1.   Examples of Dermatologic Ointments and Creams by Therapeutic Category

Preparation	Corresponding Commercial Product	Usual Percentage Strength of Active Ingredient	Use
Adrenocortical Steroids			
Alclometasone Diproprionate Cream and Ointment	Aclovate Cream and Ointment (Glaxo Dermatology)	0.05% cream and ointment	For the relief of inflammatory dermatoses.
Fluocinolone Acetonide Cream and Ointment	Synalar Cream & Ointment (Medicis)	0.025% cream and ointment	For the relief of inflammatory dermatoses.
Hydrocortisone Acetate Cream and Ointment	Cortaid Cream and Ointment (Upjohn)	0.5% and 1%	For the relief of inflammatory dermatoses.
Triamcinolone Acetonide Cream and Ointment	Aristocort A Cream and Ointment (Fujisawa)	0.1% (ointment) and 0.1%, 0.025%, and 0.5% (cream)	For the relief of inflammatory dermatoses.
Adrenocorticoid/Antifungal Combination			
Betamethasone and Clotrimazole Cream	Lotrisone Cream (Schering)	1% betamethasone and 0.05% clotrimazole	For the relief and treatment of inflammatory and pruritic manifestations that could be complicated by fungal overgrowth.
Analgesic			
Capsaicin Cream	Zostrix Cream (Genderm)	0.025%	For the relief of arthritic pain.
Antiacne			
Tretinoin Cream	Retin-A (Ortho)	0.025%, 0.05% and 0.1%	A derivative of vitamin A used for the topical treatment of acne vulgaris
Antianginal			
Nitroglycerin Ointment	Nitro-Bid Ointment (Hoechst Marion Roussel)	2%	Used for systemic nitroglycerin effects to reduce the workload of the heart by smooth muscle relaxation of peripheral arteries and veins.
Antibacterial/Anti-infectives			
Gentamicin Sulfate Cream and Ointment	Garamycin Cream and Ointment (Schering)	0.1%	For the treatment of skin infections caused by susceptible microorganisms affected by local treatment.
Nystatin Cream	Mycostatin Cream (Westwood-Squibb)	0.5% 100,000 units/g	For the treatment of skin infections caused by susceptible microorganisms affected by local treatment.
Polymyxin B Sulfate, Bacitracin Zinc and Neomycin Ointment	Neosporin Ointment (Warner Wellcome)	5,000 units/g polymyxin B; 400 units/g bacitracin zinc; and 3.5 mg/g neomycin	For the treatment of minor cuts and scrapes.

continued

Table 9.1.   Examples of Dermatologic Ointments and Creams by Therapeutic Category

Preparation	Corresponding Commercial Product	Usual Percentage Strength of Active Ingredient	Use
Antifungals			
Miconazole Nitrate Cream	Monistat-Derm Cream (Ortho)	2%	For cutaneous candidiasis and treatment of tinea infections caused by *Trichophyton sp.*
Tolnaftate Cream	Tinactin Cream (Schering-Plough)	1%	For topical treatment of tinea pedis, tinea cruris, tinea corporis and tinea manuum.
Antineoplastic			
Fluorouracil Cream	Efudex Cream (Roche)	5%	For treatment of multiple actinic or solar keratoses.
Antipruritic/Analgesic			
Lidocaine Ointment	Xylocaine Ointment	2.5%	For relief of pain and itching due to minor skin irritation and insect bites.
Astringent/Protectant			
Zinc Oxide Ointment	Desitin Ointment (Pfizer)	40%	Used topically as an astringent and protective in various skin conditions as diaper rash.
Depigmenting Agents			
Hydroquinone Cream	Eldopaque Cream (ICN Pharmaceuticals)	4%	Used in the temporary bleaching of hyperpigmented skin blemished due to freckles, old age spots, and cholasma.
Scabicide			
Crotamiton Cream	Eurax Cream (Westwood-Squibb)	10%	For eradication of scabies and symptomatic treatment of pruritus.

does not exceed 50 and if not more than 1 tube contains more than 8 such particles (2).

The USP directs that ophthalmic ointments must be packaged in collapsible ointment tubes. These tubes have an elongated narrow tip to facilitate application of a narrow band of ointment to the eye.

In preparing to apply an ointment to the eye, the patient's or caregiver's hands should be washed and dried thoroughly. Then the ointment tube is held between the thumb and the forefinger and the tip placed near to the eyelid without touching it.

The patient's head should be tilted back, and with the index finger of the opposite hand, the lower eyelid of the affected eye should be gently pulled downward. The tip of the ointment tube should be held slightly above the inside portion of the sack between the lower eyelid and eyeball. Without touching the tip to any part of the eye, a thin ribbon of ointment, approximately 1/4 to 1/2 inch, should be placed along the inside of the lower lid. The patient should face down and slowly close the eye for a few seconds. Then, any excess ointment should be wiped from the eyelids and lashes with a clean tis-

Table 9.2.   Examples of Topical Gels

Active Ingredient	Proprietary Product	Gelling Agent	Route/Use
Acetic Acid	Aci-Jel (Ortho-McNeil)	Tragacanth and acacia	Vaginal: restoration and maintenance of vagninal acidity
Becaplermin	Regranex Gel (Ortho-McNeil)	Sodium CMC	Dermatologic: recombinant human-platelet-derived growth factor used to promote healing of diabetic ulcers of the lower extremity
Benzoyl Peroxide	Desquam-X Gel (Westwood-Squibb)	Carbomer 940	Dermatologic: acne vulgaris
Clindamycin	Cleocin T Topical Gel (Pharmacia & Upjohn)	Carbomer 934P	Dermatologic: acne vulgaris
Clobetasol Propionate	Temovate Gel (Glaxo-Wellcome)	Carbomer 934P	Dermatologic: antipruritic
Cyanocobalamin	Nascobal (Schwartz)	Methylcellulose	Nasal: hematologic
Desoximetasone	Topicort Gel (Hoechst Marion Roussel)	Carbomer 940	Dermatologic: antiinflammatory/antipruritic
Metronidazole	Metro-Gel Vaginal (3M)	Carbomer 934P	Vaginal: bacterial vaginosis
Podofilox	Condylox Gel (Oclassen)	Hydroxypropyl cellulose	Rectal: anogenital warts
Progesterone	Crinone Gel (Wyeth-Ayerst)	Carbomer 934P	Vaginal: bioadhesive gel for progesterone supplementation and replacement
Timolol Maleate	Timoptic-XE (Merck)	Gelrite gellan gum	Opthalmic gel-forming solution used in treatment of elevated intraocular pressure
Tretinoin	Retin-A Gel (Ortho)	Hydroxypropyl cellulose	Dermatologic: acne vulgaris

sue. To facilitate the procedure, a patient may sit in front of a mirror with elbows stabilized or have another person administer the ointment. After use, the ointment must be capped quickly and tightly.

The patient should be advised that blurred vision will occur as the ophthalmic ointment spreads over the eye and not to be alarmed. If the ointment is to be administered only once daily it is often preferable to do so at bedtime when vision impairment will be inconsequential.

It is important to emphasize to the patient that ocular products if handled improperly can become contaminated by bacteria known to cause ocular infections which may lead to serious consequences. Thus every effort made to avoid touching the tip of the tube to the eye, eyelid, fingertip or any other surface, and, the ointment should be used by only one person. Examples of ophthalmic ointments and gels are presented in Tables 9.2 and 9.3.

Features and Use of Nasal Ointments and Gels

Among the dosage forms used in the topical treatment of the nasal mucosa are ointments and gels. Other dosage forms used include inhalants, solutions and suspensions, discussed elsewhere in this text.

The nose is a respiratory organ which is a passageway for air to the lungs. Its surface is coated with a continuous thin layer of mucous produced by subepithelial mucous glands. The ciliated epithelium of the nasal passage facilitates the movement of the mucous layer. The mucous contains lysozyme, glycoproteins and immunoglobulins which act against bacteria and protects against their entry into the lungs. The ciliary action and the sneeze reflex add further defense against external entry (15).

Drugs introduced into the nasal passage are primarily for localized effects on the mucous mem-

Table 9.3.   Examples of Opthalmic Ointments

Opthalmic Ointment	*Corresponding Commercial Product*	*% of Active Ingredient*	*Category*
Chloramphenicol Ophthalmic Ointment	Chloromycetin Ophthalmic Ointment (Parke-Davis)	1%	Antibacterial antibiotic
Dexamethasone Sodium Phosphate Ophthalmic Ointment	Decadron Phosphate Ophthalmic Ointment (Merck Sharp & Dohme)	0.05%	Anti-inflammatory adrenocortical steroid
Gentamicin Sulfate Ophthalmic Ointment	Garamycin Ophthalmic Ointment (Schering)	0.3%	Antibacterial antibiotic
Isoflurophate Ophthalmic Ointment	Floropryl Sterile Ophthalmic Ointment (Merck)	0.025%	Cholinesterase inhibitor
Neomycin Sulfate and Dexamethasone Sodium Phosphate Ophthalmic Ointment	NeoDecadron Ophthalmic Ointment (Merck)	0.35% neomycin base and 0.05% dexamethasone phosphate equivalents	Antibacterial/ antiinflammatory
Polymyxin B—Bacitracin Ophthalmic Ointment	Polysporin Ophthalmic Ointment (Burroughs Wellcome)	per g: polymyxin B sulfate, 10,000 units and bacitracin zinc, 500 units	Antimicrobial
Polymyxin B—Bacitracin—Neomycin Ophthalmic Ointment	Neosporin Ophthalmic Ointment (Burroughs Wellcome)	per g: polymyxin B sulfate, 5000 units; bacitracin, zinc, 400 units; neomycin sulfate, 5 mg	Antimicrobial
Sulfacetamide Sodium Ophthalmic Ointment	Sodium Sulamyd Ophthalmic Ointment (Schering)	10 and 30%	Antibacterial
Sulfisoxazole Diolamine Ophthalmic Ointment	Gantrisin Ophthalmic Ointment (Roche)	4%	Antibacterial
Tetracycline HCl Ophthalmic Ointment	Achromycin Ophthalmic Ointment (Lederle)	1%	Antibacterial antibiotic
Tobramycin Ophthalmic Ointment	Tobrex Ophthalmic Ointment (Alcon)	0.3%	Antibacterial antibiotic
Vidarabine Ophthalmic Ointment	Vira-A-Ophthalmic Ointment (Parke Davis)	3%	Antiviral

branes and underlying tissues (e.g., nasal decongestants). However, drug absorption to the general circulation does occur through the rich blood supply feeding the nasal lining. The nasal route of administration is used for the systemic absorption of a number of drugs including butorphanol tartrate (STADOL NS, Bristol-Myers Squibb) an analgesic, cyanocobalamin (NASCOBAL gel, Schwartz) a hematopoietic, narfaralin acetate (SYNAREL, Searle) for the treatment of endometriosis and nicotine (NICOTROL NS, McNeil) as an adjunct in smoking cessation. In addition, the nasal route holds great promise for the administration of insulin, vaccines and a number of other polypeptides and proteins.

Features and Use of Rectal Preparations

Among the dosage forms used in the topical treatment of anorectal conditions are ointments, creams and cream-like aerosol foams. Other dosage forms used are solutions (for enema or irrigation) and suppositories, discussed elsewhere in this text.

Ointments and creams are used for topical application to the perianal area and for insertion within the anal canal. They largely are used to treat local conditions of anorectal pruritus, inflammation and the pain and discomfort associated with hemorrhoids. The drugs employed include astringents (e.g., zinc oxide), protectants and lubricants (e.g., cocoa butter, lanolin), local anesthetics (e.g., pramoxine HCl), and antipruritics and anti-inflammatory agents (e.g., hydrocortisone).

The perianal area is that portion of skin immediately surrounding the anus. The anal canal is approximately 3 cm in length and connects to the rectum. Both the anal canal and rectum have mucosal linings. Healthy perianal skin and the mucosa act as barriers to infection.

Substances applied rectally may be absorbed by diffusion into the general circulation via the network of three hemorrhoidal arteries and accompanying veins in the anal canal (16). The rectal route *is* used for the systemic absorption of therapeutic levels of certain drugs (e.g., prochlorperazine as suppositories) when the oral route is unsatisfactory, as in conditions of vomiting. However, systemic effects from ointments/creams intended for localized action is usually limited due to the insolubility of certain agents (e.g., zinc oxide) and the subtherapeutic amounts absorbed of soluble drugs, which may be present in the formulation.

The bases used in anorectal ointments and creams include combinations of polyethylene glycol 300 and 3350, emulsion cream bases utilizing cetyl alcohol and cetyl esters wax, and white petrolatum and mineral oil. When antimicrobial preservatives are required, methylparaben, propylparaben, benzyl alcohol, and butylated hydroxyanisole (BHA) are frequently used.

Before applying rectal ointments and creams to the perianal skin, the affected area should be cleansed and dried by gentle patting with toilet tissue. Then a portion of the ointment or cream is placed on a tissue and a thin film is gently spread over the affected area. Products having a water-washable base are easier to spread and remove after application and tend to stain clothing less than products having an oleaginous base.

Rectal ointments and creams are co-packaged with special perforated plastic tips for products to be administered into the anus, primarily in the treatment of the pain and inflammation associated with hemorrhoids (Fig. 9.7). Before use, the rectal tip should be thoroughly cleaned, screwed onto the ointment tube in place of the cap, and lubricated with mineral oil or a lubricating jelly. With the patient lying down on the back or side, or in an otherwise comfortable position, the rectal tip is slowly and carefully inserted part way into the anus. By squeezing the tube, medication is forced through the perforations in the rectal tip and released to the inner lining of the anus. The tip is then slowly removed from the anus and any excess ointment or cream removed from the perianal area. The rectal tip should be cleaned thoroughly, the closure cap replaced on the tube and the hands washed.

Rectal aerosol foam products (e.g., Proctofoam-HC, Schwarz) also are accompanied by applicators to facilitate administration. When ready to use, the applicator is attached to the aerosol container and filled with a measured dose of product. The applicator is then inserted into the anus and the product delivered by pushing the plunger of the applicator.

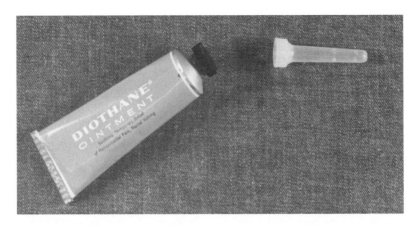

Fig. 9.7   *Example of rectal ointment with perforated inserter/applicator tip. Proper use described in text.*

After removal, the applicator and the patient's hands should be thoroughly washed.

Patient's should be instructed on the proper use of the product dispensed and, in case of rectal bleeding, advised to seek additional medical advice. Examples of rectal ointments and creams are presented in Table 9.4.

Features and Use of Vaginal Preparations

Among the dosage forms used in the topical treatment of conditions and diseases of the vulvovaginal area are ointments, creams, cream-like foams and gels. Other dosage forms used include suppositories, vaginal inserts, transdermal drug delivery systems and oral forms, discussed elsewhere in this text.

The vaginal surface is lined with squamous epithelium cells and mucous produced from various underlying glands. Topical products are used to treat vulvovaginal infections, vaginitis, conditions of endometrial atrophy and for contraception with spermatocidal agents.

The usual pathogenic organisms involved in vulvovaginal infections and vaginitis are *Trichomonas vaginalis, Candida (Monilia) albicans,* and *Hemophilus vaginalis.* Among the anti-infective agents used in the various anti-infective products are nystatin, clotrimazole, miconazole, clindamycin, and sulfonamides. Endometrial atrophy may be treated locally with the hormonal substances dien-estrol and progesterone which are used to restore the vaginal mucosa to its normal state. Contraceptive preparations containing spermicidal agents as nonoxynol-9 and octoxynol are used alone or in combination with a cervical diaphragm.

As noted previously, because products intended for use in the vulvovaginal area come into direct contact with tissues prone to infection it is important that these product be manufactured and tested to be free of offending microorganisms, yeasts and molds. Because gels are especially subject to bacterial growth, most vaginal gels are preserved with antimicrobial agents.

Ointments, creams, and gels for vaginal use are packaged in tubes; vaginal foams in aerosol canisters. Although some preparations are applied externally to the vulva (e.g., Mycelex-7 External Vulva Cream, Bayer) most are intended to be delivered into the vagina by means of inserter-applicator tips which accompany the products (Fig. 9.8).

In treating external vulvar conditions, the patient squeezes a small amount of product onto the fingers or tissue and gently spreads it over the affected area. For intravaginal treatment, the patient uses the plastic inserters-applicators some of which are prefilled and disposable and others reusable and filled by the patient immediately prior to use.

In filling applicators, the closure cap is removed from the tube, the applicator screwed on in its place, and the tube gently squeezed until the applicator is filled and the plunger rises to its predetermined stopping point. The filled applicator then is

Table 9.4. Examples of Rectal and Vaginal Creams and Ointments

Commercial Preparation	Active Ingredients	Product Type	Primary Use
RECTAL			
Anusol (Warner Wellcome)	Starch	Ointment	Hemorrhoid treatment
Tronolane (Ross)	Pramoxine HCl	Cream	Hemorrhoidal analgesic/antipruritic
VAGINAL			
Mycelex-7 (Bayer)	Clotrimazole	Cream	Antifungal
AVC (Hoechst Marion Roussel)	Sulfanilamide	Cream	Vulvovaginitis caused by *candida albicans*
Cleocin (Pharmacia & Upjohn)	Clindamycin PO$_4$	Cream	Bacterial vaginosis
Terazol 7 (Ortho)	Terconazole	Cream	Antifungal (*Candida albicans*)
Ogen (Upjohn)	Estropipate	Cream	Estrogenic for vulvar and vaginal atrophy
Premarin (Wyeth-Ayerst)	Conjugated estrogens	Cream	Atrophic vaginitis and kraurosis vulvae
Ortho-Cream (Ortho)	Nonoxynol 9	Cream	Spermicide contraceptive for use with a diaphragm

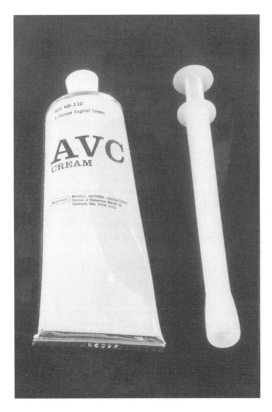

Fig 9.8. *Example of vaginal cream with inserter. Proper use described in text.*

unscrewed from the tube and replaced by the cap. Inserting intravaginal products is best accomplished with the patient lying on her back or in an otherwise comfortable position. The applicator barrel is firmly grasped and inserted into the vagina as far as possible without causing discomfort. The plunger is depressed until it stops, releasing the medication in the vagina. The applicator is carefully withdrawn for washing or discard. The patient should be instructed to wash her hands thoroughly after use.

Aerosol foams are used intravaginally in the same general manner. The aerosol package contains an inserter device that, when attached to the canister, may be filled with foam. The filled inserter is placed in the vagina and the product delivered by pushing the plunger. Vaginal foams are oil-in-water emulsions, resembling light creams. They are water-miscible and non-greasy.

When once-a-day administration is prescribed, it is best done at bedtime for reasons of medication retention, the avoidance of daytime leakage, and lessened soiling of clothing. Creams with water-washable bases are preferred over oleaginous oint-

ments. Patients who are pregnant must not use intravaginal products except with their doctor's approval and supervision. Tampons are not to be used during intravaginal treatment.

Nonmedicated lubricant jellies are used by physicians in rectal, urethral and vaginal examination procedures. All products should be tightly closed when not in use to prevent contamination. If left unsealed, gels and jellies are particularly prone to lose their water to the air and dry out. Examples of vaginal ointments, creams, and gels are presented in Tables 9.2 and 9.4.

References

1. Shah VP, Behl CR, Flynn GL, Higuchi WI, Schaefer H. Principles and criteria in the development and optimization of topical therapeutic products. Pharm Res 1992;9:1107–1112.
2. The United States Pharmacopeia. 23rd ed. Rockville, MD: United States Pharmacopeial Convention, 1995.
3. Corbo M, Schulz TW, Wong GK, Van Buskirk GA. Development and validation of in vitro release testing methods for semisolid formulations. Pharm Tech 1993; 17:112–128.
4. Shah VP, Elkins J, Hanus J, Noorizadeh C, Skelly JP. In vitro release of hydrocortisone from topical preparations and automated procedure. Pharm Res 1991;8: 55–63.
5. Forcinio H. Tubes: the ideal packaging for semisolid products. Pharm Tech 1998;22:32–36.
6. Montebello Packaging, Oak Park, IL.
7. MG America, Inc., Fairfield, NJ.
8. Black CD. Transdermal drug delivery systems. US Pharm 1982;1:49.
9. Walters KA. Percutaneous absorption and transdermal therapy. Pharm Tech 1986;10:30–42.
10. Surber C, et al. Optimization of topical therapy: partitioning of drugs into stratum corneum. Pharm Res 1990;7:1320–1324.
11. Lee VHL. Mechanisms and facilitation of corneal drug penetration. J Controlled Release 1990;11:79–90.
12. Compounding ophthalmic preparations. International Journal of Pharmaceutical Compounding 1998; 2:184–188.
13. Gourley DR, Makoid MC. Ophthalmic products. In: Handbook of nonprescription drugs. Washington DC: American Pharmaceutical Association, 1982;6: 281–292.
14. Lee JY. Sterilization control and validation for topical ointments. Pharm Tech 1992;16:104–110.
15. Cormier JF, Bryant BG. Cold and allergy products. In: Handbook of nonprescription drugs. Washington DC: American Pharmaceutical Association, 1982;6: 73–114.
16. Hodes B. Hemorrhoidal products. In: Handbook of nonprescription drugs. Washington DC: American Pharmaceutical Association, 1982;6:451–463.

10

TRANSDERMAL DRUG DELIVERY SYSTEMS

Chapter at a Glance

TRANSDERMAL DRUG delivery systems (TDDSs) facilitate the passage of therapeutic quantities of drug substances through the skin and into the general circulation for their systemic effects. The concept for the *percutaneous absorption* of drug substances was first conceived by Stoughton in 1965 (1). The first transdermal system, Transderm Scop [Ciba (now Novartis)] was approved by the Food and Drug Administration in 1979 for the prevention of nausea and vomiting associated with travel, particularly by sea.

Evidence of percutaneous drug absorption may be found through measurable blood levels of the drug, detectable excretion of the drug and/or its metabolites in the urine, and through the clinical response of the patient to the administered drug therapy. With transdermal drug delivery, the blood concentration needed to achieve therapeutic efficacy may be determined by comparative analysis of patient response to drug blood levels. For transder-

mal drug delivery, it is considered ideal if the drug penetrates through the skin to the underlying blood supply without drug buildup in the dermal layers (2). This is in direct contrast to the types of topical dosage forms discussed in the previous chapter, in which drug residence in the skin, the target organ, is desired.

As discussed in the previous chapter, the skin is comprised of the stratum corneum (the outer layer), the living epidermis, and the dermis, which together provide the skin's barrier layers to penetration by external agents (see Fig. 9.6). The film that covers the stratum corneum is comprised of sebum and sweat, but because of its varied composition and lack of continuity it is not a significant factor in drug penetration nor are the hair follicles and sweat and sebaceous gland ducts which comprise only a minor proportion of the skin's surface.

The percutaneous absorption of a drug generally results from the direct penetration of the drug through the stratum corneum, a 10 to 15 μm thick layer of flat, partially desiccated nonliving tissue (3–4). The stratum corneum is composed of approximately 40% protein (mainly keratin) and 40% water, with the balance being lipid, principally as triglycerides, free fatty acids, cholesterol, and phospholipids. The lipid content is concentrated in the extracellular phase of the stratum corneum and forms to a large extent the membrane surrounding the cells. Because a drug's major route of penetration is through the intercellular channels, the lipid component is considered an important determinant in the first step of the absorption process (5). Once through the stratum corneum, drug molecules may then pass through the deeper epidermal tissues and into the dermis. When the drug reaches the vascularized dermal layer, it becomes available for absorption into the general circulation.

The stratum corneum, being keratinized tissue, behaves as a semipermeable artificial membrane, and drug molecules penetrate by passive diffusion. It is the major rate-limiting barrier to transdermal drug transport (6). Over most of the body, the stratum corneum has 15–25 layers of flattened corneocytes with an overall thickness of about 10 μm (6). The rate of drug movement across this skin layer depends on the drug concentration in the vehicle, its aqueous solubility, and the oil/water partition coefficient between the stratum corneum and the vehicle (7). Substances that possess both aqueous and lipid solubility characteristics are good candidates for diffusion through the stratum corneum as well as through the epidermal and dermal layers.

Factors Affecting Percutaneous Absorption

Not all drug substances are suitable for transdermal drug delivery. Among the factors playing a part in percutaneous absorption are the physical and chemical properties of the drug, including its molecular weight, solubility, partitioning coefficient and pKa, the nature of the carrier-vehicle and the condition of the skin. Although general statements applicable to all possible combinations of drug, vehicle, and skin condition are difficult to draw, the consensus of the majority of research findings may be summarized as follows (2–11).

1. Drug concentration is an important factor. Generally, the amount of drug percutaneously absorbed per unit of surface area per time interval increases as the concentration of the drug substance in the TDDS is increased.

2. More drug is absorbed through percutaneous absorption when the drug substance is applied to a larger surface area (e.g., a larger size TDDS).

3. The drug substance should have a greater physicochemical attraction to the skin than to the vehicle in which it is presented for the drug to leave the vehicle in favor of the skin. Some solubility of the drug in both lipid and water is thought to be essential for effective percutaneous absorption. In essence, the aqueous solubility of a drug determines the concentration presented to the absorption site and the partition coefficient influences the rate of transport across the absorption site. Drugs generally penetrate through the skin better in their unionized form. Polar drugs tend to cross the cell barrier through the lipid-rich regions (transcellular route) whereas the nonpolar drugs favor transport between cells (intercellular route) (6).

4. Drugs with molecular weights between 100 and 800 with adequate lipid and aqueous solubility can permeate skin. The ideal molecular weight of a drug for transdermal drug delivery is believed to be 400 or less.

5. The hydration of the skin generally favors percutaneous absorption. TDDS act as occlusive moisture barriers through which the sweat from the skin cannot pass, resulting in increased skin hydration.

6. Percutaneous absorption appears to be greater when the TDDS is applied to a skin site with a thin horny layer than with one that is thick.

7. Generally, the longer the period of time the medicated application is permitted to remain in contact with the skin, the greater will be the total drug absorption.

These general statements on percutaneous absorption apply to skin in the normal state. Skin that is abraded or cut will permit drugs to gain direct access to the subcutaneous tissues and the capillary network obviating the designed function of the TDDS.

Percutaneous Absorption Enhancers

There is great interest among pharmaceutical scientists to develop chemical permeation enhancers and physical methods that can increase the percutaneous absorption of therapeutic agents.

Chemical Enhancers

By definition, a chemical skin penetration enhancer *increases skin permeability by reversibly dam-*

aging or by altering the physicochemical nature of the stratum corneum to reduce its diffusional resistance (12). Among the alterations are increased hydration of the stratum corneum and/or a change in the structure of the lipids and lipoproteins in the intercellular channels through solvent action or denaturation (4, 13–17).

Some drugs have an inherent capacity to permeate the skin without need of chemical enhancers. However, in instances in which this is not the case, chemical permeation enhancers may be effective in rendering an otherwise impenetrable substance useful in transdermal drug delivery (17). More than 275 different chemical compounds have been cited in the literature as skin penetration enhancers including acetone, azone, dimethylacetamide, dimethylformamide, dimethylsulfoxide (DMSO), ethanol, oleic acid, polyethylene glycol, propylene glycol and sodium lauryl sulfate (13–15). The selection of a permeation enhancer in developing a TDDS should be based not only on its efficacy in enhancing skin permeation, but also on its dermal toxicity (low), and its physicochemical and biocompatibility with the system's other components (16).

Iontophoresis and Sonophoresis

In addition to chemical means, there are some physical methods being used to enhance transdermal drug delivery and penetration, namely, iontophoresis and sonophoresis (6,15,18–23). *Iontophoresis* involves the delivery of charged chemical compounds across the skin membrane using an applied electrical field. A number of drugs have been the subject of such iontophoretic studies, including lidocaine (18), dexamethasone, amino acids/peptides/insulin (19–20), verapamil (6), and propranolol (21). There is particular interest to develop alternative routes for the delivery of biologically active peptides. These agents are presently delivered by injection, because of their rapid metabolism and poor absorption after oral delivery. They are also poorly absorbed from the transdermal route, because of their large molecular size, ionic character and the general impenetrability of the skin (20). However, iontophoretic-enhanced transdermal delivery has shown some promise as a means for peptide/protein administration.

Sonophoresis, or high-frequency ultrasound, is also being studied as a means to enhance transdermal drug delivery (22–23). Among the agents examined have been hydrocortisone, lidocaine, and salicylic acid in such formulations as gels, creams, and lotions. It is thought that high-frequency ultrasound can influence the integrity of the stratum corneum and thus affect its penetrability.

Percutaneous Absorption Models

Skin permeability and percutaneous absorption have been the subject of numerous studies undertaken to define the underlying principles and to optimize transdermal drug delivery. Although many experimental methods and models have been used, they tend to fall into one of two categories: 1) in vivo, and 2) in vitro studies.

In Vivo Studies

In vivo skin-penetration studies may be undertaken for one or more of the following purposes (24):

1. To verify and quantify the cutaneous bioavailability of a topically applied drug;
2. To verify and quantify the systemic bioavailability of a transdermally delivered drug;
3. To establish bioequivalence of different topical formulations of the same drug substance;
4. To determine the incidence and degree of systemic toxicologic risk following the topical application of a specific drug/drug product; and
5. To relate resultant blood levels of drug in human to systemic therapeutic effects.

The most relevant studies are performed in humans; however, animal models may be used insofar as they may be effective as predictors of human response. Animal models include the weanling pig, rhesus monkey, and hairless mouse or rat (24–25). Biological samples used in drug penetration/drug absorption studies include skin sections, venous blood from the application site, blood from the systemic circulation and excreta (urine, feces and expired air) (24–28).

In Vitro Studies

Skin permeation testing may be performed in vitro using various skin tissues (human or animal whole skin, dermis or epidermis) in a diffusion cell (29). In vitro penetration studies using human skin are limited because of difficulties of procurement, storage, expense, and variability in permeation (30). Excised animal skins may also be variable in quality and permeation. Animal skins are much more permeable than human skin. One alternative that has been shown to be effective is shed snake skin (*Elaphe obsoleta*, black rat snake), which is nonliving, pure stratum corneum, hairless, and similar to human skin, but slightly less permeable (30–31). Also, the product Living Skin Equivalent (LSE) Testskin (Organogenesis, Inc.) was developed as an alternative for dermal absorption studies. The material is an organotypic coculture of human dermal fibroblasts in a collagen-containing matrix and a stratified epidermis composed of human epidermal keratinocytes. The material may be used in cell culture studies or in standard diffusion cells.

Diffusion cell systems are employed in vitro to quantify the release rates of drugs from topical preparations (32). In these systems, skin membranes or synthetic membranes may be employed as barriers to the flow of drug and vehicle, to simulate the biologic system. The typical diffusion cell has two chambers one on each side of the test diffusion membrane. A temperature-controlled solution of the drug to be contained in the TDDS is placed in one chamber and a receptor solution in the other chamber. When skin is used as the test membrane, it separates the two solutions. Drug diffusion through the skin may be determined by periodic sampling and assay of the drug content in the receptor solution. The skin may also be analyzed for drug content to show drug permeation rates and/or drug retention in the skin (29).

The USP describes the apparatus and procedure to determine the drug dissolution (drug release) of medication from a transdermal delivery system and provides an "Acceptance Table" against which the product must conform to meet the monograph standard for a given article (33). Commercial systems are available that utilize transdermal diffusion cells and autosampling systems to determine the release rates of drugs from transdermal systems (34).

Design Features of Transdermal Drug Delivery Systems (TDDSs)

Transdermal drug delivery systems (also often called transdermal "patches") are designed to support the passage of drug substances from the surface of the skin, through its various layers and into the systemic circulation. Examples of the configuration and composition of TDDSs are described in the text, presented in Table 10.1 and shown in Figures 10.1 through 10.4. Figures 10.5 through 10.8 depict the manufacture of TDDSs. Technically, TDDSs may be categorized into two types, monolithic and membrane-controlled systems.

Monolithic systems incorporate a drug matrix layer between backing and frontal layers (Fig. 10–3). The drug-matrix layer is composed of a polymeric

material in which the drug is dispersed. The polymer matrix controls the rate at which the drug is released for percutaneous absorption. The matrix may be of two types; with or without an excess of drug with regard to its equilibrium solubility and steady-state concentration gradient at the stratum corneum (21,35). In types having no excess, drug is available to maintain the saturation of the stratum corneum only as long as the level of drug in the device exceeds the solubility limit of the stratum corneum. As the concentration of drug in the device diminishes below the skin's saturation limit, the transport of drug from device to skin gradually declines (35). In systems that have an excess amount of drug present in the matrix, a drug reserve is present to assure continued drug saturation at the stratum corneum. In these instances, the rate of drug decline is less than in the type having no drug reserve.

In the preparation of monolithic systems, the drug and the polymer are dissolved or blended together, cast as the matrix and dried (21). The gelled matrix may be produced in sheet or cylindrical form, with individual dosage units cut and assembled between the backing and frontal layers. Most TDDSs are designed to contain an excess of drug and thus have drug-releasing capacity beyond the time frame recommended for replacement. This ensures continuous drug availability and absorption as used TDDSs are replaced on schedule with fresh ones.

Membrane-controlled transdermal systems are designed to contain a drug reservoir or "pouch", usually in liquid or gel form, a rate-controlling membrane, and backing, adhesive, and protecting layers (Fig. 10–2). Transderm-Nitro (Novartis) and Transderm-Scop (Novartis) are examples of this technology. Membrane-controlled systems have the advantage over monolithic systems in that as long as the drug solution in the reservoir remains saturated, the release rate of drug through the controlling membrane remains constant (21–22). In membrane systems, a small quantity of drug is frequently placed in the adhesive layer to initiate prompt drug absorption and pharmacotherapeutic effects on skin placement. Membrane-controlled systems may be prepared by preconstructing the delivery unit, filling the drug reservoir, and sealing, or by a process of lamination, which involves a continuous process of construction, dosing and sealing (Figs. 10.5 through 10.8).

In summary, either the drug delivery device or the skin may serve as the rate-controlling mechanism in drug transport from transdermal systems.

Table 10.1. Examples of Transdermal Drug Delivery Systems (40–44, 47–51)

Therapeutic Agent	TDDS	Design/Contents	Comments
Clonidone	Catapres-TTS (Boehringer Ingelheim)	Four-layered patch: (1) a backing layer of pigmented polyester film; (2) drug reservoir of clonidine, mineral oil, polyisobutylene, and colloidal silicon dioxide; (3) a microporous polypropylene membrane controlling the rate of drug delivery; and (4) an adhesive formulation of agents noted in (2) above.	Transdermal therapeutic systems designed to deliver a therapeutic dose of the antihypertensive drug clonidine at a constant rate for 7 days, permitting once-a-week dosing. TDDS generally applied to hairless or shaven areas of upper arm or torso.
Estradiol	Estraderm (Novartis)	Four-layered patch: (1) a transparent polyester film; (2) drug reservoir of estradiol and alcohol gelled with hydroxypropyl cellulose; (3) an ethylene-vinyl acetate copolymer membrane; and (4) an adhesive formulation of light mineral oil and polyisobutylene	Transdermal system designed to release 17β-estradiol continuously. The transdermal patch is generally applied twice weekly over a cycle of 3 weeks with dosage frequency adjusted as required. The patch is generally applied to the trunk including the abdomen and buttocks, alternating sites with each application.
	Vivelle (Novartis)	Three-layered patch: (1) a translucent ethylene vinyl alcohol copolymer film; (2) estradiol in a matrix of a medical adhesive of polyisobutylene and ethylene vinylacetate copolymer; and (3) a polyester release liner which is removed prior to application.	Use and application is similar to the Estraderm TDDS.
	Climara (Berlex)	Three-layered system: (1) a translucent polyethylene film; (2) acrylate adhesive matrix containing estradiol; and (3) a protective liner of siliconized or fluoropolymer-coated polyester film which is removed prior to use.	Use and application similar to the Estraderm TDDS. System may be applied once weekly.
Fentanyl	Duragesic (Janssen)	Four-layered patch (1) a backing layer of polyester film; (2) drug reservoir of fentanyl and alcohol gelled with hydroxyethyl cellulose; (3) a rate-controlling ethylene-vinyl acetate copolymer membrane; and (4) a fentanyl-containing silicone adhesive.	Transdermal therapeutic system providing continuous 72-hour systemic delivery of fentanyl, a potent opioid analgesic. The drug is indicated in patients having chronic pain requiring opioid analgesia.

continued

Table 10.1.   Examples of Transdermal Drug Delivery Systems (40–44, 47–51)

Therapeutic Agent	TDDS	Design/Contents	Comments
Nicotine	Habitrol (Novartis Consumer)	Multi-layered round patch: (1) an aluminized backing film; (2) a pressure-sensitive acrylate adhesive; (3) methacryclic acid copolymer solution of nicotine dispersed in a pad of nonwoven viscose and cotton; (4) an acrylate adhesive layer; and (5) a protective aluminized release liner that overlays the adhesive layer and is removed prior to use.	
	NicoDerm CQ (SmithKline Beecham Consumer)	Multi-layered rectangular patch: (1) an occlusive backing of polyethylene/aluminum/polyester/ethylene-vinyl acetate copolymer; (2) drug reservoir of nicotine in an ethylene vinyl acetate copolymer matrix; (3) rate-controlling membrane of polyethylene; (4) polyisobutylene adhesive; and (5) protective liner removed prior to application.	Transdermal therapeutic systems providing continuous release and systemic delivery of nicotine as an aid in smoking cessation programs. The patches listed vary somewhat in nicotine content and dosing schedules.
	Nicotrol (McNeil Consumer)	Multi-layered rectangular patch: (1) outer backing of laminated polyester film; (2) rate-controlling adhesive, nonwoven material, and nicotine; (3) disposable liner removed prior to use.	
	Prostep (Lederle)	Multi-layered round patch: (1) beige-colored foam tape and acrylate adhesive; (2) backing foil, gelatin and low-density polyethylene coating; (3) nicotine-gel matrix; (4) protective foil with well; and (5) release liner removed prior to use.	
Nitroglycerin	Deponit (Schwarz Pharma)	A three-layer system: (1) covering foil; (2) nitroglycerin matrix with polyisobutylene adhesive, plasticizer and release membrane; and (3) protective foil removed before use.	

continued

Table 10.1. Examples of Transdermal Drug Delivery Systems (40–44, 47–51)

Therapeutic Agent	TDDS	Design/Contents	Comments
	Nitro-Dur (Key)	Nitroglycerin in a gel-like matrix composed of glycerin, water, lactose, polyvinyl alcohol, povidone and sodium citrate sealed in a polyester-foil-polyethylene laminate.	TDDSs designed to provide the controlled release of nitroglycerin for treatment of angina. Daily application to chest, upper arm or shoulder.
	Transderm-Nitro (Novartis)	Four-layered patch: (1) backing layer of aluminized plastic; (2) drug reservoir containing nitroglycerin adsorbed on lactose, colloidal silicon dioxide, and silicone medical fluid, (3) an ethylene/vinyl acetate copolymer membrane; and (4) silicone adhesive.	
Scopolamine	Transderm Scōp (Novartis Consumer)	Four-layered patch: (1) backing layer of aluminized polyester film; (2) drug reservoir of scopolamine, mineral oil, and polyisobutylene; (3) a microporous polypropylene membrane for rate delivery of scopolamine; and (4) adhesive of polyisobutylene, mineral oil, and scopolamine	TDDS for continuous release of scopolamine over a 3-day period as required for the prevention of nausea and vomiting associated with motion sickness. The patch is placed behind the ear. When repeated administration is desired, the first patch is removed and the second patch placed behind the other ear. Also FDA-approved for prevention of nausea associated with certain anesthetics and analgesics used in surgery.
Testosterone	Testoderm (Alza)	Three-layer patch: (1) backing layer of polyethylene terephthalate; (2) matrix film layer of testosterone and ethylene-vinyl acetate copolymer; and (3) adhesive strips of polyisobutylene and colloidal silicone dioxide.	The patch is placed on the scrotum in the treatment of testosterone deficiency.
	Androderm (SmithKline Beecham)	Five-layer patch: (1) backing film of ethylene vinyl acetate copolymer/polyester laminate; (2) drug reservoir gel of testosterone, alcohol, glycerin, glyceryl monooleate, methyl laurate gelled with an acrylic acid copolymer; (3) a microporous polyethylene membrane; (4) acrylic adhesive; (5) an adhesive polyester laminate.	The patch is placed on the back, abdomen, upper arms or thighs in the treatment of testosterone deficiency.

If the drug is delivered to the stratum corneum at a rate less than the absorption capacity, the *device* is the controlling factor; if the drug is delivered to the skin area to saturation, the *skin* is the controlling factor to the rate of drug absorption. Thus, the rate of drug transport in all TDDSs, monolithic and membrane, is controlled by either artificial or natural (skin) membranes.

Transdermal drug delivery systems may be constructed of a number of layers, including 1) an occlusive backing membrane to protect the system from environmental entry and from loss of drug from the system or moisture from the skin; 2) a drug reservoir or matrix system to store and release the drug at the skin-site; 3) a release liner, which is removed before application and enables drug release; and 4) an adhesive layer to maintain contact with the skin after application. TDDSs are packaged in individual sealed packets to preserve and protect them until use.

The backing layer must be occlusive to retain skin moisture and hydrate the site of application

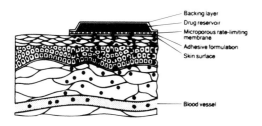

Fig. 10.1 *Depiction of a four-layered therapeutic transdermal system showing the continuous and controlled amount of medication released from the system, permeating the skin and entering the systemic circulation. (Courtesy of Alza Corporation.)*

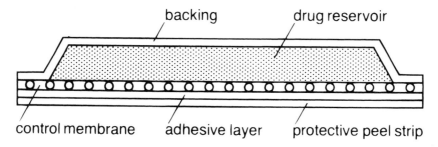

Fig. 10.2 *The Transderm-Nitro Transdermal Therapeutic System (Summit). The patch delivers nitroglycerin through the skin directly into the blood stream for 24 hours. Transderm-Nitro is used to treat and prevent angina. The system consists of a water-resistant backing layer, a reservoir of nitroglycerin, followed by a semipermeable membrane to control precisely and predictably the release of medicine, and an adhesive layer to hold the system onto the skin. The adhesive layer also contains an initial priming dose of nitroglycerin to insure prompt release and absorption of the medication. (Courtesy of Summit Pharmaceuticals [Novartis]).*

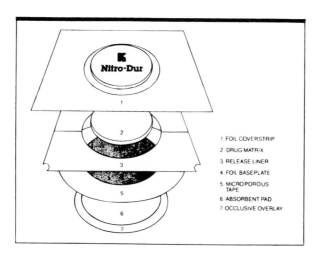

Fig. 10.3 *Nitro-Dur Transdermal Infusion System, depicting the construction of the product. (Courtesy of Key Pharmaceuticals, Inc.)*

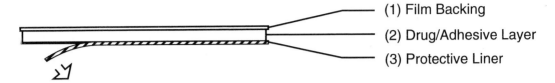

- (1) Film Backing
- (2) Drug/Adhesive Layer
- (3) Protective Liner

Fig. 10.4 *Depiction of a two-layered transdermal drug delivery system, excluding the protective liner which is removed prior to application.*

enabling increased drug penetration. Preferred backing materials are approximately 2–3 mm in thickness and have a low moisture vapor transmission rate of approximately <20 g/m²/24 hr (36). Films of polypropylene, polyethylene, and polyolefin which are transparent or pigmented are in use in TDDSs as backing liners.

The adhesive layer must be pressure sensitive, providing the ability to adhere to the skin with minimal pressure and remain in place for the intended period of wear. The adhesive should be non-irritating, allow easy peel-off after use, permit unimpeded drug flux to the skin and must be compatible with all other system components. The adhesive material is usually safety tested for skin compatibility including tests for skin irritation, skin sensitivity and cytotoxicity (37). In some TDDSs, the drug is contained within the adhesive layer. Polybutylacrylate is commonly used as the adhesive in TDDSs.

The drug release membranes are commonly made of polyethylene, with microporous structures of varying pore sizes to fit the desired specifications of the particular transdermal system.

Included among the design objectives of TDDSs are the following (2,8,35,38–39). A TDDS should do the following:

1. Deliver the drug at an optimal rate to the skin for percutaneous absorption at therapeutic levels;
2. Contain medicinal agents having the necessary physicochemical characteristics to release from the system and partition into the stratum corneum;
3. Occlude the skin to ensure the one-way flux of the drug into the stratum corneum;
4. Have a therapeutic advantage over other dosage forms and drug delivery systems;
5. Have components as adhesive, vehicle, and active agent which are not irritating or sensitizing to the skin; and
6. Adhere well to the patient's skin and have a patch-size, appearance, and site-placement that encourages patient acceptance.

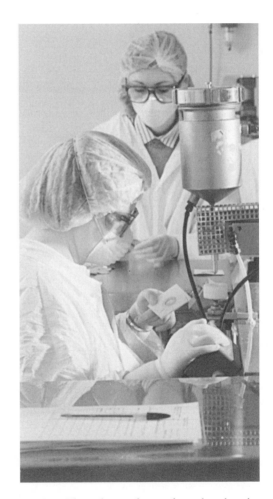

Fig. 10.5 *Pilot scale manufacture of transdermal patches. (Courtesy of Elan Corporation, plc.)*

Advantages and Disadvantages of TDDSs

Among the advantages of TDDSs are the following:

1. They can avoid gastrointestinal drug absorption difficulties caused by gastrointestinal

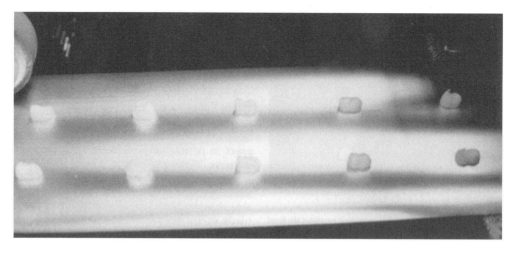

Fig. 10.6   *Measured dose for reservoir, placed on web prior to sealing into the transdermal delivery system. (Courtesy of CIBA Pharmaceutical Company.)*

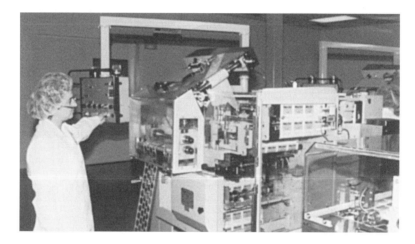

Fig. 10.7   *Equipment utilized in the cutting and packaging of transdermal drug delivery patches. (Courtesy of Schering Laboratories)*

pH, enzymatic activity and drug interactions with food, drink, or other orally administered drugs.

2. They can substitute for oral administration of medication when that route is unsuitable, as in instances of vomiting and/or diarrhea.

3. They avoid the *first-pass effect*, that is, the initial pass of a drug substance through the systemic and portal circulation following gastrointestinal absorption, thereby possibly avoiding the drug's deactivation by digestive and liver enzymes.

4. The systems are noninvasive, avoiding the inconvenience of parenteral therapy.

5. They provide extended therapy with a single application, thereby improving patient compliance

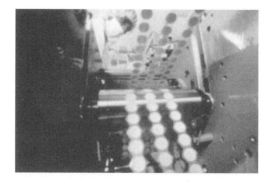

Fig. 10.8   *Rotary die-cutting pressure executes the final step in manufacturing Transderm Scōp systems prior to packaging. (Courtesy of Alza Corporation.)*

over other dosage forms requiring more frequent dose administration.

6. The activity of drugs having short half-lives is extended through the reservoir of drug present in the therapeutic delivery system and its controlled release characteristics.

7. Drug therapy may be terminated rapidly by removal of the application from the surface of the skin.

8. Ease of rapid identification of the medication in emergencies (e.g., nonresponsive, unconscious, or comatose patient) due to the physical presence, features and identifying-markings on the TDDS.

The disadvantages of TDDSs are:

1. Only relatively potent drugs are suitable candidates for transdermal delivery due to the natural limits of drug entry imposed by the skin's impermeability.

2. Some patients may develop contact dermatitis at the site of application due to one or more of the system components, necessitating discontinuation.

Examples of Transdermal Drug Delivery Systems

The following sections briefly describe some of the TDDS in current use. Table 10.1 describes the specific design components of representative examples of these systems.

Transdermal Scopolamine

As noted at the outset of this chapter, transdermal scopolamine was the first TDDS to receive FDA approval. Scopolamine, a belladonna alkaloid, is used to prevent travel-related motion sickness as well as the nausea and vomiting which results from the use of certain anesthetics and analgesics used in surgery.

The Transderm-Scop system is a circular flat patch 0.2 mm thick and 2.5 cm^2 in area (40). It is a four-layer system described in Table 10.1. The TDDS contains 1.5 mg of scopolamine and is designed to deliver approximately 1 mg of scopolamine at an approximately constant rate to the systemic circulation over the 3-day lifetime of the system. An initial priming dose of 200 mcg of scopolamine, contained in the adhesive layer of the system, saturates the skin binding sites and rapidly brings the plasma concentration to the required steady-state level. The continuous release of scopolamine through the rate-controlling microporous membrane maintains the plasma level constant. The rate of release is less than the skin's capability for absorption and thus, the membrane, not the skin, controls the delivery of the drug into the circulation.

The patch is worn in a hairless area behind the ear (Fig. 10.9). Because of the small size of the patch, the system is unobtrusive, convenient, and well-accepted by the patient. The TDDS is applied at least 4 hours before the antinausea effect is required. Only one disk should be worn at a time and may be kept in place for up to 3 days. If continued treatment is required, a fresh disk is placed behind the second ear. The most common side effects encountered are dryness of the mouth and drowsiness. Use, particularly in the geriatric population, also may result in an interference with orientation, cognition and memory. The TDDS is not intended for use in children and should be used with caution during pregnancy.

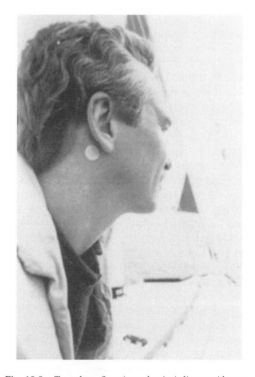

Fig. 10.9 *Transderm Scop (scopolamine) disc provides protection from the nausea and vomiting of motion sickness. (Courtesy of Alza Corporation and CIBA Consumer Pharmaceuticals).*

Transdermal Nitroglycerin

A number of nitroglycerin-containing TDDSs have been developed, including: Deponit (Schwarz), Minitran (3M Pharmaceuticals), Nitro-Dur (Key) and Transderm-Nitro (Novartis). The design of each of these systems briefly is described in Table 10.1. Each of these products maintains nitroglycerin drug delivery for 24 hours after application.

Nitroglycerin is a drug substance utilized widely in the prophylactic treatment of angina. The drug has a relatively low dose, short plasma half-life, high-peak plasma levels and inherent side-effects when taken sublingually (a popular route for its administration). It is rapidly metabolized by the liver when taken orally; this first-pass effect is obviated by the transdermal route.

The various commercially available TDDSs control the rate of drug delivery through a rate-controlling membrane and/or through controlled drug-release from the drug matrix or drug reservoir. When a TDDS is applied to the skin, nitroglycerin is absorbed continuously resulting in active drug reaching the target organs (heart, extremities) before being inactivated by the liver. Only a portion of the total nitroglycerin in the system is delivered over the usual 24 hours use-period; the remainder serves as the thermodynamic energy source to release the drug and remains in the system. For example, in the Deponit TDDS system, only 15% of the nitroglycerin content is delivered after 12 hours of use (41).

The rate of drug release is dependent upon the system. For example in the Transderm-Nitro system, 0.02 mg nitroglycerin is delivered per hour for every cm^2 of applied system size whereas in the Deponit system, each cm^2 delivers approximately 0.013 mg of nitroglycerin per hour (41–42). Systems of various surface areas and nitroglycerin content are provided to accommodate individual patient requirements. Because of different release rates, these systems cannot be used interchangeably by a patient.

The Nitro-Dur matrix is in a highly kinetic equilibrium state (43). Dissolved nitroglycerin molecules are constantly exchanging with adsorbed nitroglycerin molecules bound to the surfaces of the suspended lactose crystals. Sufficient nitroglycerin is adsorbed to the lactose in each matrix to maintain nitroglycerin in the fluid phase (aqueous glycerol) at a stable but saturated level (5 mg nitroglycerin/cm^2 matrix). When the matrix is applied to the surface of the skin, nitroglycerin molecules migrate from solution in the matrix, by diffusion, to solution in the skin. To make up for the molecules lost to the

body, there is a shift of equilibrium in the matrix such that more molecules of nitroglycerin leave the crystals than are adsorbed from solution. When balance is restored, the solution is again at a saturated level. Thus, the crystals of lactose act as a "reservoir" of drug to maintain drug saturation in the fluid phase. The Nitro-Dur matrix, in turn, acts as a saturated "reservoir" for diffusive drug input through the skin (43).

The construction of the nitroglycerin systems are not all alike. For example, the Transderm-Nitro TDDS is a four-layer drug-pouch system, as described in Table 10.1 and depicted in Figure 10.2, whereas the Deponit TDDS is a thin two-layered matrix system resembling that shown in Figure 10.4.

Patients should be given explicit instructions regarding the use of nitroglycerin transdermal systems. Generally, these TDDSs are placed on the chest, with the back, upper arms, or shoulders (Fig. 10.10). The site selected should be free of hair, clean, and dry so that the patch adheres without difficulty. The use of the extremities below the knee or elbow is discouraged as are areas that are abraded or have lesions or cuts. The patient should understand that physical exercise and elevated ambient temperatures, e.g., sauna, may increase the absorption of nitroglycerin.

Transdermal Clonidine

In 1985, the first transdermal system for hypertension, Catapres TTS (clonidine *transdermal therapeutic system*, Boehringer Ingelheim), was marketed. The drug clonidine lends itself to transdermal delivery because of its lipid solubility, high volume of distribution and therapeutic effectiveness in low plasma concentrations. The TDDS provides controlled release of clonidine for 7 days. The product is a four-layered patch as described in Table 10.1.

Catapres TTS is available in several sizes with the amount of drug released proportional to the area of the patch-size. To ensure constant release over the seven-day use period, the drug content in the system is greater than the total amount of drug delivered. The energy source of drug release derives from the concentration gradient existing between a saturated solution of drug in the system and the much lower concentration prevailing in the skin. Clonidine flows in the direction of the lower concentration at a constant rate limited by a rate-controlling membrane (44).

The system is applied to a hairless area of intact skin on the upper outer arm or chest. After appli-

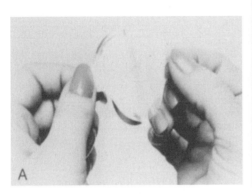
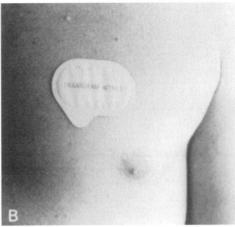

Fig. 10.10   *The Transderm-Nitro patch. Prior to applying to the skin, a plastic liner is removed exposing the adhesive side of the patch. Transderm-Nitro delivers nitroglycerin at a constant and predetermined rate through the skin directly into the bloodstream. The patch is designed to provide 24-hour protection against angina attacks. (Courtesy of Alza Corporation and CIBA Pharmaceuticals [Novartis]).*

cation, clonidine in the adhesive layer saturates the skin sites. Then, clonidine from the drug reservoir begins to flow through the rate-controlling membrane and through the skin to the systemic circulation. Therapeutic plasma clonidine levels are achieved 2 to 3 days after initial application. Application of a new system to a fresh skin site at weekly intervals maintains therapeutic plasma concentrations. If the patch is removed and not replaced with a new system, therapeutic plasma clonidine levels will persist for about 8 hours and then decline slowly over several days. Over this time period, blood pressure returns gradually to pretreatment levels. If the patient experiences localized skin irritation before completing 7 days of use, the system may be removed and replaced with a new one applied on a fresh skin site (44).

Transdermal Nicotine

Nicotine TDDSs are used as adjuncts (e.g., along with counseling) in smoking cessation programs. They have been shown to be an effective aid in quitting the smoking habit when used according to product-recommended strategies (45). In a blinded study, users of nicotine TDDSs are more than twice as likely to quit smoking than individuals wearing a placebo patch (45).

The nicotine TDDSs provide sustained blood levels of nicotine as "nicotine-replacement-therapy" to help the patient establish and sustain remission from smoking (46). Motivation to quit smoking is enhanced through the reduction of

withdrawal symptoms and by partially satisfying the nicotine craving and desired sensory feelings provided by smoking (46).

The commercially available patches contain from 7 to 22 mg of nicotine for daily application during the course of treatment ranging from about 6 to 12 weeks. Different treatment regimens are used for light versus heavy smokers. Examples of nicotine TDDSs are described in Table 10.1. A nicotine TDDS usually is applied to the arm or upper front torso, with patients advised not to smoke when wearing the system. The TDDS is replaced daily, with sites alternated. Some of the nicotine replacement programs provide a gradual reduction in nicotine dosage (patch strength) during the treatment program. Used TDDSs should be discarded properly because the retained nicotine content is poisonous to children and pets.

Nicotine replacement.

production, such as atrophic vaginitis and kraurosis vulvae.

Orally administered estradiol is rapidly metabolized by the liver to estrone and its conjugates, giving rise to higher circulating levels of estrone than estradiol. In contrast, the skin metabolizes estradiol only to a small extent. Therefore, transdermal administration produces therapeutic serum levels of estradiol with lower circulating levels of estrone and estrone conjugates than does oral therapy and requires a smaller total dose. Research has demonstrated that postmenopausal women receiving either transdermal or oral therapy will obtain the desired therapeutic effects from both dosage forms, e.g., lower gonadotropin levels, lower percentages of vaginal parabasal cells, decreased excretion of calcium and lower calcium-to-creatinine ratio. Studies have also demonstrated that systemic side effects from oral estrogens can be reduced by using the transdermal dosage form. Because estradiol has a short half-life (~1 hour), transdermal administration of estradiol allows a rapid decline in blood levels after the transdermal system is removed, e.g., in a cycling regimen (47).

Therapy is usually administered on a cyclic schedule (e.g., 3 weeks of therapy followed by 1 week without) especially in women who have not undergone a hysterectomy. The transdermal system is applied to a clean dry area of the skin on the trunk of the body, either the abdomen or upper quadrant of the buttocks. The patch should not be applied to the waistline because tight clothing may damage or dislodge the system.

The Vivelle (Novartis) and the Climara (Berlex) estradiol TDDSs are two-layered matrix systems described in Table 10.1 and resembling that shown in Figure 10.4 . The estradiol is contained in the adhesive layer (48–49). These systems are used in the same general manner as Estraderm TDDS; however, some of these systems are applied every 7 days.

Transdermal Testosterone

Testosterone transdermal systems, Testoderm (Alza) and Androderm (SmithKline Beecham), are available with various delivery rates as hormone replacement therapy in men who have an absence or deficiency of testosterone (50–51).

The Testoderm TDDS is a two-layer system as described in Table 10.1. For optimal absorption, it is applied to clean, dry scrotal skin that has been dry-shaved. Scrotal skin is reported to be at least five times more permeable to testosterone than other skin sites (50). The TDDS is placed on the scrotum

by stretching the scrotal skin with one hand and pressing the adhesive side of the TDDS against the skin with the other hand, holding it in place for about 10 seconds. The TDDS is applied daily, usually in the morning to mimic endogenous testosterone release (52). Optimum serum levels are reached within 2 to 4 hours after application. The patch is worn 22 to 24 hours daily for 6 to 8 weeks.

The Androderm TDDS is designed to be applied nightly to a clean, dry, unabraded area of the skin of the back, abdomen, upper arms or thighs. It should not be applied to the scrotum (51). The five-layer system is described in Table 10.1.

Other Transdermal Therapeutic Systems

In addition to the drugs currently incorporated into TDDSs, others are under study, including: diltiazem, isosorbide dinitrate, propranolol, nifedipine, mepindolol and verapamil, cardiovascular agents; levonorgestrel/estradiol for hormonal contraception, physostigmine and xanomeline for Alzheimer's disease therapy, naltrexone and methadone for substance addiction, buspirone for anxiety, bupropion for smoking cessation, and papaverine for male impotence.

General Clinical Considerations in the Use of TDDSs

The patient should be advised of the following general guidelines as well as product-specific instructions in the use of TDDSs (53–54).

1. Percutaneous absorption may vary according to the site of application. There is a preferred general application site stated in the literature/ package insert for each product. The patient should be advised of the importance of using the recommended site and rotating locations within that site in the application of replacement patches. Rotating locations is important to allow the skin beneath a patch to regain its normal permeability characteristics after being occluded and also to prevent the possibility of skin irritation. Skin sites may be reused after a week.
2. TDDSs should be applied to clean dry skin areas that are relatively free of hair and not oily, irritated, inflamed, broken or calloused. Wet or moist skin can accelerate drug permeation beyond that which is intended. Oily skin can affect the adhesion of the patch. If hair is present at the intended site, it should be carefully cut and not

wet-shaven nor should a depilatory agent be used since the latter can remove the outermost layers of the stratum corneum and affect the designed rate and extent of drug permeation.

3. Use of skin lotions should be avoided at the application site because they affect skin hydration and also can alter the partition coefficient between the drug in the TDDS and the skin.

4. TDDDs should not be physically altered by cutting (as in an attempt to reduce the dose) since this would destroy the integrity of the system.

5. A TDDS should be removed from its protective package, being careful not to tear or cut into the unit. The protective backing should be removed to expose the adhesive layer while being careful not to touch the adhesive surface (which sometimes contains drug) to the fingertips. The TDDS should be pressed firmly against the skin-site with the heal of the hand for about 10 seconds to assure uniform contact and adhesion.

6. A TDDS should be placed at a site that is not subject to being rubbed off by clothing or movement (as the belt line). TDDSs generally may be left on when showering, bathing or swimming. Should a TDDS prematurely dislodge, an attempt may be made to reapply it, or it may be replaced with a fresh system, the latter being worn for a full time period before it is replaced.

7. A TDDS should be worn for the full period of time stated in the product's instructions. Following that period, it should be removed and replaced with a fresh system as directed.

8. The patient or caregiver should be instructed to cleanse the hands thoroughly before and after applying a TDDS. Care should be taken not to rub the eyes or touch the mouth during handling of the system.

9. If the patient exhibits sensitivity or intolerance to a TDDS or if undue skin irritation results, the patient should seek reevaluation.

10. Upon removal, a used TDDS should be folded in half with the adhesive layer together so that it cannot be reused. The used patch, which contains residual drug, should be placed in the replacement patch's package pouch and discarded in a manner safe to children and pets.

References

1. Stoughton RD. Percutaneous absorption. Toxicol Appl Pharmacol 1965;7:1–8.

2. Black CD. Transdermal drug delivery systems. US Pharm 1982;1:49.

3. Shah VP, Behl CR, Flynn GL, et al. Principles and criteria in the development and optimization of topical therapeutic products. Pharm Res 1992;9:1107–1111.

4. Walters KA. Percutaneous absorption and transdermal therapy. Pharm Tech 1986;10:30–42.

5. Hadgraft J. Structure activity relationships and percutaneous absorption. J Controlled Release 1991;25: 221–226.

6. Ghosh TK, Banga AK. Methods of enhancement of transdermal drug delivery: part I, physical and biochemical approaches. Pharm Tech 1993;17:72–98.

7. Surber C, et al. Optimization of topical therapy: partitioning of drugs into stratum corneum. Pharm Res 1990; 7:1320–1324.

8. Cleary GW. Transdermal concepts and perspectives. Miami, FL: Key Pharmaceuticals, 1982.

9. Melendres JL, et al. In vivo percutaneous absorption of hydrocortisone: multiple-application dosing in man. Pharm Res 1992;9:1164.

10. Barr M. Percutaneous absorption. J Pharm Sci 1962; 51:395–409.

11. Idson B. Percutaneous absorption. J Pharm Sci 1975; 64:901–924.

12. Shah VP, Peck CC, Williams RL. Skin penetration enhancement: clinical pharmacological and regulatory considerations. In: Walters KA and Hadgraft J, eds. Pharmaceutical skin penetration enhancement. New York: Dekker, 1993.

13. Osborne DW, Henke JJ. Skin penetration enhancers cited in the technical literature. Pharm Tech 1997;21: 50–66.

14. Idson B. Percutaneous absorption enhancers. Drug Cosmetic Ind 1985;137:30.

15. Rolf D. Chemical and physical methods of enhancing transdermal drug delivery. Pharm Tech 1988;12: 130–139.

16. Ghosh TK, Banga AK. Methods of enhancement of transdermal drug delivery: part IIA, chemical permeation enhancers. Pharm Tech 1993;17:62–90.

17. Ghosh TK, Banga AK. Methods of enhancement of transdermal drug delivery: part IIB, chemical permeation enhancers. Pharm Tech 1993;17:68–76.

18. Riviere JE, Monteiro-Riviere NA, Inman AO. Determination of lidocaine concentrations in skin after transdermal iontophoresis: effects of vasoactive drugs. Pharm Res 1992; 9:211–219.

19. Green PG, Hinz RS, Cullander C, Yamane G, Guy RH. Iontophoretic delivery of amino acids and amino acid derivatives across the skin in vitro. Pharm Res 1991;8:1113–1120.

20. Choi HK, Flynn GL, Amidon GL. Transdermal delivery of bioactive peptides: the effect of n-decylmethyl sulfoxide, pH, and inhibitors on enkephalin metabolism and transport. Pharm Res 1990;7:1099–1106.

21. D'Emanuele A, Staniforth JN. An electrically modulated drug delivery device III: factors affecting drug stability during electrophoresis. Pharm Res 1992;9: 312–315.

22. Bommannan D, Okuyama H, Stauffer P, Guy RH. Sonophoresis I: the use of high-frequency ultrasound to enhance transdermal drug delivery. Pharm Res 1992;9:559–564.

23. Bommannan D, Menon GK, Okuyama H, Elias PM, Guy RH. Sonophoresis II: examination of the mechanism(s) of ultrasound-enhanced transdermal drug delivery. Pharm Res 1992;9:1043–1047.

24. Shah VP, et al. In vivo percutaneous penetration/absorption. Pharm Res 1991;8:1071–1075.

25. Bronaugh RL, Stewart RF, Congdon ER. Methods for in vitro percutaneous absorption studies II. Animal models for human skin. Toxicol Appl Pharmacol 1982; 62:481–488.

26. Nugent FJ, Wood JA. Methods for the study of percutaneous absorption. Canadian J Pharm Sci 1980;15: 1–7.

27. Addicks W, et al. Topical drug delivery from thin applications: theoretical predictions and experimental results. Pharm Res 1990;7:1048–1054.

28. Kushla GP, Zatz JL. Evaluation of a noninvasive method for monitoring percutaneous absorption of lidocaine in vivo. Pharm Res 1990;7:1033–1037.

29. Chaisson D. Dissolution performance testing of transdermal systems. Dissolution Technologies 1995; 2:8–11.

30. Itoh T, Magavi R, Casady RL, Nishihata T, Rytting JH. A method to predict the percutaneous permeability of various compounds: shed snake skin as a model membrane. Pharm Res 1990;7:1302–1306.

31. Itoh T, Wasinger L, Turunen TM, Rytting JH. Effects of transdermal penetration enhancers on the permeability of shed snakeskin. Pharm Res 1992;9: 1168–1172.

32. Rolland A, Demichelis G, Jamoulle JC, Shroot B. Influence of formulation, receptor fluid, and occlusion, on in vitro drug release from topical dosage forms, using an automated flow-through diffusion cell. Pharm Res 1992;9:82–86.

33. United States Pharmacopeia, 23rd ed. Rockville, MD: United States Pharmacopeial Convention, Inc., 1995.

34. Microette Transdermal Diffusion Cell Autosampling System. Chattsworth CA: Hanson Research Corporation, 1992.

35. Good WR. Transdermal drug-delivery systems. Medical Device & Diagnostic Ind 1986;8:37–42.

36. Godbey KL. Development of a novel transdermal drug delivery backing film with a low moisture vapor transmission rate. Pharm Tech 1997;21:98–107.

37. 3M transdermal drug delivery components. St. Paul, MN: 3M,1996.

38. Fara JW. Short- and long-term transdermal drug delivery systems. In: Drug delivery systems, Pharm Tech. Springfield, OR: Aster Publishing Corporation, 1983:33–40.

39. Shaw JE, Chadrasekaran SK. Controlled topical delivery of drugs of systemic action. Drug Metab Rev 1978;8:223.

40. Transderm-Scop Transdermal Therapeutic System: professional literature. Summit, NJ: Novartis Consumer Pharmaceuticals, 1998.

41. Deponit Nitroglycerin Transdermal Delivery System: professional literature. Milwaukee, WI: Schwarz Pharma, 1998.

42. Transderm-Nitro Transdermal Therapeutic System: professional literature. East Hanover, NJ: Novartis Pharmaceuticals, 1998.

43. Nitro-Dur Transdermal Infusion System: professional literature. Kenilworth, NJ: Key Pharmaceuticals, 1998.

44. Catapress-TTS: professional literature. Ridgefield, CT: Boehringer Ingelheim Pharmaceuticals, 1998.

45. Fiore MC, Smith SS, Jorenby DE, Baker TB. The effectiveness of the nicotine patch for smoking cessation. JAMA 1994;271:1940–1947.

46. Wongwiwatthananukit S, Jack HM, Popovich NG. Smoking cessation: part 2—pharmacologic approaches. JAPhA 1998;38:339–353.

47. Estraderm Estradiol Transdermal System: professional literature. East Hanover, NJ: Novartis Pharmaceuticals, 1998.

48. Vivelle Estradiol Transdermal System: professional literature. East Hanover, NJ: Novartis Pharmaceuticals, 1998.

49. Climara Estradiol Transdermal System: professional literature. Wayne, NJ: Berlex Laboratories, 1998.

50. Testoderm Testosterone Transdermal System: professional literature. Palo Alto, CA: Alza Pharmaceuticals, 1998.

51. Androderm Testosterone Transdermal System: professional literature. Philadelphia, PA: SmithKline Beecham Pharmaceuticals, 1998.

52. Levien T, Baker DE. Reviews of transdermal testosterone and liposomal doxorubicin. Hosp Pharm 1996;31:973–988.

53. Black CD. A pharmacists guide to the use of transdermal medication. Washington DC: The American Pharmaceutical Association, 1996

54. Berba J, Banakar U. Clinical efficacy of current transdermal drug delivery systems: a retrospective evaluation. Am Pharm 1990;NS30:33–41.

SUPPOSITORIES AND INSERTS

Chapter at a Glance

Suppositories

SUPPOSITORIES ARE solid dosage forms intended for insertion into body orifices where they melt, soften, or dissolve and exert localized or systemic effects. The derivation of the word *suppository* is from the Latin *supponere,* meaning "to place under," as derived from *sub* (under) and *ponere* (to place) (1). Thus, suppositories are meant both linguistically and therapeutically to be placed "under" the body, as into the rectum.

Suppositories are commonly used rectally, vaginally, and occasionally urethrally. They have various shapes and weights (Fig. 11.1). The shape and size of a suppository must be such that it is capable of being easily inserted into the intended body orifice without causing undue distension, and once in-

serted, it must be retained for the appropriate period. Rectal suppositories are inserted with the fingers, but certain vaginal suppositories, particularly the vaginal "inserts" or vaginal tablets prepared by compression, may be inserted high in the vaginal tract with the aid of a special insertion appliance.

Rectal suppositories are usually about 32 mm (1½ inches) in length, are cylindrical, and have one or both ends tapered. Some rectal suppositories are shaped like a bullet, a torpedo, or the little finger. Depending on the density of the base and the medicaments present in the suppository, the weight of rectal suppositories may vary. Adult rectal suppositories weigh about 2 g when cocoa butter (theobroma oil) is employed as the suppository base. Rectal suppositories for use by infants and children are about half the weight and size of the

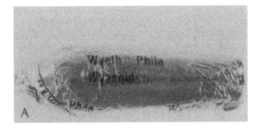

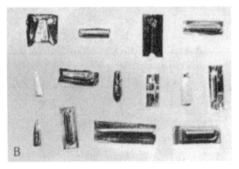

Fig. 11.1 *A, Close-up of a commercially prepared and packaged rectal suppository (Courtesy of Wyeth-Ayerst Laboratories); B, Examples of a variety of commercially available rectal and vaginal suppositories wrapped in paper, foil, and plastic.*

adult suppositories and assume a more pencil-like shape. Vaginal suppositories, also called *pessaries,* are usually globular, oviform, or cone-shaped and weigh about 5 g when cocoa butter is the base. However, depending on the base and the individual manufacturer's product, the weights of vaginal suppositories may vary widely. Urethral suppositories, also called *bougies,* are slender, pencil-shaped suppositories intended for insertion into the male or female urethra. Male urethral suppositories may be 3 to 6 mm in diameter and approximately 140 mm in length, although this may vary. When cocoa butter is employed as the base, these suppositories weigh about 4 g. Female urethral suppositories are about half the length and weight of the male urethral suppository, being about 70 mm in length and weighing about 2 g when made of cocoa butter.

Local Action

Once inserted, the suppository base melts, softens, or dissolves, distributing the medicaments it carries to the tissues of the region. These medicaments may be intended for retention within the cavity for localized drug effects, or they may be intended to be absorbed for the exertion of systemic effects. Rectal suppositories intended for localized action are most frequently used to relieve constipation or the pain, irritation, itching, and inflammation associated with hemorrhoids or other anorectal conditions. Antihemorrhoidal suppositories frequently contain a number of components, including local anesthetics, vasoconstrictors, astringents, analgesics, soothing emollients, and protective agents. A popular laxative, glycerin suppositories promote laxation by the local irritation of the mucous membranes, probably by the dehydrating effect of the glycerin on those membranes. Vaginal suppositories or inserts intended for localized effects are employed mainly as contraceptives, antiseptics in feminine hygiene, and as specific agents to combat an invading pathogen. Most commonly, the drugs used are nonoxynol-9 for contraception, and trichomonacides to combat vaginitis caused by *Trichomonas vaginalis, Candida (Monilia) albicans,* and other microorganisms. Urethral suppositories may be used as antibacterials and as a local anesthetic preparative to urethral examination.

Systemic Action

For systemic effects, the mucous membranes of the rectum and vagina permit the absorption of many soluble drugs. Although the rectum is used frequently as the site for the systemic absorption of drugs, the vagina is not as frequently used for this purpose.

Among the advantages over oral therapy of the rectal route of administration for achieving systemic effects are these: a) drugs destroyed or inactivated by the pH or enzymatic activity of the stomach or intestines need not be exposed to these destructive environments; b) drugs irritating to the stomach may be given without causing such irritation; c) drugs destroyed by portal circulation may bypass the liver after rectal absorption (drugs enter the portal circulation after oral administration and absorption); d) the route is convenient for administration of drugs to adult or pediatric patients who may be unable or unwilling to swallow medication; and e) it is an effective route in the treatment of patients with vomiting episodes.

Examples of drugs administered rectally in the form of suppositories for their systemic effects include a) prochlorperazine, and chlorpromazine for the relief of nausea and vomiting and as a tranquilizer; b) oxymorphone HCl for narcotic anal-gesia; c) ergotamine tartrate, for the relief of migraine syndrome, d) indomethacin, a non-steroidal anti-inflammatory analgesic and antipyretic, and e) ondansetron for the relief of nausea and vomiting.

Some Factors of Drug Absorption from Rectal Suppositories

The dose of a drug administered rectally may be greater than or less than the dose of the same drug given orally, depending on such factors as the constitution of the patient, the physicochemical nature of the drug and its ability to traverse the physiologic barriers to absorption, and the nature of the suppository vehicle and its capacity to release the drug and make it available for absorption.

The factors that affect the rectal absorption of a drug administered in the form of a suppository may be divided into two main groups: 1) physiologic factors, and 2) physicochemical factors of the drug and the base (2,3).

Physiologic Factors

The human rectum is approximately 15 to 20 cm in length. When empty of fecal material, the rectum contains only 2 to 3 mL of inert mucous fluid. In the resting state, the rectum is nonmotile; there are no villi or microvilli on the rectal mucosa (3). However, there is abundant vascularization of the submucosal region of the rectum wall with blood and lymphatic vessels.

Among the physiologic factors that affect drug absorption from the rectum are the colonic contents, circulation route, and the pH and lack of buffering capacity of the rectal fluids.

Colonic Content

When systemic effects are desired from the administration of a medicated suppository, greater absorption may be expected from a rectum that is void than from one that is distended with fecal matter. A drug will obviously have greater opportunity to make contact with the absorbing surface of the rectum and colon in the absence of fecal matter. Therefore, when deemed desirable, an evacuant enema may be administered and allowed to act before the administration of a suppository of a drug to be absorbed. Other conditions such as diarrhea, colonic obstruction due to tumorous growths, and tissue dehydration can all influence the rate and degree of drug absorption from the rectal site.

Circulation Route

Drugs absorbed rectally, unlike those absorbed after oral administration, bypass the portal circulation during their first pass into the general circulation, thereby enabling drugs otherwise destroyed in the liver to exert systemic effects. The lower hemorrhoidal veins surrounding the colon receive the absorbed drug and initiate its circulation throughout the body, bypassing the liver. Lymphatic circulation also assists in the absorption of rectally administered drugs.

pH and Lack of Buffering Capacity of the Rectal Fluids

Because rectal fluids are essentially neutral in pH (7–8) and have no effective buffer capacity, the form in which the drug is administered will not generally be chemically changed by the rectal environment.

The suppository base employed has a marked influence on the release of active constituents incorporated into it. While cocoa butter melts rapidly at body temperature, because of its immiscibility with fluids, it fails to release fat-soluble drugs readily. For systemic drug action using a cocoa butter base, it is preferable to incorporate the ionized (salt form) rather than the unionized (base) form of a drug to maximize bioavailability. Although unionized drugs partition out of water-miscible bases such as glycerinated gelatin and polyethylene glycol more readily, the bases themselves tend to dissolve slowly and thus retard the release of the drug.

Physicochemical Factors of the Drug and Suppository Base

Physicochemical factors include such properties as the relative solubility of the drug in lipid and in water and the particle size of a dispersed drug. Physicochemical factors of the base include its ability to melt, soften, or dissolve at body temperature, its ability to release the drug substance, and its hydrophilic or hydrophobic character.

Lipid-water Solubility

The lipid-water partition coefficient of a drug (discussed in Chapter 3) is an important consideration in the selection of the suppository base and in anticipating drug release from that base. A lipophilic drug that is distributed in a fatty suppository base in low concentration has less of a tendency to escape to the surrounding aqueous fluids than would a hydrophilic substance present in a fatty base to an extent approaching its saturation. Water soluble bases—for example, polyethylene glycols—which dissolve in the anorectal fluids, release for absorption both water-soluble and oil-soluble drugs. Naturally, the more drug a base contains, the more drug will be available for potential absorption. However, if the concentration of a drug in the intestinal lumen is above a particular amount, which varies with the drug, the rate of absorption is not changed by a further increase in the concentration of the drug.

Particle Size

For drugs present in a suppository in the undissolved state, the size of the drug particle will influence its rate of dissolution and its availability for absorption. As indicated many times previously, the smaller the particle size, the more readily the dissolution of the particle and the greater the chance for rapid absorption.

Nature of the Base

As indicated earlier, the base must be capable of melting, softening, or dissolving to release its drug components for absorption. If the base interacts with the drug inhibiting its release, drug absorption will be impaired or even prevented. Also, if the base is irritating to the mucous membranes of the rectum, it may initiate a colonic response and prompt a bowel movement, negating the prospect of complete drug release and absorption.

In a study of the bioavailability of aspirin from five brands of commercial suppositories, absorption rates varied, and even with the best product, only about 40% of the dose was absorbed when the retention time in the bowel was limited to 2 hours. Thus, the absorption rates were considered exceedingly low, especially when compared with orally administered aspirin, and of dubious dependability (4).

Because of the possibility of chemical and/or physical interactions between the medicinal agent and the suppository base, which could affect the stability and/or bioavailability of the drug, the absence of any drug interaction between the two agents should be ascertained before or during formulation.

Long-acting or slow-release suppositories are also prepared. Morphine sulfate in slow release suppositories are prepared by compounding pharmacists. The base includes a material such as alginic acid, which will prolong the release of the drug over several hours (5–7).

Suppository Bases

Analogous to the ointment bases, suppository bases play an important role in the release of the medication they hold and therefore in the availability of the drug for absorption for systemic effects or for localized action. Of course, one of the first requisites for a suppository base is that it remains solid at room temperature but softens, melts, or dissolves readily at body temperature so that the drug it contains may be made fully available soon after insertion. Certain bases are more efficient in drug relase than others. For instance, cocoa butter (theobroma oil) melts quickly at body temperature, but because the resulting oil is immiscible with the body fluids, fat-soluble drugs tend to remain in the oil and have little tendency to enter the aqueous physiologic fluids. For water-soluble drugs incorporated in cocoa butter, the reverse is usually true, and good release results. Fat-soluble drugs seem to be released more readily from bases of glycerinated gelatin or polyethylene glycol, both of which dissolve slowly in body fluids. When irritation or inflammation is to be relieved, as in the treatment of anorectal disorders, cocoa butter appears to be the superior base because of its emollient or soothing, spreading action.

Classification of Suppository Bases

For most purposes, it is convenient to classify suppository bases according to their physical characteristics into two main categories and a third miscellaneous group: 1) fatty or oleaginous bases, 2) water-soluble or water-miscible bases, and 3) miscellaneous bases, generally combinations of lipophilic and hydrophilic substances.

Fatty or Oleaginous Bases

Fatty bases are perhaps the most frequently employed suppository bases, principally because cocoa butter is a member of this group of substances. Among the other fatty or oleaginous materials used in suppository bases are many hydrogenated fatty acids of vegetable oils such as palm kernel oil and cottonseed oil. Also, fat-based compounds containing compounds of glycerin with the higher molecular weight fatty acids, such as palmitic and stearic acids, may be found in fatty suppository bases. Such compounds as glyceryl monostearate and glyceryl monopalmitate are examples of this type of agent. The suppository bases in many commercial products employ various and varied combinations of these types of materials to achieve a base possessing the desired hardness under conditions of shipment and storage and the desired quality of submitting to the temperature of the body to release their medicaments. In some instances, suppository bases are prepared with the fatty materials emulsified or with an emulsifying agent present to prompt emulsification when the suppository makes contact with the aqueous body fluids. These types of bases are arbitrarily placed in the third, or "miscellaneous" group of suppository bases.

Cocoa Butter, NF, is defined as the fat obtained from the roasted seed of *Theobroma cacao.* At room temperature it is a yellowish, white solid having a faint, agreeable chocolate-like odor. Chemically, it is a triglyceride (combination of glycerin and one or different fatty acids) primarily of oleopalmitostearin and oleodistearin. Because cocoa butter melts between 30° to 36°C, it is an ideal suppository base, melting just below body temperature and yet maintaining its solidity at usual room temperatures. However, because of its triglyceride content, cocoa butter exhibits marked *polymorphism,* or the property of existing in several different crystalline forms. Because of this, when cocoa butter is hastily or carelessly melted at a temperature greatly exceeding the minimum required temperature and then quickly chilled, the result is a metastable crystalline form (α crystals) with a melting point much lower than the original cocoa butter. In fact, the melting point may be so low that the cocoa butter will not solidify at room temperature. However, since the crystalline form represents a metastable condition, there is a slow transition to the more stable β form of crystals having the greater stability and the higher melting point. This transition may require several days. Consequently if suppositories that have been prepared by melting cocoa butter for the base do not harden soon after molding, they will be useless to the patient and a loss of time, materials, and prestige to the pharmacist. Cocoa butter must be slowly and evenly melted, preferably over a water bath of warm water, to avoid the formation of the unstable crystalline form and ensure the retention in the liquid of the more stable β crystals that will constitute nuclei upon which the congealing may occur during chilling of the liquid.

Substances such as phenol and chloral hydrate have a tendency to lower the melting point of cocoa butter when incorporated with it. If the melting point is lowered to such an extent that it is not feasible to prepare a solid suppository using cocoa butter alone as the base, solidifying agents like cetyl esters wax (about 20%) or beeswax (about 4%) may be melted with the cocoa butter to compensate for the softening effect of the added substance. However, the addition of hardening agents must not be so excessive as to prevent the melting of the base after the suppository has been inserted into the body, nor must the waxy material interfere with the therapeutic agent in any way so as to alter the efficacy of the product.

Other bases in this category include commercial products such as Fattibase (triglycerides from palm, palm kernel, and coconut oils with self-emulsifying glyceryl monostearate and polyoxyl stearate) and the Wecobee bases (triglycerides derived from coconut oil), Witepsol bases (triglycerides of saturated fatty acids C12-C18 with varied portions of the corresponding partial glycerides).

Water-soluble and Water-miscible Bases

The main members of this group are bases of glycerinated gelatin and bases of polyethylene glycols.

Glycerinated gelatin suppositories may be prepared by dissolving granular gelatin (20%) in glycerin (70%) and adding a solution or suspension of the medication (10%). A glycerinated gelatin base is most frequently used in the preparation of vaginal suppositories, where the prolonged localized action of the medicinal agent is usually desired. The glycerinated gelatin base is slower to soften and mix with the physiologic fluids than is cocoa butter and therefore provides a more prolonged release.

Because glycerinated gelatin-based suppositories have a tendency to absorb moisture due to the hygroscopic nature of glycerin, they must be protected from atmospheric moisture for them to maintain their shape and consistency. Due also to the hygroscopicity of the glycerin, the suppository may have a dehydrating effect and be irritating to the tissues upon insertion. The water present in the formula for the suppositories minimizes this action; however, if necessary, the suppositories may be moistened with water prior to their insertion to reduce the initial tendency of the base to draw water from the mucous membranes and irritate the tissues.

Urethral suppositories may be prepared from a glycerinated gelatin base of a formula somewhat different from the one indicated above. For urethral suppositories, the gelatin constitutes about 60% of the weight of the formula, the glycerin about 20%, and the medicated aqueous portion about 20%. Urethral suppositories of glycerinated gelatin are much more easily inserted than suppositories with a cocoa butter base, owing to the brittleness of cocoa butter and its rapid softening at body temperature.

Polyethylene glycols are polymers of ethylene oxide and water, prepared to various chain lengths, molecular weights, and physical states. They are available in a number of molecular weight ranges, the more commonly used being polyethylene glycol 300, 400, 600, 1000, 1500, 1540, 3350, 4000, 6000, and 8000. The numerical designations refer to the average molecular weights of each of the polymers. Polyethylene glycols having average molecular weights of 300, 400, and 600 are clear, colorless liquids. Those having average molecular weights of greater than 1000 are wax-like, white solids with the hardness increasing with an increase in the molecular weight. Example melting ranges for the polyethylene glycols include the 300 (−15 to −18°C), 400 (4–8°C), 600 (20–25°C), 1000 (37–40°C), 1450 (43–46°C), 3350 (54–58°C), 4600 (57–61°C), 6000 (56–63°C) and for the 8000 (60–63°C). Various combinations of these polyethylene glycols may be combined by fusion, using two or more of the various types to achieve a suppository base of the desired consistency and characteristics.

Pharmacists have been called on in recent years to prepare progesterone vaginal suppositories extemporaneously. These suppositories, used in premenstrual syndrome, are commonly prepared by molding using a polyethylene glycol base. Formulas for these suppositories are presented later in this chapter.

Polyethylene glycol suppositories do not melt at body temperature but rather dissolve slowly in the body's fluids. Therefore, the base need not be formulated to melt at body temperature. Thus it is possible, and in fact routine, to prepare suppositories from polyethylene glycol mixtures having melting points considerably higher than that of body temperature. Not only does this property permit a slower release of the medication from the base once the suppository has been inserted, but it also permits the convenient storage of these suppositories without need of refrigeration and without danger of their softening excessively in warm weather. Their solid nature also permits them to be inserted slowly without the fear that they will melt in the fingertips (as cocoa butter suppositories sometimes do). Because they do not melt at body temperature, but mix with mucous secretions upon their dissolution, polyethylene glycol-based suppositories do not "leak" from the orifice as do many cocoa butter-based suppositories. If the polyethylene glycol suppositories do not contain at least 20% of water to avoid the irritation of the mucous membranes after insertion, they should be dipped in water just before use. This procedure prevents moisture being drawn from the tissues after insertion and the "stinging" sensation.

Miscellaneous Bases

In the miscellaneous group of bases are included those which are mixtures of the oleaginous and water-soluble or water-miscible materials. These materials may be chemical or physical mixtures. Some are preformed emulsions, generally of the w/o type, or they may be capable of dispersing in aqueous fluids. One of these substances is polyoxyl 40 stearate, a surface-active agent that is employed in a number of commercial suppository bases. Polyoxyl 40 stearate is a mixture of the monostearate and distearate esters of mixed polyoxyethylene diols and the free glycols, the average polymer length being equivalent to about 40 oxyethylene units. The substance is a waxy, white to light tan solid that is water-soluble. Its melting point is generally between 39°C and 45°C. Other surface active agents useful in the preparation of suppository bases also fall into this broad grouping. Mixtures of many fatty bases (including cocoa butter) with emulsifying agents capable of forming w/o emulsions have been prepared. These bases have the ability to hold water or aqueous solutions and are sometimes referred to as "hydrophilic" suppository bases.

Preparation of Suppositories

Suppositories are prepared by three methods: 1) *molding* from a melt, 2) *compression,* and 3) *hand rolling* and *shaping*. The method most frequently employed in the preparation of suppositories both on a small scale and on an industrial scale is molding.

Preparation by Molding

Basically, the steps in molding include a) the melting of the base, b) incorporating of any required medicaments, c) pouring the melt into molds, d) allowing the melt to cool and congeal into suppositories, and e) removing the formed suppositories from the mold. Suppositories of cocoa butter, glycerinated gelatin, polyethylene glycol, and most other suppository bases are suitable for preparation by molding.

Suppository Molds

Suppository molds are commercially available with the capability of producing individual or large numbers of suppositories of various shapes and sizes. Individual plastic suppository molds may be obtained to form a single suppository. Other molds, as those most commonly found in the community pharmacy, are capable of producing 6, 12, or more suppositories in a single operation (Fig. 11.2). Industrial molds produce hundreds of suppositories from a single batch (Figs. 11.3, 11.4).

Molds in common use today are made from stainless steel, aluminum, brass, or plastic. The molds, which separate into sections, generally longitudinally, are opened for cleaning before and after the preparation of a batch of suppositories, closed when the melt is poured, and opened again to remove the cold, molded suppositories. Care must be exercised in cleaning the molds, as any scratches on the molding surfaces will take away from the desired smoothness of the resulting suppositories. Plastic molds are especially prone to scratching.

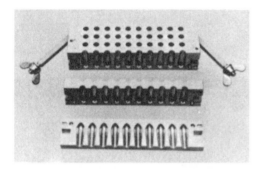

Fig. 11.2 *Partially opened suppository mold capable of producing 50 torpedo-shaped suppositories in a single molding. (Courtesy of Chemical and Pharmaceutical Industry Co., Inc.)*

Although satisfactory reusable and disposable molds are commercially available for the preparation of suitable rectal, vaginal, and urethral suppositories, if necessary in the extemporaneous preparation of suppositories, temporary molds may be successfully formed by pressing heavy aluminum foil about an object having the shape of the desired suppository, then carefully removing the object, and filling the shaped foil with the melt. For instance, glass stirring rods may be used to form molds for urethral suppositories, cylindrical pencils or pens may be used to form molds for rectal suppositories, and any cone-shaped object may be used to form vaginal suppositories.

Lubrication of the Mold

Depending on the formulation, suppository molds may require lubrication before the melt is poured to facilitate the clean and easy removal of the molded suppositories. Lubrication is seldom necessary when the suppository base is cocoa butter or polyethylene glycol, as these materials contract sufficiently on cooling within the mold to separate from the inner surfaces and allow their easy

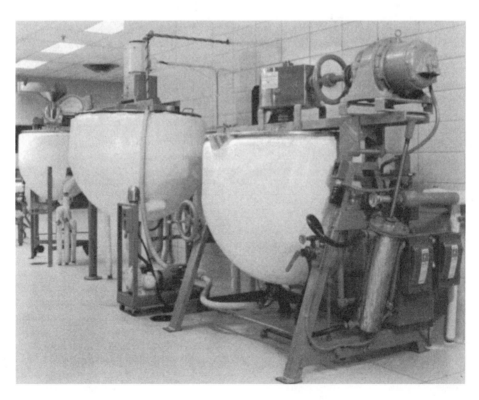

Fig. 11.3 *Large, heated tanks for the preparation of the melt in the commercial production of suppositories by molding. (Courtesy of Wyeth-Ayerst Laboratories.)*

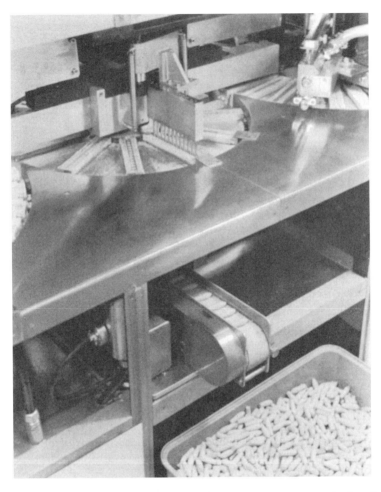

Fig. 11.4 *Highly automated large-scale production of molded suppositories. Molding operation (at the right) is followed by the removal of the suppositories from the molds, dropping them onto a conveyor belt and into a collection basket. (Courtesy of Wyeth-Ayerst Laboratories.)*

removal. Lubrication is usually necessary when glycerinated gelatin suppositories are prepared. A thin coating of mineral oil applied with the finger to the molding surfaces usually suffices to provide the necessary lubrication. It should be stressed, however, that any materials which might cause irritation to the mucous membranes should not be employed as a mold lubricant.

Calibration of the Mold

Each individual mold is capable of holding a specific volume of material in each of its openings. If the material is cocoa butter, the weight of the resulting suppositories will differ from the weight of suppositories prepared in the same mold with a mixture of polyethylene glycols as the base because of the difference in the densities of the materials.

Similarly, any added medicinal agent would further alter the densities of the bases, and the weights of the resulting suppositories would be different from those prepared with base material alone.

The pharmacist should calibrate each of his suppository molds for the suppository bases that he usually uses (usually cocoa butter and a polyethylene glycol base) in order that he may prepare medicated suppositories each having the proper quantity of medicaments.

The first step in the calibration of a mold is to prepare molded suppositories from base material alone. After removal from the mold, the suppositories are weighed, and the total weight and the average weight of each suppository are recorded (for the particular base used). To determine the volume of the mold, the suppositories are then carefully melted in a calibrated beaker, and the volume of the melt is determined for the total number as well as for the average of one suppository.

Determination of the Amount of Base Required

In his prescriptions for medicated suppositories to be prepared extemporaneously by the pharmacist, the prescribing physician indicates the amount of a medicinal substance that he desires in each suppository, but he leaves the amount of base to the discretion of the pharmacist. Generally, in filling such prescriptions, the pharmacist calculates the amounts of materials needed for the preparation of one or two more suppositories than the number prescribed to compensate for the inevitable loss of some material and to ensure having enough material to prepare the last required suppository.

In determining the amount of base to be incorporated with the medicaments, the pharmacist must be certain that the required amount of drug is provided in each suppository. Because the volume of the mold is known (from the determined volume of the melted suppositories formed from the base), the volume of the drug substances subtracted from the total volume of the mold will give the volume of base required. In instances in which the added amounts of medicaments are slight, they may be considered to be negligible, and no deduction from the total volume of base may be deemed necessary. However, if considerable quantities of substances are to be incorporated into the suppository, the volumes of these materials are important and should be used to calculate the amount of base actually required to completely fill the mold. The total volumes of these materials are subtracted from the volume of the mold, and the appropriate amount of base is added. Because the suppository bases are solids at room temperature, the volume of base determined may be converted to weight from the density of the material. For example, if 12 mL of cocoa butter are required to fill a suppository mold and if the medicaments in the formula have a collective volume of 2.8 mL, then 9.2 mL of the cocoa butter will be required. By multiplying 9.2 mL times the density of cocoa butter, 0.86 g/mL, it may be calculated that 7.9 g of cocoa butter will be required. After adjusting for the preparation of an extra suppository or two, the calculated amount is weighed.

Another method for the determination of the amount of base in the preparation of medicated suppositories requires the following steps: a) weigh the active ingredient for the preparation of a single suppository; b) dissolve it or mix it (depending on its solubility in the base) with a portion of melted base insufficient to fill one cavity of the mold, and add the mixture to a cavity; c) add additional melted base to the cavity to fill it completely; d) allow the suppository to congeal and harden; and e) remove the suppository from the mold and weigh it. The weight of the active ingredients present, subtracted from the weight of the suppository, yields the weight of the amount of base used. This amount of base multiplied by the number of suppositories to be prepared in the mold is the total amount of base required.

A third method involves the placing of all of the required medicaments for the preparation of the total number of suppositories (including one extra) in a calibrated beaker. To this is added a portion of the melted base and the drug substances incorporated. Then sufficient additional melted base is added until the volume of mixture is reached that is required for the preparation of the necessary suppositories, based on the original calibration of the volume of the mold.

A summary of density calculations for the preparation of suppositories by molding is found in the accompanying Physical Pharmacy Capsule.

Preparing and Pouring the Melt

Using the least possible heat, the weighed suppository base material is melted, generally over a water bath, since a great deal of heat is not usually required. A porcelain casserole, which is a dish having a pouring lip and a handle, is perhaps the best utensil to use, since it later permits the convenient pouring of the melt into the cavities of the mold. Medicinal substances are usually incorporated into a portion of the melted base by mixing on a glass or porcelain tile with a spatula. After incorporation, this material is added with stirring to the remaining base which has been allowed to cool almost to its congealing point. Any volatile materials or heat labile substances should be incorporated at this point with thorough stirring.

The melt is poured carefully and continuously into each cavity of the mold, which has been previously equilibrated to room temperature. If any undissolved or suspended materials in the mixture are of greater density than the base so that they have a tendency to settle, constant stirring, even during pouring, is required, else the last filled cavity will contain a disproportionate share of the undissolved materials. The solid materials remain suspended if the pouring is performed just above the congealing point and not when the base is too fluid. If the melt is not near the congealing point

Physical Pharmacy Capsule 11.1   **Density (Dose Replacement) Calculations for Suppositories**

In the preparation of suppositories, it is generally assumed that if the quantity of active drug is less than 100 mg, then the volume occupied by the powder is insignificant and need not be considered. This is usually based on a 2 gram suppository weight. Obviously, if a suppository mold of less than 2 grams is used, the powder volume may need to be considered.

The density factors of various bases and drugs need to be known to determine the proper weights of the ingredients to be used. Density factors relative to cocoa butter have been determined. If the density factor of a base is not known, it is simply calculated as the ratio of the blank weight of the base and cocoa butter. Density factors for a selected number of ingredients are shown in Table 1.

Table 1.   Density Factors for Cocoa Butter Suppositories

Alum	1.7	Morphine HCl	1.6
Aminophylline	1.1	Opium	1.4
Aspirin	1.3	Paraffin	1.0
Barbital	1.2	Peruvian Balsam	1.1
Belladonna extract	1.3	Phenobarbital	1.2
Benzoic Acid	1.5	Phenol	0.9
Bismuth carbonate	4.5	Potassium bromide	2.2
Bismuth salicylate	4.5	Potassium iodide	4.5
Bismuth subgallate	2.7	Procaine	1.2
Bismuth subnitrate	6.0	Quinine HCl	1.2
Boric Acid	1.5	Resorcinol	1.4
Castor oil	1.0	Sodium bromide	2.3
Chloral hydrate	1.3	Spermaceti	1.0
Cocaine HCl	1.3	Sulfathiazole	1.6
Digitalis leaf	1.6	Tannic acid	1.6
Glycerin	1.6	White wax	1.0
Ichthammol	1.1	Witch hazel fluid extract	1.1
Iodoform	4.0	Zinc oxide	4.0
Menthol	0.7	Zinc sulfate	2.8

Three different methods of calculating the quantity of base that the active medication will occupy and the quantities of ingredients required will be illustrated here: 1) dosage replacement factor, 2) density factor, and 3) occupied volume methods.

DETERMINATION OF THE DOSAGE REPLACEMENT FACTOR METHOD

$$f = \frac{100\ (E - G)}{(G)(X)} + 1$$

where E = the weight of the pure base suppositories, and

G = the weight of suppositories with X% of the active ingredient.

Cocoa butter is arbitrarily assigned a value of 1 as the standard base. Examples of other dosage replacement factors are shown in Table 2.

EXAMPLE 1

Prepare a suppository containing 100 mg of phenobarbital (f = 0.81) using cocoa butter as the base. The weight of the pure cocoa butter suppository is 2.0 g. Since 100 mg of phenobarbital is to be contained in an approximately 2.0 g suppository, it will be about 5% phenobarbital. What will be the total weight of each suppository?

$$0.81 = \frac{100\ (2 - g) + 1}{(g)(5)} \quad g = 2.019$$

Physical Pharmacy Capsule 11.1   **Density (Dose Replacement) Calculations for Suppositories (Continued)**

Table 2. Dosage Replacement Factors for Selected Drugs

Balsam Peru	0.83	Phenol	0.9
Bismuth subgallate	0.37	Procaine HCl	0.8
Bismuth subnitrate	0.33	Quinine HCl	0.83
Boric Acid	0.67	Resorcin	0.71
Camphor	1.49	Silver protein, mild	0.61
Castor oil	1.0	Spermaceti	1.0
Chloral hydrate	0.67	White/yellow wax	1.0
Ichthammol	0.91	Zinc oxide	0.15–0.25
Phenobarbital	0.81		

DETERMINATION OF DENSITY FACTOR METHOD

1. Determine the average blank weight, A, per mold using the suppository base of interest.
2. Weigh the quantity of suppository base necessary for 10 suppositories.
3. Weigh 1.0 g of medication.

   The weight of medication per suppository, B, is then equal to 1 g/10 supp = 0.1 g/supp.

4. Melt the suppository base and incorporate the medication, mix, pour into molds, cool, trim, and remove from the molds.
5. Weigh the 10 suppositories and determine the average weight (C).
6. Determine the density factor as follows:

$$\text{Density factor} = \frac{B}{A - C + B}$$

where
     A = average weight of blank,
     B = weight of medication per suppository, and
     C = average weight of medicated suppository.

7. Take the weight of the medication required for each suppository and divide by the density factor of the medication to find the replacement value of the suppository base.
8. Subtract this quantity from the blank suppository weight.
9. Multiply by the number of suppositories required to obtain the quantity of suppository base required for the prescription.
10. Multiply the weight of drug per suppository by the number of suppositories required to obtain the quantity of active drug required for the prescription.

EXAMPLE 2

Prepare 12 acetaminophen 300 mg suppositories using cocoa butter, where the average weight of the cocoa butter blank is 2 g and the average weight of the medicated suppository is 1.8 g.

$$DF = \frac{0.3}{2 - 1.8 + 0.3} = 0.6$$

From step 7:   (0.3 gm)/0.6 = 0.5 (the replacement value of the base)

From step 8:   2.0 gm − 0.5 g = 1.5 g

From step 9:   12 × 1.5 g = 18 g cocoa butter required

From step 10:   12 × 0.3 g = 3.6 g acetaminophen

Physical Pharmacy Capsule 11.1   **Density (Dose Replacement) Calculations for Suppositories (Continued)**

DETERMINATION OF OCCUPIED VOLUME METHOD

1. Determine the average weight per mold (blank) using the suppository base of interest.
2. Weigh the quantity of suppository base necessary for 10 suppositories.
3. Divide the density of the active drug by the density of the suppository base to obtain a ratio.
4. Divide the total weight of active drug required for the total number of suppositories by the ratio obtained in step 3 (this will give the amount of suppository base displaced by the active drug).
5. Subtract the amount obtained in step 4 from the total weight of the prescription (number of suppositories multiplied by the weight of the blanks) to obtain the weight of suppository base required.
6. Multiply the weight of active drug per suppository times the number of suppositories to be prepared to obtain the quantity of active drug required.

EXAMPLE 3

Prepare 10 suppositories, each containing 200 mg of a drug with a density of 3.0. The suppository base has a density of 0.9 and a prepared blank weighs 2.0 g. Using the "determination of occupied volume method," prepare the requested suppositories.

From step 1:   The average weight per mold is 2.0 g.

From step 2:   The quantity required for 10 suppositories would be 2 g $\times$ 10 supp = 20 g.

From step 3:   The density ratio is 3.0/0.9 = 3.3.

From step 4:   The amount of suppository base displaced by the active drug is 2.0 g/3.3 = 0.6 g.

From step 5:   The weight of the suppository base required is 20 g $-$ 0.6 g = 19.4 g.

From step 6:   The quantity of active drug required is 0.2 g $\times$ 10 = 2.0 g.

The required weight of the suppository base is 19.4 g and the active drug is 2 g.

---

when poured, the solids may settle within each cavity of the mold to reside at the tips of the suppositories, with the result that the suppositories may be broken when removed from the mold. Alternatively, a small quantity of silica gel (about 25 mg per suppository) can be incorporated into the formula to aid in keeping the active drug suspended. In filling each suppository cavity, the pouring must be continuous to prevent *layering*, which may lead to a product easily broken on handling. To ensure a completely filled mold upon congealing, the melt is poured excessively over each opening, actually rising above the level of the mold. The excessive material may actually form a continuous ribbon along the top of the mold above the cavities. This use of extra suppository material prevents the

formation of recessed dips in the ends of the suppositories and justifies the preparation of extra suppository melt. When solidified, the excess material is evenly scraped off of the top of the mold with a spatula (the spatula can be warmed by dipping into a beaker of warm water—this will make a smooth surface on the back of the suppository during trimming). The mold is usually placed in the refrigerator to hasten the hardening of the suppositories.

When the suppositories are hard, the mold is removed from the refrigerator and allowed to come to room temperature. Then the sections of the mold are separated, and the suppositories are dislodged with the pressure being exerted principally on their ends and only if needed on the tips. Generally, little, if any, pressure is required, and the suppositories simply fall out of the mold when it is opened.

Preparation by Compression

Suppositories may be prepared by forcing the mixed mass of the suppository base and the medicaments into special molds using suppository-making machines. In preparation for compression into the molds, the suppository base and the other formulative ingredients are combined by thorough mixing, the friction of the process causing the base to soften into a pastelike consistency. On a small scale, a mortar and pestle may be used. If the mortar is heated in warm water before use and then dried, the softening of the base and the mixing process is greatly facilitated. On a large scale, a similar process may be used, employing mechanically operated kneading mixers and a warmed mixing vessel.

The process of compression is especially suited for the making of suppositories containing medicinal substances that are heat labile and for suppositories containing a great deal of substances insoluble in the base. In contrast to the molding method, there is no likelihood of insoluble matter settling during the preparation of suppositories by compression. The disadvantage to the process is that the special suppository machine is required and there is some limitation as to shapes of suppositories that can be made from the available molds.

In preparing suppositories with the compression machine, the suppository mass is placed into a cylinder which is then closed, and pressure is applied from one end, mechanically, or by turning a wheel, and the mass is forced out of the other end into the suppository mold or die. When the die is filled with the mass, a movable end plate at the back of the die is removed and when additional pressure is applied to the mass in the cylinder, the formed suppositories are ejected. The end plate is returned, and the process is repeated until all of the suppository mass has been used. Various sizes and shapes of dies are available. It is possible to prepare suppositories of uniform circumference by extrusion through a perforated plate and by cutting the extruded mass to the desired length.

Preparation by Hand Rolling and Shaping

With the ready availability of suppository molds of accommodating shapes and sizes, there is little requirement for today's pharmacist to shape suppositories by hand. Hand rolling and shaping is a historic part of the art of the pharmacist; a description of the method may be found in the third edition of this text or in pharmacy compounding texts.

Rectal Suppositories

Examples of rectal suppositories are presented in Table 11.1. As noted earlier, drugs as aspirin given for pain, ergotamine tartrate for treating migraine headaches, theophylline as a smooth muscle relaxant in treating asthma, and chlorpromazine and prochlorperazine, which act as antiemetics and tranquilizers, are intended to be absorbed into the general circulation to provide systemic drug effects. The rectal route of administration is especially useful in instances in which the patient is unwilling or unable to take medication by mouth.

Suppositories are also intended to provide local action within the perianal area. Local anesthetic suppositories are commonly employed to relieve *pruritus ani* of various causes, and the pain sometimes associated with hemorrhoids. Many of the commercial hemorrhoidal suppositories contain a number of medicinal agents including astringents, protectives, anesthetics, lubricants, and others, intended to relieve the discomfort of the condition. Cathartic suppositories are contact-type agents that act directly on the colonic mucosa to produce normal peristalsis. Because the contact action is restricted to the colon, the motility of the small intestine is not appreciably affected. Cathartic suppositories are more rapid-acting than orally administered medication. Suppositories of bisacodyl are usually effective in 15 minutes to an hour, and glycerin suppositories usually within a few minutes following insertion.

Some commercially prepared suppositories are available for both adult and pediatric use. The difference is in the shape and drug content. Pediatric suppositories are more narrow and pencil-shaped than the typical bullet-shaped adult suppository. Glycerin suppositories are commonly available in each type.

A formula for glycerin suppositories is as follows:

Glycerin	91 g
Sodium Stearate	9 g
Purified Water	5 g
To make about	100 g

In the preparation of this suppository, the glycerin is heated in a suitable container to about 120°F.

Table 11.1. Examples of Rectal Suppositories

Suppository	Corresponding Commercial Product	Active Constituent per Suppository	Type of Effect	Category and Comments
Bisacodyl Suppositories	Dulcolax Suppositories (Novartis)	10 mg	Local	Cathartic. See text for additional discussion. Base: hydrogenated vegetable oil.
Chlorpromazine Suppositories	Thorazine Suppositories (SmithKline Beecham)	25 and 100 mg	Systemic	Anti-emetic; tranquilizer. Base: glycerin, glyceryl monopalmitate and monostearate, and hydrogenated fatty acids of coconut and palm kernel oils.
Hydrocortisone Suppositories	Anusol-HC Suppositories (Warner-Lambert)	25 mg	Local	For use in pruritis ani, inflamed hemorrhoids, and other inflammatory conditions of the anorectum. Base: hydrogenated glycerides.
Hydromorphone Suppositories	Dilaudid Suppositories (Knoll)	3 mg	Systemic	Analgesic. Base: Cocoa butter with silicone dioxide.
Indomethacin Suppositories	Indocin Suppositories (Merck & Co.)	50 mg	Systemic	Nonsteroidal antiinflammatory analgesic indicated in various forms of arthritis. The rate of rectal absorption from suppositories is more rapid than from orally administered capsules. Base: polyethylene glycols 3350 and 8000.
Mesalamine Suppositories	Rowasa (Solvay)	500 mg	Local	Antiinflammatory. Base: Hard fat.
Oxymorphone Suppositories	Numorphan Suppositories (Endo)	5 mg	Systemic	Analgesic. Base: Polyethylene glycols 1000 and 3350.
Prochlorperazine Suppositories	Compazine Suppositories (SmithKline Beecham)	2.5, 5 and 25 mg	Systemic	Anti-emetic. Base: glycerin, glyceryl monopalmitate and monostearate, and hydrogenated fatty acids of coconut and palm kernel oils.
Promethazine HCl Suppositories	Phenergan Suppositories (Wyeth-Ayerst)	12.5, 25 and 50 mg	Systemic	Antihistamic, antiemetic and sedative actions: used to manage conditions of allergic origin; for preoperative or postoperative sedation or nausea and vomiting; and for motion sickness. Base: cocoa butter and white wax.

Then the sodium stearate is dissolved with stirring in the hot glycerin, the purified water added, and the mixture immediately poured into the suppository mold. It is recommended that if the mold is of metal, that it also be heated prior to the addition of the glycerin mixture. After cooling to solidification, the suppositories are removed. From the above formula, about fifty adult suppositories may be prepared. Approximately the same formulation is used in pharmaceutical and cosmetic "stick" type products, such as deodorants and antiperspirants.

Glycerin, a hygroscopic material, contributes to the laxative effect of the suppository by drawing water from the intestine and also from its irritant action on the mucous lining. The sodium stearate, a soap, is the solidifying agent in the suppository and may also contribute to the laxative action. Because of the hygroscopic nature of glycerin, the suppositories attract moisture and should be maintained in tight containers, preferably at temperatures below 25°C.

The pharmacist should relate several helpful items

of information about the proper use of suppositories. If they must be stored in the refrigerator, suppositories should be allowed to warm to room temperature before insertion. The patient should be advised to rub cocoa butter suppositories gently with the fingers to melt the surface to provide lubrication for insertion. Glycerinated gelatin or polyethylene glycol suppositories should be moistened with water to enhance lubrication. If the polyethylene glycol suppository formulation does not contain at least 20% water, dipping it into water just prior to insertion prevents moisture from being drawn from rectal tissues after insertion and decreases subsequent irritation. The shape of the suppository determines how it will be inserted. Bullet-shaped rectal suppositories should be inserted point-end first. When the patient is instructed to use one-half suppository, the patient should be told to cut the suppository in half lengthwise with a clean razor blade. Most suppositories are dispensed in paper, foil, or plastic wrappings, and the patient must be instructed to completely remove the wrapping before insertion.

Vaginal Suppositories

Examples of vaginal suppository and tablets are presented in Table 11.2. These preparations are employed principally to combat infections occurring in the female genitourinary area, to restore the vaginal mucosa to its normal state, and for contraception. In combating vaginal infections, the usual pathogenic organisms involved are *Trichomonas vaginalis, Candida* (*Monilia*) *albicans* or other species, and *Hemophilus vaginalis.* Among the anti-infective agents found in commercial vaginal preparations are: nystatin, clotrimazole, butoconazole nitrate, terconazole, and miconazole (antifungals) and triple

sulfas, sulfanilamide, povidone-iodine, clindamycin phosphate, metronidazole and oxytetracycline (antibacterials). Nonoxynol-9, a spermicide, is employed for vaginal contraception. Estrogenic substances as dienestrol are found in vaginal preparations to restore the vaginal mucosa to its normal state.

In the preparation of vaginal suppositories, the most commonly used base consists of combinations of the various molecular weight polyethylene glycols. To this base is frequently added surfactants and preservative agents, commonly the parabens. Many of the vaginal suppositories and other types of vaginal dosage forms are buffered to an acid pH, usually around pH 4.5 which resembles that of the normal vagina. This acidity discourages pathogenic organisms and at the same time provides a favorable environment for eventual recolonization by the acid-producing bacilli normally found in the vagina.

The polyethylene glycol-based vaginal suppositories are water-miscible and are generally sufficiently firm for the patient to handle and insert without great difficulty. However, to make the task even easier, many manufacturers provide plastic insertion devices with their products which are used to hold the suppository or vaginal tablet during insertion for proper placement within the vagina (Fig. 11.5).

As noted earlier, pharmacists frequently are called on to prepare progesterone vaginal suppositories. Formulas for the extemporaneous preparation of these suppositories have been presented in the professional literature (8,9). Micronized progesterone powder is used in a base of polyethylene glycol, although in some formulas cocoa butter is employed. The suppositories are prepared by adding the progesterone to a melt of the base and molding. Some representative formulas are:

Table 11.2. Examples of Vaginal Suppositories and Tablets

Product/Manufacturer	Active Constituents	Category and Comments
AVC Suppositories (Hoechst Marion Roussel)	Sulfanilamide 1.05 g	For the treatment of *Candida albicans* infections.
Monistat 7 Suppositories (Advanced Care Products)	Miconazole nitrate 200 mg	Antifungal for treatment of localized vulvo-vaginal candidiasis (moniliasis)
Mycelex-G Vaginal Tablets (Bayer)	Clotrimazole, 500 mg	Treatment of vulvo-vaginal yeast (Candida) infections.
Semicid Vaginal Contraceptive Inserts (Robins Healthcare)	Nonoxynol-9, 100 mg	Non-systemic, reversible method of birth control.
Sultrin Vaginal Tablets (Ortho-McNeil)	Sulfathiazole, sulfacetamide and sulfabenzamide, 500 mg total	Treatment of *Haemophilus vaginalis* vaginitis.
Terazol 3 Vaginal Suppositories (Ortho-McNeil)	Terconazole, 80 mg	Treatment of vulvovaginal candidiasis (moniliasis)

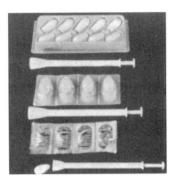

Fig. 11.5 *Dosage forms used intravaginally, including suppositories (top and middle), vaginal tablets packaged in foil (bottom), vaginal cream, and corresponding insert devices.*

Rx

Progesterone, micronized powder .... q.s.
Polyethylene Glycol 400 .... 60%
Polyethylene Glycol 8000 .... 40%

Rx

Progesterone, micronized powder .... q.s.
Polyethylene Glycol 1000 .... 75%
Polyethylene Glycol 3350 .... 25%

Rx

Progesterone, micronized powder .... q.s.
Cocoa Butter 100%

The amount of progesterone prescribed per suppository ranges from 25 to 600 mg. The suppositories are used in treating luteal phase defect, premenstrual syndrome, luteal phase spotting, and in the preparation of the endometrium for implantation (9).

The pharmacist should share several helpful hints with a woman who is about to use a vaginal suppository product. She should first be told to read the patient instructions included with the product. Throughout the entire course of therapy, the suppository should be inserted high into the vagina with the provided applicator. The patient should not discontinue therapy when the symptoms abate. Further, she should notify her physician if burning, irritation, or any signs of an allergic reaction occur. When vaginal inserts (i.e., compressed tablets) are prescribed, the pharmacist should instruct the woman to dip the tablet into water quickly before insertion. Because these dosage forms are usually administered at bedtime and can be somewhat messy if formulated into an oleaginous base, the pharmacist should suggest that the woman wear a

sanitary napkin to protect her nightwear and bed linens.

Quality control procedures listed in the USP 23/NF 18 for manufactured suppositories include identification, assay and in some cases loss on drying, disintegration and dissolution. Also, stability considerations in dispensing practice for suppositories include observation for excessive softening and oil stains on packaging (10). Compounded suppositories can be checked for calculations of theoretical and actual weight and weight variation, color, hardness, surface texture and overall appearance.

Packaging and Storage

Glycerin suppositories and glycerinated gelatin suppositories are packaged in tightly closed glass containers to prevent a moisture change in the content of the suppositories. Suppositories prepared from a cocoa butter base are usually individually wrapped or otherwise separated in compartmentalized boxes to prevent contact and adhesion. Suppositories containing light-sensitive drugs are individually wrapped in an opaque material such as a metallic foil. In fact, most commercially available suppositories are individually wrapped in either foil or a plastic material. Some are packaged in a continuous strip with suppositories being separated by tearing along perforations placed between suppositories. Suppositories are also commonly packaged in slide boxes or in plastic boxes.

Since suppositories are adversely affected by heat, it is necessary to maintain them in a cool place. Suppositories having cocoa butter as the base must be stored below 30°C/86°F, and preferably in a refrigerator (2–8°C/36–46°F). Glycerinated gelatin suppositories are best stored at temperatures below 35°F and can routinely be stored at controlled room temperature (20–25°C/68–77°F). Suppositories made from a base of polyethylene glycol may be stored at usual room temperatures without the requirement of refrigeration.

Suppositories stored in environments of high humidity may absorb moisture and tend to become spongy, whereas suppositories stored in places of extreme dryness may lose moisture and become brittle.

Inserts

Vaginal Inserts

Vaginal tablets are more widely used nowadays than are vaginal suppositories. The tablets are easier to manufacture, more stable, and less messy to handle in use. Vaginal tablets, frequently referred to as *vaginal inserts,* are usually ovoid in shape and are accompanied in their packaging with a plastic inserter, a device for easy placement of the tablet within the vagina. Vaginal tablets contain the same types of antiinfective and hormonal substances as the vaginal suppositories. They are prepared by tablet compression, and are commonly formulated to contain lactose as the base or filler, a disintegrating agent, as starch, a dispersing agent, as polyvinylpyrrolidone, and a tablet lubricant, as magnesium stearate. The tablets are intended to disintegrate within the vagina releasing their medication. Examples of vaginal tablets are presented in Table 11.2.

Some vaginal inserts are capsules of gelatin containing medication to be released intravaginally. Capsules may also be used rectally, especially in pediatrics to administer medication to children unwilling or unable to tolerate the drug orally. Capsule insertion into the rectum can be facilitated by first lightly wetting the capsule with water. Holes may be punched into these capsules prior to moistening and insertion to facilitate fluid movement into the capsule, if desired. Drugs are absorbed from the rectum, but frequently at unpredictable rates and in varying amounts as has been previously noted in this chapter. Drugs that do not dissolve rapidly and which are irritating to mucous membranes should not be placed in direct contact with such membranes.

References

1. Merkus FWHM. The Correct Application of Suppositories. Editorial. Pharmacy International, December 1980.
2. Anschel J, Lieberman HA. Suppositories. Drug Cosmetic Ind 1965;97:341.
3. Moolenaar F, Schoonen AJM. Biopharmaceutics of the rectal administration of drugs. Pharmacy International 1980;1:444–146.
4. Gibaldi M, Grundhofer B. Bioavailability of aspirin from commercial suppositories. J Pharm Sci 64:1064–1066.
5. Morgan DJ, McCormick Y, Cosolo W, et al. Prolonged release of morphine alkaloid from a lipophilic suppository base in vitro and in vivo. Int J Clin Pharmacol Ther Toxicol 1991;30:576–581.
6. Cole L, Hanning CD, Robertson S, Quinn K. Further development of a morphine hydrogel suppository. Br J Clin Pharmacol 1990;30:781–786.
7. Moolenaar F, Meyuler P, Frijlink E, et al. Rectal absorption of morphine from controlled release suppositories. Int J Pharmaceut 1994;114:170–120.
8. Roffe BD, Zimmer RA, Derewicz HJ. Preparation of progesterone suppositories. Am J Hosp Pharm 1977; 34:1334.
9. Allen LV, Stiles ML. Progesterone suppositories. U.S. Pharmacist 1988;13:16–19.
10. Anon. United States Pharmacopeia 23/National Formulary 18. Rockville MD, U.S. Pharmacopeial Convention, Inc., 1995;1957–1959.

SOLUTIONS

Chapter at a Glance

IN PHYSICOCHEMICAL terms, solutions may be prepared from any combination of solid, liquid, and gas, the three states of matter. For example, a solid solute may be dissolved in either another solid, a liquid, or a gas, and with the same being true for a liquid solute and for a gas, nine types of homogeneous mixtures are possible. In pharmacy, however, interest in solutions is for the most part limited to preparations of a solid, a liquid, and less frequently a gas solute dissolved in a liquid solvent.

In pharmaceutical terms, *solutions* are "liquid preparations that contain one or more chemical substances dissolved in a suitable solvent or mixture of mutually miscible solvents" (1). Because of a particular pharmaceutical solution's use, it may be classified as an *oral solution, otic solution, ophthalmic solution,* or *topical solution.* Still other solutions, because of their composition or use, may be classified as other pharmaceutical dosage forms. For example, aqueous solutions containing a sugar are classified as *syrups;* sweetened hydroalcoholic (combinations of water and ethanol) solutions are termed *elixirs;* solutions of aromatic materials are termed *spirits* if the solvent is alcoholic or *aromatic waters* if the solvent is aqueous. Solutions prepared by extracting active constituents from crude drugs are termed *tinctures* or *fluid extracts,* depending on their method of preparation and their concentration. *Tinctures* may also be solutions of chemical substances dissolved in alcohol or in a hydroalcoholic solvent. Certain solutions prepared to be sterile and pyrogen-free and intended for parenteral administration are classified as *injections.* Although other examples could be cited, it is apparent that a solution, as a distinct type of pharmaceutical preparation, is much further defined than is the physicochemical definition of the term *solution.*

Oral solutions, syrups, elixirs, spirits and tinctures are prepared and used for the specific effects of the medicinal agents present. In these preparations, the medicinal agents are intended to provide systemic effects. The fact that they are administered in solution form usually means that their absorption from the gastrointestinal tract into the systemic circulation may be expected to occur more rapidly than from suspension or solid dosage forms of the same medicinal agent.

Solutes other than the medicinal agent are usually present in orally administered solutions. These additional agents usually are included to provide color, flavor, sweetness, or stability to the solution. In formulating or compounding a pharmaceutical solution, the pharmacist must utilize information on the solubility and stability of each of the solutes present with regard to the solvent or solvent system employed. Combinations of medicinal or pharmaceutic agents that will result in chemical or physical interactions affecting the therapeutic quality or pharmaceutic stability of the product must be avoided.

For single-solute solutions and especially for multiple-solute solutions, the pharmacist must be aware of the solubility characteristics of the solutes and the features of the common pharmaceutical solvents. Each chemical agent has its own solubility in a given solvent. For many medicinal agents, their solubilities in the usual solvents are stated in the USP as well as in other reference books.

Solubility

Attractive forces between atoms lead to the formation of molecules and ions. The intermolecular forces, which are developed between like molecules, are responsible for the physical state (i.e., solid, liquid, or gas) of the substance under given conditions, as temperature and pressure. Under ordinary conditions, most organic compounds, and thus most drug substances, form molecular solids.

When molecules interact, attractive forces and repulsive forces are in effect. The attractive forces cause the molecules to cohere, whereas the repulsive forces prevent molecular interpenetration and destruction. When the attractive and repulsive forces are equal, the potential energy between two molecules is minimum and the system is most stable.

Dipolar molecules frequently tend to align themselves with other dipolar molecules such that the negative pole of one molecule points toward the positive pole of the other. Large groups of molecules may be associated through these weak attractions known as *dipole-dipole* or van der Waals forces. In addition to the dipolar interactions, other attractions occur between polar and nonpolar molecules and ions. These include ion-dipole forces and hydrogen bonding. The latter is of particular interest. Because of small size and large electrostatic field, the hydrogen atom can move in close to an electronegative atom, forming an electrostatic type of association referred to as a *hydrogen bond* or *hydrogen bridge.* Hydrogen bonding involves strongly electronegative atoms as oxygen, nitrogen, and fluorine. Such a bond exists in water, represented by the dotted lines:

Water

Hydrogen bonds also exist between some alcohol molecules, esters, carboxylic acids, aldehydes, and polypeptides.

When a solute dissolves, the substance's intermolecular forces of attraction must be overcome by forces of attraction between the solute and solvent molecules. This involves breaking the solute-solute forces and the solvent-solvent forces to achieve the solute-solvent attraction.

The *solubility* of an agent in a particular solvent indicates the *maximum* concentration to which a solution may be prepared with that agent and that solvent. When a solvent, at a given temperature, has dissolved all of the solute it can, it is said to be *saturated.* To emphasize the possible variation in solubility between two chemical agents and therefore in the amounts of each required to prepare a saturated solution, two official aqueous saturated solutions are cited as examples, Calcium Hydroxide Topical Solution, USP, and Potassium Iodide Oral Solution, USP. The first solution, prepared by agitating an excess amount of calcium hydroxide with purified water, contains only about 140 mg of dissolved solute per 100 mL of solution at 25°C, whereas the latter solution contains about 100 g of solute per 100 mL of solution, over 700 times as much solute as present in the calcium hydroxide topical solution. It is apparent from this comparison that the maximum possible concentration to which a pharmacist may prepare a solution varies greatly and is dependent, in part, on the chemical constitution of the solute. Through selection of a different solubilizing agent or a different chemical salt form of the medicinal agent, alteration of the pH of a solution, or substitution, in part or in whole, of the solvent, a pharmacist can in certain instances dissolve greater quantities of a solute than would otherwise be possible. For example, iodine granules are soluble in water only to the extent of 1 g in about 3000 mL of water. Using only these two agents, the maximum concentration possible would be approximately 0.03% of iodine in aqueous solution. However, through the use of an aqueous solution of potassium or sodium iodide as the solvent, much larger amounts of iodine may be dissolved as the result of the formation of a water-soluble complex with the iodide salt. This reaction is taken advantage of, for example, in Iodine Topical Solution, USP, prepared to contain about 2% of iodine and 2.4% of sodium iodide.

Temperature is an important factor in determining the solubility of a drug and in preparing its solution. Most chemicals absorb heat when they are dissolved and are said to have a *positive heat of solution,* resulting in increased solubility with an increase in temperature. A few chemicals have a *negative heat of solution* and exhibit a decrease in solubility with a rise in temperature. Other factors, in addition to temperature, affect solubility. These include the various chemical and other physical properties of both the solute and the solvent, factors of pressure, the acidity or basicity of the solution, the state of subdivision of the solute, and the physical agitation applied to the solution during the dissolving process. The solubility of a pure chemical substance at a given temperature and pressure is constant; however, its *rate of solution,* that is, the speed at which it dissolves, depends on the particle size of the substance and the extent of agitation. The finer the powder, the greater the surface area that comes in contact with the solvent, and the more rapid the dissolving process. Also, the greater the agitation, the more unsaturated solvent passes over the drug, and the faster the formation of the solution.

The solubility of a substance in a given solvent may be determined by preparing a saturated solution of it at a specific temperature and determining by chemical analysis the amount of chemical dissolved in a given weight of solution. By simple calculation, the amount of solvent required to dissolve the amount of solute can be determined. The solubility may then be expressed as grams of solute dissolving in milliliters of solvent—for example, "1 g of sodium chloride dissolves in 2.8 mL of water." When the exact solubility has not been determined, general expressions of relative solubility may be used. These terms are defined in the USP as presented in Table 12.1 (2).

A great many of the important organic medicinal agents are either weak acids or weak bases, and their solubility is dependent to a large measure on the pH of the solvent. These drugs react either with strong acids or strong bases to form water-soluble salts. For instance, the weak bases, including many of the alkaloids (atropine, codeine, and morphine), antihistamines (diphenhydramine and tripelennamine), local anesthetics (cocaine, procaine, and tetracaine), and other important drugs are not very water-soluble, but they are soluble in dilute solutions of acids. Pharmaceutical manufacturers have prepared many acid salts of these organic bases to enable the preparation of aqueous solutions. It must be recognized, however, that if the pH of the aqueous solutions of these salts is changed by the addition of alkali, the free base may separate from solution unless it has adequate solubility in water. Organic medicinals that are weak acids include the barbiturate drugs (as phenobarbital and pentobarbital) and the sulfonamides (as sulfadiazine and sulfacetamide). These and other weak acids form water-soluble salts in basic solution and may separate from solution by a lowering of the pH. Table 12.2 presents the comparative solubilities of some typical examples of weak acids and weak bases and their salts.

Table 12.1. Relative Terms of Solubility (2)

Descriptive Term	Parts of Solvent Required for 1 Part of Solute
Very soluble	Less than 1
Freely soluble	From 1 to 10
Soluble	From 10 to 30
Sparingly soluble	From 30 to 100
Slightly soluble	From 100 to 1000
Very slightly soluble	From 1000 to 10,000
Practically insoluble or insoluble	10,000 and over

Table 12.2. Water and Alcohol Solubilities of Some Selected Weak Acids, Weak Bases, and Their Salts

Drug	Number of mL of Solvent Required to Dissolve 1 g of Drug	
	Water	Alcohol
Atropine	455	2
Atropine sulfate	0.5	5
Codeine	120	2
Codeine sulfate	30	1,280
Codeine phosphate	2.5	325
Morphine	5,000	210
Morphine sulfate	16	565
Phenobarbital	1,000	8
Phenobarbital sodium	1	10
Procaine	200	soluble
Procaine hydrochloride	1	15
Sulfadiazine	13,000	sparingly soluble
Sodium sulfadiazine	2	slightly soluble

Although there are no exact rules for predicting unerringly the solubility of a chemical agent in a particular liquid, experienced pharmaceutical chemists can estimate the general solubility of a chemical compound based on its molecular structure and functional groups. The information gathered on a great number of individual chemical compounds has led to the characterization of the solubilities of groups of compounds, and though there may be an occasional inaccuracy with respect to an individual member of a group of compounds, the generalizations nonetheless serve a useful function. As demonstrated by the data in Table 12.2 and other similar data, salts of organic compounds are more soluble in water than are the corresponding organic bases. Conversely, the organic bases are more soluble in organic solvents, including alcohol, than are the corresponding salt forms. Perhaps the most written guideline for the prediction of solubility is that "like dissolves like," meaning that a solvent having a chemical structure most similar to that of the intended solute will be most likely to dissolve it. Thus, organic compounds are more soluble in organic solvents than in water. Organic compounds may, however, be somewhat water-soluble if they contain polar groups capable of forming hydrogen bonds with water. In fact, the greater the number of polar groups present, the greater will likely be the organic compound's solubility in water. Polar groups include OH, CHO, COH, CHOH, CH_2OH, COOH, NO_2, CO, NH_2, and SO_3H. The introduction of halogen atoms into a molecule tends to decrease water-solubility because of an increase in the molecular weight of the compound without a proportionate increase in polarity. An increase in the molecular weight of an organic compound without a change in polarity results in decreased solubility in water. Table 12.3 demonstrates some of these generalities through the use of specific chemical examples.

As with organic compounds, the pharmacist is aware of some general patterns of solubility that apply to inorganic compounds. For instance, most salts of monovalent cations such as sodium, potassium, and ammonium are water soluble, whereas the divalent cations like calcium, magnesium, and barium usually form water-soluble compounds with nitrate, acetate, and chloride anions but not with carbonate, phosphate, or hydroxide anions. To be sure, there are certain combinations of anion and cation that would seem to be similar in make-up but that do not have similar solubility characteristics. For instance, magnesium sulfate (Epsom salt) is soluble, but calcium sulfate is only slightly soluble; barium sulfate is very insoluble (1 g dissolves in about 400,000 mL of water) and is used as an opaque media for x-ray observation of the intestinal tract, but barium sulfide and barium sulfite are not as insoluble, and their oral use can result in poisoning; mercurous chloride (HgCl) is insoluble and was formerly used as a cathartic, but mercuric chloride ($HgCl_2$) is soluble in water and is a deadly poison if taken internally. There are many instances in which solubilities of certain drugs and their differentiation from other drugs are critical to the pharmacist in order that he or she might avoid compounding failures or therapeutic disasters.

Table 12.3. Solubilities of Selected Organic Compounds in Water as a Demonstration of Chemical Structure-Solubility Relationship

Compound	Formula	Number of mL of Water Required to Dissolve 1 g of Compound
Benzene	C_6H_6	1430
Benzoic acid	C_6H_5COOH	275
Benzyl alcohol	$C_6H_5CH_2OH$	25
Phenol	C_6H_5OH	15
Pyrocatechol	$C_6H_4(OH)_2$	2.3
Pyrogallol	$C_6H_3(OH)_3$	1.7
Carbon tetrachloride	CCl_4	2,000
Chloroform	$CHCl_3$	200
Methylene chloride	CH_2Cl_2	50

For organic as well as for inorganic solutes, the ability of a solvent to dissolve them depends on its effectiveness in overcoming the electronic forces that hold the atoms of the solute together and the corresponding lack of resolute on the part of the atoms themselves to resist the solvent action. During the dissolution process, the molecules of the solvent and the solute become uniformly mixed and cohesive forces of the atoms are replaced by new forces due to the attraction of the solute and solvent molecules for one another.

The student may find the following general rules of solubility useful.

Inorganic Molecules

1. If *both* the cation and anion of an ionic compound are *monovalent,* the solute-solute attractive forces are usually easily overcome, and therefore, these compounds are generally water soluble. (Examples, NaCl, LiBr, KI, NH_4NO_3, $NaNO_2$)
2. If only one of the two ions in an ionic compound is *monovalent,* the solute-solute interactions are also usually easily overcome and the compounds are water soluble. (Examples: $BaCl_2$, MgI_2, Na_2SO_4, Na_3PO_4)
3. If *both* the cation and anion are *multivalent,* the solute-solute interaction may be too great to be overcome by the solute-solvent interaction and the compound may have poor water solubility. (Examples: $CaSO_4$, $BaSO_4$, $BiPO_4$; Exceptions: $ZnSO_4$, $FeSO_4$)
4. Common salts of alkali metals (Na, K, Li, Cs, Rb) are usually water soluble. (Exception: Li_2CO_3)
5. Ammonium and quaternary ammonium salts are water soluble.
6. Nitrates, nitrites, acetates, chlorates, and lactates are generally water soluble. (Exceptions: silver and mercurous acetate)
7. Sulfates, sulfites, and thiosulfates are generally water soluble. (Exceptions: calcium and barium salts)
8. Chlorides, bromides, and iodides are water soluble. (Exceptions: salts of silver and mercurous ions)
9. Acid salts corresponding to an insoluble salt will be more water soluble than the original salt.
10. Hydroxides and oxides of compounds other than alkali metal cations and the ammonium ion are generally water insoluble.

11. Sulfides are water insoluble except for their alkali metal salts.
12. Phosphates, carbonates, silicates, borates, and hypochlorites are water insoluble except for their alkali metal salts and ammonium salts.

Organic Molecules

1. Molecules having one polar functional group are usually soluble to total chain lengths of five carbons.
2. Molecules having branched chains are more soluble than the corresponding straight-chain compound.
3. Water solubility decreases with an increase in molecular weight.
4. Increased structural similarity between solute and solvent is accompanied by increased solubility.

It is the pharmacist's knowledge of the chemical characteristics of drugs that permits the selection of the proper solvent for a particular solute. However, in addition to the factors of solubility, the selection is based on such additional solvent characteristics as clarity, low toxicity, viscosity, compatibility with other formulative ingredients, chemical inertness, palatability, odor, color, and economy. In most instances, and especially for solutions to be taken orally, used ophthalmically, or injected, water is the preferred solvent because it comes closer to meeting the majority of the above criteria than the other available solvents. In many instances, when water is used as the primary solvent, an auxiliary solvent is also employed to augment the solvent action of water or to contribute to a product's chemical or physical stability. Alcohol, glycerin, and propylene glycol, perhaps the most used auxiliary solvents, have been quite effective in contributing to the desired characteristics of pharmaceutical solutions and in maintaining their stability.

Other solvents, such as acetone, ethyl oxide, and isopropyl alcohol, are too toxic to be permitted in pharmaceutical preparations to be taken internally, but they are useful as reagent solvents in organic chemistry and in the preparatory stages of drug development, as in the extraction or removal of active constituents from medicinal plants. For purposes such as this, certain solvents are officially recognized in the compendia. A number of fixed oils, such as corn oil, cottonseed oil, peanut oil, and sesame oil, serve useful solvent functions particularly in the preparation of oleaginous injections and are recognized in the official compendia for this purpose.

Some Solvents For Liquid Preparations

The following agents find use as solvents in the preparation of solutions.

Alcohol, USP (Ethyl Alcohol, Ethanol, C_2H_5OH)

Next to water, alcohol is the most useful solvent in pharmacy. It is used as a primary solvent for many organic compounds. Together with water it forms a hydroalcoholic mixture that dissolves both alcohol-soluble and water-soluble substances, a feature especially useful in the extraction of active constituents from crude drugs. By varying the proportion of the two agents, the active constituents may be selectively dissolved and extracted or allowed to remain behind according to their particular solubility characteristics in the menstruum. Alcohol, USP, is 94.9 to 96.0% C_2H_5OH by volume (i.e., v/v) when determined at 15.56°C, the U.S. Government's standard temperature for alcohol determinations. *Dehydrated Alcohol,* USP, contains not less than 99.5% C_2H_5OH by volume and is utilized in instances in which an essentially water-free alcohol is desired.

Alcohol has been well recognized as a solvent and excipient in the formulation of oral pharmaceutical products. Certain drugs are insoluble in water and must be dissolved in an alternate vehicle. Alcohol is often preferred because of its miscibility with water and its ability to dissolve many water-insoluble ingredients, including drug substances, flavorants, and antimicrobial preservatives. Alcohol is frequently used with other solvents, as glycols and glycerin, to reduce the amount of alcohol required. It also is used in liquid products as an antimicrobial preservative alone or as a copreservative with parabens, benzoates, sorbates, and other agents.

However, aside from its pharmaceutic advantages as a solvent and preservative, concern has been expressed over the undesired pharmacologic and potential toxic effects of alcohol when ingested in pharmaceutical products particularly by children. Thus, the FDA has proposed that manufacturers of OTC oral drug products restrict, insofar as possible, the use of alcohol and include appropriate warnings in the labeling. For OTC oral products intended for children under 6 years of age, the recommended alcohol-content limit is 0.5%; for products intended for children 6 to 12 years of age, the recommended limit is 5%; and for products recommended for children over 12 years of age and for adults, the recommended limit is 10%.

Diluted Alcohol, NF

Diluted Alcohol, NF, is prepared by mixing equal volumes of Alcohol, USP, and Purified Water, USP. The final volume of such mixtures is not the sum of the individual volumes of the two components, but due to contraction of the liquids upon mixing, the final volume is generally about 3% less than what would normally be expected. Thus when 50 mL of each component is combined, the resulting product measures approximately 97 mL. It is for this reason that the strength of Diluted Alcohol, NF, is not exactly half that of the more concentrated alcohol, but slightly greater, approximately 49%. Diluted alcohol is a useful hydroalcoholic solvent in various pharmaceutical processes and preparations.

Alcohol, Rubbing

Rubbing Alcohol contains about 70% of ethyl alcohol by volume, the remainder consisting of water, denaturants with or without color additives and perfume oils, and stabilizers. In each 100 mL, it must contain not less than 355 mg of sucrose octaacetate or 1.4 mg of denatonium benzoate, bitter substances that discourage accidental or abusive oral ingestion. The denaturants employed in rubbing alcohol are according to the Internal Revenue Service, U.S. Treasure Department, Formula 23-H, which is composed of 8 parts by volume of acetone, 1.5 parts by volume of methyl isobutyl ketone, and 100 parts by volume of ethyl alcohol. The use of this denaturant mixture makes the separation of ethyl alcohol from the denaturants a virtually impossible task with ordinary distillation apparatus. This discourages the illegal removal and use as a beverage of the alcoholic content of rubbing alcohol.

The product is volatile and flammable and should be stored in tight containers remote from fire. It is employed as a rubefacient externally and as a soothing rub for bedridden patients, a germicide for instruments, and a skin cleanser prior to injection. It is also used as a vehicle for topical preparations. Synonym: Alcohol Rubbing Compound.

Glycerin, USP (Glycerol), $CH_2OH \cdot CHOH \cdot CH_2OH$

Glycerin is a clear syrupy liquid with a sweet taste. It is miscible both with water and alcohol. As a solvent, it is comparable with alcohol, but because of its viscosity, solutes are slowly soluble in it unless it is rendered less viscous by heating. Glycerin has preservative qualities and is often used as a stabilizer and as an auxiliary solvent in conjunction with water or alcohol. It is used in many internal preparations.

Isopropyl Rubbing Alcohol

Isopropyl Rubbing Alcohol is about 70% by volume isopropyl alcohol, the remainder consisting of water with or without color additives, stabilizers, and perfume oils. It is used externally as a rubefacient and soothing rub and as a vehicle for topical products. This preparation and a commercially available 91% isopropyl alcohol solution are commonly employed by diabetic patients in preparing needles and syringes for hypodermic injections of insulin and for disinfecting the skin.

Propylene Glycol, USP, $Ch_3CH(OH)CH_2OH$

Propylene glycol, a viscous liquid, is miscible with water and alcohol. It is a useful solvent with a wide range of applications and is frequently substituted for glycerin in modern pharmaceutical formulations.

Purified Water, USP, H_2O

Naturally occurring water exerts its solvent effect on most substances it contacts and thus is impure and contains varying amounts of dissolved inorganic salts, usually sodium, potassium, calcium, magnesium, and iron, chlorides, sulfates, and bicarbonates, as well as dissolved and undissolved organic matter and microorganisms. Water found in most cities and towns where water is purified for drinking purposes usually contains less than 0.1% of total solids, determined by evaporating a 100 mL sample of water to dryness and weighing the residue (which would weigh less than 100 mg). Drinking water must meet the United States Public Health Service regulations with respect to bacteriological purity. Acceptable drinking water should be clear, colorless, odorless, and neutral or only slightly acid or alkaline, the deviation from neutral being due to the nature of the dissolved solids and gases (carbon dioxide contributing to the acidity and ammonia to the alkalinity of water).

Ordinary drinking water obtained from the tap is not generally acceptable for the manufacture of most aqueous pharmaceutical preparations or for the extemporaneous compounding of prescriptions because of the chemical incompatibilities that may result from the combination of dissolved solids present and the medicinal agents being added. Signs of such incompatibilities are precipitation, discoloration, and occasionally effervescence. Its use is permitted in the washing and in the extraction of crude vegetable drugs, in the preparation of certain products for external use, and in other instances in which the difference between the use of water and purified water is of no consequence. Naturally, when large volumes of water are required to clean pharmaceutical machinery and equipment, tap water may be economically employed so long as a residue of solids is prevented by using purified water as the final rinse or by wiping the water dry with a meticulously clean cloth.

Purified Water, USP is obtained by distillation, ion-exchange treatment, reverse osmosis, or other suitable process. It is prepared from water complying with the federal Environmental Protection Agency with respect to drinking water. Compared with ordinary drinking water, Purified Water, USP is more free of solid impurities. When evaporated to dryness, it must not yield greater than 0.001% of residue (1 mg of total solids per 100 mL of sample evaporated). Thus purified water is 100 times more free of dissolved solids than is water. Purified Water, USP is intended for use in the preparation of aqueous dosage forms, *except* those intended for parenteral administration (injections). For the latter purpose, Water for Injection, USP, Bacteriostatic Water for Injection, USP, or Sterile Water for Injection, USP, are utilized. These are discussed in Chapter 14.

The main methods used in the preparation of purified water are distillation and ion-exchange; these methods are described briefly as follows.

Distillation Method

To prepare purified water, there are many commercially available stills in various sizes and styles with various capacities of from about one-half to 100 gallons of distillate per hour. Generally the first portion of aqueous distillate (about the first 10 to 20%) must be discarded, since it contains many foreign volatile substances usually found in urban drinking water, the usual starting material in the preparation of purified water. Also, the last portion of water (about 10% of the original volume of water) remaining in the distillation apparatus must be discarded and not subjected to further distillation because distillation to dryness would undoubtedly result in the decomposition of the remaining solid impurities to

volatile substances that would distill and contaminate the previously collected portion of distillate.

Ion-Exchange Method

On a large or small scale, the ion-exchange method for the preparation of purified water offers a number of advantages over the distillation method. For one thing, the requirement of heat is eliminated and with it costly and troublesome maintenance frequently encountered in the operation of the more complex distillation apparatus. Because of the simpler equipment and the nature of the method, the ion-exchange process permits ease of operation, minimal maintenance, and a more mobile facility. Many pharmacies and small laboratories that purchase large volumes of distilled water from commercial suppliers for use in their work would no doubt benefit financially and in convenience through the installation of an ion-exchange demineralizer in the work area.

The ion-exchange equipment in use today generally involves the passage of water through a column of cation and anion exchangers, consisting of water-insoluble, synthetic, polymerized phenolic, carboxylic, amino, or sulfonated resins of high molecular weight. These resins are mainly of two types: a) the cation, or acid exchangers, which permit the exchange of the cations in solution (in the tap water) with hydrogen ion from the resin; b) the anion, or base exchange resins, which permit the removal of anions. These two processes are successively or simultaneously employed to remove both cations and anions from water. The processes are indicated as follows, with M^+ indicating the metal or cation (as Na^+) and the X-indicating the anion (as Cl^-).

Cation Exchange

$$H\text{-Resin} + M^+ + X^- + H_2O \rightarrow M\text{-Resin} + H^+ + X^- + H_2O \text{ (pure)}$$

Anion Exchange

$$Resin\text{-}NH_2 + H^+ + X^- + H_2O \rightarrow Resin\text{-}NH_2 \cdot HX + H_2O \text{ (pure)}$$

Water purified in this manner is referred to as *demineralized* or *de-ionized water*, and may be used in any pharmaceutical preparation or prescription calling for distilled water.

Reverse Osmosis

This is one of the processes referred to in the industry as crossflow (or tangential flow) membrane filtration (3). In this process, a pressurized stream of water is passed *parallel to* the inner side of a filter membrane core. A portion of the feed water, or influent, permeates the membrane as filtrate, while the balance of the water sweeps tangentially along the membrane to exit the system without being filtered. The filtered portion is called the *permeate* because it has permeated the membrane. The water that has passed through the system is referred to as the *concentrate,* because it contains the concentrated contaminants rejected by the membrane. Whereas, in *osmosis,* the flow through a semi-permeable membrane is from a less concentrated solution to a more concentrated solution, the flow in this crossflow system is from a more concentrated to a less concentrated solution—thus the term *reverse osmosis.* Depending on their pore size, crossflow filter membranes can remove particles defined in the range of *microfiltration* (0.1 to 2 microns, e.g., bacteria); *ultrafiltration* (0.01 to 0.1 microns, e.g., virus); *nanofiltration* (0.001 to 0.01 microns, e.g., organic compounds in the molecular weight range of 300 to 1000); and *reverse osmosis* (particles smaller than 0.001 microns). Reverse osmosis removes virtually all virus, bacteria, pyrogens, organic molecules, and 90–99% of all ions (3).

Preparation of Solutions

Most pharmaceutical solutions are unsaturated with solute. Thus the amounts of solute to be dissolved are usually well below the capacity of the volume of solvent employed. The strengths of pharmaceutical preparations are usually expressed in terms of % *strength,* although for very dilute preparations, expressions of *ratio strength* may be used. These expressions and examples are shown in Table 12.4.

The term %, when used without qualification (as with w/v, v/v, or w/w) means % weight-in-volume for solutions or suspensions of solids in liquids; % weight-in-volume for solutions of gases in liquids; % volume-in-volume for solutions of liquids in liquids; and weight-in-weight for mixtures of solids and semisolids.

Some chemical agents that may be soluble in a given solvent are only slowly soluble and require an extended time for dissolving. To hasten the dissolution process, a pharmacist may employ one or several techniques; such as applying heat, reducing the particle size of the solute, utilizing a solubilizing agent, or subjecting the ingredients to rigorous agitation during the preparation of the solution. Normally, most chemical agents are more soluble in solvents at elevated temperatures than at room temperature or below because an endothermic reaction between the solute and the solvent utilizes the energy of the heat to enhance the dissolution process. However, elevated temperatures cannot be maintained for pharmaceuticals, and the net effect of heat is simply an increase in the *rate* of solution rather than an increase in solubility. An increased rate is satisfactory to the pharmacist, because most of his solutions are unsaturated anyway and do not require the presence of solute above the normal capacity of the solvent at room temperature. Pharmacists are reluctant to use heat to facilitate solution, and when they do, they are careful not to exceed the minimally required tem-

Table 12.4. Common Methods of Expressing the Strengths of Pharmaceutical Preparations

Expression	Abbreviated Expression	Meaning and Example
Percent weight-in-volume	% w/v	number of grams of a constituent in 100 mL of preparation (e.g., 1% w/v = 1 g of constituent in 100 mL of preparation).
Percent volume-in-volume	% v/v	number of mL of a constituent in 100 mL of preparation (e.g., 1% v/v 1 mL of constituent in 100 mL of preparation).
Percent weight-in-weight	% w/w	number of grams of a constituent in 100 g of preparation (e. g., 1% w/w = 1 g of constituent in 100 g of preparation).
Ratio strength, weight-in-volume	——:—— w/v	number of grams of constituent in stated number of mL of preparation (e.g., 1:1000 w/v = 1 g of constituent in 1000 mL of preparation).
Ratio strength, volume-in-volume	——:—— v/v	number of mL of constituent in stated number of mL of preparation (e.g., 1:1000 v/v = 1 mL of constituent in 1000 mL of preparation).
Ratio strength, weight-in-weight	——:—— w/w	number of grams of constituent in stated number of grams of preparation (e.g., 1:1000 w/w = 1 g of constituent in 1000 g of preparation).

perature, for many medicinal agents are destroyed at elevated temperatures, and the advantage of rapid solution may be completely offset by drug deterioration. If volatile solutes are to be dissolved or if the solvent is volatile (as alcohol), the heat would encourage the loss of these agents to the atmosphere and must therefore be avoided. Pharmacists are aware that certain chemical agents, particularly calcium salts, undergo exothermic reactions as they dissolve and give off heat. For such materials the use of heat would actually discourage the formation of a solution. The best pharmaceutical example of this type of chemical is calcium hydroxide, which is used in the preparation of Calcium Hydroxide Topical Solution, USP. This solute is soluble in water to the extent of 140 mg per 100 mL of solution at 25°C (about 77°F) and 170 mg per 100 mL of solution at 15°C (about 59°F). Obviously the temperature at which the solution is prepared or stored can affect the concentration of the resultant solution.

In addition to, or instead of, raising the temperature of the solvent to increase the rate of solution, a pharmacist may choose to decrease the particle size of the solute. This may be accomplished by the *comminution* (grinding a solid to a fine state of subdivision) of the solute with a mortar and pestle on a small scale or industrial micronizer on a large scale. The reduced particle size causes an increase in the surface area of the substance exposed to the solvent. If the powder is placed in a suitable vessel (as a beaker, graduate cylinder, or bottle) with a portion of the solvent and is stirred or shaken, as suited to the container, the rate of solution may be increased due to the continued circulation of fresh solvent to the drug's surface and the constant removal of newly formed solution from the drug's surface.

Most solutions are prepared by simple solution of the solutes in the solvent or solvent mixture. On an industrial scale, solutions are prepared in large mixing vessels with ports for mechanical stirrers to effect solution (Fig. 12.1). When heat is desired, thermostatically controlled mixing tanks may be used.

Oral Solutions and Preparations for Oral Solution

Solutions intended for oral administration usually contain flavorants and colorants to make the

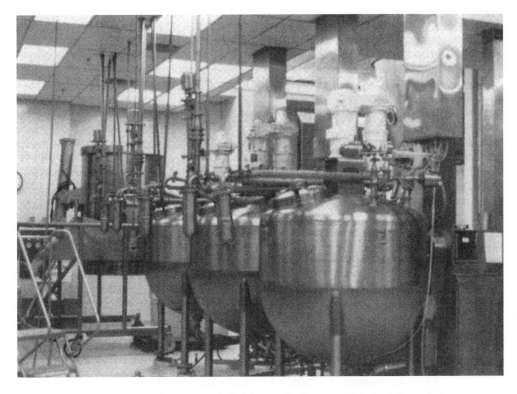

Fig. 12.1 *Large scale pharmaceutical mixing vessels. (Courtesy of Schering Laboratories.)*

medication more attractive and palatable for the patient. When needed, they may also contain stabilizers to maintain the chemical and physical stability of the medicinal agents and preservatives to prevent the growth of microorganisms in the solution. The formulation pharmacist must be wary of chemical interactions which may occur between the various components of a solution which may result in an alteration in the preparation's stability and/or potency. For instance, it has been demonstrated that esters of p-hydroxybenzoic acid (methyl-, ethyl-, propyl-, and butylparabens), frequently used preservatives in oral preparations, have a tendency to partition into certain flavoring oils (4). This partitioning effect could reduce the effective concentration of the preservatives in the aqueous medium of a pharmaceutical product below the level needed for preservative action.

Liquid pharmaceuticals for oral administration are usually formulated such that the patient receives the usual dose of the medication in a conveniently administered volume, as 5 mL (one teaspoonful), 10 mL, or 15 mL (one tablespoonful). A few solutions have unusually large doses, as Magnesium Citrate Oral Solution, USP with a usual adult dose of 200 mL. On the other hand many solutions used in pediatric patients are given by drop, utilizing a calibrated dropper usually furnished by the manufacturer in the product package.

Dry Mixtures for Solution

A number of medicinal agents, particularly certain antibiotics, have insufficient stability in aqueous solution to meet extended shelf-life periods. Thus, commercial manufacturers of these products provide them to the pharmacist in dry powder or granule form for reconstitution with a prescribed amount of purified water immediately before dispensing to the patient. The dry powder mixture contains all of the formulative components including drug, flavorant, colorant, buffers, and others, except for the solvent. Once reconstituted by the pharmacist the resultant solutions remain stable when stored in the refrigerator for the labeled periods, usually from 7 to 14 days depending upon the preparation. This is a sufficient period of time for the patient to complete the volume of medication usually prescribed. However, if medication remains after the patient completes the course of therapy, instructions should be explained to discard the remaining portion which would be unfit for use at a later date.

Examples of dry powder mixtures intended for reconstitution to oral solutions are the following:

Cloxacillin Sodium for Oral Solution, USP (Teva); an antiinfective antibiotic

Oxacillin Sodium for Oral Solution, USP [Prostaphlin (Teva)]; an antiinfective antibiotic

Penicillin V Potassium for Oral Solution, USP [Pen-Vee K (Wyeth-Ayerst)]; an antiinfective antibiotic

Potassium Chloride for Oral Solution, USP [K-LOR (Abbott)]; a potassium supplement

Oral Solutions

In the practice of pharmacy, the pharmacist may be called on to dispense a commercially prepared oral solution; dilute the concentration of a solution, as in the preparation of a pediatric form of an adult product; prepare a solution through the reconstitution of a dry powder mixture; or extemporaneously compound an oral solution from bulk components.

In each instance, the pharmacist should be sufficiently knowledgeable of the dispensed product to expertly advise the patient of the proper use, dosage, method of administration, and storage of the product. Knowledge of the solubility and stability characteristics of the medicinal agents and the solvents employed in the commercial products is useful to the pharmacist in informing the patient of the advisability of mixing the solution with juice, milk, or other beverages upon administration. Information regarding the solvents used in each commercial product appears on the product label and in the accompanying package insert. Table 12.5 presents examples of some oral solutions. Some solutions of special pharmaceutical interest are described later in this chapter.

Oral Rehydration Solutions

Rapid fluid loss associated with diarrhea can lead to dehydration and ultimately death in some patients, particularly infants. More than five million children younger than 4 years of age die due to diarrheal illnesses each year worldwide (5). Diarrhea is characterized by an increased frequency of loose, watery stools, and because there is an intensive fluid loss, dehydration can be an outcome. During diarrhea, the small intestine secretes far above the normal amount of fluid and electrolytes, and this simply exceeds the ability of the large intestine to reabsorb it. This fluid loss occurs mostly from the body's extracellular fluid compartment and can lead to a progressive loss of blood volume culminating in hypovolemic shock.

Table 12.5. Examples of Oral Solutions by Category

Oral Solution	Some Representative Commercial Products	Concentration of Commercial Product	Comments
Antidepressants			
Nortriptyline HCl Oral Solution	Pamelor Oral Solution (Novartis)	10 mg nortriptyline/5 mL	Tricyclic antidepressant
Fluoxetine HCl	Prozac Liquid (Dista)	20 mg fluoxetine/5 mL	Used in the treatment of depression and for obsessive-compulsive disorder.
Antiperistaltic			
Diphenoxylate HCl and Atropine Sulfate Oral Solution	Lomotil Liquid (Searle)	2.5 mg of diphenoxylate HCl and 0.025 mg of atropine sulfate/5 mL	This preparation is indicated in the management of diarrhea. Diphenoxylate is related structurally and pharmacologically to the narcotic meperidine. Atropine sulfate is added to the solution in subtherapeutic amounts to discourage (by virtue of side effects) deliberate overdosage.
Loperamide HCl Oral Solution	Imodium A-D Liquid (McNeil Consumer Products)	1 mg of loperamide HCl per 5 mL	This preparation is indicated for the treatment of diarrhea for both adults and children 6 years of age and older. Loperamide is structurally related to haloperidol.
Antipsychotics			
Haloperidol Oral Solution	Haldol Concentrate (Ortho-McNeil)	2 mg haloperidol/mL	These solutions are used primarily in severe neuropsychiatric conditions when oral medication is preferred and other oral dosage forms (as tablets and capsules) are considered impractical. The concentrated solutions are employed by adding the desired amount of the concentrate by calibrated dropper to soup or a beverage as tomato or fruit juices, milk, coffee, tea or carbonated beverages.
Perphenazine Oral Solution	Trilafon Concentrate (Schering)	16 mg perphenazine/5 mL	
Thiothixene HCl Oral Solution	Navane concentrate (Pfizer)	equivalent of 5 mg thiothixene/mL	
Bronchodilator			
Theophylline Oral Solution	Theophylline Oral Solution (Roxane)	80 mg of theophylline per 15 mL	This alcohol-free solution is used for the treatment of bronchial asthma and reversible bronchospasm associated with chronic bronchitis and emphysema.
Cathartics			
Magnesium Citrate Oral Solution, USP	—	amount of magnesium citrate equivalent to between 1.55 g and 1.9 g/100 mL of magnesium oxide	Discussed in text
Sodium Phosphate Oral Solution	Phospho-Soda (Fleet)	2.4 g monobasic sodium phosphate and 0.9 g dibasic sodium phosphate per 5 mL.	Works as laxative within 1 hour when taken before meals or overnight when taken at bedtime. Usual dose is 10 to 20 mL of solution, best taken diluted with one-half glass of water and followed with a full glass of water.

continued

Table 12.5.   Examples of Oral Solutions by Category

Oral Solution	Some Representative Commercial Products	Concentration of Commercial Product	Comments
Corticosteroid			
Prednisolone Sodium Phosphate Oral Liquid	Pediapred Oral Solution (Medeva)	5 mg prednisolone (as sodium phosphate) per 5 mL	Synthetic adrenocortical steroid with predominantly glucocorticoid properties indicated in the treatment of endocrine, rheumatic, collagen, allergic, and other disorders.
Dental Caries Protectant			
Sodium Fluoride Oral Solution	Pediaflor Drops (Boss)	0.5 mg/mL	Prophylaxis of dental caries; intended for use when community water supplies are inadequately fluoridated.
Electrolyte Replenisher			
Potassium Chloride Oral Solution	KaoChlor 10% Liquid (Savage)	20 mEq of KCl/15 mL, in a flavored aqueous vehicle	Used in conditions of hypopotassemia (low level of potassium in the blood). Condition may be prompted by severe or chronic diarrhea, a low level of potassium intake in the diet, increased renal excretion of potassium, and other causes. The solution is diluted with water or fruit juice before taking.
Fecal Softener			
Docusate Sodium Solution	Colace Syrup (Roberts)	10 mg docusate sodium/mL	Usually 50 to 200 mg of the drug is measured by calibrated dropper and mixed with milk, fruit juice, or other liquid (to mask the taste) before administration. The drug softens the fecal mass by lowering the surface tension, thus permitting normal bowel habits, particularly in geriatric, pediatric cardiac, obstetric, and surgical patients. Dosage is taken for several days or until bowel movements are normal.
Hematinic			
Ferrous Sulfate Oral Solution	Fer-In-Sol Drops (Mead Johnson Nutritional)	15 mg ferrous sulfate/ 0.6 mL	Used for prevention and treatment of iron deficiency anemias. Usual prophylactic dose of 0.3 or 0.6 mL measured by calibrated dropper and mixed with water, fruit juice, or vegetable juice before administration. Dosage form intended primarily for infants and children.
Histamine H$_2$ Antagonist			
Cimetidine HCl Liquid	Tagamet HCl Liquid (SmithKline Beecham)	300 mg of cimetidine HCl per 5 mL	This preparation is indicated to treat peptic ulcer disease and pathological hypersecretory conditions, e.g., Zollinger-Ellison syndrome.
Narcotic Agonist Analgesic			
Methadone HCl Oral Solution	Methadone HCL (Roxane)	1 or 2 mg/mL	For relief of severe pain; detoxification and maintenance treatment of narcotic addiction.
Vitamin D Source			
Ergocalciferol Solution	Calciferol Drops (Schwarz)	8,000 units/mL	A solution of water-insoluble ergocalciferol (vitamin D$_2$) in propylene glycol. The usual prophylactic dose of ergocalciferol is about 400 units and the therapeutic dose may be as high as 200,000 to 500,000 units daily in treating rickets.

Diarrhea is a normal physiologic body response to rid itself of a noxious or toxic substance, e.g., *Rotavirus, Escherichia coli*. Thus, the treatment approach is to allow the diarrhea to proceed and not to terminate it too quickly, but promptly replace the fluid and electrolytes that are lost to prevent dehydration. The loss of fluid during diarrhea is accompanied by a depletion of sodium, potassium and bicarbonate ions, which if severe can result, as mentioned, in hypovolemic shock, as well as acidosis, hyperpnea and vomiting. If continuous, bouts of vomiting and diarrhea can cause malnutrition as well. Consequently, the goal is to replace lost fecal water with an oral rehydration solution and utilize nutritional foods such as soybean formula and bran.

Oral rehydration solutions are usually effective in treatment of patients with mild volume depletion of 5 to 10% of body weight. These are available over-the-counter, are relatively inexpensive and their use has diminished the incidence of complications associated with parenterally-administered electrolyte solutions. Therapy with these solutions is based on the observation that glucose is actively absorbed from the small intestine, even during bouts of diarrhea. This active transport of glucose is advantageous because it is coupled with sodium absorption. Almost like in domino fashion, sodium absorption promotes anion absorption which in turn promotes water absorption to short circuit dehydration. To produce maximal absorption of sodium and water, studies have demonstrated that the optimal concentrations of glucose and sodium in an isotonic solution are 110 mM (2%) glucose and 60 mEq/L of sodium ion, respectively. Bicarbonate and/or citrate ions are also included in these solutions to help correct the subsequent metabolic acidosis which is caused by diarrhea and dehydration.

A typical oral rehydration solution contains 45 mEq Na^+, 20 mEq K^+, 35 mEq Cl^-, 30 mEq citrate, and 25 g of dextrose per liter. These formulations are available in liquid or powder/packet form for reconstitution. It is important that the user add the specific amount of water needed to prepare the powder forms. Further, these products should not be mixed with or given with other electrolyte-containing liquids, such as milk or fruit juices. Otherwise, there is no method to calculate how much electrolyte the patient actually received. Commercially available, ready-to-use oral electrolyte solutions to prevent dehydration or achieve rehydration include Pedialyte Solution (Ross), and Rehydrate Solution (Ross). These products also contain dextrose or glucose. Ricelyte Oral Solution (Mead Johnson) contains electrolytes in a syrup of rice solids. The rice-based formula produces a lower osmotic effect than the dextrose- or glucose-based formulas and is thought to be more effective in reducing stool output and shortening the duration of diarrhea. The pharmacist must discourage the production of homemade versions of electrolyte solutions. The success of the commercial solutions is based on the accuracy of the formulation. If prepared incorrectly, homemade preparations could cause hypernatremia or cause the diarrhea to worsen.

Oral Colonic Lavage Solution

Traditionally, the preparation of the bowel for procedures such as a colonoscopy have consisted of the administration of clear liquid diets for 24 to 48 hours preceding the procedure, the administration of oral laxatives, e.g., magnesium citrate or bisacodyl, the night before, and cleansing enemas administered 2 to 4 hours prior to procedure commencement. Typically, to circumvent the cost of having to hospitalize the patient the night before the procedure, patients were allowed to perform this regimen at home. However, while the results have been satisfactory, that is, the bowel is cleared for the procedure, poor patient compliance with and acceptance of this regimen can cause problems during the procedure. Further, additive effects of malnutrition and poor oral intake prior to the procedure can cause more patient problems.

Consequently, an alternative method to prepare the gastrointestinal tract has been devised. This procedure requires less time and dietary restriction and obviates the need for cleansing enemas. This method involves the oral administration of a balanced solution of electrolytes with polyethylene glycol (PEG-3350). Prior to its dispensing to the patient, the pharmacist reconstitutes this powder with water creating an iso-osmotic solution having a mildly salty taste. The polyethylene glycol acts as an osmotic agent within the gastrointestinal tract and the balanced electrolyte concentration results in virtually no net absorption or secretion of ions. Thus, a large volume of this solution can be administered without a significant change in water or electrolyte balance.

The formulation of this oral colonic lavage solution is as follows:

Polyethylene Glycol 3350	236.00 g
Sodium Sulfate	22.74 g
Sodium Bicarbonate	6.74 g
Sodium Chloride	5.86 g
Potassium Chloride	2.97 g

In 4800 mL disposable container.

The recommended adult dosage of this product is 4 L of solution before the gastrointestinal procedure. The patient is instructed to drink 240 mL of solution every 10 minutes until about 4 L are consumed. The patient is advised to drink each portion quickly rather than sipping it continuously. Usually, the first bowel movement will occur within 1 hour. Several regimens are utilized, and one method is to schedule patients for a midmorning procedure, allowing the patient 3 hours for drinking and a 1-hour waiting period to complete bowel evacuation.

To date, this approach to bowel evacuation has been associated with a low incidence of side effects, primarily nausea, transient abdominal fullness, bloating, and occasionally, cramps and vomiting. Ideally, the patient should not have taken any food 3 to 4 hours before beginning the administration of the solution. In no case should solid foods be taken by the patient for at least 2 hours before the solution is administered. No foods, except clear liquids, are permitted after this product is administered and prior to the examination. The product must be stored in the refrigerator after reconstitution, and this aids somewhat in decreasing the salty taste of the product.

Magnesium Citrate Oral Solution

Magnesium citrate oral solution is a colorless to slightly yellow, clear, effervescent liquid having a sweet, acidulous taste and a lemon flavor. It is commonly referred to as "Citrate" or as "Citrate of Magnesia." It is required to contain an amount of magnesium citrate equivalent to between 1.55 and 1.9 g of magnesium oxide in each 100 mL.

The solution is prepared by reacting official magnesium carbonate with an excess of citric acid (equation 1), flavoring and sweetening the solution with lemon oil and syrup, filtering with talc, and then carbonating it by the addition of either potassium or sodium bicarbonate (equation 2). The solution may be further carbonated by the use of carbon dioxide under pressure.

$$(1) \ (MgCO_3)_4 \cdot Mg(OH)_2 + 5H_3C_6H_5O_7 \rightarrow$$
$$5MgHC_6H_5O_7 + 4CO_2 + 6H_2O$$

$$(2) \ 3KHCO_3 + H_3C_6H_5O_7 \rightarrow K_3C_6H_5O_7$$
$$+ 3CO_2 + 3H_2O$$

The solution provides an excellent medium for the growth of molds, and any mold spores present during the manufacture of the solution must be killed if the preparation is to remain stable. For this reason, during the preparation of the solution the liquid is heated to boiling (prior to carbonation), boiled water is employed to bring the solution to its proper volume, and boiling water is used to rinse the final container. The final solution may be sterilized.

Magnesium citrate solution has always been troublesome because it has a tendency to deposit a crystalline solid upon standing. Apparently this is due to the formation of some almost insoluble, normal magnesium citrate (rather than the exclusively dibasic form as in equation 1). The cause of the problem has largely been attributed to the indefinite composition of the official magnesium carbonate, which by definition is "a basic hydrated magnesium carbonate or a normal hydrated magnesium carbonate" (see equation 1). It contains the equivalent of 40 to 43.5% of magnesium oxide. Apparently, solutions prepared from magnesium carbonates with differing equivalents of magnesium oxide vary in stability, with the most stable ones being prepared from samples of magnesium carbonate having the lower equivalent of magnesium oxide. The formula for the preparation of 350 mL of magnesium citrate solution calls for the use of 15 g of official magnesium carbonate, which corresponds to approximately 6.0 to 6.47 g of magnesium oxide.

In carbonating the solution, the bicarbonate may be added in tablet form rather than as a powder in order to delay the effervescence resulting from its contact with the citric acid. If the powder were used, the reaction would be immediate and violent, and it would be virtually impossible to close the bottle in time to prevent the loss of carbon dioxide or solution. The solution may be further carbonated by the use of CO_2 under pressure. Most of the magnesium citrate solutions prepared commercially today are packaged in the same type of bottles as "soft drink" carbonated beverages. The solution is packaged in bottles of 300 mL. Since the solution is carbonated, it loses some of its character if allowed to stand for a period of time after the container has been opened. Magnesium citrate solution is stored in a cold place, preferably in a refrigerator, keeping the bottle on its side so the cork or rubber liners of the caps are kept moist and swollen, thereby maintaining the airtight seal between the cap and the bottle.

The solution is employed as a saline cathartic, with the citric acid, lemon oil, syrup, carbonation, and the low temperature of the refrigerated solution all contributing to the patient's acceptance of the large volume of medication. For many patients it represents a pleasant way of taking an otherwise bitter saline cathartic.

Sodium Citrate and Citric Acid Oral Solution

This official solution contains 100 mg of sodium citrate and 67 mg of citric acid in each mL of aqueous solution. The solution is administered orally in doses of 10 to 30 mL as frequently as four times daily as a systemic alkalinizer. Systemic alkalinization is useful in patients having conditions in which long term maintenance of an alkaline urine is desirable, such as patients with uric acid and cystine calculi of the urinary tract. The solution is also a useful adjuvant when administered with uricosuric agents in gout therapy since urates tend to crystallize out of an acid urine.

Syrups

Syrups are concentrated, aqueous preparations of a sugar or sugar-substitute with or without added flavoring agents and medicinal substances. Syrups containing flavoring agents but not medicinal substances are called *nonmedicated* or *flavored vehicles* (syrups). Some official, previously official and examples of commercially available nonmedicated syrups are presented in Table 12.6. These syrups are intended to serve as pleasant-tasting vehicles for medicinal substances to be added in the extemporaneous compounding of prescriptions or in the preparation of a standard formula for a *medicated syrup,* which is a syrup containing a therapeutic agent. Due to the inability of some children and elderly people to swallow solid dosage forms, it is not unusual today for a pharmacist to be asked to prepare an oral liquid dosage form of a medication available in the pharmacy only as tablets or capsules. In doing so, considerations of drug solubility, stability, and bioavailability must be considered case by case (6,7). The liquid dosage form selected for compounding may be a solution or a suspension, depending upon the chemical and physical characteristics of the particular drug and its solid dosage form. Vehicles are commercially available for this purpose (7).

Medicated syrups are commercially prepared from the starting materials; that is, by combining each of the individual components of the syrup, as sucrose, purified water, flavoring agents, coloring agents, the therapeutic agent, and other necessary and desirable ingredients. Naturally, medicated syrups are employed in therapeutics for the value of the medicinal agent present in the syrup.

Syrups provide a pleasant means of administering a liquid form of a disagreeable tasting drug. They are particularly effective in the administration of drugs to youngsters, since their pleasant taste usually dissipates any reluctance on the part of the child to take the medicine. The fact that syrups contain little or no alcohol adds to their favor among parents.

Any water-soluble drug that is stable in aqueous solution may be added to a flavored syrup. However care must be exercised to ensure the compati-

Table 12.6. Examples of Nonmedicated Syrups (Vehicles)

Nonmedicated Syrup	*Comments*
Cherry Syrup	A sucrose-based syrup containing about 47% by volume of cherry juice. The syrup's tart and fruit flavor is attractive to most patients and the acidic pH of the syrup makes it useful as a vehicle for drugs requiring an acid medium.
Cocoa Syrup	This syrup is a suspension of cocoa powder in an aqueous vehicle sweetened and thickened with sucrose, liquid glucose, and glycerin, and flavored with vanilla and sodium chloride. The syrup is particularly effective in administering bitter tasting drugs to children.
Orange Syrup	This sucrose-based syrup utilizes sweet orange peel tincture, and citric acid as the source of flavor and tartness. The syrup resembles orange juice in taste and is a good vehicle for drugs stable in an acidic medium.
Ora-Sweet and Ora-Sweet SF (Paddock Laboratories)	Commercially available vehicles for the extemporaneous compounding of syrups. Both vehicles have a pH between 4 and 4.5 and are alcohol free. Ora-Sweet SF syrup is sugar free.
Raspberry Syrup	A sucrose-based syrup containing about 48% by volume of raspberry juice. It is a pleasantly flavored vehicle used to disguise the salty or sour taste of saline medicaments.
Syrup	This is an 85% solution of sucrose in purified water. This "simple syrup" may be used as the basis for the preparation of flavored or medicated syrups.

bility between the medicinal drug substance and the other formulative components of the syrup. Also, certain flavored syrups have an acidic medium, whereas others may be neutral or slightly basic and the proper selection must be made to insure the stability of any added medicinal agent. Perhaps the most frequently found types of medications administered as medicated syrups are antitussive agents and antihistamines. This is not to imply that other types of drugs are not formulated into syrups; a variety of medicinal substances can be found in syrup form and among the many commercial products. Examples of medicated syrups are presented in Table 12.7.

Components of Syrups

Most syrups contain the following components in addition to the purified water and any medicinal agents present: 1) the sugar, usually sucrose, or sugar-substitutes used to provide sweetness and viscosity, 2) antimicrobial preservatives, 3) flavorants, and 4) colorants. Also, many syrups, especially those prepared commercially, contain special solvents, solubilizing agents, thickeners, or stabilizers.

Sucrose and Non-Sucrose Based Syrups

Sucrose is the sugar most frequently employed in syrups, although in special circumstances it may be replaced in whole or in part by other sugars, as dextrose, or non-sugars as sorbitol, glycerin and propylene glycol. In some instances, all glycogenetic substances (materials converted to glucose in the body), including those agents mentioned above, are replaced by nonglycogenetic substances such as methylcellulose or hydroxyethylcellulose. These two materials are not hydrolyzed and absorbed into the blood stream, and their use results in an excellent syrup-like vehicle for medications intended for use by diabetic patients and others whose diets must be controlled and restricted to nonglycogenetic substances. The viscosity resulting from the use of these cellulose derivatives is much like that of a sucrose syrup. The addition of one or more artificial sweeteners usually produces an excellent facsimile of a true syrup.

The characteristic "body" that the sucrose and the alternative agents seek to impart to the syrup is essentially the result of attaining the proper viscosity. This quality, together with the sweetness and the flavorants added, results in a type of pharmaceutical preparation that masks the taste of added medicinal agents. When the syrup is swallowed, only a

portion of dissolved drug actually makes contact with the taste buds, the remainder of the drug being carried past them and down the throat in the containment of the viscous syrup. This type of physical concealment of the taste is not possible for a solution of a drug in an unthickened, mobile, aqueous preparation. In the case of antitussive syrups, the thick sweet syrup has a soothing effect on the irritated tissues of the throat as it passes over them.

Most syrups contain a high proportion of sucrose, usually 60 to 80%, not only because of the desirable sweetness and viscosity of such solutions but also because of their inherent stability in contrast to the unstable character of dilute sucrose solutions. The aqueous sugar medium of dilute sucrose solutions is an efficient nutrient medium for the growth of microorganisms, particularly yeasts and molds. On the other hand, concentrated sugar solutions are quite resistant to microbial growth, due to the unavailability of the water required for the growth of microorganisms. This aspect of syrups is best demonstrated by the simplest of all syrups, Syrup NF, which has the synonym of "simple syrup" and is prepared by dissolving 85 g of sucrose in enough purified water to make 100 mL of syrup. The resulting preparation requires no additional preservation; in fact, preservatives may not be added to this official syrup. When properly prepared and maintained, the syrup is inherently stable and resistant to the growth of microorganisms. An examination of this syrup reveals its concentrated nature and the relative absence of available water for microbial growth. Syrup has a specific gravity of about 1.313, which means that each 100 mL of syrup weighs 131.3 g. Because 85 g of sucrose are present, the difference between 85 g and 131.3 g or 46.3 g, represents the weight of the purified water present. Thus, 46.3 g, or mL, of purified water are used to dissolve the 85 g of sucrose. The solubility of sucrose in water is 1 g in 0.5 mL of water; therefore, to dissolve 85 g of sucrose, about 42.5 mL of water would be required. Thus, only a very slight excess of water (about 3.8 mL per 100 mL of syrup) is employed in the preparation of syrup. Although not enough to be particularly amenable to the growth of microorganisms, the slight excess of water permits the syrup to remain physically stable under conditions of varying temperatures. If the syrup were completely saturated with sucrose, under cool storage conditions some sucrose might crystallize from solution and, by acting as nuclei, initiate a type of chain reaction that would result in the separation of an amount of sucrose dispropor-

Table 12.7. Examples of Medicated Syrups by Category

Syrup	Some Representative Commercial Products	Concentration of Commercial Product*	Comments
Analgesic			
Meperidine HCl Syrup	Demerol Syrup (Sanofi)	50 mg meperidine HCl/5 mL	Narcotic analgesic indicated for relief of moderate to severe pain and as an adjunct to general anethesia.
Anticholinergics			
Dicyclomine HCl Syrup	Bentyl Syrup (Hoechst Marion Roussel)	10 mg dicyclomine HCl/5 mL	Used as adjunctive therapy in treatment of peptic ulcer.
Oxybutynin Chloride Syrup	Ditropan Syrup (Hoechst Marion Roussel)	5 mg of oxybutynin chloride per 5 mL	Used for the relief of symptoms associated with voiding in patients with uninhibited neurogenic and reflex neurogenic bladder.
Antiemetics			
Chlorpromazine HCl Syrup	Thorazine Syrup (SmithKline Beecham)	10 mg chlorpromazine HCl/5 mL	Used to control nausea and vomiting.
Dimenhydrinate Syrup	Childrens Dramamine Liquid (Pharmacia & Upjohn)	12.5 mg dimenhydrinate/ 5 mL	Used to control nausea, vomiting, and motion sickness.
Prochlorperazine Edisylate Syrup	Compazine Syrup (SmithKline Beecham)	5 mg prochlorperazine edisylate/5 mL	Used to control nausea and vomiting.
Promethazine HCl Syrup	Phenergan Syrup (Wyeth-Ayerst)	6.25 mg and 25 mg promethazine HCl/5 mL	Used to control nausea, vomiting, motion sickness, and allergic reactions.
Anticonvulsant			
Sodium Valproate Syrup	Depakene Syrup (Abbott)	250 mg of valproic acid (as sodium salt) per 5 mL	Used as the sole or adjunctive therapy in simple (petit mat) and complex absence seizure disorders.
Antihistamines			
Chlorpheniramine Maleate Syrup	Chlor-Trimeton Allergy Syrup (Schering-Plough)	2 mg chlorpheniramine maleate/5 mL	
Cyproheptadine HCl Syrup	Periactin Syrup (Merck & Co.)	2 mg cyproheptadine HCl/5 mL	All of the antihistamines listed are used for prevention and treatment of allergic reactions.
Hydroxyzine HCl Syrup	Atarax Syrup (Pfizer)	10 mg hydroxyzine HCl/5 mL	
Antipsychotic			
Lithium Citrate Syrup	Lithium Citrate Syrup (Roxane)	8 mEq lithium/5mL	Used in the management of psychotic disorders.
Antitussives			
Dextromethorphan Syrup	Benylin Adult Cough Formula (Warner-Lambert Consumer)	15 mg dextromethrophan/ 5 mL	For relief of cough.
Diphenhydramine Syrup	Benylin Allergy Liquid Medication (Warner-Lambert Consumer)	12.5 mg of diphenhydramine HCl per 5 mL	Used for the control of coughs due to colds or allergy.
Antiviral			
Amantadine HCl Syrup	Symmetrel Syrup (Endo)	50 mg amantadine HCl/ 5 mL	Prevention of respiratory infections caused by A_2 (Asian) viral strains. Treatment of idiopathic Parkinson's disease.

continued

Table 12.7.   Examples of Medicated Syrups by Category

Syrup	Some Representative Commercial Products	Concentration of Commercial Product*	Comments
Bronchodilators			
Albuterol Sulfate Syrup	Proventil Syrup (Schering) Ventolin Syrup (Allen & Hanburys)	2 mg of albuterol sulfate per 5 mL	Used for the relief of bronchospasm in patients with obstructive airway disease, and for the prevention of exercise induced bronchospasm.
Metaproterenol Sulfate Syrup	Alupent Syrup (Boehringer Ingelheim)	10 mg of metaproterenol sulfate per 5 mL	
Cathartic			
Lactulose Syrup	Chronulac Syrup (Hoechst Marion Roussel)	10 g of lactulose per 15 mL	Dose is 15 to 30 ml, daily as a laxative.
Cholinergic			
Pyridostigmine Bromide Syrup	Mestinon Syrup (ICN Pharmaceuticals)	60 mg pyridostigmine bromide/5 mL	Used in treatment of myasthenia gravis.
Decongestant			
Pseudoephedrine Hydrochloride Syrup	Children's Sudafed Liquid (Warner-Lambert)	15 mg of pseudoephedrine hydrochloride per 5 mL	Used for the temporary relief of nasal congestion due to the common cold, hay fever or other upper respiratory allergies, and nasal congestion associated with sinusitis.
Emetic			
Ipecac Syrup	Ipecac Syrup (Roxane)	21 mg ether-soluble alkaloids of ipecac/15 mL	Used to induce vomiting in poisoning. The dose of 15 ml, may be repeated in 20 minutes if vomiting does not occur. If after the second dose, vomiting does not occur, the stomach should be emptied by gastric lavage.
Expectorant			
Guaifenesin Syrup	Guaifenesin Syrup (Roxane)	100 mg guaifenesin/5 mL	For symptomatic relief of respiratory conditions associated with cough and bronchial congestion.
Fecal Softener			
Docusate Sodium Syrup	Colace Syrup (Roberts)	20 mg docusate sodium/5 mL	Stool softener by surface-action.
Gastrointestinal Stimulant			
Metoclopramide Syrup	Reglan Syrup (Robins)	5 mg of metoclopramide HCl per 5 mL	Used to provide relief of symptoms associated with diabetic gastroparesis (gastric stasis) and gastroesophageal reflux.
Hemostatic			
Aminocaproic Acid Syrup	Amicar Syrup (Immunex)	1.25 g aminocaproic acid/5 mL	Used in treatment of excessive bleeding resulting from systemic hyperfibrinolysis and urinary fibrinolysis.
Hypnotic/Sedative			
Chloral Hydrate Syrup	Chloral Hydrate Syrup (Pharmaceutical Associates)	500 mg chloral hydrate/5 mL	Sedative in doses of 250 mg and hypnotic to induce sleep at doses of 500 mg. Alcoholic beverages should be avoided when taking this syrup. The syrup is usually diluted with water or other beverage before taking.

*The amount per stated volume of syrup constitutes a usual single dose of the medication unless otherwise stated.

tionate to its solubility at the storage temperature. The syrup would then be very much unsaturated and probably suitable for microbial growth. As formulated, the official syrup is both stable and resistant to crystallization as well as to microbial growth. However, many of the other official syrups and a host of commercial syrups are not intended to be as nearly saturated as Syrup, NF, and therefore must employ added preservative agents to prevent microbial growth and to ensure their stability during their period of use and storage.

As noted earlier, sucrose-based syrup may be substituted in whole or in part by other agents in the preparation of medicated syrups. A solution of a polyol, as sorbitol, or a mixture of polyols, as sorbitol and glycerin, are commonly used. Sorbitol Solution, USP, which contains 64% by weight of the polyhydric alcohol sorbitol is employed as shown in the following example formulations for medicated syrups (8):

Antihistamine Syrup

Chlorpheniramine Maleate..........	0.4 g
Glycerin	25.0 mL
Syrup..	83.0 mL
Sorbitol Solution	282.0 mL
Sodium Benzoate...........................	1.0 g
Alcohol...	60.0 mL
Color and flavor	q.s.
Purified Water, to make	1000.0 mL

Ferrous Sulfate Syrup

Ferrous Sulfate	135.0 g
Citric Acid......................................	12.0 g
Sorbitol Solution	350.0 mL
Glycerin.	50.0 mL
Sodium Benzoate...........................	1.0 g
Flavor	q.s.
Purified Water, to make	1000.0 mL

Acetaminophen Syrup

Acetaminophen	24.0 g
Benzoic Acid..................................	1.0 g
Disodium Calcium EDTA.............	1.0 g
Propylene Glycol...........................	150.0 mL
Alcohol...	150.0 mL
Saccharin Sodium..........................	1.8 g
Purified Water...............................	200.0 mL
Flavor	q.s.
Sorbitol Solution, to make	1000.0 mL

Cough-Cold Syrup

Dextromethorphan Hydrobromide...........................	2.0 g
Guaifenesin	10.0 g
Chlorpheniramine Maleate..........	0.2 g
Phenylephrine Hydrochloride	1.0 g
Sodium Benzoate...........................	1.0 g
Saccharin Sodium.........................	1.9 g

Citric Acid......................................	1.0 g
Sodium Chloride...........................	5.2 g
Alcohol...	50.0 mL
Sorbitol Solution	324.0 mL
Syrup..	132.0 mL
Liquid Glucose	44.0 mL
Glycerin	50.0 mL
Color	q.s.
Flavor	q.s.
Purified Water, to make	1000.0 mL

All materials used in the extemporaneous compounding and manufacturing of pharmaceuticals should be of USP/NF quality and obtained from FDA-approved sources.

Antimicrobial Preservative

The amount of a preservative required to protect a syrup against microbial growth varies with the proportion of water available for growth, the nature and inherent preservative activity of some formulative materials (as many flavoring oils that are inherently sterile and possess antimicrobial activity), and the capability of the preservative itself. Among the preservatives commonly used in the preservation of syrups with the usually effective concentrations are benzoic acid (0.1 to 0.2%), sodium benzoate (0.1 to 0.2%), and various combinations of methyl-, propyl-, and butylparabens (totaling about 0.1%). Frequently alcohol is used in the preparation of syrups to assist in the dissolving of alcohol-soluble ingredients, but normally it is not present in the final product in amounts that would be considered to be adequate for preservation (15 to 20%). See accompanying Physical Pharmacy Capsule 12.1, Preservation of Syrups.

Flavorant

Most syrups are flavored with synthetic flavorants or with naturally occurring materials as volatile oils (e.g. orange oil), vanillin, and others, to render the syrup pleasant tasting. Because syrups are aqueous preparations, these flavorants must possess sufficient water-solubility. However, sometimes a small amount of alcohol is added to a syrup to ensure the continued solution of a poorly (water) soluble flavorant.

Colorant

To enhance the appeal of the syrup, a coloring agent is used that correlates with the flavorant employed (i.e. green with mint, brown with chocolate,

Physical Pharmacy Capsule 12.1   **Preservation of Syrups**

Syrups can be preserved by 1) storage at low temperature, 2) adding preservatives such as glycerin, benzoic acid, sodium benzoate, methyl paraben or alcohol in the formulation, or 3) by the maintenance of a high concentration of sucrose as a part of the formulation. High sucrose concentrations will usually protect an oral liquid dosage form from growth of most microorganisms. A problem arises, however, when pharmacists must add other ingredients to syrups that can result in a decrease in the sucrose concentration. This may cause a loss of the preservative effectiveness of the sucrose. This can be overcome, however, by calculating the quantity of a preservative (such as alcohol) to add to the formula to maintain the preservative effectiveness of the final product.

EXAMPLE

Rx Active drug	5 mL volume occupied
Other drug solids	3 mL volume occupied
Glycerin	15 mL
Sucrose	25 g
Ethanol	95% q.s.
Purified Water q.s.	100 mL

How much alcohol would be required to preserve this prescription? We will use the "free water" method to calculate the quantity of alcohol required.

Simple syrup contains 85 g of sucrose per 100 mL of solution, which weighs 131.3 g (Sp. Gr. = 1.313). It takes 46.3 mL of water to prepare the solution (131.3 − 85 = 46.3) and the sucrose occupies a volume of (100 − 46.3 = 53.7) 53.7 mL.

1. Since this solution is preserved, 85 g of sucrose preserves 46.3 mL of water and 1 g of sucrose preserves 0.54 mL of water. With 25 g of sucrose present, the amount of water preserved is:

$$25 \times 0.54 = 13.5 \text{ mL}$$

2. Since 85 g of sucrose occupies a volume of 53.7 mL, 1 g of sucrose will occupy a volume of 0.63 mL. The volume occupied by the sucrose in this prescription is:

$$25 \times 0.63 = 15.75 \text{ mL}$$

3. The active drug and other solids occupy 8 mL (5 + 3) volume.
4. Each mL of glycerin can preserve an equivalent quantity of volume (2 × 15 = 30), so 30 mL would be preserved.
5. The volume taken care of so far is 13.5 + 15.75 + 8 + 30 = 67.25 mL. The quantity of "free water" remaining is:

$$100 - 67.25 = 32.75 \text{ mL}$$

6. Since it requires about 18% alcohol to preserve the water,

$$0.18 \times 32.75 = 5.9 \text{ mL of alcohol (100\%) would be required.}$$

7. If 95% ethanol is used, then 5.9/0.95 = 6.21 mL would be required.

To prepare the prescription, about 6.21 mL of 95% ethanol can be added, with sufficient purified water to make 100 mL of the final solution.

etc.). The colorant used is generally water soluble, nonreactive with the other syrup components, and color-stable at the pH range and under the intensity of light that the syrup is likely to encounter during its shelf-life.

Preparation of Syrups

Syrups are most frequently prepared by one of four general methods, depending on the physical and chemical characteristics of the ingredients.

Broadly stated, these methods are 1) solution of the ingredients with the aid of heat, 2) solution of the ingredients by agitation without the use of heat, or the simple admixture of liquid components, 3) addition of sucrose to a prepared medicated liquid or to a flavored liquid, and 4) by percolation of either the source of the medicating substance or of the sucrose. In certain instances a syrup may be successfully prepared by more than one of the above methods, and the selection may simply be a matter of preference on the part of the pharmacist.

For many of the official syrups there is no officially designated method for preparation. This is due to the fact that most official syrups are available on a commercial basis and are not prepared extemporaneously by the pharmacist.

Solution with the Aid of Heat

Syrups are prepared by this method when it is desired to prepare the syrup as quickly as possible and when the syrup's components are not damaged or volatilized by heat. In this method the sugar is generally added to the purified water, and heat is applied until solution is effected. Then, other required heat-stable components are added to the hot syrup, the mixture is allowed to cool, and its volume is adjusted to the proper level by the addition of purified water. In instances in which heat-labile agents or volatile substances, as volatile flavoring oils and alcohol, are to be added, they are generally added to the syrup after the solution of the sugar is effected by heat, and the solution is rapidly cooled to room temperature.

The use of heat facilitates the rapid solution of the sugar as well as certain other components of syrups; however, caution must be exercised against becoming impatient and using excessive heat. Sucrose, a disaccharide, may be hydrolyzed into monosaccharides, dextrose (glucose), and fructose (levulose). This hydrolytic reaction is referred to as *inversion*, and the combination of the two monosaccharide products is *invert sugar*. When heat is applied in the preparation of a sucrose syrup, some inversion of the sucrose is almost certain. The speed of inversion is greatly increased by the presence of acids, the hydrogen ion acting as a catalyst to the reaction. Should inversion occur, the sweetness of the syrup is altered, because invert sugar is sweeter than sucrose; and the normally colorless syrup darkens due to the effect of heat on the levulose portion of the invert sugar. When the syrup is greatly overheated, it becomes amber colored due to the caramelization of the sucrose. Syrups so decomposed are more susceptible to fermentation and to microbial growth than the stable, nondecomposed syrups. Because of the prospect of decomposition by heat, syrups cannot be sterilized by autoclaving. The use of boiled purified water in the preparation of a syrup can enhance its permanency, and the addition of preservative agents, when permitted, can protect it during its shelf life. Storage in tight containers is a requirement for all syrups.

Solution by Agitation without the Aid of Heat

To avoid heat-induced inversion of sucrose, a syrup may be prepared without heat by agitation. On a small scale, sucrose and other formulative agents may be dissolved in purified water by placing the ingredients in a vessel of greater capacity than the volume of syrup to be prepared, thus permitting the thorough agitation of the mixture. This process is more time-consuming than that utilizing heat to facilitate the solution of sucrose, but the product has maximum stability. Huge glass-lined or stainless steel tanks affixed with mechanical stirrers or agitators are employed in the large-scale preparation of syrups.

Sometimes simple syrup or some other nonmedicated syrup, rather than sucrose, is employed as the sweetening agent and vehicle. In instances such as this, other liquids that are soluble in the syrup or miscible with it may be added and thoroughly mixed to form a uniform product. When solid agents are to be added to a syrup, it is best to dissolve them in a minimal amount of purified water and then incorporate the resulting solution into the syrup. When solid substances are added directly to a syrup, they dissolve slowly because the viscous nature of the syrup does not permit the solid substance to distribute readily throughout the syrup to the available solvent and also because a limited amount of available water is present in concentrated syrups.

Addition of Sucrose to a Medicated Liquid or to a Flavored Liquid

Occasionally a medicated liquid, as a tincture or fluidextract, is employed as the source of medication in the preparation of a syrup. Many such tinctures and fluidextracts contain alcohol-soluble constituents and are prepared with alcoholic or hydroalcoholic vehicles. If the alcohol-soluble components are desired medicinal agents to be present in the corresponding syrup, some means of rendering them water-soluble is employed. However, if the alcohol-soluble components are undesirable or unnecessary components of the corresponding syrup, they are generally removed by mixing the tincture or fluidextract with water, allowing the mixture to stand until separation of the water-insoluble agents is complete, and filtering them from the mixture. The filtrate then represents the medicated liquid to which the sucrose is added in the preparation of the syrup. In other instances when the tincture or fluidextract is miscible with aqueous preparations, it may be added directly to simple syrup or to a flavored syrup to medicate it.

Percolation

In the percolation method, either sucrose may be percolated to prepare the syrup, or the source of the medicinal component may be percolated to form an extractive to which sucrose or syrup may be added. This latter method really involves two separate procedures: first the preparation of the extractive of the drug and then the preparation of the syrup.

An example of a syrup prepared by percolation is ipecac syrup. Ipecac syrup is prepared by adding glycerin and syrup to an extractive of powdered ipecac obtained by percolation. The drug ipecac consists of the dried rhizome and roots of *Cephaëlis ipecacuanha* and contains the medicinally active alkaloids, emetine, cephaeline, and psychotrine. These alkaloids are extracted from the powdered ipecac by percolation with a hydroalcoholic solvent.

The syrup is categorized as an emetic with a usual dose of 15 mL. This amount of syrup is commonly used in the management of poisoning in children when the evacuation of the stomach contents is desirable. About 80% of children given this dose will vomit within a half hour. For a household emetic in event of poisoning, 1-oz. bottles of the syrup may be sold without the requirement of a prescription. Ipecac syrup also has some application as a nauseant expectorant, in doses smaller than the emetic dose.

Evidence indicates that many bulimics—most commonly young women in their late teens to early 30s—use syrup of ipecac to bring on attacks of vomiting in an attempt to lose more weight (9). Pharmacists must be aware of this misuse of syrup of ipecac and warn these individuals because one of the active ingredients besides ipecac in the syrup is emetine. With continual use of the syrup, emetine builds up toxic levels within body tissues and in 3 to 4 months

can do irreversible damage to heart muscles resulting in symptoms mimicking a heart attack. Shortness of breath is the most common symptom in patients who misuse syrup of ipecac, but some persons may describe low blood pressure-related symptoms and irregularities of heart beat.

Elixirs

Elixirs are clear, sweetened, hydroalcoholic solutions intended for oral use, and are usually flavored to enhance their palatability. *Nonmedicated* elixirs are employed as vehicles and *medicated* elixirs for the therapeutic effect of the medicinal substances they contain. Compared with syrups, elixirs are usually less sweet and less viscous because they contain a lower proportion of sugar and consequently are less effective than syrups in masking the taste of medicinal substances. However, because of their hydroalcoholic character, elixirs are better able than aqueous syrups to maintain both water-soluble and alcohol-soluble components in solution. Also because of their stable characteristics and the ease which they are prepared (by simple solution), from a manufacturing standpoint, elixirs are preferred over syrups.

The proportion of alcohol present in elixirs varies widely since the individual components of the elixirs have different water and alcohol solubility characteristics. Each elixir requires a specific blend of alcohol and water to maintain all of the components in solution. Naturally, for those elixirs containing agents which have poor water-solubility the proportion of alcohol required is greater than for elixirs prepared from components having good water solubility. In addition to alcohol and water, other solvents, such as glycerin and propylene glycol, are frequently employed in elixirs as adjunct solvents.

Although many elixirs are sweetened with sucrose or with a sucrose-syrup, some utilize sorbitol, glycerin and/or artificial sweeteners. Elixirs having a high alcoholic content usually utilize an artificial sweetener, such as saccharin, which is required only in small amounts, rather than sucrose which is only slightly soluble in alcohol and requires greater quantities for equivalent sweetness.

All elixirs contain flavoring materials to increase their palatability and most elixirs have coloring agents to enhance their appearance. Elixirs containing over 10 to 12% of alcohol are usually self-preserving and do not require the addition of an antimicrobial agent for their preservation.

Although the USP monographs for medicated elixirs provide standards, they do not generally provide official formulas. Formulations are left up to the individual manufacturers. Example formulations for some medicated elixirs are as follows (8):

Phenobarbital Elixir

Phenobarbital	4.00 g
Orange Oil	0.25 mL
Propylene Glycol	100.00 mL
Alcohol	200.00 mL
Sorbitol Solution	600.00 mL
Color	q.s.
Purified Water, to make	1000.00 mL

Theophylline Elixir

Theophylline	5.3 g
Citric Acid	10.0 g
Liquid Glucose	44.0 g
Syrup	132.0 mL
Glycerin	50.0 mL
Sorbitol Solution	324.0 mL
Alcohol	200.00 mL
Saccharin Sodium	5.0 g
Lemon Oil	0.5 g
FDC Yellow No. 5	0.1 g
Purified Water, to make	1000.0 mL

Medicated elixirs are formulated such that a patient receives the usual adult dose of the drug in a convenient measure of elixir. For most elixirs, one or two teaspoonfuls (5 or 10 mL) provide the usual adult dose of the drug. One advantage of elixirs over their counterpart drugs in solid dosage forms is the flexibility and ease of dosage administration to patients who have difficulty swallowing solid forms.

A disadvantage of elixirs for children and for adults who choose to avoid alcohol is their alcoholic content. The reader may wish to refer to the discussion of alcohol as a solvent earlier in this chapter for FDA-recommended limits on alcohol content for OTC oral products.

Because of their usual content of volatile oils and alcohol, elixirs should be stored in tight, light-resistant containers and protected from excessive heat.

Preparation of Elixirs

Elixirs are usually prepared by simple solution with agitation and/or by the admixture of two or more liquid ingredients. Alcohol-soluble and water-soluble components are generally dissolved separately in alcohol and in purified water, respectively. Then the aqueous solution is added to the alcoholic solution, rather than the reverse, in order to maintain the highest possible alcoholic strength at all times so that minimal separation of the alcohol-soluble components occurs. When the two solutions are completely mixed the mixture is made to volume with the specified solvent or vehicle. Frequently the final mixture will not be clear, but cloudy, due principally to the separation of some of the flavoring oils by the reduced alcoholic concentration. If this occurs, the elixir is usually permitted to stand for a prescribed number of hours, to ensure the saturation of the hydroalcoholic solvent and to permit the oil globules to coalesce so that they may be more easily removed by filtration. Talc, a frequent filter aid in the preparation of elixirs, has the ability to absorb the excessive amounts of oils and therefore assist in their removal from the solution. The presence of glycerin, syrup, sorbitol, and propylene glycol in elixirs generally contributes to the solvent effect of the hydroalcoholic vehicle, assists in the dissolution of the solute, and enhances the stability of the preparation. However, the presence of these materials adds to the viscosity of the elixir and slows the rate of their filtration.

Nonmedicated Elixirs

Nonmedicated elixirs may be useful to the pharmacist in the extemporaneous filling of prescriptions involving: 1) the addition of a therapeutic agent to a pleasant tasting vehicle, and 2) the dilution of an existing medicated elixir. In selecting a liquid vehicle for a drug substance, the pharmacist should be concerned with the solubility and stability of the drug substance in water and alcohol. If a hydroalcoholic vehicle is selected, the proportion of alcohol present should be only slightly above that amount which is needed to effect and maintain the drug's solution. When a pharmacist is called on to dilute an existing medicated elixir, the nonmedicated elixir he or she selects as the diluent should have the approximate alcoholic concentration as the elixir being diluted. Also, the flavor and color characteristics of the diluent should not be in conflict with the medicated elixir and all components should be chemically and physically compatible.

In years past, when pharmacists were called on more frequently than today to compound prescriptions, the three most commonly used nonmedicated elixirs were: Aromatic Elixir, Compound Benzaldehyde Elixir, and Iso-Alcoholic Elixir.

Medicated Elixirs

As noted previously, medicated elixirs are employed for the therapeutic benefit of the medicinal agent present. In most instances, the official and commercial elixirs contain a single therapeutic agent. The main advantage of having only a single therapeutic agent present is that the dosage taken of that single drug may be increased or decreased by simply taking more or less of the elixir, whereas when two or more therapeutic agents are present in the same preparation, it is impossible to increase or decrease the amount taken of one without an automatic and corresponding adjustment in the dose taken of the other; a change which may not be desired. Thus, for patients required to take more than a single medication, many physicians prefer them to take separate preparations of each drug so that if an adjustment in the dosage of one is desired, it may be accomplished without the concomitant adjustment of the other. Table 12.8 presents some examples of medicated elixirs. Some of these are briefly discussed below.

Antihistamine Elixirs

As indicated in Table 12.8, antihistamines are useful primarily in the symptomatic relief of certain allergic disorders. In their action, they suppress symptoms caused by histamine, one of the chemical agents released during the antigen-antibody reaction of the allergic response. Although only minor differences exist in the properties of most antihistamines, one or another may be preferred by a prescriber through his experience in managing a specific type of allergic reaction. A prescriber's preference may also be based on the incidence of adverse effects that may be expected to occur. The incidence and severity of these effects do vary somewhat with the drug and the dose of each drug. The most common untoward effect is sedation, and patients taking antihistamines should be warned against engaging in activities requiring mental alertness, as driving an automobile or tractor or operating machinery. Other common adverse effects include dryness of the nose, throat, and mouth, dizziness and disturbed concentration. Included among the most sedating antihistamines are diphenhydramine, doxylamine, and methapyrilene. In fact, diphenhydramine is used as a sleep aid in numerous over-the-counter products for its ability to cause drowsiness.

Most antihistaminic agents are basic amines. By forming salts through interaction with acid, the compounds are rendered water soluble. These salt forms are used in elixirs and thus the elixirs of the antihistamines are not required to contain a large proportion of alcohol. Because the acid salts of the antihistamines are used, the pH of these elixirs is on the acid side and must remain so if the drugs are to remain freely soluble in water. A pharmacist should keep this in mind when utilizing one of these elixirs in the compounding of a prescription involving adding or mixing other components.

Barbiturate Sedative/Hypnotic Elixirs

The barbiturates are sedative/hypnotic agents that are used to produce various degrees of central nervous system depression. As the dose of these drugs is increased, the effects go from sedation to hypnosis to respiratory depression, the latter being the cause of death in fatal barbiturate overdosage.

Barbiturates are administered in small doses in the daytime hours as sedatives to reduce restlessness and emotional tension. The appropriate dose for this purpose is that amount which alleviates anxiety or tension but does not produce drowsiness or lethargy. Greater doses of the barbiturates may be given before bedtime as hypnotics to relieve insomnia.

Barbiturates have been classified according to the duration of their (hypnotic) effects; that is, *long-acting, intermediate-acting, short-acting,* or *ultrashort-acting* agents. The long-acting barbiturates including phenobarbital are considered most useful in maintaining daytime sedation and in treating some convulsive states and least useful in acting as hypnotics. The intermediate-acting barbiturates include amobarbital and are used primarily for short-term daytime sedation and are effective in treating insomnia. The barbiturates classified as short-acting include pentobarbital and secobarbital and are used similarly to the intermediate-acting barbiturates. The ultrashort-acting barbiturates, as thiopental, are given intravenously to induce anesthesia.

The most common untoward effect noticed in patients taking barbiturates is drowsiness and lethargy. Large doses may produce residual sedation resembling the hangover following alcohol intoxication. Prolonged use of barbiturates may lead to psychic or physical dependence. This dependence, in susceptible individuals, leads to compulsive abuse of the drug with severe withdrawal symptoms following abstinence. In heavy chronic users, abrupt withdrawal may lead to convulsions, delirium, and occasionally to coma and death. Some pharmaceutic aspects of Phenobarbital Elixir are presented below.

Phenobarbital Elixir

Phenobarbital elixir is formulated to contain 0.4% of phenobarbital, which provides about 20 mg of drug per teaspoonful (5 mL) of elixir. The elixir is commonly flavored with orange oil, colored

Table 12.8.   Examples of Medicated Elixirs by Category

Elixir	Some Representative Commercial Products	Usual Adult Dose of Drug/Volume of Commercial Elixir	Comments
Adrenocortical Steroid			
Dexamethasone Elixir	Decadron Elixir (Merck & Co.)	500 µg/5 mL	Dexamethasone is a synthetic analogue of hydrocortisone that is considered to be about 30 times more potent than the latter drug. The commercial dexamethasone elixir is packaged with a calibrated dropper for the accurate measurement of small doses and is intended primarily for children, but also has utility for adults who may have trouble swallowing tablets. The elixir is used for many indications, including the treatment of rheumatoid arthritis, skin diseases, allergies and inflammatory conditions. The commercial product contains 5% alcohol.
Analgesic/Antipyretic			
Acetaminophen Elixir	Children's Tylenol Elixir (McNeil)	160 mg/5 mL	Use for reduction of pain and lowering of fever particularly in patients sensitive to or unable to take aspirin. Elixir especially useful for pediatric patients, and is alcohol-free.
Anticholinergic/Antispasmodic			
Hyoscyamine Sulfate Elixir	Levsin Elixir (Schwarz)	0.125 mg hyoscyamine sulfate/5 mL	Used to control gastric secretion, visceral spasm, hypermotility, and abdominal cramps. The commercial product contains 20% alcohol.
Antihistamine			
Diphenhydramine HCl Elixir	Benadryl Elixir (Warner-Lambert)	12.5 mg/5 mL	Antihistamine elixirs are employed for a variety of allergic reactions including: perennial and seasonal allergic rhinitis, vasomotor rhinitis, allergic skin manifestations of urticaria, reactions to insect bites, and others. The commercial product contains 5.6% alcohol.
Antipsychotic			
Fluphenazine HCl Elixir	Fluphenazine HCl Elixir (Pharmaceutical Associates)	2.5 mg/5 mL	Used in the management of psychotic disorders.
Cardiotonic			
Digoxin Elixir	Lanoxin Pediatric Elixir (Glaxo Wellcome)	50 µg/mL	Among other effects, digoxin increases the force of myocardial contraction. Used in congestive heart failure, atrial fibrillation and other cardiac conditions. See text for additional discussion. The commercial product contains 10% alcohol.
Sedative/Hypnotics			
Butabarbital Sodium Elixir	Butisol Sodium Elixir (Wallace)	30 mg/5 mL	The barbiturate elixirs are utilized in low dosage as sedatives and in higher dosage as hypnotics. The butabarbital sodium elixir contains 7% alcohol and the phenobarbital elixir contains 14% alcohol. See text for additional discussion.
Phenobarbital Elixir	Phenobarbital Elixir (Roxane)	20 mg/5 mL	

red with an FDA-approved colorant, and sweetened with syrup. The official elixir contains about 14% of alcohol, which is used to dissolve the phenobarbital. However, this amount represents almost the very minimum required to keep the phenobarbital in solution. Thus glycerin is often added to enhance the solubility of phenobarbital.

Phenobarbital is a long-acting barbiturate with a duration of action of about 4 to 6 hours and a usual adult dose as a sedative of about 30 mg and a hypnotic dose of about 100 mg. The strength of the elixir permits the convenient adjustment of dosage to achieve the proper degree of sedation in the treatment of infants, children, and certain adult patients. The elixir is commercially available from a variety of manufacturers under its nonproprietary name.

Digoxin Elixir

No official method of preparation is indicated for Digoxin Elixir USP; however, it is required to contain 4.50 mg to 5.25 mg of digoxin per 100 mL of elixir or about 0.25 mg per 5 mL teaspoonful. The usual oral adult dose of digoxin as a cardiotonic agent is about 1.5 mg on initial therapy and about 0.5 mg for maintenance therapy.

Digoxin is a cardiotonic glycoside obtained from the leaves of *Digitalis lanata.* It is a white crystalline powder that is insoluble in water, but soluble in dilute alcohol solutions. The official elixir contains about 10% of alcohol. Digoxin is a poisonous drug, and its dose must be carefully determined and administered to each individual patient. Adults generally take digoxin tablets rather than the elixir, which must be measured by the highly variable household teaspoon. The elixir is generally employed in pediatric practice, and the commercial product available for this purpose is packaged with a calibrated dropper to facilitate accurate dosage measurements.

Digoxin is one of many drugs that is available to the prescriber in more than a single type of dosage form. The prescriber frequently has the choice of selecting a solid dosage form, as a tablet or capsule, or a liquid form of the medication for his patient. The advantages of each have been noted previously but it is important here to point out again that drugs administered in different dosage forms may exhibit different bioavailability characteristics with varying patterns of drug release and rates and extents of drug absorption. Such differences have been noted for digoxin, between tablets from different manufacturers, as well as between tablets

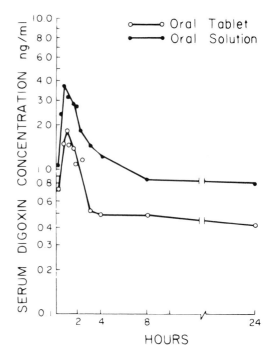

Fig. 12.2   *Serum digoxin concentrations following administration of 0.5 mg of digoxin by oral tablet and elixir-like oral solution. (Adapted from Huffman DH, Azarnoff DL. Absorption of orally given digoxin preparations. JAMA 1972;222: 957.)*

and oral liquid dosage forms. Figure 12.2 shows the differences noted in one study of the serum digoxin levels following administration of 0.5 mg of digoxin by oral tablet and oral solution having an elixir-like vehicle. It can be readily seen that the serum digoxin levels following administration of the oral solution were considerably greater than from the oral tablet.

A patient taking a drug known to exhibit bioavailability problems, and whose therapeutic dosage regimen has been successfully established with a particular drug product, should not be changed to another product.

Tinctures

Tinctures are alcoholic or hydroalcoholic solutions prepared from vegetable materials or from chemical substances. They vary in their method of preparation, the strength of their active ingredient, their alcoholic content, and their intended use in medicine or pharmacy. When they are prepared from chemical substances (e.g., iodine, thimerosal, etc.) tinctures are prepared by simple solution of the chemical agent in the solvent.

Depending on the preparation, tinctures contain alcohol in amounts ranging from approximately 15 to 80%. The alcoholic content protects against microbial growth and keeps the alcohol-soluble extractives in solution. In addition to alcohol, other solvents, as glycerin, may be employed. The solvent mix of each tincture is important in maintaining the integrity of the product. Tinctures cannot be mixed successfully with liquids too diverse in solvent character without the likelihood of inducing the precipitation of the solute. For example, compound benzoin tincture, prepared with alcohol as the sole menstruum, contains alcohol-soluble principles that are immediately expelled from solution upon the addition of water.

Because of the alcoholic content, tinctures must be tightly stoppered and not exposed to excessive temperatures. Also, because many of the constituents found in tinctures undergo a photochemical change upon exposure to light, many tinctures must be stored in light-resistant containers and protected from sunlight.

Medicated tinctures taken orally include paregoric, or camphorated tincture of opium. Usually, patients requiring oral medication nowadays would prefer to take a tablet or capsule or a pleasant-tasting elixir or syrup. Tinctures have a rather high alcoholic content and some physicians and patients alike prefer other forms of medication.

Proper Administration and Use of Liquid Peroral Dosage Forms

The dosage forms discussed in this chapter are all to be administered by mouth. Conveniently, these can be measured in a spoon, i.e., teaspoon, tablespoon, depending on the desired dosage and swallowed. Preferably, however, these medicines should be measured out in calibrated devices for administration. These devices assure the patient that the correct dose will be received because teaspoons, for example, can vary dramatically in the volume they deliver. Even though these are liquids, it is recommended that the patient follow the administration of the liquid dosage form with a glassful of water.

The pharmacist must be careful in the selection of liquid products given the patient's history and other concurrent medicines. For example, some syrups contain sucrose or another sugar as an ingredient, and the pharmacist must recall that such syrups would not be optimal for use in an oral pre-

scription intended for a diabetic patient. Similarly, a product that is formulated as an elixir would not be advantageous to use in a patient who receives concurrent medicines that possess an antabuse-like activity, i.e., the patient may get violently ill from the concurrent ingestion of alcohol. Metronidazole and chlorpropramide are two drugs that have been implicated to cause this reaction when mixed with alcohol. Further, if the patient is receiving another drug that causes drowsiness the pharmacist must make a decision to intervene and contact the prescribing physician to determine whether the prescribed elixir could be harmful to the patient.

Topical Solutions and Tinctures

Topical Solutions

Generally, the topical solutions employ an aqueous vehicle, whereas the topical tinctures characteristically employ an alcoholic vehicle. As required, co-solvents or adjuncts to enhance stability or the solubility of the solute are employed.

Most topical solutions and tinctures are prepared by simple solution of the solutes in the solvent. However, certain solutions are prepared by chemical reaction and these in particular are discussed later in this section. Of the tinctures for topical use, one, Compound Benzoin Tincture, is prepared by maceration of the natural components in the solvent; the others are prepared by simple solution.

Because of the nature of the active constituents or the solvents, many of the topical solutions and tinctures are self-preserved. Those that are not may contain suitable preservatives. Topical solutions and tinctures should be packaged in containers that make them convenient to use. Those that are used in small volume, as the anti-infectives, are usually packaged in glass bottles having an applicator tip as a part of the cap assembly, or in plastic squeeze bottles which deliver the medication in drops. Many of the anti-infective solutions and tinctures contain a dye to delineate the area of application to the skin. In contrast to aqueous solutions, when the alcoholic tinctures are applied to abraded or broken skin, they cause a stinging sensation.

Sprays

Sprays may be defined as aqueous or oleaginous solutions in the form of coarse droplets or as finely divided solids to be applied topically, most usually to the nasal-pharyngeal tract or to the skin. Many commercially available sprays are used intranasally to relieve nasal congestion and inflammation and to combat infection and contain antihistamines, sympathomimetic agents, and antibiotic substances. Because of the noninvasive nature and quickness with which nasal sprays can deliver medication systemically, the future will demonstrate the administration of several drugs by this route that typically have been administered by other routes of administration. Most notably, insulin and glucagon will be administered in this fashion. Research has demonstrated that the administration of glucagon, for example, via a nasal spray can relieve hypoglycemic symptoms within 7 minutes, a definite advantage over conventional emergency intravenous glucose or intramuscular glucagon.

Other sprays are employed against sunburn and heat burn and contain local anesthetics, antiseptics, skin protectants, and antipruritics. Throat sprays containing antiseptics, deodorants, and flavorants may be effectively employed to relieve conditions such as halitosis, sore throat, or laryngitis. Other sprays may be employed to treat athlete's foot and other fungal infections. Numerous other medicinal and cosmetic uses of sprays are commonly available in pharmacies.

To achieve the breaking up of a solution into small particles so that it may be effectively sprayed or to facilitate the spraying of a powder, several mechanical devices have been developed and are commonly employed. The plastic spray bottle, which is gently squeezed to issue a spray of its contents, is familiar to most persons. It is commonly used for nasal decongestant sprays as well as cosmetically, especially for body deodorant products. Recently, one-way pump sprays have been developed to deliver medication into the nose. These sprays are used for both legend, e.g., Nasalide (Syntex), and nonlegend, e.g., Nostrilla (Boehringer Ingelheim), medicines. The advantage of these over the conventional sprays is that its design prevents drawback contamination of nasal fluids into the bottle after administration, a definite advantage for someone trying to cope with viruses associated with the common cold. Pharmacists are familiar with medicinal *atomizers,* which are employed for the issuance of a medicated solution to the patient in the form of fine droplets (Fig. 12.3). One type of atomizer operates by the squeezing of a rubber bulb at the end of the apparatus, which causes a flow of air partially to enter the glass reservoir in which the solution is held and partially to exit from the opposite end of the system. The air forced into

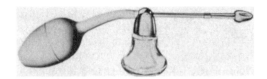

Fig. 12.3 *A common type of atomizer for the administration of a spray of liquid medication. The model shown has an adjustable tip for directing the spray upward or downward to reach otherwise inaccessible areas of the throat. (Courtesy of The DeVilbiss Co.)*

the reservoir causes the liquid to rise in a small dip tube, which is maintained below the level of the liquid, forcing the solution up and into the stream of air exiting the system. The air and the solution are forced through a jet opening and the liquid is broken up into a spray, the droplets being carried by the airstream. In other similar apparatuses, the stream of air caused by the depression of the bulb does not enter the reservoir of solution, but passes swiftly over it, creating a pressure change that causes a sucking up of the liquid into the dip tube and into the airstream in which it exits the system. Examples of solutions and tinctures intended for application to the skin are presented in Tables 12.9 and 12.10. As shown in these tables, the majority of these preparations are used as anti-infective agents. All medication intended for external use should be clearly labeled "FOR EXTERNAL USE ONLY" and kept out of the reach of children. In addition to their listing in Table 12.9, the following topical solutions are discussed because of their particular pharmaceutic interest.

Aluminum Acetate Topical Solution

The solution is colorless and has a faint acetous odor and a sweetish, astringent taste. It is widely applied topically as an astringent wash or wet dressing after dilution with 10 to 40 parts of water. It is frequently used as an ingredient in various types of dermatological preparations, as lotions, creams, and pastes. Commercial premeasured tablets and packets of powders are available for the preparation of this solution.

Synonym: Burow's Solution

Aluminum Subacetate Topical Solution

The requirement for the amount of acetic acid differentiates Aluminum Acetate Topical Solution from Aluminum Subacetate Topical Solution. In the latter solution the ratio of aluminum oxide to acetic acid is 1:2.35, whereas in aluminum acetate topical solution the ratio is 1:3.52. Aluminum Subacetate

Table 12.9. Examples of Solutions Applied Topically to the Skin

Solution	Corresponding Commercial Product	Percent Active Constituent in Commercial Solution	Vehicle	Category and Comments
Aluminum Acetate Topical Solution	—	5%	Aqueous	Astringent. See text for additional discussion.
Aluminum Subacetate Topical Solution	—	Approximately 2.45% aluminum oxide and 5.8% acetic acid	Aqueous	Astringent. See text for additional discussion.
Calcium Hydroxide Topical Solution (Limewater)	—	0.14%	Aqueous	Astringent. See text for additional discussion.
Chlorhexidine Gluconate Solution	Hibiclens Skin Cleanser (Stuart)	4%		Used topically as a skin wound and general skin cleanser, a surgical scrub, and preoperative skin preparation. Effectiveness encompasses gram-positive and gram-negative bacteria such as *Pseudomonas aeruginosa*.
Clindamycin Phosphate Topical Solution	Cleocin T topical Solution (Pharmacia & Upjohn)	1%	Isopropyl Alcohol/ Water	Used in treatment of acne vulgaris.
Clotrimazole Topical Solution	Lotrimin Solution (Schering)	1%	PEG 400	Antifungal
Coal Tar Topical Solution (Liquor Carbonis Detergens; LCD)	—	20%	Alcohol	Antieczematic; antipsoriatic. See text for additional discussion.
Erythromycin Topical Solution	Erymax Topical Solution (Allergan Herbert)	2%	Polyethylene glycol/ acetone/ alcohol	Used in treatment of acne vulgaris
Fluocinolone Acetonide Topical Solution	Synalar Topical Solution (Medicis)	0.01%	Propylene glycol	Adrenocortical steroid (topical anti-inflammatory)
Fluorouracil Topical Solution	Efudex Topical Solution (Roche)	2 and 5%	Propylene glycol	Antineoplastic (actinic keratoses).
Hydrogen Peroxide Topical Solution	—	3%	Aqueous	Topical anti-infective. See text for additional discussion.
Hydroquinone Topical Solution	Melanex Topical Solution (Neutrogena Dermatologies)	3%	Water/alcohol/ propylene glycol	Indicated in the temporary bleaching of hyperpigmented skin in conditions as chloasma and melasma.
Minoxidil Solution	Rogaine Topical Solution (Pharmacia & Upjohn)	2% and 5%	Alcohol/water/ propylene glycol	Long-term topical treatment of male pattern baldness by stimulating hair regrowth.
Povidone-Iodine Topical Solution	Betadine Solution (Purdue Frederick)	7.5% and 10%	Aqueous	Topical anti-infective. See text for additional discussion.
Tolnaftate Topical Solution	Tinactin Solution (Schering-Plough)	1%	Polyethylene glycol	Topical anti-fungal.

Table 12.10.   Examples of Tinctures Applied Topically to the Skin

Tincture	Percent Active Constituent in Commercial Tincture	Vehicle	Category and Comments
Green Soap Tincture	65%	Alcohol	Detergent. Also contains 2% lavender oil as perfume.
Iodine Tincture	2%	Alcohol-water	Topical anti-infective. See text for additional discussion.
Compound Benzoin Tincture	10% benzoin; 2% aloe; 8% storax; 4% tolu balsam	Alcohol	Topical protectant. Prepared by maceration of the ingredients in alcohol. See text for additional discussion.

Topical Solution is the stronger solution and is used in the preparation of the Aluminum Acetate Topical Solution. The solution, diluted first with 20 to 40 parts of water, is used externally as an astringent wash and wet dressing (modified Burow's Solution).

Calcium Hydroxide Topical Solution

Calcium hydroxide topical solution, commonly referred to as *limewater,* must contain not less than 140 mg of $Ca(OH)_2$ in each 100 mL of solution. Calcium hydroxide is less soluble in hot than in cold water, and, in the preparation of this solution cool purified water is employed as the solvent. The solution is intended to be saturated with solute, and to ensure saturation, an excess of calcium hydroxide, 300 mg for each 100 mL of solution to be prepared, is agitated with the purified water, vigorously and repeatedly, during a period of 1 hour. After this time, the excess calcium hydroxide is allowed to settle and remain at the bottom of the container. This permits the solution to remain saturated should a portion of the dissolved solute at the solution's surface react with the carbon dioxide of the air to form insoluble calcium carbonate:

$$Ca(OH)_2 + CO_2 \rightarrow CaCO_3 + H_2O$$

The calcium carbonate settles to the bottom of the container and by appearance is indistinguishable from the remaining excess of calcium hydroxide. The calcium hydroxide reserve dissolves as calcium is removed from solution in the form of the carbonate and in this way continually maintains the saturation of the solution. After the solution stands for an appreciable length of time, the undissolved material in the bottom of the container is composed of varying proportions of calcium hydroxide and calcium carbonate. Because of the uncertainty

of the residue's composition, additional quantities of calcium hydroxide solution may not be prepared by adding more purified water to the solution.

The solution should be stored in well-filled, tightly stoppered containers to deter the absorption of carbon dioxide and should be kept in a cool place to maintain an adequate concentration of dissolved solute. Only the clear supernatant liquid is dispensed. This is best accomplished by the use of a siphoning apparatus assembled so as to avoid the entrainment of the residue in the siphoning tubes.

The solution is categorized as an astringent. For this purpose it is generally employed in combination with other ingredients in dermatological solutions and lotions to be applied topically. Synonyms: Lime Water; Liquor Calcis.

Coal Tar Topical Solution

Coal tar topical solution is an alcoholic solution containing 20% of coal tar and 5% of polysorbate 80. It is prepared by mixing the coal tar with two and a half times its weight of washed sand, adding the polysorbate 80 and most of the alcohol, and then macerating the mixture for 7 days in a closed vessel with frequent agitation followed by filtration and adjustment to the proper volume with alcohol. The final alcoholic content is between 81 and 86% ethyl alcohol.

Coal tar is a nearly black, viscous liquid having a characteristic naphthalene-like odor and a sharp, burning taste. It is the tar obtained as a by-product during the destructive distillation of bituminous coal. It is slightly soluble in water and partially soluble in most organic solvents, including alcohol. In the preparation of the official solution, the coal tar is mixed with the sand in order to distribute it mechanically and create a large surface area of tar exposed to the solvent action of the alcohol. During the period of maceration, or soaking, the alcohol-soluble components of the tar dissolve, leaving the undissolved portion clinging to the sand. Filtration removes the sand and the insoluble tar components from the solution. The container in which the solution was prepared should be rinsed with alcohol, and the washings should be passed through the filter paper in the adjustment of the final volume of the solution.

In the extemporaneous compounding of prescriptions and in the therapeutic application of this preparation onto the skin, the solution is frequently mixed with aqueous preparations or simply diluted with water. Because coal tar is only slightly soluble in water, in instances such as this it would separate from the solution were it not for the presence of the polysorbate 80 in the preparation. This agent, commercially available as Tween 80 (ICI Americas) and as other brand-name products, is an oily liquid that is a nonionic surfactant. It is quite effective in dispersing the water-insoluble components of coal tar upon its admixture with an aqueous preparation.

Coal tar is a local antieczematic. The solution is used in the external treatment of a wide variety of chronic skin conditions after dilution with about 9 volumes of water, or in combination with other agents in various lotions, ointments or solutions. Synonyms: Liquor Carbonis Detergens: Liquor Picis Carbonis; LCD

Hydrogen Peroxide Topical Solution

Hydrogen Peroxide Topical Solution contains between 2.5 and 3.5% (w/v) of hydrogen peroxide, H_2O_2. Suitable preservatives, totaling not more than 0.05%, may be added.

One method of preparation involves the action of either phosphoric or sulfuric acid on barium peroxide:

$$BaO_2 + H_2SO_4 \rightarrow BaSO_4 + H_2O_2$$

Another method involves the electrolytic oxidation of a cold solution of concentrated sulfuric acid to form persulfuric acid, which when hydrolyzed liberates hydrogen peroxide:

$$2H_2SO_4 \rightarrow H_2S_2O_8 + H_2$$
$$H_2S_2O_8 + 2H_2O \rightarrow 2H_2SO_4 + H_2O_2$$

A solution prepared by this method usually contains about 30% of hydrogen peroxide and is capable of liberating 100 times its volume of oxygen. A solution of this strength is commonly referred to as "100 volume peroxide." The dilute solution, which contains about 3% hydrogen peroxide and liberates 10 times its volume of oxygen, may be prepared from the concentrated solution.

The solution is a clear, colorless liquid that may be odorless or may have the odor of ozone. It usually deteriorates upon long standing with the formation of oxygen and water. Preservative agents, as acetanilide, which have been found to retard the solution's decomposition are usually added in the amount stated above. Decomposition is enhanced by light and by heat, and for this reason the solution should be preserved in tight, light-resistant containers, preferably at a temperature not exceeding 35°C (95°F). The solution is also decomposed by practically all organic matter and other reducing agents and reacts with oxidizing agents to liberate oxygen and water; metals, alkalies, and other agents can catalyze its decomposition.

Hydrogen peroxide solution is categorized as a local anti-infective for use topically on the skin and mucous membranes. Its germicidal activity is based on the release of nascent oxygen on contact with the tissues. However, because of the short duration of this release, the chief value of the preparation in the reduction of infection is probably its ability to cleanse wounds by mechanical action through the effervescence and frothing caused by the release of oxygen.

Synonym: Peroxide.

Chlorhexidine Gluconate Solution

Since 1957 chlorhexidine gluconate has been employed extensively as a broad spectrum antiseptic in clinical and veterinarian medicine. Its spectrum encompasses gram-positive and gram-negative bacteria, including *Pseudomonas aeruginosa*. In a concentration of 4% (Hibiclins, Stuart) it is used as a surgical scrub, hand wash and as a skin wound and general skin cleanser. Procedures are established for all of these purposes to maximize the effectiveness of the chlorhexidine. Experience has demonstrated that irritation, dermatitis and/or photosensitivity associated with the topical use of chlorhexidine are rare.

In 1987, the FDA and the Council of Dental Therapeutics of the American Dental Association approved chlorhexidine gluconate, 0.12% (Peridex, Procter & Gamble) as the first prescription only antiplaque/antigingivitis drug with antimicrobial activity. When used as a mouth rinse, microbiologic sampling of plaque has shown a reduction of aerobic and anaerobic bacteria, ranging from 54 to 97% through 6 months of use. The oral rinse should be used twice daily for 30 seconds, morning and night after tooth brushing. Usually a 15 mL dose of undiluted solution is used, and expectorated after rinsing. The most common side effect of chlorhexidine is the formation of an extrinsic yellow-brown stain on the teeth and tongue, after only a few days use. The amount of stain that appears depends on the concentration of chlorhexidine and individual susceptibility. Increased consumption of tannin containing substances, e.g., tea, red wine, port wine, will increase the level of discoloration. The developed stain can be periodically removed with a dental prophylaxis.

Povidone-Iodine Topical Solution

The agent povidone-iodine is a chemical complex of iodine with polyvinylpyrrolidone, the latter agent being a polymer having an average molecular weight of about 40,000. The povidone-iodine complex contains approximately 10% of available iodine and slowly releases it when applied to the skin.

The preparation is employed topically as a surgical scrub and nonirritating antiseptic solution with its effectiveness directly attributable to the presence and the release of iodine from the complex.

Commercial product: Betadine Solution (Purdue Frederick).

Thimerosal Topical Solution

Thimerosal is a water-soluble, organic, mercurial, antibacterial agent used topically for its bacteriostatic and mild fungistatic properties. It is used mainly to disinfect skin surfaces and as an application to wounds and abrasions. In certain instances it has been applied to the eye, nose, throat, and urethra in dilutions of 1:5000. It is also used as a preservative for various pharmaceutical preparations, including many vaccines and other biological products.

Thimerosal Topical Solution contains 0.1% thimerosal. Also present are ethylene diamine solution and sodium borate to maintain the alkalinity (usually pH 9.8 to 10.3) required for the solution's stability. Monoethanolamine is used as an additional stabilizer. The solution is affected by light and must be maintained in light-resistant containers.

Commercial Product: Merthiolate Solution (Lilly).

Vaginal and Rectal Solutions

Vaginal Douches

Solutions may be prepared from powders as indicated above or from liquid solutions or liquid concentrates. In using liquid concentrates, the patient is instructed to add the prescribed amount of concentrate (usually a teaspoonful or bottle-capful)

with a certain amount of warm water (frequently a quart). The resultant solution then contains the appropriate amount of chemical agents in proper strength. The agents present are similar to the ones described above for douche powders. Examples are shown in Figure 12.4.

Powders are used to prepare solutions for vaginal *douche,* that is, for the irrigative cleansing of the vagina. The powders themselves may be prepared and packaged in bulk or as unit packages. A unit package is designed to contain the appropriate amount of powder to prepare the specified volume of douche solution. The bulk powders are utilized by the teaspoonful or tablespoonful amounts in the preparation of the desired solution. The user simply adds the prescribed amount of powder to the appropriate volume of warm water and stirs until dissolved. Among the components of douche powders are the following:

a. Boric acid or sodium borate.
b. Astringents, as potassium, alum, ammonium alum, zinc sulfate.
c. Antimicrobials, as oxyquinoline sulfate, povidone-iodine.
d. Quaternary ammonium compounds, as benzethonium chloride.
e. Detergents, as sodium lauryl sulfate.
f. Oxidizing agents, as sodium perborate.
g. Salts, as sodium citrate, sodium chloride.
h. Aromatics, as menthol, thymol, eucalyptol, methyl salicylate, phenol.

Douche powders are used for their hygienic effects. A few douche powders, containing specific therapeutic anti-infective agents as those mentioned previously in the discussion of vaginal sup-

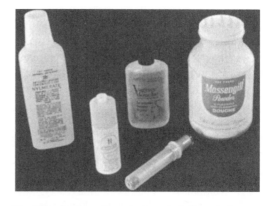

Fig. 12.4 *Products for vaginal use, including solution concentrates, powder, and aerosol foam with insert device.*

positories, are used against Monilial and Trichomonal infections.

Retention Enemas

A number of solutions are administered rectally for the local effects of the medication (e.g., hydrocortisone) or for systemic absorption (e.g., aminophylline). In the case of aminophylline, the rectal route of administration minimizes the undesirable gastrointestinal reactions associated with oral therapy. Clinically effective blood levels of the agents are usually obtained within 30 minutes following rectal instillation. Corticosteroids are administered as retention enemas or continuous drip as adjunctive treatment of some patients with ulcerative colitis.

Evacuation Enemas

Rectal enemas are used to cleanse the bowel. Commercially, many enemas are available in disposable plastic squeeze bottles containing a premeasured amount of enema solution. The agents present are solutions of sodium phosphate and sodium biphosphate, glycerin and docusate potassium, and light mineral oil.

Patient instruction from a pharmacist is advantageous to ensure that the patient correctly uses these products. The patient should be advised to gently insert the rectal tip of the product with steady pressure and be told that it is not absolutely necessary to squeeze all of the contents out of the disposable plastic bottle. Lastly, the patient should be told that the product will most probably work within 5 to 10 minutes.

Topical Tinctures

Examples of tinctures for topical application to the skin are presented in Table 12.10. Those of particular pharmaceutic interest are discussed briefly as follows.

Iodine Tincture

Iodine Tincture is prepared by dissolving 2% of iodine crystals and 2.4% of sodium iodide in an amount of alcohol equal to half the volume of tincture to be prepared and the diluting the solution to volume with sufficient purified water. The sodium iodide reacts with the iodine to form sodium triiodide:

$$I_2 + NaI \leftrightarrow NaI_3$$

This reaction prevents the formation of ethyl iodide from the interaction between iodine and the alcohol, which would result in the loss of the antibacterial activity of the tincture. An added benefit of the triiodide form of iodine is its water solubility which is important should the tincture, which contains between 44 and 50% alcohol, be diluted with water during use.

The tincture is a popular local anti-infective agent applied topically to the skin in general household first-aid procedures. The reddish-brown color, which produces a stain on the skin, is useful in delineating the application over the affected skin area. The tincture should be stored in tight containers to prevent loss of alcohol.

Compound Benzoin Tincture

Compound Benzoin Tincture is prepared by the maceration in alcohol of 10% benzoin and lesser amounts of aloe, storax and tolu balsam totaling about 24% of starting material. The drug mixture is best macerated in a wide-mouthed container, since it is difficult to introduce storax, a semi-liquid, sticky material into a narrow-mouthed container. Generally, it is advisable to weigh the storax in the container in which it will be macerated to avoid possible loss through a transfer of the material from one container to another.

The tincture is categorized as a protectant. It is used to protect and toughen skin in the treatment of bedsores, ulcers, cracked nipples, and fissures of the lips and anus. It is also commonly used as an inhalant in bronchitis and other respiratory conditions, one teaspoonful commonly being added to a pint of boiling water. The volatile components of the tincture travel with the steam vapor and are inhaled by the patient. Because of the incompatibility of the alcoholic tincture and water, mixture of the two produces a milky product with some separation of resinous material. Alcohol or acetone may be used as necessary to remove the residue from the vaporizer after use.

Compound tincture of benzoin serves as a delivery vehicle of podophyllum in the treatment of venereal warts. It is important that podophyllum not be systemically absorbed after application because the drug can effect peripheral neuropathy characterized by paresthesias, loss of sensation and loss of deep tendon reflexes in the extremities, in addition to neuropathy involving the central nervous system, e.g., lethargy, confusion, coma. Secondly, the podophyllum is teratogenic and should be administered only when the risk to benefit ratio is extremely low in a pregnant woman suffering from venereal warts. Thus, the nonocclusive compound tincture of benzoin is preferred to the occlusive flexible collodion.

Compound Benzoin Tincture is best stored in tight, light-resistant containers. Exposure to direct sunlight or to excessive heat should be avoided.

The tincture originated in the fifteenth or sixteenth century and through the years probably has acquired more synonyms than any other official preparation. A few of these are indicated as follows.

Synonyms: Friar's Balsam; Turlington's Drops; Persian Balsam; Swedish Balsam; Jerusalem Balsam; Wade's Drops; Turlington's Balsam of Life.

Thimerosal Tincture

The same general remarks made during the discussion of Thimerosal Topical Solution apply to thimerosal Tincture except that sodium chloride and sodium borate are absent from the tincture and the vehicle of the tincture is composed of water, acetone, and about 50% alcohol. A number of metals, notably copper, cause the decomposition of the tincture, and for this reason it must be manufactured and stored in glass or suitably resistant containers. Monoethanolamine and ethylenediamine are used as stabilizers in the official solution and tincture and are thought to be effective because of their chelating action on traces of metallic impurities that may be present at the time of preparation or may later gain access to the preparation.

The commercial preparation is colored orange red and has a greenish fluorescence. The red stain it leaves on the skin defines the area of application. The preparation is a commonly used household antiseptic for application topically on the skin in abrasions and cuts and also in the preoperative preparation of patients for surgery.

Special Application Solutions

Nasal Preparations

The vast majority of preparations intended for intranasal use contain adrenergic agents and are employed for their decongestant activity on the nasal mucosa. Most of these preparations are in solution-form, and are administered as nose drops or sprays; however, a few are available as nasal jellies. Examples of products for intranasal use are shown in Figure 12.5 and presented in Table 12.11.

Nasal Decongestant Solutions

Most nasal decongestant solutions are aqueous preparations, rendered isotonic to nasal fluids (approximately equivalent to 0.9% sodium chloride), buffered to maintain drug stability while approximating the normal pH range of the nasal fluids (pH 5.5 to 6.5), and stabilized and preserved as required. The antimicrobial preservatives used are the same as those used in preserving ophthalmic solutions. The concentration of adrenergic agent in the majority of nasal decongestant solutions is quite low, ranging from about 0.05 to 1.0%. Certain commercial solutions which are available for both pediatric and adult use, are available in two strengths, the pediatric strength being approximately one-half of the adult strength.

Nasal decongestant solutions are employed in the treatment of rhinitis of the common cold and for vasomotor and allergic rhinitis including hay fever, and for sinusitis. Their frequent use or their use for prolonged periods may lead to chronic edema of the nasal mucosa, i.e., *rhinitis medicamentosa,* aggravat-

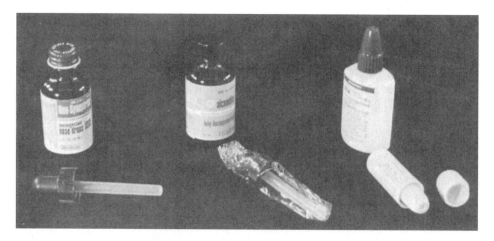

Fig. 12.5   *Examples of commercial packaging of nasal solutions, showing drop and spray containers and a nasal inhaler.*

Table 12.11.   Examples of Some Commercial Nasal Preparations

Product Name	Manufacturer	Active Ingredient	Use/Indications
Afrin Nasal Spray and Afrin Nose Drops	Schering-Plough	oxymetazole HCl (0.05%)	Nasal adrenergic/decongestant
Beconase AQ Nasal Spray	Glaxo Wellcome	beclomethasone diproprionate (0.042%)	Synthetic corticosteroid indicated for the relief of symptoms of seasonal or perennial allergic or vasomotor rhinitis
Diapid Nasal Spray	Sandoz	lopressin (0.185 mg/mL)	Antidiuretic; for control or prevention of diabetes insipidus due to deficiency of endogenous posterior pituitary antidiuretic hormone.
Nasalcrom Nasal Spray	McNeil	cromolyn sodium (4%)	Prevention and treatment of symptoms of allergic rhinitis
Nasalide Nasal Solution	Dura	flunisolide (0.025%)	Indicated in the treatment of symptoms of seasonal or perennial rhinitis
Neo-Synephrine Nose Drops/ Spray	Bayer Consumer	phenylephrine HCl (0.125 to 1.0%)	Nasal adrenergic/decongestant
Neo-Synephrine Maximum Strength 12 Hour	Bayer Consumer	oxymetazoline HCl (0.05%)	Nasal adrenergic/decongestant
Ocean Mist	Fleming	isotonic sodium chloride	To restore moisture and relieve dry, crusted and inflamed nasal membranes.
Privine HCl Nasal Solution	Novartis	naphazoline HCl (0.05 and 0.1%)	Nasal adrenergic/decongestant
Syntocinon Nasal Spray	Sandoz	oxytocin (40 units/mL)	Synthetic oxytocin hormone. Employed for initial milk let-down preparatory to breast feeding.
Tyzine Pediatric Nose Drops	Key	tetrahydrozoline HCl (0.05%)	Nasal adrenergic/decongestant

ing the symptom that they are intended to relieve. Thus, they are best used for short periods (no longer than 3 to 5 days) with the patients advised not to exceed the recommended dosage and frequency of use.

The easiest but least comfortable approach to treat rebound congestion is to completely withdraw application of the topical vasoconstrictor. Unfortunately, this approach will promptly result in bilateral vasodilation with almost total nasal obstruction. A more acceptable method is to withdraw application of drug in only one nostril, and have the patient continue using the medication in the other nostril. Once the rebound congestion subsides in the drug-free nostril, about 1 to 2 weeks, a total withdrawal is then instituted. Another approach is the substitution of a topical saline solution or spray *in lieu* of the topical vasoconstrictor. This effectively keeps the nasal mucosa moist and provides psychologic assistance to patients who are dependent upon placing medication into their nostrils.

Most of the adrenergic drugs used in nasal decongestant solutions are synthetic compounds similar in chemical structure, pharmacologic activity, and side effects to the parent compound, naturally occurring epinephrine. Epinephrine as a pure chemical substance was first isolated from suprarenal gland in 1901 and was called both *Suprarenin* and *Adrenalin*. Synthetic epinephrine was prepared just a few years later.

Most solutions for nasal use are packaged in dropper bottles or in plastic spray bottles, usually containing 15 to 30 mL of medication. The products should be determined to be stable in the containers used and the packages tightly closed during periods of nonuse. The patient should be advised that should the solution become discolored or contain precipitated matter, it should be discarded.

The patient should also understand that there is a difference in the duration of the effect of topical decongestants. For example, phenylephrine should be used every 3 to 4 hours, whereas oxymetazoline, which is longer acting, should only be used every 12 hours.

Inhalation Solutions

Inhalations are drugs or solutions of drugs administered by the nasal or oral respiratory route. The drugs may be administered for their local action on the bronchial tree or for their systemic effects through absorption from the lungs. Certain gases, as oxygen and ether, are administered by inhalation as are finely powdered drug substances and solutions of drugs administered as fine mists. Sterile Water for Inhalation, USP and Sodium Chloride Inhalation, USP may be used as vehicles for inhalation solutions.

As discussed in Chapter 13, a number of drug substances are administered through pressure packaged *inhalation aerosols*. For the inhaled drug substance or solution to reach the bronchial tree, the inhaled particles must be just a few microns in size.

A widely used instrument capable of producing fine particles for inhalation therapy is the *nebulizer*. This apparatus, shown in Figure 12.6, contains an atomizing unit within a curved, glass, bulb-like chamber. A rubber bulb at the end of the apparatus is depressed and the medicated solution is drawn up a narrow glass tube and broken into fine particles by the passing airstream. The fine particles produced range between 0.5 and 5 microns. The larger, heavier droplets of the mist do not exit the apparatus but fall back into the reservoir of medicated liquid. The lighter particles do escape with the airstream and are inhaled by the patient who operates the nebulizer with the exit orifice in his mouth, inhaling as he depresses the rubber bulb.

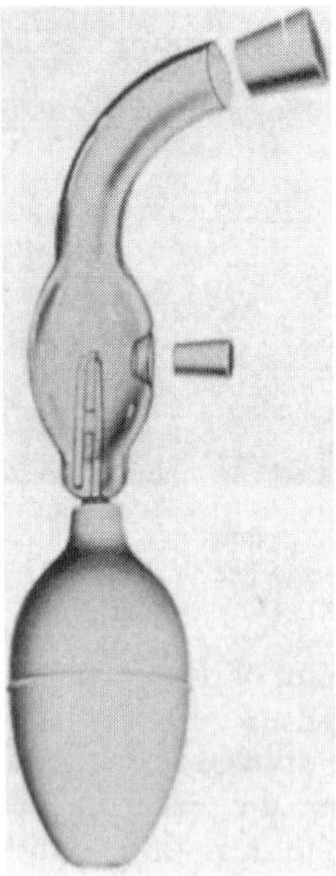

The pharmacist should advise the patient on the proper technique to use the nebulizer and provide additional patient instructions, e.g., do not exceed physician's instructions and use the smallest amount of product necessary to afford relief. The pharmacist could also advise on how to cope with dryness of the mouth that might occur. Further, the pharmacist should emphasize the need to clean the nebulizer after its use and explain how to do it.

The common household *vaporizer*, as the one depicted in Figure 12.7, produces a fine mist of steam that may be used to humidify a room. When a volatile medication is added to the water in the chamber or to a special medication cup present in some models, the medication volatilizes and is also inhaled by the patient. *Humidifiers*, as shown in Figure 12.8, are used to provide a cool mist to the air in a room. Moisture in the air is important to prevent mucous membranes of the nose and throat

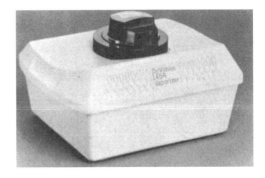

Fig. 12.7 *Example of commercially available vaporizer. (Courtesy of The DeVilbiss Co.)*

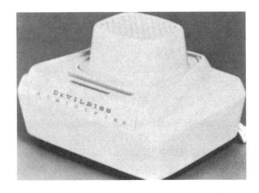

Fig. 12.8 *Example of a commercially available humidifier. (Courtesy of The DeVilbiss Co.)*

Fig. 12.6 *Example of a nebulizer used in inhalation therapy. See text for description of operation. (Courtesy of The DeVilbiss Co.)*

from becoming dry and irritated. Vaporizers and humidifiers are commonly used in the adjunctive treatment of colds, coughs, and chest congestion.

The pharmacist can help a patient select a vaporizer or humidifier depending upon one's needs. Both devices have advantages and disadvantages. Manufacturing guidelines and legal regulations, e.g., lock tops, have made vaporizers more safe today than in the years past. So the possibility of scalding due to an overturned vaporizer is less with newer models. Further, the heat generated in a vaporizer kills the mold and bacteria that may be in the water tank. Humidifiers are more costly, but use less electricity than vaporizers. In addition, compared to vaporizers, humidifiers are noisier during operation, can leave a deposition of minerals on woodwork and furniture, and can effectively cool down a room by 1° to 3° (a problem with young children). The patient should learn about these subtle differences from the pharmacist.

Ultrasonic humidifiers are also available, and while they are effective and operate at an almost noiseless level, they apparently pose a health problem. While these are highly efficient at nebulizing water into fine droplets, they are also efficient at nebulizing up to 90% of water contaminants as well. These contaminants include mold, bacteria, lead, and dissolved organic gases, which could ultimately cause acute respiratory irritation to chronic lung problems in unsuspecting patients. Thus, patients should either be advised to run water through a high-grade demineralization filter before filling their ultrasonic humidifier, or buy a humidifier with a built-in filter that works.

Examples of Medicated Inhalation Solutions

A number of inhalations are pressure packaged as inhalation aerosols and are discussed in Chapter 13. Several other inhalations used in medicine are solutions intended to be administered by nebulizer or other apparatus. Among these are: isoetharine inhalation solution (Bronkosol, Sanofi) and isoproterenol inhalation solution (Isuprel Solution, Sanofi), both used for the relief of bronchial spasms in the treatment of bronchial asthma and related conditions.

Inhalants

Inhalants are drugs or combinations of drugs that by virtue of their high vapor pressure can be carried by an air current into the nasal passage where they exert their effect. The device in which the drug or drugs is contained and from which they are administered is termed an *inhaler.*

Certain nasal decongestants may be employed in the form of inhalants. For instance the drug propylhexedrine (Benzedrex, Menley & James Labs) is a liquid which volatilizes slowly at room temperature. This quality enables it to be effective as an inhalant. The inhalers in which the drug is held contain cylindrical rolls of fibrous material impregnated with the volatile drug substance. The medication which has an amine-like odor is usually masked with added aromatic agents. The inhaler is placed in the nostril and vapor inhaled to relieve nasal congestion. As with the other nasal adrenergic agents, excessive or too frequent use can result in nasal edema and increased rather than decreased congestion. The inhalers are effective so long as the volatile drug remains present. To ensure that the drug does not escape during periods of nonuse, the caps on the inhalers should be tightly closed.

Amyl Nitrite Inhalant

Amyl nitrite is a clear, yellowish, volatile liquid that acts as a vasodilator when inhaled. The drug is prepared in sealed glass vials that are covered with a protective gauze cloth (Fig. 12.9). Upon use, the glass vial is broken in the fingertips and the cloth soaks up the liquid which is then inhaled. The vials generally contain 0.3 mL of the drug substance. The effects of the drug are rapid and are used in the treatment of anginal pain.

Propylhexedrine Inhalant

Propylhexedrine is a liquid adrenergic (vasoconstrictor) agent that volatilizes slowly at room temperature. This quality enables it to be effectively used as an inhalant. The official inhalant consists of cylindrical rolls of suitable fibrous material impregnated with propylhexedrine, usually aromatized to mask its amine-like odor, and contained in a suitable inhaler. The vapor of the drug is inhaled into the nostrils when needed to relieve nasal congestion due to colds and hay fever. It may also be employed to relieve ear block and the pressure pain in air travelers.

Each plastic tube of the commercial product contains 250 mg of propylhexedrine with aromatics. The containers should be tightly closed after each opening to prevent loss of the drug vapors. The counterpart commercial product is Benzedrex Inhaler (Menley & James Labs).

Proper Administration and Use of Nasal Drops and Sprays

To minimize the possibility of contamination, the pharmacist should point out to the patient that the nasal product only be used by one person and kept

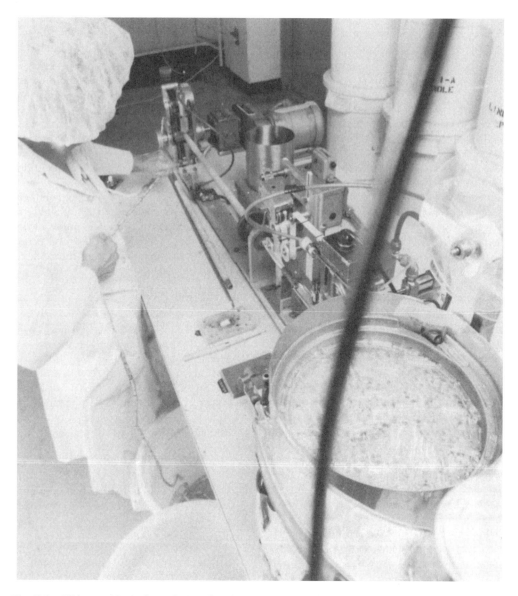

Fig. 12.9 *Silking operation in the production of amyl nitrate Vaporole. (Courtesy of Burroughs Wellcome Company.)*

out of the reach of children. If the nasal product is intended for a child the directions should be clear to the patient. If an over-the-counter product is used, the parent should note the directions on the label.

Before using the drops, the patient should be advised to gently blow the nose and wash his/her hands thoroughly with soap and water. For maximum penetration with drops, a patient should lie down on a flat surface, such as a bed, hanging the head over the edge, and then tilting the head back as far as comfortable. The prescribed number of drops are then gently placed into the nostrils, and to allow the medication to spread in the nose, the patient should remain in this position for a few minutes. After this, the dropper should be replaced in the bottle and tightened.

Before using the spray the patient should be advised to gently blow the nose to clear the nostrils and wash his/her hands thoroughly with soap and water. The patient should be told not to shake the plastic squeeze bottle for use, but be sure to remove the plastic cap. While holding the head upright the patient should insert the nose-piece into the nostril, pointing it slightly backward, and close the other nostril with one finger. The patient should then spray the prescribed or recommended amount, squeezing the bottle sharply and firmly while sniffing through the nose. Sprays should always be administered with the patient in an upright position. Spraying medicine into the nostrils should not be performed with the head over the edge of a bed (the preferred procedure for administration of nasal drops) because it could result in the systemic absorption of the drug, rather than a local effect.

The patient should be advised not to overuse the product. For example, some decongestant medicines such as oxymetazoline and xylometazoline can predispose the patient to rebound congestion if used for more than 3 to 5 consecutive days. The patient should also understand the normal time frame in which to see results and be advised that after a certain number of days if relief is not achieved to consult the physician. Lastly, patients should realize not to share their medicated spray with another person to prevent the possibility of cross-contamination between individuals. Certain nasal medications (e.g., Vancenase, Schering [beclomethasone diproprionate]) are available for administration through aerosol inhalers.

Nasal Route for Systemic Effects

The nasal route for drug delivery is of current interest because of the need to develop a non-oral, nonparenteral route for newly developed synthetic biologically active peptides and polypeptides (10–15). Polypeptides, such as insulin, that are subject to destruction by the gastrointestinal fluids are currently administered by injection. However, the nasal mucosa has been shown to be amenable to the systemic absorption of certain peptides, as well as to nonpeptide drug molecules including scopolamine, hydralazine, progesterone, and propranolol (13–14). The nasal route is advantageous for nonpeptide drugs that are poorly absorbed orally.

The adult nasal cavity has about a 20 mL capacity, with a large surface area (about 180 cm^2) for drug absorption afforded by the microvilli present along the pseudostratified columnar epithelial cells of the nasal mucosa (12,14). The nasal tissue is highly vascularized, providing an attractive site for rapid and efficient systemic absorption. One great advantage to nasal absorption is that it avoids first-pass metabolism by the liver. However, the identification of metabolizing enzymes in the nasal mucosa of certain animal species suggests the same possibility in humans and the potential for some intranasal drug metabolism (12).

For some peptides and small molecular compounds, intranasal bioavailability has been comparable to that of injections. However, bioavailability decreases as the molecular weight of a compound increases, and for proteins composed of more than 27 amino acids bioavailability may be low (11). Various pharmaceutic techniques and formulation adjuncts, as surface-active agents, have been shown to be capable of enhancing the nasal absorption of large molecules (11,14).

Pharmaceuticals currently on the market or in various stages of clinical investigation for nasal delivery include lypressin (Diapid, Sandoz), oxytocin (Syntocinon, Sandoz), desmopressin (DDAVP, Rhone-Poulenc Rorer), vitamin B-12 (Ener-B Gel, Nature's Bounty), progesterone, insulin, calcitonin, propranolol, and butorphanol (10,11).

Otic Solutions

Otic preparations are sometimes referred to as *ear* or *aural* preparations. Solutions are most frequently used in the ear, with suspensions and ointments also finding some application. Ear preparations are usually placed in the ear canal by drops or in small amounts for the removal of excessive cerumen (ear wax) or for the treatment of ear infections, inflammation, or pain. Because the outer ear is a skin-covered structure and susceptible to the same dermatologic conditions as other parts of the body's surface, skin conditions which arise are treated using the variety of topical dermatological preparations previously discussed in Chapter 9.

Cerumen-Removing Solutions

Cerumen is a combination of the secretions of the sweat and sebaceous glands of the external auditory canal. The secretions, if allowed to dry, form a sticky semisolid which holds shed epithelial cells, fallen hair, dust and other foreign bodies that make their way into the ear canal. Excessive accumulation of cerumen in the ear may cause itching, pain, impaired hearing and is a deterrent to otologic examination. If not removed periodically, the cerumen may become impacted and its removal made more difficult and painful.

Through the years, light mineral oil, vegetable oils, and hydrogen peroxide have been commonly used agents to soften impacted cerumen for its removal. Recently, solutions of synthetic surfactants have been developed for their *cerumenolytic* activity in the removal of ear wax. One of these agents, tri-ethanolamine polypeptide oleate-condensate, commercially formulated in propylene glycol, is used to emulsify the cerumen thereby facilitating its removal [Cerumenex Drops (Purdue Frederick)]. Another commercial product utilizes carbamide peroxide in glycerin/propylene glycol [Debrox Drops (SmithKline Beecham)]. On contact with the cerumen, the carbamide peroxide releases oxygen which disrupts the integrity of the impacted wax, allowing its easy removal.

In removing cerumen, the procedure usually involves placing the otic solution in the ear canal with the patient's head tilted at a 45° angle, inserting a cotton plug to retain the medication in the ear for 15 to 30 minutes, followed by gentle flushing of the ear canal with lukewarm water using a soft rubber ear syringe.

Anti-infective, Anti-inflammatory, and Analgesic Ear Preparations

Drugs used topically in the ear for their anti-infective activity include such agents as chloramphenicol, colistin sulfate, neomycin, polymyxin B sulfate, and nystatin, the latter agent used to combat fungal infections. These agents are formulated into ear drops (solutions or suspensions) in a vehicle of anhydrous glycerin or propylene glycol. These viscous vehicles permit maximum contact time between the medication and the tissues of the ear. In addition, their hygroscopicity causes them to draw moisture from the tissues thereby reducing inflammation and diminishing the moisture available for the life process of the microorganisms present. To assist in relieving the pain which frequently accompanies ear infections, a number of anti-infective otic preparations also contain analgesic agents as antipyrine and local anesthetics as lidocaine, dibucaine, and benzocaine.

Topical treatment of ear infections is frequently considered adjunctive, with concomitant systemic treatment with orally administered antibiotics also undertaken.

Liquid ear preparations of the anti-inflammatory agents hydrocortisone and dexamethasone sodium phosphate are prescribed for their effects against the swelling and inflammation which frequently accompany allergic and irritative manifestations of the ear as well as for the inflammation and pruritus which sometimes follow treatment of ear infections. In the latter instance, some physicians prefer the use of corticosteroids in ointment form, pack-aged in ophthalmic tubes. These packages allow the placement of small amounts of ointment in the ear canal with a minimum of waste. Many of the commercially available products used in this manner are labeled "eye-ear" to indicate their dual use.

Aside from the antibiotic-steroid combinations that are used to treat otitis externa, which is known synonymously as swimmer's ear, acetic acid (2%) in aluminum acetate solution and boric acid (2.75%) in isopropyl alcohol are used. These drugs help to re-acidify the ear canal and the vehicles serve to help dry the ear canal. By drying the ear canal, the growth medium for the offending microorganisms, usually *Pseudomonas aeruginosa,* is kept in check. Pharmacists may also be called on to extemporaneously prepare a solution of acetic acid, 2 to 2.5% in rubbing alcohol (70% isopropyl alcohol or ethanol), propylene glycol or anhydrous glycerin. The source of the acetic acid can be glacial acetic acid but usually distilled white vinegar (5% acetic acid) is used. Boric acid, 2 to 5%, dissolved in either ethanol or propylene glycol has also been recommended for use in the ear. This substance, however, may be absorbed from broken skin and be toxic. Thus, its use is usually limited, especially in children with burst ear drums.

Pain in the ear frequently accompanies ear infection or inflamed or swollen ear tissue. Frequently, the pain is far out of proportion to the actual condition. Because the ear canal is so narrow, even a slight inflammation can cause intense pain and discomfort for the patient. Topical analgesic agents generally are employed together with internally administered analgesics, as aspirin, and other agents, as anti-infectives, to combat the cause of the problem.

Topical analgesics for the ear are usually solutions and frequently contain the analgesic antipyrine and the local anesthetic benzocaine in a vehicle of propylene glycol or anhydrous glycerin (e.g., Auralgan Otic Solution, Wyeth-Ayerst). Again, these hygroscopic vehicles reduce the swelling of tissues (and thus some pain) and the growth of microorganisms by drawing moisture from the swollen tissues into the vehicle. These preparations are commonly employed to relieve the symptoms of acute otitis media. Examples of some commercial otic preparations are presented in Table 12.12.

As determined on an individual product basis, some liquid otic preparations require preservation against microbial growth. When preservation is required, such agents as chlorobutanol (0.5%), thimerosal (0.01%), and combinations of the

Table 12.12. Examples of Some Commercial Otic Preparations

Product Name	Manufacturer	Active Ingredient	Vehicle	Use/Indications
Americaine Otic	Medeva	benzocaine	glycerin, polyethylene, glycol 300	Local anesthetic for relief of ear pain and pruritis in otitis media, swimmer's ear, and similar conditions
Auralgan Otic Solution	Ayerst-Wyeth	antipyrine, benzocaine	dehydrated glycerin	Acute otitis media
Cerumenex Ear Drops	Purdue Frederick	triethanolamine poly-peptide oleate-condensate	propylene glycol	Cerumenolytic agent to remove impacted earwax
Chloromycetin Otic	Parke-Davis	chloramphenicol	propylene glycol	Antiinfective
Cortisporin Otic Solution	Glaxo Wellcome	polymyxin B sulfate, neomycin sulfate, hydrocortisone	glycerin, propylene glycol, water for injection	Superficial bacterial infections
Debrox Drops	SmithKline Beecham	carbamide peroxide	anhydrous glycerin	Ear wax removal
PediOtic Suspension	Monarch	polymyxin B sulfate, neomycin sulfate, hydrocortisone	mineral oil, propylene glycol, water for injection	Superficial bacterial infections
Metreton Ophthalmic/ Otic Solution	Schering-Plough	prednisolone sodium phosphate	aqueous	Antiinflammatory
Otobiotic Otic Solution	Schering-Plough	polymyxin B sulfate, hydrocortisone	propylene glycol, glycerin, water	Superficial bacterial infections
VoSol Otic Solution	Wallace	acetic acid	propylene glycol	Antibacterial/antifungal

parabens are commonly used. Antioxidants, as sodium bisulfite, and other stabilizers are also included in otic formulations, as required. Ear preparations are usually packaged in small (5 to 15 mL) glass or plastic containers with a dropper.

Proper Administration and Use of Otic Drops

When ear drops are prescribed, it is important for the pharmacist to first determine how the drops are to be used. For example, ear wax removal drops should be instilled and then removed by the patient with an ear syringe. Alternatively, drops intended to treat external otitis infection are intended to be instilled and left in the ear.

The pharmacist should make sure the patient or parent understands that administration is intended for the ear and the frequency of application. To facilitate patient acceptance the pharmacist should point out that the bottle or container of medication should first be warmed in the hands, and if the product is a suspension, shaken prior to withdrawal into the dropper. The pharmacist should

also explain the need to store the medication in a safe place out of the reach of children and away from extremes of temperature.

When instilled into the ear, to allow the drops to run in deeper, the earlobe should be held up and back. For a child, the earlobe should be held down and back. For convenience it is probably easier to have someone other than the patient to administer the drops.

Some ear drops by virtue of their formulation, i.e., low pH, may cause stinging upon administration. Thus, parents and children should be forewarned especially if a child, for example, has tympanostomy tubes in the ear. The patient should also understand the length, in days, to use the product. For antibiotic ear drops it is not necessary to finish the entire bottle because therapy could last 20 to 30 days depending upon the dosage regimen. Therefore, patients should be instructed to continue using the drops for 3 days beyond the time ear symptoms disappear. Products for otitis externa may take up to 7 to 10 days to demonstrate efficacy.

If a child is prone to develop ear infections as a result of swimming or showering, it might be advisable to recommend the parents to consult a physician for prophylactic medication to use during swimming season, and consider using form-fitting ear plugs that fit snugly in the ear when swimming or showering. Further, after the child emerges from the water or shower, the parents can be advised to use a home hair blow dryer on a low setting to dry out the ear. It will dry out the ear quickly without trauma. The dryer should not be placed too close to the child's ear.

Topical Oral (Dental) Solutions

A variety of medicinal substances are employed topically in the oral cavity for a number of purposes and in a wide range of dosage forms. Among the drugs and preparations included in this group are the following:

Benzocaine—Topical anesthetic. Indicated for temporary relief of pain, soreness, and irritation in the mouth associated with teething, orthodontic appliances, new or poorly fitting dentures, and canker sores.

Camphorated Parachlorophenol—Dental anti-infective. A eutectic liquid composed of 65% camphor and 35% parachlorophenol, used in dentistry for the sterilization of deep root canals.

Carbamide Peroxide Topical Solution—Dental anti-infective. Acts as a chemomechanical cleansing and debriding agent through the release of bubbling oxygen. The commercial product (Gly-Oxide Liquid, Smith Kline Beecham) contains 10% carbamide in flavored anhydrous glycerin.

Cetylpyridinium Chloride Solution and Cetylpyridinium Chloride Lozenges—Local anti-infective. Commercial counterparts (Cepacol Mouthwash/Gargle and Cepacol Lozenges) contain 1:2000 w/v and 1:1500 w/v of cetylpyridinium chloride respectively. Used primarily as a freshening mouth cleanser. Lozenges have benzyl alcohol present to act as a local anesthetic in soothing throat irritations.

Erythrosine Sodium Topical Solution and Erythrosine Sodium Soluble Tablets—Diagnostic aid (dental disclosing agent). Solution applied topically to the teeth to reveal plaque left by inadequate brushing. Tablets chewed for the same purpose and are not to be swallowed.

Eugenol—Dental analgesic. Applied topically to dental cavities and dental protectives. Eugenol is a pale yellow liquid having an aromatic odor of clove and a spicy taste.

Lidocaine Oral Spray—Topical dental anesthetic. Applied through metered spray in the amounts of 10 mg per spray; 20 mg per quadrant of gingiva and oral mucosa is usually employed. [Xylocaine Oral Spray (Astra)]

Nystatin Oral Suspension—Antifungal. May be employed for oral fungal infections by retaining in the mouth as long as possible before swallowing.

Saliva Substitutes—These contain electrolytes in a carboxymethylcellulose base and are indicated for the relief of dry mouth and throat in xerostomia.

Sodium Fluoride Oral Solution, and Sodium Fluoride Tablets—Dental caries prophylactic. Solution applied to the teeth or, when drinking water does not contain adequate fluoride, a dilute solution may be swallowed. Tablets containing 1.1 or 2.2 mg of sodium fluoride are chewed or swallowed as required.

Sodium Fluoride and Phosphoric Acid Gel and Sodium Fluoride and Phosphoric Acid Topical Solution—Dental caries prophylactic. Gel and solution applied to the teeth; each contains 1.23% of fluoride ion and 1% of phosphoric acid.

Triamcinolone Acetonide Dental Paste—Topical anti-inflammatory agent. Applied to the oral mucous membranes as a 0.1% paste.

Zinc Oxide-Eugenol Mixture—A temporary filling mix.

In addition to the above-named drugs and preparations, a host of other products for oral use are commercially available. Some of these products are medicated, as teething lotions and toothache drops, whereas others are used for hygienic purposes, as dentifrices, denture products, and many of the mouthwashes. Among the variety of products is a like variety of physical forms, as solutions, emulsions, ointments, pastes, aerosols, etc., with the manufacture of each following the same general procedures as has been previously outlined in this text. One type of dosage form for oral use, the lozenge, has not been previously described.

Miscellaneous Solutions

Aromatic Waters

Aromatic waters are clear, aqueous solutions saturated with volatile oils or other aromatic or volatile substances. Aromatic waters are no longer in wide-spread use. In years past, aromatic waters were prepared from a number of volatile substances including the following: orange flower oil, peppermint oil, rose oil, anise oil, spearmint oil, wintergreen oil, camphor and chloroform. Naturally, the odors and tastes of aromatic waters are of the volatile substances from which they are prepared.

Most of the aromatic substances in the preparation of aromatic waters have very low solubilities in water, and even though a water may be saturated, its concentration of aromatic material is still rather small. Aromatic waters may be used for perfuming and/or flavoring.

Diluted Acids

Diluted acids are aqueous solutions prepared by diluting the corresponding concentrated acids with purified water. The strength of a diluted acid is generally expressed on a per cent weight-to-volume (% w/v) basis, that is, the weight in grams of solute per 100 mL of solution, whereas the strength of a concentrated acid is generally expressed in terms of per cent weight-to-weight (% w/w), which indicates the number of grams of solute per 100 g of solution. In order to prepare a diluted acid from a concentrated one, it is first necessary to calculate the amount of solute required in the diluted product. Then, the amount of concentrated acid required to supply the needed amount of solute can be determined.

To illustrate, concentrated hydrochloric acid contains not less than 35 g and not more than 38 g of solute (absolute HCl) per 100 g of acid and therefore is considered to be, on the average, 36.5% w/w in strength. Diluted hydrochloric acid contains between 9.5 and 10.5 g of solute per 100 mL of solution and is therefore considered to be approximately 10% w/v in strength. If, for example, one wished to prepare 100 mL of the diluted acid from the concentrated acid, he would require 10 g of solute. The amount of concentrated hydrochloric acid required to supply this amount of solute may be calculated by the following proportion:

$$\frac{36.5 \text{ g (solute)}}{100 \text{ g (conc. acid)}} = \frac{10 \text{ g (solute)}}{x \text{ (g conc. acid)}}$$

solving for x:

$$36.5x = 1000 \text{ g}$$
$$x = 27.39 \text{ g (conc. acid)}$$

Thus, 27.39 g of concentrated acid are required to supply 10 g of solute needed for the preparation of 100 mL of the diluted acid. Although the required amount of concentrated acid may be accurately weighed, it is a cumbersome task, and as a rule pharmacists prefer to measure liquids volumetrically. Therefore, in the preparation of diluted acids, the calculations are generally carried one step further to determine the *volume* of concentrated acid that corresponds with the calculated weight. Because this additional step requires the use of the concentrated acid's specific gravity, a brief review of specific gravity seems appropriate.

By definition, specific gravity is a ratio, expressed decimally, of the weight of a substance to the weight of an equal volume of a standard, both substances having the same temperature or the temperature of each being known. Water is used as the standard for liquids and solids; hydrogen or air, for gases. In pharmacy, specific gravity calculations mainly involve liquids and solids, and water is an excellent choice for a standard, because it is readily available and easily purified.

At 4°C, the density of water is 1 g per cubic centimeter (cc). Because the USP states that 1 mL may be considered the equivalent of 1 cc, in pharmacy, water is assumed to weigh 1 g per mL. By the following equation, used to calculate specific gravity, a substance having a density the same as water would have a specific gravity of 1.0:

$$\text{sp gr} = \frac{\text{weight of a substance}}{\text{weight of an equal volume of water}}$$

In solving this equation, the same units of weight must be used in each part of the ratio. These units cancel out, and the ratio is expressed decimally.

Specific gravity indicates the relative weight of a substance compared to an equal volume of water. For example, if 10 mL of a liquid weigh 20 g, an equal volume of water would weigh 10 g, and the ratio in the equation would be 20 g/10 g yielding a specific gravity of 2.0. This would indicate that the liquid is twice as heavy as water in equal volume. By the same token, a liquid having a specific gravity of 0.5 would be half as heavy as water; a liquid with a specific gravity of 0.8 would be eight-tenths as heavy as water, etc.

If both the volume of a liquid and its specific gravity are known, its weight may be calculated. For instance, if concentrated hydrochloric acid has a specific gravity of 1.17, it is that number times as heavy as water, and 100 mL of the acid would weigh 1.17 times as much as 100 mL of water. Since 100 mL of water weigh 100 g, 100 mL of the acid would weigh 1.17 times that or 117 g.

If one knows the weight of a liquid and its specific gravity, the volume of the liquid may be determined.

For example, a liquid that is twice as heavy as water would have a specific gravity of 2.0 and would occupy half the volume that an equal weight of water would occupy. If one had 100 g of this liquid and substituted in the above equation as indicated below, the volume of the liquid could be arrived at:

$$2.0 = \frac{100 \text{ g}}{\text{weight of an equal volume of water}}$$

$$\text{weight of an equal volume of water} = \frac{100 \text{ g}}{2.0}$$

$$= 50 \text{ g}$$

Since 50 g is the weight of an equal volume of water, it follows that the water must measure 50 mL. Since the volume of the water is an "equal volume" to the other liquid, that liquid must also measure 50 mL.

The volume represented by 27.39 g of the concentrated hydrochloric acid may be similarly determined by dividing the specific gravity of the concentrated acid into its weight and equating the answer of weight of an equal volume of water to the volume of the acid:

$$\frac{27.39 \text{ g}}{1.17} = 23.41 \text{ g, weight of equal volume of water.}$$

Thus, because 23.41 g of water measures 23.41 mL and because it is equal in volume to the concentrated acid, the latter also measures 23.41 mL and would be required to prepare 100 mL of the 10% w/v diluted acid.

Once the aforementioned is thoroughly understood, the following simplified formula can be used to calculate the amount of a concentrated acid required in the preparation of a specific volume of the corresponding diluted acid:

$$\frac{\text{Percentage strength} \quad \text{Volume of diluted}}{\text{(w/v) of diluted acid} \times \text{acid to be prepared}}$$
$$\overline{\text{Percentage strength (w/w)} \times \text{Specific gravity of}}$$
$$\text{of concentrated acid} \qquad \text{concentrated acid}$$

$$= \text{Volume of concentrated acid to use}$$

Recalculating the preparation of 100 mL of diluted hydrochloric acid from the concentrated acid gives the following:

$$\frac{10 \times 100 \text{ mL}}{36.5 \times 1.17} = \frac{23.41 \text{ mL of concentrated}}{\text{acid to use.}}$$

Most diluted acids have a strength of 10% w/v, with the exception of diluted acetic acid which is 6% w/v. The strengths of these acids are commen-surate with the concentrations generally used for medicinal or pharmaceutical purposes. The concentrations of the corresponding concentrated acids vary widely from one acid to another, depending upon various properties of the solute such as solubility, stability, and ease of preparation. For instance, concentrated sulfuric acid is generally between 95 and 98% w/w, nitric acid between 69 and 71% w/w, and concentrated phosphoric acid between 85 and 88% w/w. As a result, the amounts of each concentrated acid required to prepare the corresponding diluted acid vary widely and must be calculated on an individual basis.

There is very little use of diluted acids in medicine today. However, because of its antibacterial effects, acetic acid finds application as 1% solutions in surgical dressings, as an irrigating solution to the bladder in 0.25% concentration, and also as a spermatocidal in some proprietary contraceptive preparations.

Spirits

Spirits are alcoholic or hydroalcoholic solutions of volatile substances. Generally, the alcoholic concentration of spirits is rather high, usually over 60%. Because of the greater solubility of aromatic or volatile substances in alcohol than in water, spirits can contain a greater concentration of these materials than the corresponding aromatic waters. When mixed with water or with an aqueous preparation, the volatile substances present in spirits generally separate from solution and form a milky preparation.

Spirits may be used pharmaceutically as flavoring agents and medicinally for the therapeutic value of the aromatic solute. As flavoring agents they are used to impart the flavor of their solute to other pharmaceutical preparations. For medicinal purposes, spirits may be taken orally, applied externally, or used by inhalation, depending upon the particular preparation. When taken orally, they are generally mixed with a portion of water to reduce the pungency of the spirit. Depending on the materials utilized, spirits may be prepared by simple solution, solution by maceration, or distillation. The spirits most recently official in the USP/NF were aromatic ammonia spirit, camphor spirit, compound orange spirit, and peppermint spirit.

Nonaqueous Solutions

Liniments

Liniments are alcoholic or oleaginous solutions or emulsions of various medicinal substances intended for external application to the skin with rubbing. Liniments with an alcoholic or hydroalcoholic vehicle are useful in instances in which rubefacient, counterirritant, or penetrating action is desired; oleaginous liniments are employed primarily when massage is desired. By their nature, oleaginous liniments are less irritating to the skin than alcoholic liniments. Liniments are not applied to skin areas that are broken or bruised because excessive irritation might result. The vehicle for a liniment should therefore be selected on the basis of the type of action desired (rubefacient, counterirritant, or just massage) and also on the solubility of the desired components in the various solvents. For oleaginous liniments, the solvent may be a fixed oil such as almond oil, peanut oil, sesame oil, or cottonseed oil or a volatile substance such as wintergreen oil or turpentine, or it may be a combination of fixed and volatile oils.

All liniments should bear a label indicating that they are suitable only for external use and must never be taken internally. Liniments that are emulsions or that contain insoluble matter must be shaken thoroughly before use to ensure an even distribution of the dispersed phase, and for these preparations a "Shake Well" label is indicated. Liniments should be stored in tight containers. Depending on their individual ingredients, liniments are prepared in the same manner as solutions, emulsions, or suspensions, as the case may warrant.

Collodions

Collodions are liquid preparations composed of pyroxylin dissolved in a solvent mixture usually composed of alcohol and ether with or without added medicinal substances. Pyroxylin (soluble gun cotton, collodion cotton) is obtained by the action of a mixture of nitric and sulfuric acids on cotton and consists chiefly of cellulose tetranitrate. It has the appearance of raw cotton when dry but is harsh to the touch. It is frequently available commercially moistened with about 30% alcohol or other similar solvent.

One part of pyroxylin is slowly but completely soluble in 25 parts of a mixture of 3 volumes of ether and 1 volume of alcohol. It is also soluble in acetone and glacial acetic acid. Pyroxylin is precipitated from solution in these solvents upon the addition of water. Pyroxylin, like collodions, is exceedingly flammable and must be stored away from flame in well-closed containers, protected from light.

Collodions are intended for external use. When applied to the skin with a fine camel's hair brush or glass applicator, the solvent rapidly evaporates, leaving a filmy residue of pyroxylin. This provides an occlusive protective coating to the skin, and when the collodion is medicated it leaves a thin layer of that medication firmly placed against the skin. Naturally, collodions must be applied to dry tissues to effect adhesion to the skin's surface. The products must be clearly labeled "For External Use Only" or with words of similar effect.

Collodion

Collodion is a clear or slightly opalescent, viscous liquid prepared by dissolving pyroxylin (4% w/v) in a 3:1 mixture of ether and alcohol. The resulting solution is highly volatile and flammable and should be preserved in tight containers at a temperature not exceeding 30°C remote from fire.

The product is capable of forming a protective film on application to the skin and the volatilization of the solvent. The film is useful in holding the edges of an incised wound together. However, its presence on the skin is uncomfortable due to its inflexible nature. The following product, which is flexible, has a greater appeal when a nonpliable film is not required.

Flexible Collodion

Flexible Collodion is prepared by adding 2% of camphor and 3% of castor oil to collodion. The castor oil renders the product flexible, permitting its comfortable use over skin areas that are normally moved, such as fingers and toes. The camphor makes the product waterproof. Physicians frequently apply the coating over bandages or stitched incisions to make them waterproof and to protect them from external stress.

Salicylic Acid Collodion

Salicylic Acid Collodion is a 10% solution of salicylic acid in flexible collodion. It is used for its keratolytic effects, especially in the removal of corns from the toes. Patients who use such products should be advised about their proper use. The product should be applied one drop at a time onto the corn or wart allowing time to dry before the next drop is added. Because salicylic acid can be irritating to normal, healthy skin every attempt must be made to ensure application directly onto the corn or wart. A useful preventive measure is to line the adjacent healthy skin with some white petrolatum prior to application of the product. Lastly, proper tightening and storage of the product after use is an absolute necessity because of the volatility of the vehicle.

Extraction Methods for Preparing Solutions

Certain pharmaceutical preparations are prepared by the process of *extraction*—that is, by the withdrawal of desired constituents from crude drugs through the use of selected solvents in which the desired constituents are soluble. *Crude drugs* are vegetable or animal drugs that have undergone no other processes than collection, cleaning, and drying. Because each crude drug contains a number of constituents that may be soluble in a given solvent, the products of extraction, termed *extractives,* do not contain just a single constituent but rather varying numbers of constituents, depending upon the drug used and the conditions of the extraction. *Tinctures, fluidextracts* and *extracts* are the pharmaceutical products most commonly prepared from extractives.

Plant materials are composed of heterogeneous mixtures of constituents, some of which are pharmacologically active and others that are pharmacologically inactive and considered inert. Among the varied plant constituents are sugars, starches, mucilages, proteins, albumins, pectins, cellulose, gums, inorganic salts, fixed and volatile oils, resins, tannins, coloring materials, and a number of very active constituents such as alkaloids and glycosides. The solvent systems used in extraction are selected on the basis of their capacity to dissolve the maximum amount of desired active constituents and the minimum amount of undesired constituents.

In many instances, the *active* constituents of a plant drug are of the same general chemical type, have similar solubility characteristics and can be simultaneously extracted with a single solvent or a single solvent-mixture. The process of extraction concentrates the active constituents of a crude drug and removes from it the extraneous matter. In drug extraction, the solvent or solvent-mixture is referred to as the *menstruum,* and the plant residue, which is exhausted of active constituents, is termed the *marc.*

The selection of the menstruum to use in the extraction of a crude drug is based primarily on the relative solubility in it of the active constituents. Although water and alcohol and, to a lesser extent, glycerin are probably the most frequently employed solvents in drug extraction, acetic acid and organic solvents like ether may be used for special purposes.

Because of its ready availability, cheapness, and good solvent action for many plant constituents, water has some use in drug extraction, particularly in combination with other solvents. However, as a sole solvent it has many disadvantages and is infrequently used alone. For one thing, most active plant constituents are complex organic chemical compounds that are less soluble in water than in alcohol. Although water has a great solvent action on such plant constituents as sugars, gums, starches, coloring principles, and tannins, most of these are not particularly desirable components of an extracted preparation. Water also tends to extract plant principles that, upon standing in the extractive, later separate leaving an undesired residue. Finally, unless preserved, aqueous preparations serve as excellent growth media for molds, yeasts, and bacteria. When water alone is employed as the menstruum, alcohol is frequently added to the extractive or to the final preparation as an antimicrobial preservative.

Hydroalcoholic mixtures are perhaps the most versatile and most widely employed menstruums. They combine the solvent effects of both water and alcohol, and the complete miscibility of these two agents permits a flexible combining of the two agents to form solvent mixtures most suited to the extraction of the active principles from a particular drug. A hydroalcoholic menstruum generally provides inherent protection against microbial contamination and helps to prevent the separation of extracted material on standing. Alcohol is used alone as a menstruum only when necessary because it is more expensive than hydroalcoholic mixtures.

Glycerin, a good solvent for many plant substances, is occasionally employed as a cosolvent with water or alcoholic menstruums because of its ability to extract and then prevent inert materials from precipitating upon standing. It is especially useful in this regard in preventing the separation of tannin and tannin oxidation products in extractives. Because glycerin has preservative action, depending upon its concentration in the final product, it may contribute to the stability of a pharmaceutical extractive.

Methods of Extraction

The principal methods of drug extraction are maceration and percolation. Generally, the method of extraction selected for a given drug depends on several factors, as the nature of the crude drug, its adaptability to each of the various extraction methods, and the interest in obtaining complete or near-complete extraction of the drug.

Frequently a combination of maceration and percolation is actually employed in the extraction of a crude drug. The drug is macerated first to soften the plant tissues and to dissolve much of the active constituents, and the percolation process is then conducted to achieve the separation of the extractive from the marc.

Maceration

The term *maceration* comes from the Latin *macerare,* meaning "to soak." It is a process in which the properly comminuted drug is permitted to soak in the menstruum until the cellular structure is softened and penetrated by the menstruum and the soluble constituents are dissolved.

In the maceration process, the drug to be extracted is generally placed in a wide-mouth container with the prescribed menstruum, the vessel is stoppered tightly, and the contents are agitated repeatedly over a period usually ranging from 2 to 14 days. The agitation permits the repeated flow of fresh solvent over the entire surface area of the comminuted drug. An alternative to this repeated shaking is to place the drug in a porous cloth bag that is tied and suspended in the upper portion of the menstruum, much the same as a tea bag is suspended in water in the preparation of a cup of tea. As the soluble constituents dissolve in the menstruum, they tend to settle to the bottom because of an increase in the specific gravity of the liquid due to its added weight. Occasional dipping of the drug bag may facilitate the speed of the extraction. The extractive is separated from the marc by expressing the bag of drug and washing it with additional fresh menstruum, the washings being added to the extractive. If the maceration is performed with an unbagged drug, the marc may be removed by straining and/or filtration, with the marc being washed free of extractive by the additional passage of menstruum through the strainer or filter into the total extractive.

For drugs containing little or no cellular material, such as benzoin, aloe and tolu, which dissolve almost completely in the menstruum, maceration is the most efficient method of extraction.

Maceration is usually conducted at a temperature of between 15° to 20°C for a period of 3 days or until the soluble matter is dissolved.

Percolation

The term *percolation,* from the Latin *per,* meaning "through," and *colare,* meaning "to strain," may be described generally as a process in which a comminuted drug is extracted of its soluble constituents by the slow passage of a suitable solvent through a column of the drug. The drug is packed in a special extraction apparatus termed a *percolator,* with the extractive collected called the *percolate.* Most drug extractions are performed by percolation.

In the process of percolation the flow of the menstruum over the drug column is generally downward to the exit orifice, drawn by the force of gravity as well as the weight of the column of liquid. In certain specialized and more sophisticated percolation apparatus, additional pressure on the column is exerted with positive air pressure at the inlet and suction at the outlet or exit.

Percolators for drug extraction vary greatly as to their shape, capacities, composition, and, most important, their utility. Percolators employed in the large-scale industrial preparation of extractives are generally made of stainless steel or are glass-lined large metal vessels that vary greatly in size and in operation. Percolators used to extract leaves, for instance, may be 6 to 8 feet in diameter and 12 to 18 feet high (Fig. 12.10). Percolators employed to extract other vegetable parts like seeds that are greater in density than leaves and would pack too tightly in percolators of such large dimensions are extracted in much smaller percolators. Some special industrial percolators are designed to percolate with hot menstruums; in others pressure is utilized to force the menstruum through the drug columns.

Percolation on a small scale generally involves the use of glass percolators of various shapes for extraction of small amounts (perhaps up to 1000 g) of crude drug. The shape of percolators in common laboratory and small-scale use are a) cylindrical, with little if any taper except for the lower orifice; b) cylindrical-like, but with a definite taper downward; and c) conical, or funnel-shaped. Each type has a special utility in drug extraction.

The cylindrical percolator is particularly suited to the complete extraction of drugs with a minimal expenditure of menstruum. By the passage of the menstruum over the drug contained in a high, narrow column (rather than in a lower, wider column), each drug particle is more repeatedly exposed to passing solvent. A funnel-shaped percolator is useful for the percolation of drugs that swell a great deal during the maceration process, since the large upper surface permits the expansion of the drug column with little risk of a too tightly packed column or breakage of a glass percolator.

Example Preparations Prepared by Extraction Processes

Fluidextracts

Fluidextracts are liquid preparations of vegetable drugs, prepared by percolation. They contain alcohol

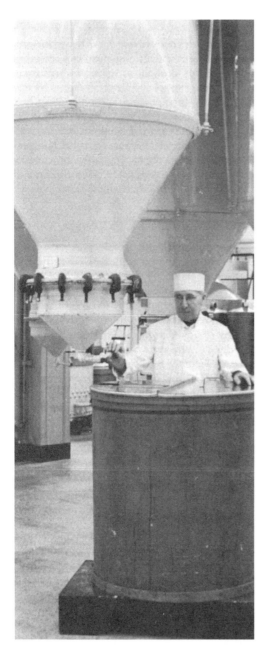

Fig. 12.10 *Large industrial percolators used in extracting crude drugs to make fluidextracts, tinctures, and powdered extracts.*

as a solvent or as a preservative, or both, and are made so that each mL contains the therapeutic constituents of 1 g of the standard drug that it represents. Because of their concentrated nature, many fluidextracts are considered too potent to be taken

safely in self-administration by the patient and their use per se is almost nonexistent in medical practice. Also, many fluidextracts are simply too bitter tasting or otherwise unpalatable to be accepted by the patient. Therefore, most fluidextracts today are either modified by the addition of flavoring or sweetening agents before use, or are used pharmaceutically as the drug source component of other liquid dosage forms, such as syrups.

Extracts

Extracts are concentrated preparations of vegetable or animal drugs obtained by removal of the active constituents of the respective drugs with suitable menstrua, evaporation of all or nearly all of the solvent, and adjustment of the residual masses or powders to the prescribed standards.

Extracts are potent preparations, usually between two and six times as potent on a weight basis as the crude drug used as the starting material. They contain primarily the active constituents of the crude drug, with a great portion of the inactive constituents and structural components of the crude drug having been removed. Their function is to provide in small amounts and in convenient, stable physical form the medicinal activity and character of the more bulky plants that they represent. As such, they have use in product formulation.

In the manufacture of most extracts, percolation is employed to remove the active constituents from the drug, with the percolates generally being reduced in volume by evaporation of the solvent by distillation under reduced pressure, the latter being used to reduce the degree of heat and to protect the drug substances against thermal decomposition. The extent of the removal of the solvent determines the final physical character of the extract. Extracts are made in three forms: a) *semiliquid extracts* or those of a syrupy consistency prepared without the intent of removing all or even most of the menstruum, b) *pilular* or *solid extracts* of a plastic consistency prepared with nearly all of the menstruum removed, and c) *powdered extracts* prepared to be dry by the removal of all of the menstruum insofar as is feasible or practical. Pilular and powdered extracts differ only by the slight amount of remaining solvent in the former preparation, but each has its pharmaceutical advantage because of its physical form. For instance, the pilular extract is preferred in compounding a plastic dosage form such as an ointment or paste or one in which a pliable material facilitates compounding, whereas the powdered form is preferred in the compounding of such dosage forms as powders, capsules, and tablets.

References

1. United States Pharmacopeia 23/National Formulary 18, United States Pharmacopeial Convention, Inc., Rockville, MD, 1995;1947.
2. United States Pharmacopeia 23/National Formulary 18, United States Pharmacopeial Convention, Inc., Rockville, MD, 1995;10.
3. Pure Water Handbook. Minnetonka, MN: Osmonics, Inc., 1991.
4. Chemburkar PB, Joslin RS. Effect of flavoring oils on preservative concentrations in oral liquid dosage forms. J Pharm Sci 1975;64:414–441.
5. Gossel TA. Oral rehydration solutions. US Pharmacist 1987;12:90–98.
6. Handbook on Extemporaneous Formulations. American Society of Hospital Pharmacists, Bethesda, MD, 1987.
7. Pesko LJ. Compounding: Oral liquids. Am Druggist 1993;208:49.
8. Oral Liquid Pharmaceuticals. ICI Americas, Inc., Wilmington, DE, 1975.
9. Murphy D. Ipecac misuse by bulimics: APhA launches educational campaign. Am Pharm 1985; NS25:264–265.
10. Nudelman I. Nasal delivery: A revolution in drug administration. Drug Delivery Systems. Eugene, OR: Aster Publishing Corp., 1987; 43–48.
11. Longenecker JP. New drug delivery systems: Intranasal delivery: A novel route for protein therapeutics. Wellcome Trends Pharm 1989;11:7–9.
12. Sarkar MA. Drug metabolism in the nasal mucosa. Pharm Res 1992;9:1–9.
13. Fu RCC, Whatley JL, Fleitman JS. Intranasal delivery of RS-93522, a dihydropyridine-type calcium-channel antagonist. Pharm Res 1991;8:134–138.
14. Donovan MD, Flynn GL, Amidon GL. The molecular weight of nasal absorption: The effect of absorption enhancers. Pharm Res 1990;8: 808–815.
15. Schipper NGM, Verhoef JC, Merkus FWHM. The nasal mucociliary clearance: Relevance to nasal drug delivery. Pharm Res 1991;8:812–814.

DISPERSE SYSTEMS

Chapter at a Glance

THIS CHAPTER includes the main types of liquid preparations containing undissolved or immiscible drug distributed throughout a vehicle. In these preparations, the substance distributed is referred to as the *dispersed phase* and the vehicle is termed the *dispersing phase* or *dispersion medium.* Together, they produce a *dispersed system.*

The particles of the dispersed phase are usually solid materials that are insoluble in the dispersion medium. In the case of emulsions, the dispersed phase is a liquid substance which is neither soluble nor miscible with the liquid of the dispersing phase. The emulsification process results in the dispersion of liquid drug as fine droplets throughout the dispersing phase. In the case of an aerosol, the dispersed phase may be air that is present as small bubbles throughout a solution or an emulsion. Dispersions also consist of droplets of a liquid (solution or suspension) in air.

The particles of the dispersed phase vary widely in size, from large particles visible to the naked eye down to particles of colloidal dimension, falling between 1.0 nm and 0.5 μm in size. Dispersions containing coarse particles, usually 10–50 μm in size, are referred to as *coarse dispersions* and include the *suspensions* and *emulsions.* Dispersions containing particles of smaller size are termed *fine dispersions* (0.5–10 μm), and, if the particles are in the colloidal range, *colloidal dispersions. Magmas* and *gels* represent such fine dispersions.

Largely because of their greater size, dispersed particles in a coarse dispersion have a greater tendency to separate from the dispersion medium than do the particles of a fine dispersion. Most solids in dispersion tend to settle to the bottom of the container because of their greater density than the dispersion medium, whereas most emulsified liquids for oral use are oils and generally have a lesser density than the aqueous medium in which they are dispersed and tend to rise toward the top of the preparation. Complete and uniform redistribution of the dispersed phase is essential to the accurate administration of uniform doses. For a properly prepared dispersion, this should be accomplished by the moderate agitation of the container.

The focus of this chapter is on dispersions of drugs administered orally or topically. The same basic pharmaceutical characteristics apply to those dispersion systems administered by other routes of administration. Included among these are ophthalmic suspensions, and sterile suspensions for injection.

Suspensions

Suspensions may be defined as preparations containing finely divided drug particles (referred to as the *suspensoid*) distributed somewhat uniformly throughout a vehicle in which the drug exhibits a minimum degree of solubility. Some suspensions are available in ready-to-use form—that is, already distributed through a liquid vehicle with or without stabilizers and other pharmaceutical additives (Fig. 13.1). Other preparations are available as dry powders intended for suspensions in liquid vehicles. This type of product generally is a powder mixture containing the drug and suitable suspending and dispersing agents, which upon dilution and agitation with a specified quantity of vehicle (generally purified water) results in the formation of a suspension suitable for administration. Figure 13.2 demonstrates the preparation of this type of product. Drugs that are unstable if maintained for extended periods of time in the presence of an aqueous vehicle (for example, many antibiotic drugs) are most frequently supplied as dry powder mixtures for reconstitution at the time of dispensing. This type of preparation is designated in the USP by a title of the form ". . . for Oral Suspension." Prepared suspensions not requiring reconstitution at the time of dispensing are simply designated as ". . . Oral Suspension."

Reasons for Suspensions

There are several reasons for preparing suspensions. For one thing, certain drugs are chemically unstable when in solution but stable when suspended. In instances such as this, the suspension insures chemical stability while permitting liquid therapy. For many patients, the liquid form is preferred over the solid form of the same drug because of the ease of swallowing liquids and the flexibility in the administration of a range of doses. This is particularly advantageous for infants, children and the elderly. The disadvantage of a disagreeable taste of certain drugs

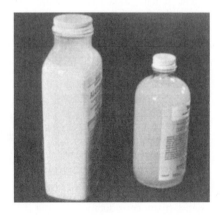

Fig. 13.1   *Examples of some commercial oral suspensions.*

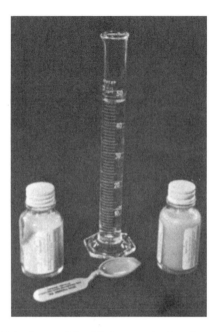

Fig. 13.2 *Commercial antibiotic preparation for oral suspension following reconstitution with purified water. On the left is the dry powder mixture, and on the right the suspension after reconstitution with the specified amount of purified water.*

when given in solution form is overcome when the drug is administered as undissolved particles of an oral suspension. In fact, chemical forms of certain poor-tasting drugs have been specifically developed for their insolubility in a desired vehicle for the sole purpose of preparing a palatable liquid dosage form. For example, the water-insoluble ester form of chloramphenicol, chloramphenicol palmitate, was developed to prepare a palatable liquid dosage form of the chloramphenicol, the result being the development of Chloramphenicol Palmitate Oral Suspension, USP. By the creation of insoluble forms of drugs for use in suspensions, the difficult taste-masking problems of developmental pharmacists are greatly reduced, and the selection of the flavorants to be used in a given suspension may be based on taste preference rather than on a particular flavorant's ability to act as a masking agent for an unpleasant tasting drug. For the most part, oral suspensions are aqueous preparations with the vehicle flavored and sweetened to suit the anticipated taste preferences of the intended patient.

Features Desired in a Pharmaceutical Suspension

There are many considerations in the development and preparation of a pharmaceutically ele-

gant suspension. In addition to therapeutic efficacy, chemical stability of the components of the formulation, permanency of the preparation, and esthetic appeal of the preparation—desirable qualities in all pharmaceutical preparations—a few other features apply more specifically to the pharmaceutical suspension:

1. A properly prepared pharmaceutical suspension should settle slowly and should be readily redispersed upon the gentle shaking of the container.
2. The characteristics of the suspension should be such that the particle size of the suspensoid remains fairly constant throughout long periods of undisturbed standing.
3. The suspension should pour readily and evenly from its container.

These main features of a suspension, which depend on the nature of the dispersed phase, the dispersion medium, and pharmaceutical adjuncts, will be discussed briefly.

Sedimentation Rate of the Particles of a Suspension

The various factors involved in the rate of velocity of settling of the particles of a suspension are embodied in the equation of Stokes' law, which is presented in the accompanying Physical Pharmacy Capsule.

Stokes' equation was derived for an ideal situation in which uniform, perfectly spherical particles in a very dilute suspension settle without effecting turbulence in their downward course, without collision of the particles of the suspensoid, and without chemical or physical attraction or affinity for the dispersion medium. Obviously, Stokes' equation does not apply precisely to the usual pharmaceutical suspension in which the suspensoid is irregularly shaped, of various particle diameters, and not spherical, in which the fall of the particles *does* result in both turbulence and collision, and also in which there may be a reasonable amount of affinity of the particles for the suspension medium. However, the basic concepts of the equation do give a valid indication of the factors that are important to the suspension of the particles and a clue to the possible adjustments that can be made to a formulation to decrease the rate of particle sedimentation.

From the equation it is apparent that the velocity of fall of a suspended particle is greater for larger particles than it is for smaller particles, all other factors remaining constant. By reducing the particle size of the dispersed phase, one can expect a slower *rate* of descent of the particles. Also, the greater the

Physical Pharmacy Capsule 13.1   **Sedimentation Rate & Stokes' Equation**

Stokes' Equation:

$$\frac{dx}{dt} = \frac{d^2(\rho_i - \rho_e)g}{18\eta}$$

where

    dx/dt is the rate of settling,
    d is the diameter of the particles,
    ρ_i is the density of the particle,
    ρ_e is the density of the medium,
    g is the gravitational constant, and
    η is the viscosity of the medium.

A number of factors can be adjusted to enhance the physical stability of a suspension, including the diameter of the particles and the density and viscosity of the medium. The effect of changing these is illustrated in the following example.

EXAMPLE 1
A powder has a density of 1.3 g/cc and is available as a powder with an average particle diameter of 2.5 microns (assuming the particles to be spheres). According to Stoke's Equation, this powder will settle in water (viscosity of 1 cps assumed) at a rate of:

$$\frac{(2.5 \times 10^{-4})^2(1.3 - 1.0)(980)}{18 \times 0.01} = 1.02 \times 10^{-4} \text{ cm/sec}$$

If the particle size of the powder is reduced to 0.25 μ and water is still used as the dispersion medium, the powder will now settle at a rate of:

$$\frac{(2.5 \times 10^{-5})^2(1.3 - 1.0)(980)}{18 \times 0.01} = 1.02 \times 10^{-6} \text{ cm/sec}$$

As is evident, a decrease in particle size by a factor of 10 results in a reduction in the rate of settling by a factor of 100. This enhanced effect is a result of the "d" factor in Stokes Equation being squared.

Now, if a different dispersion medium, such as glycerin, is used in place of water, a further decrease in settling will result. Glycerin has a density of 1.25 g/cc and a viscosity of 400 cps.

The larger particle size powder (2.5 μ) will settle at a rate of:

$$\frac{(2.5 \times 10^{-4})^2(1.3 - 1.25)(980)}{18.4} = 4.25 \times 10^{-8} \text{ cm/sec}$$

The smaller particle size (0.25 μ) powder will now settle at a rate of:

$$\frac{(2.5 \times 10^{-5})^2(1.3 - 1.25)(980)}{18 \times 4} = 4.25 \times 10^{-10} \text{ cm/sec}$$

A summary of these results is shown in the following table:

Condition	Rate of Settling (cm/sec)
2.5 μ powder in water	1.02×10^{-4}
0.25 μ powder in water	1.02×10^{-6}
2.5 μ powder in glycerin	4.25×10^{-8}
0.25 μ powder in glycerin	4.25×10^{-10}

As is evident from this table, a change in dispersion medium results in the greatest change in the rate of settling of particles. Particle size reduction also can contribute significantly to suspension stability. These factors are important in the formulation of physically stable suspensions.

density of the particles, the greater the rate of descent, provided the density of the vehicle is not altered. Because aqueous vehicles are used in pharmaceutical oral suspensions, the density of the particles is generally greater than that of the vehicle, a desirable feature, for if the particles were less dense than the vehicle, they would tend to float, and floating particles would be quite difficult to distribute uniformly in the vehicle. The rate of sedimentation may be appreciably reduced by increasing the viscosity of the dispersion medium, and within limits of practicality this may be done. However, a product having too high a viscosity is not generally desirable, because it pours with difficulty and it is equally difficult to redisperse the suspensoid. Therefore, if the viscosity of a suspension is increased, it is done so only to a modest extent to avoid these difficulties.

The viscosity characteristics of a suspension may be altered not only by the vehicle used, but also by the solids content. As the proportion of solid particles is increased in a suspension, so is the viscosity. The viscosity of a pharmaceutical preparation may be determined through the use of a Brookfield Viscometer, which measures viscosity by the force required to rotate a spindle in the fluid being tested (Fig. 13.3).

For the most part, the physical stability of a pharmaceutical suspension appears to be most appropriately adjusted by an alteration in the dispersed phase rather than through great changes in the dispersion medium. In most instances, the dispersion medium is supportive to the adjusted dispersed phase. These adjustments mainly are concerned with particle size, uniformity of particle size, and separation of the particles so that they are not likely to become greatly larger or to form a solid cake on standing.

Physical Features of the Dispersed Phase of a Suspension

Probably the most important single consideration in a discussion of suspensions is the size of the drug particles. In most good pharmaceutical suspensions, the particle diameter is between 1 and 50 μm.

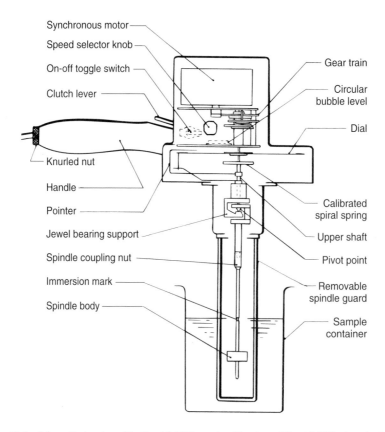

Fig. 13.3   *Schematic drawing of the Brookfield Viscometer. (Courtesy of Brookfield Engineering Laboratories.)*

Particle size reduction is generally accomplished by dry-milling prior to the incorporation of the dispersed phase into the dispersion medium. One of the most rapid, convenient, and inexpensive methods of producing fine drug powders of about 10 to 50 μm size is *micropulverization*. Micropulverizers are high-speed, attrition or impact mills which are efficient in reducing powders to the size acceptable for most oral and topical suspensions. For still finer particles, under 10 μm, the process of *fluid energy* grinding, sometimes referred to as *jet-milling* or *micronizing*, is quite effective. By this process, the shearing action of high velocity compressed air streams on the particles in a confined space produces the desired ultrafine or micronized particles. The particles to be micronized are swept into violent turbulence by the sonic and supersonic velocity of the air streams. The particles are accelerated into high velocities and collide with one another, resulting in fragmentation and a decrease in the size of the particles. This method may be employed in instances in which the particles are intended for parenteral or ophthalmic suspensions. Particles of extremely small dimensions may also be produced by *spray-drying* techniques. A spray dryer is a cone-shaped piece of apparatus into which a solution of a drug is sprayed and rapidly dried by a current of warmed, dry air circulating in the cone. The resulting dry powder is then collected. It is not possible for a community pharmacist to achieve the same degree of particle-size reduction with such simple comminuting equipment as the mortar and pestle. However, many micronized drugs are commercially available and when needed may be purchased by the pharmacist in bulk quantities.

As shown by Stokes' equation, the reduction in the particle size of a suspensoid is beneficial to the stability of the suspension in that the rate of sedimentation of the solid particles is reduced as the particles are decreased in size. The reduction in particle size produces slow, more uniform rates of settling. However, one should avoid reducing the particle size to too great a degree of fineness, since fine particles have a tendency to form a compact cake upon settling to the bottom of the container. The result may be that the cake resists breakup upon shaking, and forms rigid aggregates of particles which are of larger dimension and less suspendable than the original suspensoid. The particle shape of the suspensoid can also affect caking and product stability. It has been shown that symmetrical barrel-shaped particles of calcium carbonate produced more stable suspensions than did asymmetrical needle-shaped particles of the same agent.

The needle-shaped particles formed a tenacious sediment-cake on standing which could not be redistributed whereas the barrel-shaped particles did not cake on standing (1).

To avoid the formation of a cake, measures must be taken to prevent the agglomeration of the particles into larger crystals or into masses. One common method of preventing the rigid cohesion of small particles of a suspension is through the intentional formation of a less rigid or loose aggregation of the particles held together by comparatively weak particle-to-particle bonding forces. Such an aggregation of particles is termed a *floc* or a *floccule*, with flocculated particles forming a type of lattice structure that resists complete settling (although flocs settle more rapidly than fine, individual particles) and thus are less prone to compaction than unflocculated particles. The flocs settle to form a higher sediment volume than unflocculated particles, the loose structure of which permits the aggregates to break up easily and distribute readily with a small amount of agitation.

There are several methods of preparing flocculated suspensions, the choice depending on the type of drug involved and the type of product desired. For instance, in the preparation of an oral suspension of a drug, clays such as diluted bentonite magma are commonly employed as the flocculating agent. The structure of the bentonite magma and of other clays used for this purpose also assists the suspension by helping to support the floc once formed. When clays are unsuitable as agents, as in a parenteral suspension, frequently a floc of the dispersed phase can be produced by an alteration in the pH of the preparation (generally to the region of minimum drug solubility). Electrolytes can also act as flocculating agents, apparently by reducing the electrical barrier between the particles of the suspensoid and forming a bridge so as to link them together. The carefully determined concentration of nonionic and ionic surface-active agents (surfactants) can also induce the flocculation of particles in suspension and increase the sedimentation volume.

Dispersion Medium

Oftentimes, as with highly flocculated suspensions, the particles of a suspension settle too rapidly to be consistent with what might be termed a pharmaceutically elegant preparation. The rapid settling hinders the accurate measurement of dosage and from an esthetic point of view produces too unsightly a supernatant layer. In many of the commercial suspensions, suspending agents are added to the dispersion medium to lend it a structure to assist in the suspension of the dispersed phase. Carboxymethylcellulose, methylcellulose, microcrystalline cellulose, polyvinyl pyrrolidone, xanthan gum, and bentonite are a few of the agents employed to thicken the dispersion medium and help suspend the suspensoid. When polymeric substances and hydrophilic colloids are used as suspending agents, appropriate tests must be performed to show that the agent does not interfere with the availability for therapeutic effects of the suspension's medicinal substance. These materials can bind certain medicinal agents, rendering them unavailable or more slowly available for their therapeutic function. Also, the amount of the suspending agent must not be such to render the suspension too viscous to agitate (to distribute the *suspensoid*) or to pour. The study of the flow characteristics is termed rheology. A summary of the concepts of rheology is found in the accompanying Physical Pharmacy Capsule 13.2.

Support of the suspensoid by the dispersion medium may depend on several factors: the density of the suspensoid, whether it is flocculated, and the amount of material requiring support.

The solid content of a suspension intended for oral administration may vary considerably, depending on the dose of the drug to be administered, the volume of product desired to be administered, and also on the ability of the dispersion medium to support the concentration of drug while maintaining desirable features of viscosity and flow. The usual adult oral suspension is frequently designed to supply the dose of the particular drug in a convenient measure of 5 mL or one teaspoonful. Pediatric suspensions are formulated to deliver the appropriate dose of drug by administering a dose-calibrated number of drops. Figure 13.4 shows commonly packaged oral suspensions administered as pediatric drops. Some are accompanied by a calibrated drop-

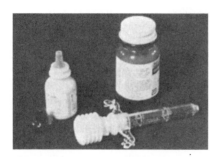

Fig. 13.4 *Examples of oral pediatric suspensions showing package designs of a built-in dropper device and a calibrated dropper accompanying the medication container.*

per, whereas other packages have the drop capability built into the container. On administration the drops may be placed directly into the infant's mouth or mixed with a small portion of food. Because many of the suspensions of antibiotic drugs intended for pediatric use are prepared in a highly flavored, sweetened, colored base, they are frequently referred to by their manufacturers and also popularly as "syrups," even though in fact they are suspensions.

Preparation of Suspensions

In the preparation of a suspension, the pharmacist must be acquainted with the characteristics of both the intended dispersed phase and the dispersion medium. In some instances the dispersed phase has an affinity for the vehicle to be employed and is readily "wetted" by it upon its addition. Other drugs are not penetrated easily by the vehicle and have a tendency to clump together or to float on top of the vehicle. In the latter case, the powder must first be wetted by a so-called "wetting agent" to make the powder more penetrable by the dispersion medium. Alcohol, glycerin, and other hygroscopic liquids are employed as wetting agents when an aqueous vehicle is to be used as the dispersion phase. They function by displacing the air in the crevices of the particles, dispersing the particles, and subsequently allowing the penetration of dispersion medium into the powder. In the large-scale preparation of suspensions the wetting agents are mixed with the particles by an apparatus such as a colloid mill; on a small scale in the pharmacy, they are mixed with a mortar and pestle. Once the powder is wetted, the dispersion medium (to which have been added all of the formulation's soluble components such as colorants, flavorants, and preservatives) is added in portions to the powder, and the mixture is thoroughly blended before subsequent additions of vehicle. A portion of the vehicle is used to wash the mixing equipment free of suspensoid, and this portion is used to bring the suspension to final volume and insure that the suspension contains the desired concentration of solid matter. The final product is then passed through a colloid mill or other blender or mixing device to insure uniformity.

Whenever appropriate, suitable preservatives should be included in the formulation of suspensions to preserve against bacterial and mold contamination.

An example formula for an oral suspension follows (2). In the example, the suspensoid is the antacid aluminum hydroxide, the preservatives are methylparaben and propylparaben, with syrup and sorbitol solution providing the viscosity as well as the sweetness.

Physical Pharmacy Capsule 13.2   **Rheology**

Rheology is the study of flow and involves the viscosity characteristics of powders, fluids, and semisolids. Materials are divided into two general categories depending upon their flow characteristics: Newtonian and non-Newtonian. Newtonian flow is characterized by a constant viscosity, regardless of the shear rates applied. Non-Newtonian flow is characterized by a change in viscosity characteristics with increasing shear rates. Non-Newtonian flow includes plastic, pseudoplastic and dilatant flow.

Newton's Law of Flow relates parallel layers of liquid, with the bottom layer fixed, when a force is placed on the top layer and the top plane moves at constant velocity and each lower layer moves with a velocity directly proportional to its distance from the stationary bottom layer. The velocity gradient, or rate of shear (dv/dr), is the difference of velocity dv between two planes of liquid separated by the distance dr. The force (F'/A) applied to the top layer that is required to result in flow (rate of shear, G) is called the shearing stress (F). The relationship can be expressed.

$$\frac{F'}{A} = \eta \frac{dv}{dr}$$

where η is the viscosity coefficient, or viscosity. This relationship is often written

$$\eta = \frac{F}{G}$$

where $F = F'/A$ and $G = dv/dr$. The higher the viscosity of a liquid, the greater the shearing stress required to produce a certain rate of shear. A plot of F vs G yields a rheogram. A Newtonian fluid will plot as a straight line with the slope of the line being η. The unit of viscosity is the *poise*, which is the shearing force required to produce a velocity of 1 cm/sec between two parallel planes of liquid, each 1 cm^2 in area and separated by a distance of 1 cm. The most convenient unit to use is the centipoise, or cp (equivalent to 0.01 poise).

These basic concepts can be illustrated in the following two graphs.

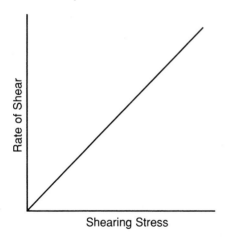

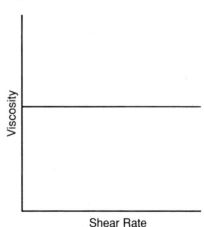

EXAMPLE 1

What is the shear rate when an oil is rubbed into the skin with a relative rate of motion between the fingers and the skin of about 10 cm/sec and the film thickness is about 0.02 cm?

$$G = \frac{10 \text{ cm/sec}}{0.02} = 500 \text{ sec}^{-1}$$

Rheology   (Continued)

The viscosity of Newtonian materials can be easily determined using a capillary viscometer, such as the Ostwald Pipet, and the following relationship:

$$\eta' = ktd$$

where η' = viscosity,
   k = a coefficient, including such factors as the radius and length of the capillary, volume of the liquid flowing, pressure head, etc,
   t = time, and
   d = density of the material.

The official compendia, the USP-NF, utilize Kinematic Viscosity, which is the absolute viscosity divided by the density of the liquid, as follows:

$$\text{Kinematic viscosity} = \eta'/\rho$$

The relative viscosity of a liquid can be obtained by utilizing a capillary viscometer and comparing data with a second liquid of known viscosity, provided the densities of the two liquids are known, as follows:

$$\eta'/\eta'_o = (\rho t)/(\rho_o t_o)$$

EXAMPLE 2

At 25°C, water has a density of 1.0 g/cc and a viscosity of 0.895 cps. The time of flow of water in a capillary viscometer is 15 sec. A 50% aqueous solution of glycerin has a flow time of 750 sec. The density of the glycerin solution is 1.216 g/cc. What is the viscosity of the glycerin solution?

$$\eta' = \frac{(0.895)(750)(1.216)}{(1)(15)} = 54.4 \text{ cps}$$

EXAMPLE 3

The time of flow between marks on an Ostwald viscometer using water (ρ = 1) was 120 sec at 20°C. The time for a liquid (ρ = 1.05) to flow through the same viscometer was 230 sec. What is the absolute and relative viscosity of the liquid?

$$\eta = (0.01)\frac{(1.05)(230)}{(1.0)(120)}$$

$$\eta = 0.020 \text{ poise} = 2.0 \text{ centipoise}$$

Viscosity is related to temperature according to:

$$\eta' = Ae^{Ev/RT}$$

where A = a constant depending on the molecular weight and molar volume of the material, Ev = the activation energy required to initiate flow between molecules, R = the gas constant, and T = the absolute temperature.

Viscosity is additive in ideal solutions, as follows:

$$\frac{1}{\eta} = \frac{1}{\eta}V_1 + \frac{1}{\eta}V_2$$

where η = the viscosity of the solutions, and V_1 and V_2 = the volume fractions of the pure liquids.

EXAMPLE 4

What is the viscosity of the liquid resulting from mixing 300 mL of liquid A (η = 1.0 cp) and 200 mL of liquid B (η = 3.4 cp)?

$$\frac{1}{\eta} = \frac{1(0.6)}{1.0} + \frac{1(0.4)}{3.4}$$

$$\eta = 1.4 \text{ cps}$$

Rheology   (Continued)

Non-Newtonian substances are those that fail to follow Newton's Equation of Flow. Example materials include colloidal solutions, emulsions, liquid suspensions, and ointments. There are three general types of non-Newtonian materials: plastic, pseudoplastic, and dilatant.

Substances that exhibit plastic flow are called *Bingham bodies*. Plastic flow does not begin until a shearing stress, corresponding to a certain yield value, is exceeded. The flow curve intersects the shearing stress axis and does not pass through the origin. The materials are "elastic" below the yield value.

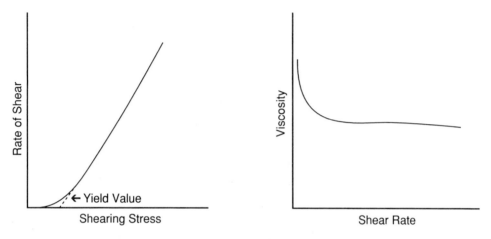

Pseudoplastic substances begin flow when a shearing stress is applied; therefore, they exhibit no yield value. With increasing shearing stress, the rate of shear increases; consequently, these materials are also called "shear-thinning" systems. It is postulated that this occurs as the molecules, primarily polymers, align themselves along the long axis and slip or slide past each other.

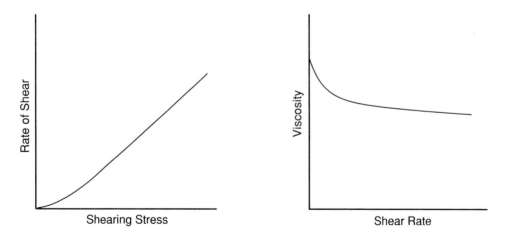

Dilatant materials are those that increase in volume when sheared, and the viscosity increases with increasing shear rate. These are also called "shear thickening" systems. Dilatant systems are usually characterized by having a high percentage of solids in the formulation.

Rheology   (Continued)

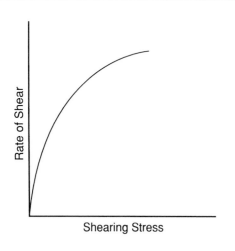

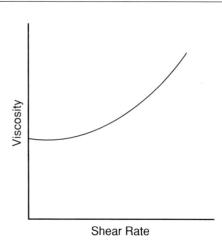

The viscosity of non-Newtonian materials is determined using a viscometer capable of producing differing shear rates, measuring the shear stress, and plotting the results. Other types of flow not detailed here include *thixotropic, antithixotropic,* and *rheopexic*. Thixotropic flow is used in some pharmaceutical formulations to advantage. It is a reversible gel-sol transformation. Upon setting, a network gel is formed that provides a rigid matrix that will stabilize suspensions and gels. When stressed (by shaking), the matrix relaxes and forms a sol, with the characteristics of a liquid dosage form for ease of use. All these unique flow types can be characterized by studying their respective rheograms.

Aluminum Hydroxide Compressed	
Gel	326.8 g
Sorbitol Solution	282.0 mL
Syrup	93.0 mL
Glycerin	25.0 mL
Methylparaben	0.9 g
Propylparaben	0.3 g
Flavor	q.s.
Purified Water, to make	1000.0 mL

In preparing a formula such as this, the parabens are dissolved in a heated mixture of the sorbitol solution, glycerin, syrup, and a portion of the water. The mixture is then cooled and the aluminum hydroxide added with stirring. The flavor is added and sufficient purified water to volume. The suspension is then homogenized, using a hand homogenizer, homomixer, or colloid mill. An example of a high-speed, industrial-size mixer used to prepare dispersions of various types including suspensions and emulsions is shown in Fig. 13.5. A large storage holding tank with a liquid filling unit in the process of filling large mouth suspension bottles is shown in Figure 13.6.

Sustained-Release Suspensions

The formulation of liquid oral suspensions having sustained-release capabilities has resulted in only limited success due to the difficulty in maintaining the stability of sustained-release particles when present in liquid dispersal systems (3). Product development research has centered around the same types of technologies used in preparing sustained-release tablets and capsules (i.e., coated beads, drug impregnated wax matrix, microencapsulation, ion-exchange resins, etc.). The use of a combination of ion-exchange resin complex and particle coating *has* resulted in product success via the so-called Pennkinetic system. By this technique, ionic drugs are complexed with ion-exchange resins and the drug-resin complex particles coated with ethyl cellulose (3). In liquid formulations (suspensions) of the coated particles, the drug remains adsorbed onto the resin, but is slowly released by the ion-exchange process when taken into the gastrointestinal tract. An example of this product type is hydrocodone polistirex [Tussionex Pennkinetic Extended-Release Suspension (Medeva)].

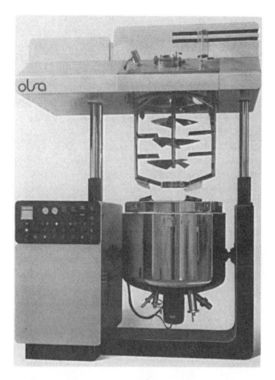

Fig. 13.5 *Example of an industrial mixer for the manufacture of disperse systems including suspensions and emulsions. (Courtesy of Key International, Inc.)*

Extemporaneous Compounding of Suspensions

Unfortunately, not all medicines are available in a convenient, easy to take liquid dosage form. Consequently, patients who are not able to swallow solid medicines, e.g., infants, the elderly, may present a special need. Thus, the pharmacist may have to use a solid dosage form, e.g., tablet, capsule, of the drug and extemporaneously compound a liquid product. A difficulty that confronts the pharmacist is a lack of ready information of stability of a drug when it is incorporated into a liquid vehicle. It is known that drugs in liquid form have faster decomposition rates than when in solid form, and some are affected by the pH of the medium. Leucovorin calcium when compounded from crushed tablets or the injectable form is most stable in milk or antacid and is unstable in acidic solutions.

To overcome this information gap, the pharmacist can attempt to contact the pharmaceutical manufacturer of the solid dosage form to attain stability information. A number of extemporaneous formulations have appeared in the professional literature, e.g., for prednisone oral suspension(4) and keto-

conazole suspension(5) and some manufacturers provide within the package insert a formula for the preparation of an oral liquid form, e.g., Rifadin (Hoechst Marion Roussel). Further, the Committee on Extemporaneous Formulations, an American Society of Hospital Pharmacy special interest group, has compiled and published a listing of extemporaneous formulations in a text titled, *Handbook of Extemporaneous Formulations.* It is a compilation of formulations based upon documented stability data and unpublished data compiled by pharmaceutical manufacturers and practitioners.

Typically, when formulating an extemporaneous suspension, the contents of a capsule are emptied into a mortar or the tablets of the drug crushed in a mortar with a pestle. The selected vehicle is then slowly added to and mixed with the powder to create a paste and then diluted to the desired volume. The selected vehicle can be commercially available for this purpose, e.g., Roxane's Diluent (Flavored) for Oral Use (Roxane) or the"Ora"family of preparations (Ora-Sweet, Ora-Sweet SF, Ora-Plus [Paddock]).

The extent of the formulation depends upon the patient for whom the product is intended. For example, a liquid suspension for a neonate does not necessitate the inclusion of preservatives, colorings, flavorings and alcohol because of the potential for each of these to cause either acute or long-term adverse effects. Because this liquid product will probably be administered through a tube feeding threaded through the mouth into the stomach, and because taste sensation is usually underdeveloped in the neonate a flavoring agent is not required.

In the neonate, alcohol can alter liver function, cause gastric irritation and effect neurologic depression. So unless it is absolutely necessary it should be omitted from an extemporaneous formulation. Pharmacists must be cautious because some vehicles such as Aromatic Elixir, NF contain a significant amount of alcohol, i.e., 21 to 23%, and would not be preferable for use in this patient type. The same problem would hold for liquid formulations for the elderly or any patient who may be receiving another medication that depresses the central nervous system.

Preservatives have been implicated for deleterious adverse effects in preterm infants. Benzyl alcohol should be omitted from neonate formulations because this agent can cause a gasping syndrome characterized by a deterioration of multiple organ systems and eventually death. Propylene glycol has also been implicated to cause problems, i.e., seizures, stupor, in some preterm infants. Thus, formulations for neonates should be purposely kept simple, and not compounded to supply more than just a few days of medicine.

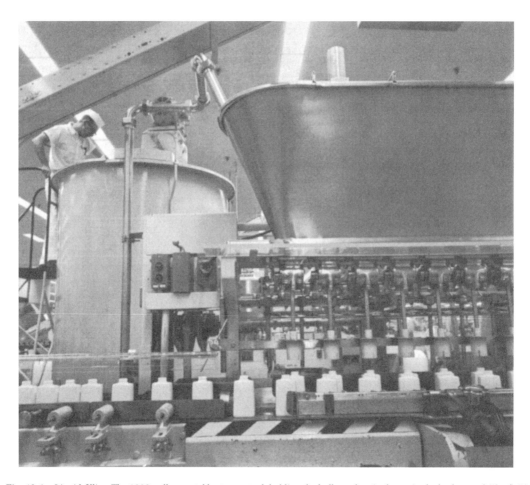

Fig. 13.6 *Liquid filling. The 1000-gallon portable storage tank holding the bulk product is shown in the background. The fluid preparation is pumped from the bottom of the tank through sanitary piping to the large stainless steel hopper located in the foreground. Immediately below the hopper are eight piston-type filling cylinders. Extending from the filling heads are eight filling tubes, each with a bottle-centering bell. On the left, bottles are shown being conveyed after cleaning. As they pass through an indexing worm, the bottles are then spaced accurately for transfer by a pusher bar to the filling position. After filling, incoming bottles push those filled onto the conveyor to the bottle-capping operation. (Courtesy of The Upjohn Company.)*

To minimize stability problems of the extemporaneously prepared product, it should be placed in air-tight, light-resistant containers by the pharmacist and subsequently stored in the refrigerator by the patient. Because it is a suspension, the patient should be instructed to shake it well prior to use and on a daily basis watch for any color change or consistency change that might indicate a stability problem with the formulation.

Packaging and Storage of Suspensions

All suspensions should be packaged in wide mouth containers having adequate airspace above the liquid to permit adequate shaking and ease of pouring. Most suspensions should be stored in tight containers protected from freezing, excessive heat, and light. It is important that suspensions be shaken before each use to ensure a uniform distribution of solid in the vehicle and thereby uniform and proper dosage.

Examples of Oral Suspensions

Examples of official and commercial oral suspensions are presented in Table 13.1. Antacid and antibacterial suspensions are briefly discussed below as examples of this dosage form.

Table 13.1.   Examples of Oral Suspensions by Category

Oral Suspension	Some Representative Commercial Products	Concentration of Respective Drug in Commercial Oral Suspension	Comments
Antacids			
Alumina, Magnesia, and Simethicone Oral Suspension	Mylanta Liquid (Johnson & Johnson Merck)	Aluminum hydroxide, 200 mg; magnesium hydroxide, 200 mg; and simethicone, 20 mg/5 mL	These preparations are used to counteract gastric hyperacidity and to relieve distress in the upper gastrointestinal tract. See text for additional discussion.
Magaldrate Oral Suspension	Riopan Oral Suspension (Whitehall)	540 mg of hydroxymagnesium aluminate, a chemical entity of aluminum and magnesium hydroxides	
Magnesia and Alumina Oral Suspension	Maalox Suspension (Novartis Consumer Health)	225 mg of aluminum hydroxide and 200 mg of magnesium hydroxide/5 mL	
Aluminum Hydroxide and Magnesium Carbonate Oral Suspension Gaviscon Liquid	Antacid (SmithKline Beecham Consumer)	Aluminum hydroxide, 95 mg, magnesium carbonate, 358 mg/15 mL, and sodium alginate	
Anthelmintics			
Pyrantel Pamoate Oral Suspension	Antiminth Oral Suspension (Pfizer)	250 mg/5 mL	Employed to rid the body of worm infections. See text for additional discussion.
Thiabenzadole Oral Suspension	Mintezol Oral Suspension (Merck & Company)	500 mg/5 mL	
Antibacterials (Antibiotics)			
Chloramphenicol Palmitate Oral Suspension	Chloromycetin Palmitate Oral Suspension (Parke-Davis)	150 mg/5 mL	A broad-spectrum antibiotic reserved for serious infections by susceptible organisms when less potentially hazardous agents are ineffective or contraindicated. The tasteless palmitate ester of chloramphenicol is hydrolyzed in the gut to chloramphenicol before absorption.
Erythromycin Estolate Oral Suspension	Ilosone Oral Suspension (Dista)	125 and 250 mg/5 mL	Broad-spectrum macrolide antibiotic having bacteriostatic and bacteriocidal activity.
Antibacterials (Non-antibiotic Anti-infectives)			
Methenamine Mandelate Oral Suspension	Mandelamine Suspension and Mandelamine Suspension Forte (Various)	500 mg/5 mL	Methenamine mandelate oral suspension is prepared with an oleaginous vehicle. Methenamine mandelate is a chemical combination of approximately equal parts of methenamine and mandelic acid which is effective in destroying most of the pathogens commonly found to infect the urinary tract. An acid urine is essential for the activity of the drug, with maximum efficacy occurring at pH 5.5. The methenamine component of the drug in an acid urine is hydrolyzed to ammonia and the bactericidal agent, formaldehyde.

continued

Table 13.1.   Examples of Oral Suspensions by Care by Category

Oral Suspension	Some Representative Commercial Products	Concentration of Respective Drug in Commercial Oral Suspension	Comments
			The mandelic acid component meantime exerts its antibacterial action and contributes to the acidification of the urine. The usual dose of the drug is 1 g, up to four times a day.
			The suspension form of the drug is especially useful in treating pediatric patients as well as those adults who cannot or will not swallow a tablet (also official and commercially available).
Sulfamethoxazole and Trimethoprim Suspension	Bactrim Suspension (Roche), Septra Suspension (Glaxo Wellcome)	40 mg of trimethoprim and 200 mg of sulfamethoxazole per 5 mL	This suspension is used to treat acute middle ear infection (otitis media) in children and urinary tract infections due to susceptible microorganisms.
Sulfamethoxazole Oral Suspension	Gantanol Suspension (Roche)	500 mg/5 mL	These sulfa-drug suspensions are bacteriostatic agents particularly useful in the treatment of urinary tract infections. Sulfonamides competitively inhibit bacterial synthesis of folic acid and para-aminobenzoic acid.
Sulfisoxazole Acetyl Oral Suspension	Gantrisin Syrup and Gantrisin Pediatric Suspension (Roche)	500 mg/5 mL	
Anticonvulsants			
Primidone Oral Suspension	Mysoline Suspension (Wyeth-Ayerst)	250 mg/5 mL	This drug is useful in the management of grand mal epilepsy and psychomotor attacks.
Antidiarrheal			
Bismuth Subsalicylate Suspension	Pepto-Bismol Liquid (Procter & Gamble)	262 mg/15 mL	For indigestion without causing constipation, nausea, and control of diarrhea. An unlabeled use has been for the prevention and treatment of traveler's (enterotoxigenic *Escherichia coli*) diarrhea, but in neither case is it the first line of therapy.
Antiflatulent			
Simethicone Oral Suspension	Mylicon Drops (Johnson & Johnson Merck)	40 mg/0.6 mL	Used for the symptomatic treatment of gastrointestinal distress due to entrapment of gas. The drug acts by reducing the surface tension of gas bubbles, enabling them to coalesce and to be released through belching or passing flatus.
Antifungals			
Nystatin Oral Suspension	Nystatin Oral Suspension (Teva, Lederle Standard Products)	100,000 units/mL	Mycostatin is an antibiotic with antifungal activity. The suspension is held in the mouth as long as possible before swallowing in the treatment of infections of the oral cavity caused by Candida (Monilia) albicans and other Candida species.
Griseofulvin Oral Suspension	Grifulvin V Oral Suspension (Ortho)	125 mg/5 mL	Microsize griseofulvin acts systemically as an antifungal (fungistatic).

continued

Table 13.1.   Examples of Oral Suspensions by Care by Category

Oral Suspension	Some Representative Commercial Products	Concentration of Respective Drug in Commercial Oral Suspension	Comments
Antihypertensive			
Methyldopa Oral Suspension	Aldomet Oral Suspension (Merck & Co.)	250 mg/5 mL	Antihypertensive agent useful in lowering high blood pressure.
Antipsychotics, Sedatives, Antiemetics			
Hydroxyzine Pamoate Oral Suspension	Vistaril Oral Suspension (Pfizer)	25 mg/5 mL	Used in the management of anxiety, tension, and psychomotor agitation.
Thioridazine Oral Suspension	Mellaril-S Oral Suspension (Sandoz)	25 mg/5 mL	For the management of manifestations of psychotic disorders and short-term treatments of moderate to marked depression with variable degrees of anxiety in adults.
Diuretic			
Chlorothiazide Oral Suspension	Diuril Oral Suspension (Merck & Co.)	250 mg/5 mL	Acts as a diuretic by interfering with the renal tubular mechanism of electrolyte reabsorption (increases excretion of sodium and chloride).
Nonsteroidal Anti-inflammatory			
Indomethacin Oral Suspension	Indocin Oral Suspension (Merck & Co.)	25 mg/5 mL	For the active treatment of moderate to severe rheumatoid arthritis (including acute flares of chronic illness), moderate to severe osteoarthritis, acute painful shoulder (bursitis or tendinitis), and acute gouty arthritis.

Antacid Oral Suspensions

Antacids are intended to counteract the effects of gastric hyperacidity and as such are employed by persons, as peptic ulcer patients, who must reduce the level of acidity in the stomach. They are also widely employed and sold over-the-counter to patients suffering from conditions popularly referred to as "acid indigestion," "heartburn," and "sour stomach." Many patients belch or otherwise reflux acid from the stomach to the esophagus and take antacids to counter the acid brought to the esophagus and throat.

Most antacid preparations are composed of water-insoluble materials that act within the confines of the gastrointestinal tract to counteract the acid and/or soothe the irritated or inflamed linings of the gastrointestinal tract. There are a few water-soluble agents employed, as sodium bicarbonate, but for the most part, water-insoluble salts of aluminum, calcium, and magnesium are employed, as aluminum hydroxide, aluminum phosphate, dihydroxyaluminum aminoacetate, calcium carbonate, calcium phosphate, magaldrate, magnesium carbonate, magnesium oxide and magnesium hydroxide. The ability of each of these to neutralize gastric acid varies with the chemical agent. For instance, sodium bicarbonate, calcium carbonate, and magnesium hydroxide neutralize acid effectively, whereas magnesium trisilicate and aluminum hydroxide do so less effectively and much more slowly. In selecting an antacid, it is also important to consider the possible adverse effects of each agent in relation to the individual patient being treated. Each agent has its own peculiar potential for adverse effects. For instance, sodium bicarbonate possesses the capability for sodium overload and systemic alkalosis which is of potential hazard to patients on sodium-restricted diets. Magnesium preparations may lead to diarrhea and are dangerous to patients with diminished renal function due to the patients' inability to excrete all of the magnesium which may be absorbed (the gastric acid converts insoluble magnesium hydroxide to magnesium chloride which is water-soluble and is partially absorbed). Calcium carbonate carries the potential for inducing hypercalcemia and stimulation of gastric secretion and acid production, the latter effect known as "acid rebound." Excessive use of aluminum hydroxide may lead to constipation and phosphate depletion with consequent muscle weakness, bone resorption, and hypercalciuria.

The use to which an antacid is to be put is a major consideration in its selection. For instance, in the occasional treatment of heartburn, or other infrequent episodes of gastric distress, a single dose of sodium bicarbonate or a magnesium hydroxide preparation may be desired, but for the treatment of acute peptic ulcer or duodenal ulcer in which the therapeutic regimen includes the frequent administration of antacids, sodium bicarbonate would provide too great an amount of sodium and the magnesium hydroxide would induce diarrhea. Thus, in the treatment of ulcerative conditions, a combination of magnesium hydroxide and aluminum hydroxide is frequently used because the latter agent possesses some constipating effects which counter the diarrhea effects of the magnesium hydroxide.

In instances in which frequent dosage administration is required, and in cases in which gastroesophageal reflux is being treated, liquid antacids generally are preferred over tablet forms. For one thing, the liquid suspensions assert more immediate action—they do not require the time needed for tablets to disintegrate. It is important that an antacid preparation have a reasonably fast onset of action because its presence in the stomach may not last long due to gastric emptying into the intestines. It has been shown by endoscopic studies that on a fasting stomach very little antacid remains in the stomach 1 hour after administration. It is for this reason that the FDA has set the requirement that antacid tablets that are not intended to be chewed upon administration must disintegrate within 10 minutes in simulated gastric conditions. Frequent food snacks generally prolong the time an antacid remains in the stomach and can prolong its action.

Because many antacid materials, especially aluminum and calcium-containing products, interfere with the absorption of other drugs, especially the tetracycline group of antibiotics, pharmacists must caution their patients against taking such drugs concomitantly.

In addition to the suspension forms of antacids, a number of liquid antacid preparations of the magma and gel type are official and commercially available and will be mentioned later in this chapter. All of these liquid forms are usually pleasantly flavored (generally with peppermint) to enhance their palatability and patient appeal. Because liquid antacid preparations characteristi-

cally contain a large amount of solid material, they must be shaken vigorously to redistribute the antacid prior to administration. Also, a large dose of antacids is frequently required. Thus, many patients would prefer to swallow one or two tablespoonfuls of a liquid antacid preparation than to swallow whole or chew the corresponding number of tablets (commonly 3 to 6) for the equivalent dose of drug.

Antibacterial Oral Suspensions

The antibacterial oral suspensions include preparations of antibiotic substances (e.g., chloramphenicol palmitate, erythromycin derivatives, and tetracycline and its derivatives), sulfonamides (e.g., sulfamethoxazole, sulfisoxazole acetyl), other chemotherapeutic agents (e.g., methenamine mandelate and nitrofurantoin), or combinations of these (e.g., sulfamethoxazole-trimethoprim).

Many antibiotic materials are unstable when maintained in solution for an appreciable length of time and therefore, from a stability standpoint, insoluble forms of the drug substances in aqueous suspension or as dry powders for reconstitution (discussed next) are attractive to pharmaceutical manufacturers. The antibiotic oral suspensions, including those prepared by reconstitution, provide a convenient way to administer dosages to infants and children as well as to adult patients who may prefer liquid preparations to solid dosage forms. Many of the oral suspensions that are intended primarily for infants are packaged with a calibrated dropper to assist in the delivery of the prescribed dose. Examples of some commercial pediatric antibiotic oral suspensions are pictured in Figure 13.4, and examples of calibrated droppers in Figure 13.7.

The dispersing phase of antibiotic suspensions is aqueous, and usually colored, sweetened and flavored to render the liquid more appealing and palatable. As noted previously, the palmitate form of chloramphenicol was selected for the suspension dosage form not only because of its water-insolubility, but also because of its quality of being flavorless, thereby eliminating the formulating problem of trying to mask the otherwise bitter taste of the chloramphenicol base.

Examples of Other Suspensions

Otic Suspensions

Pharmacists must be aware that there may be subtle differences in the formulation of some otic suspensions that could be potentially bothersome

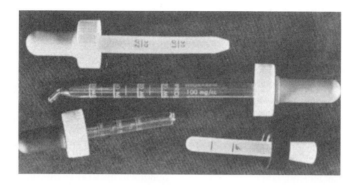

Fig. 13.7 *Examples of calibrated droppers utilized in the administration of pediatric medications.*

to the patient. This is especially so as it relates to inactive or inert ingredient differences between formulations from manufacturers which are considered equivalent on the basis of active ingredient(s) and strength. For example, several suspension combinations of polymyxin B sulfate, neomycin sulfate and hydrocortisone have been shown to be more acidic, i.e., pH 3.0 to 3.5, compared to the standard product, i.e., Cortisporin Otic Suspension (Monarch), which possesses a higher pH range, i.e., 4.8 to 5.1. Consequently, there is a risk that when drops are legally substituted, a burning and stinging sensation can occur when the drops are introduced into the ear of young children, especially those with tympanostomies. Further, it has been demonstrated that with time, the pH of these formulations, including Cortisporin, becomes more acidic, e.g., pH 3.0. Thus, if stored on the shelf for a period of time, it is conceivable that if used again, the acidity could cause irritation to the ear canal. For this reason, this antibiotic-hydrocortisone combination has been formulated into a new suspension product, i.e., PediOtic (Monarch), which has a minimum pH of 4.1.

Rectal Suspensions

Barium Sulfate for Suspension, USP may be employed orally or rectally for the diagnostic visualization of the gastrointestinal tract. Mesalamine (i.e., 5-aminosalicylic acid) suspension was introduced onto the market in 1988 as Rowasa (Solvay) for treatment of Crohn's disease, distal ulcerative colitis, proctosigmoiditis, and proctitis.

Dry Powders for Oral Suspension

A number of official and commercial preparations consist of dry powder mixtures or granules,

which are intended to be suspended in water or some other vehicle prior to oral administration. As indicated previously, these official preparations have "for Oral Suspension" in their official title to distinguish them from already prepared suspensions.

The majority of drugs prepared as a dry mix for oral suspension are antibiotics. The dry products are prepared commercially to contain the antibiotic drug, colorants (FD&C dyes), flavorants, sweeteners (as sucrose or sodium saccharin), stabilizing agents (as citric acid, sodium citrate), suspending agents (as guar gum, xanthan gum, methylcellulose), and preserving agents (as methylparaben, sodium benzoate) that may be needed to enhance the stability of either the dry powder or granule mixture or the ultimate liquid suspension. When called on to "reconstitute" and dispense one of these products, the pharmacist loosens the powder at the bottom of the container by lightly tapping it against a hard surface, and then adds the label-designated amount of purified water, usually in portions, and shakes until all of the dry powder has been suspended (Fig. 13.2). It is important for the pharmacist to add precisely the prescribed amount of purified water to the dry mixture if the proper drug concentration per dosage unit is to be achieved. Also, the use of purified water rather than tap water is needed to avoid the addition of possible offending impurities which could adversely affect the stability of the resulting preparation. Generally, manufacturers provide the dry powder or granule mixture in a slightly oversized container to permit the adequate shaking of the contents after the entire amount of purified water has been added. Pharmacists must realize that an oversized bottle is provided with each of these products and they must carefully measure out the required amount of purified water. They should not "eyeball" the amount of water to be added or mistakenly fill up the bottle with purified water. Among the official antibiotic drugs for oral suspension are the following:

Amoxicillin for Oral Suspension, USP
  [Amoxil for Oral Suspension (SmithKline Beecham)]
Ampicillin for Oral Suspension, USP
  [Omnipen for Oral Suspension (Wyeth-Ayerst)]
Bacampicillin for Oral Suspension, USP
  [Spectrobid for Oral Suspension (Roerig)]
Cefaclor for Oral Suspension, USP
  [Ceclor for Oral Suspension (Lilly)]
Cefixime for Oral Suspension, USP
  [Suprax Powder for Oral Suspension (Lederle)]
Cephadrine for Oral Suspension, USP
  [Velosef for Oral Suspension (Squibb)]
Cephalexin for Oral Suspension, USP
  [Keflex for Oral Suspension (Dista)]
Dicloxacillin Sodium for Oral Suspension, USP
  [Pathocil for Oral Suspension (Wyeth-Ayerst)]
Doxycycline for Oral Suspension, USP
  [Vibramycin Monohydrate for Oral Suspension (Pfizer)]
Erythromycin Ethylsuccinate for Oral Suspension, USP
  [E.E.S. Granules for Oral Suspension (Abbott)]
Penicillin V for Oral Suspension, USP

There are also several official combinations of antibiotics for oral suspension combined with other drugs. For example, the combination of erythromycin ethylsuccinate and acetylsulfisoxazole granules for oral suspension is indicated for the treatment of acute middle ear infection caused by susceptible strains of *Hemophilus influenzae.* Probenecid is combined with ampicillin for reconstitution and ultimate use for the treatment of uncomplicated infections (urethral, endocervical or rectal) caused by *Neisseria gonorrhoeae* in adults.

Among the official drugs other than antibiotics prepared as dry powder mixtures for reconstitution to oral suspension are the following: cholestyramine [Questran (Bristol-Myers Squibb)], a drug used in the management of high cholesterol levels; and barium sulfate [Barosperse (Mallinckrodt)], used orally or rectally as a radiopaque contrast medium to visualize the gastrointestinal tract as an aid to diagnosis. Barium sulfate was introduced into medicine about 1910 as a contrast medium in the roentgen-ray examination of the gastrointestinal tract. It is practically insoluble in water and thus

its administration, even in the large doses required, is safe because it is not absorbed from the gastrointestinal tract. The pharmacist must be careful not to confuse "barium sulfate," with other forms of barium as the *sulfide* and *sulfite,* which are soluble salts and *are* poisonous. Barium sulfate is a fine, nongritty, white, odorless and tasteless powder. When prepared into a suspension and administered orally, it is used to diagnose conditions of the hypopharynx, esophagus, stomach, small intestine and colon. The barium sulfate renders the gastrointestinal tract opaque to the x ray so that it may be photographed, revealing any abnormality in the anatomic features of the tract. When administered rectally, the barium sulfate allows visualization of the features of the rectum and colon. Mesalamine (i.e., 5-aminosalicylic acid) suspension was introduced onto the market in 1988 as Rowasa (Solvay) for treatment of Crohn's disease, distal ulcerative colitis, proctosigmoiditis, and proctitis.

Commercially, barium sulfate for diagnostic use is available as a bulk powder containing the required suspending agents for effective reconstitution to an oral suspension or enema prior to administration. Enema units, which contain prepared suspension in a ready-to-use and disposable bag, are also available.

Emulsions

An emulsion is a dispersion in which the dispersed phase is composed of small globules of a liquid distributed throughout a vehicle in which it is immiscible (Fig. 13.8). In emulsion terminology, the dispersed phase is referred to as the *internal phase,* and the dispersion medium as the *external* or *continuous phase.* Emulsions having an oleaginous internal phase and an aqueous external phase are referred to as *oil-in-water* emulsions, and are commonly designated as "o/w" emulsions. Conversely, emulsions having an aqueous internal phase and an oleaginous external phase are termed *water-in-oil* emulsions and are referred to as "w/o" emulsions. Because the external phase of an emulsion is continuous, an oil-in-water emulsion may be diluted or extended with water or an aqueous preparation, and a water-in-oil emulsion with an oleaginous or oil-miscible liquid. Generally, to prepare a stable emulsion, a third phase is necessary, that being an *emulsifying agent.* Depending on their constituents, the viscosity of emulsions can vary greatly, and pharmaceutical emulsions may be prepared as liquids or semisolids. Based on the constituents and the intended application, liquid emulsions may

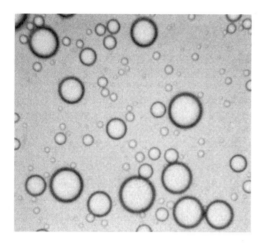

Fig. 13.8 *Mineral oil in water emulsion. The largest oil globule in the photograph measures approximately 0.04 mm. (Courtesy of James C. Price, Ph.D., College of Pharmacy, The University of Georgia.)*

be employed orally, topically, or parenterally; semisolid emulsions, topically. Many pharmaceutical preparations that may actually be emulsions may not be classified as such because they fit some other pharmaceutical category more appropriately. For instance, certain lotions, liniments, creams, ointments, and commercial vitamin drops may be emulsions but may be referred to in the terms indicated and will be discussed in this book under these various designations.

Purpose of Emulsions and of Emulsification

Pharmaceutically, the process of emulsification enables the pharmacist to prepare relatively stable and homogeneous mixtures of two immiscible liquids. It permits the administration of a liquid drug in the form of minute globules rather than in bulk. For orally administered emulsions, the oil-in-water type of emulsion permits the palatable administration of an otherwise distasteful oil by dispersing it in a sweetened, flavored aqueous vehicle in which it may be carried past the taste buds and into the stomach. The reduced particle size of the oil globules may render the oil more digestible and more readily absorbed, or if that is not the intent, more effective in its task, as for example the increased efficacy of mineral oil as a cathartic when in the emulsified form.

Emulsions to be applied externally to the skin may be prepared as o/w or w/o emulsions, de-

pending on such factors as the nature of the therapeutic agents to be incorporated into the emulsions, the desirability for an emollient or tissue softening effect of the preparation, and the condition of the skin surface. Medicinal agents that are irritating to the skin generally are less irritating if present in the internal phase of an emulsified topical preparation than in the external phase from which direct contact with the skin is more prevalent. Naturally, the miscibility or the solubility in oil and in water of a medicinal agent to be used in an emulsified preparation would dictate to a great extent the vehicle in which it must be present, and its nature would in turn suggest the phase of the emulsion that the resulting solution should become. On the unbroken skin, a water-in-oil emulsion can usually be applied more evenly because the skin is covered with a thin film of sebum, and this surface is more readily wetted by oil than by water. A water-in-oil emulsion is also more softening to the skin, because it resists drying out and is resistant to removal by contact with water. On the other hand, if it is desirable to have a preparation that is more easily removed from the skin with water, an oil-in-water emulsion would be preferred. As for absorption, absorption through the skin (percutaneous absorption) may be enhanced by the diminished particle size of the internal phase. Other aspects of topical preparations are discussed in Chapter 9 and 10.

Theories of Emulsification

Many theories have been advanced in an attempt to explain how emulsifying agents act in promoting emulsification and in maintaining the stability of the resulting emulsion. Although certain of these theories apply rather specifically to certain types of emulsifying agents and to certain conditions (as the pH of the phases of the system and the nature and relative proportions of the internal and external phases), they may be viewed in a general way to describe the manner in which emulsions may be produced and stabilized. Among the most prevalent theories are the *surface-tension theory,* the *oriented-wedge theory,* and the *plastic* or *interfacial film theory.*

All liquids have a tendency to assume a shape having the least amount of surface area exposed. For a drop of a liquid, that shape is spherical. In a spherical drop of liquid, there are internal forces that tend to promote the association of the molecules of the substance to resist the distortion of the drop into a less spherical form. If two or more drops of the same liquid come into contact with one another, the tendency is for them to join or to *coalesce,* making one larger drop having a lesser surface area than the total surface area of the individual drops. This tendency of liquids may be measured quantitatively, and when the surrounding of the liquid is air, it is referred to as the liquid's surface tension. When the liquid is in contact with a second liquid in which it is insoluble and immiscible, the force causing each liquid to resist breaking up into smaller particles is called interfacial tension. Substances that can promote the lowering of this resistance to breakup can encourage a liquid to be reduced to smaller drops or particles. These tension-lowering substances are referred to as *surface-active* (surfactants) or *wetting agents.* According to the *surface-tension theory* of emulsification, the use of these substances as emulsifiers and stabilizers results in the lowering of the interfacial tension of the two immiscible liquids, reducing the repellent force between the liquids and diminishing each liquid's attraction for its own molecules. Thus the surface-active agents facilitate the breaking up of large globules into smaller ones, which then have a lesser than usual tendency to reunite or coalesce.

The *oriented-wedge* theory assumes monomolecular layers of emulsifying agent curved around a droplet of the internal phase of the emulsion. The theory is based on the presumption that certain emulsifying agents orient themselves about and within a liquid in a manner reflective of their solubility in that particular liquid. In a system containing two immiscible liquids, presumably the emulsifying agent would be preferentially soluble in one of the phases and would be embedded more deeply and tenaciously in that phase than the other. Since many molecules of substances upon which this theory is based (for example, soaps) have a hydrophilic or water-loving portion and a hydrophobic or water-hating portion (but usually lipophilic or oil-loving), the molecules will position or orient themselves into each phase. Depending upon the shape and size of the molecules, their solubility characteristics, and thus their orientation, the wedge-shape arrangement envisioned for the molecules will cause the surrounding of either oil globules or water globules. Generally an emulsifying agent having a greater hydrophilic character than hydrophobic character will promote an oil-in-water emulsion, and a water-in-oil emulsion results through the use of an emulsifying agent that is more hydrophobic than hydrophilic. Putting it another way, the phase in which the emulsifying agent is more soluble will become the continuous

or external phase of the emulsion. Although this theory may not represent a totally accurate depiction of the molecular arrangement of the emulsifier molecules, the concept that water-soluble emulsifiers generally do form oil-in-water emulsions is important and is generally found in practice.

The *plastic-* or *interfacial-film theory* places the emulsifying agent at the interface between the oil and water, surrounding the droplets of the internal phase as a thin layer of film adsorbed on the surface of the drops. The film prevents the contact and coalescing of the dispersed phase; the tougher and more pliable the film, the greater the stability of the emulsion. Naturally, enough of the film-forming material must be available to coat the entire surface of each drop of internal phase. Here again, the formation of an oil-in-water or a water-in-oil emulsion is dependent upon the degree of solubility of the agent in the two phases, with water-soluble agents encouraging oil-in-water emulsions and oil-soluble emulsifiers the reverse.

In actuality, it is unlikely that a single theory of emulsification may be used to explain the means by which the many and varied emulsifiers promote emulsion formation and stability. It is more than likely that even within a given emulsion system, more than one of the aforementioned theories of emulsification is applicable and plays a part. For instance, lowering of the interfacial tension is important in the initial formation of an emulsion, but the formation of a protective wedge of molecules or film of emulsifier is important for continued emulsion stability. No doubt certain emulsifiers are capable of both tasks.

Preparation of Emulsions

Emulsifying Agents

The initial step in preparation of an emulsion is the selection of the emulsifier. To be useful in a pharmaceutical preparation, the emulsifying agent must possess certain qualities. For one thing, it must be compatible with the other formulative ingredients and must not interfere with the stability or efficacy of the therapeutic agent. It should be stable and not deteriorate in the preparation. The emulsifier should be nontoxic with respect to its intended use and the amount to be consumed by the patient. Also, it should possess little odor, taste, or color. Of prime importance is the capability of the emulsifying agent to promote emulsification and to maintain the stability of the emulsion for the intended shelf life of the product.

Various types of materials have been used in pharmacy as emulsifying agents, with hundreds, if not thousands, of individual agents tested for their emulsification capabilities. Although no attempt will be made here to try to discuss the merits of each of these agents in pharmaceutical emulsion, it would be well to point out the types of materials that are commonly used and their general application. Among the emulsifiers and stabilizers for pharmaceutical systems are the following:

1. Carbohydrate materials such as the naturally occurring agents acacia, tragacanth, agar, chondrus, and pectin. These materials form hydrophilic colloids when added to water and generally produce o/w emulsions. Acacia is perhaps the most frequently used emulsifier in the preparation of extemporaneous emulsions by the community pharmacist. Tragacanth and agar are commonly employed as thickening agents in acacia-emulsified products. Microcrystalline cellulose is employed in a number of commercially prepared suspensions and emulsions as a viscosity regulator to retard particle settling and provide dispersion stability.
2. Protein substances such as gelatin, egg yolk, and casein. These substances produce o/w emulsions. The disadvantage of gelatin as an emulsifier is that the emulsions prepared from it frequently are too fluid and become more fluid upon standing.
3. High molecular weight alcohols such as stearyl alcohol, cetyl alcohol, and glyceryl monostearate. These are employed primarily as thickening agents and stabilizers for o/w emulsions of certain lotions and ointments used externally. Cholesterol and cholesterol derivatives may also be employed in externally used emulsions and promote w/o emulsions.
4. Wetting agents, which may be anionic, cationic, or nonionic. These agents contain both hydrophilic and lipophilic groups, with the lipophilic protein of the molecule generally accounting for the surface-activity of the molecule. In anionic agents, this lipophilic portion is negatively charged, but in the cationic agent it is positively charged. Owing to their opposing ionic charges, anionic and cationic agents tend to neutralize each other if present in the same system and are thus considered incompatible with one another. Nonionic emulsifiers show no inclination to ionize. Depending upon their individual nature, certain of the members of these groups form o/w emulsions and others w/o

emulsions. Anionic emulsifiers include various monovalent, polyvalent, and organic soaps such as triethanolamine oleate and sulfonates such as sodium lauryl sulfate. Benzalkonium chloride, known primarily for its bactericidal properties, may be employed as a cationic-type of emulsifier. Agents of the nonionic type include the sorbitan esters and the polyoxyethylene derivatives, some of which appear in Table 13.2.

The ionic nature of a surfactant is of prime consideration in the selection of a surfactant to utilize in forming an emulsion. Nonionic surfactants are effective over pH range 3 to 10; cationic surfactants are effective over pH range 3 to 7; and, anionic surfactants require a pH of greater than 8 (6).

5. Finely divided solids such as colloidal clays including bentonite, magnesium hydroxide, and aluminum hydroxide. These generally form o/w emulsions when the insoluble material is added to the aqueous phase if there is a greater volume of the aqueous phase than of the oleaginous phase. However, if the powdered solid is added to the oil and the oleaginous phase volume predominates, a substance like bentonite is capable of forming a w/o emulsion.

The relative volume of internal and external phases of an emulsion is important, regardless of the type of emulsifier used. As the internal concentration of an emulsion is increased, there is an increase in the viscosity of the emulsion to a certain point, after which the viscosity decreases sharply. At this point, the emulsion has undergone *inversion;* that is, it has changed from an o/w emulsion to a w/o, or vice versa. In practice, emulsions may be prepared without inversion with as much as about 75% of the volume of the product being internal phase.

The HLB System

Generally, each emulsifying agent has a hydrophilic portion and a lipophilic portion with one or the other being more or less predominant and influencing in the manner already described the type of emulsion. A method has been devised (7) whereby emulsifying or surface-active agents may be categorized on the basis of their chemical make-up as to their hydrophile-lipophile balance or "HLB." By this method, each agent is assigned an HLB value or number which is indicative of the substance's polarity. Although the numbers have been assigned up to about 40, the usual range is between 1 and 20. Materials that are highly polar or hydrophilic have been assigned higher numbers than materials that are less polar and more lipophilic. Generally, those surface-active agents having an assigned HLB value of from 3 to 6 are greatly lipophilic and produce water-in-oil emulsions, and those agents have HLB values of from about 8 to 18 produce oil-in-water emulsions. Examples of some assigned HLB values for some selected surfactants are shown in Table 13.2. The type of activity to be expected from surfactants of assigned HLB numbers is presented in Table 13.3.

In the HLB system, in addition to assigning values to the emulsifying agents, values are also assigned to oils and oil-like substances. In using the HLB concept in the preparation of an emulsion, one selects emulsifying agents having the same or nearly the same HLB value as the oleaginous phase of the intended emulsion. For example, mineral oil

Table 13.2.   Examples of HLB Values for Selected Emulsifiers

Agent	HLB
Ethylene glycol distearate	1.5
Sorbitan tristearate (Span 65*)	2.1
Propylene glycol monostearate	3.4
Triton X-15†	3.6
Sorbitan monooleate (Span 80*)	4.3
Sorbitan monostearate (Span 60*)	4.7
Diethylene glycol monolaurate	6.1
Sorbitan monopalmitate (Span 40*)	6.7
Sucrose dioleate	7.1
Acacia	8.0
Amercol L-101‡	8.0
Polyoxyethylene lauryl ether (Brij 30*)	9.7
Gelatin	9.8
Triton X-45†	10.4
Methylcellulose	10.5
Polyoxyethylene monostearate (Myrj 45*)	11.1
Triethanolamine oleate	12.0
Tragacanth	13.2
Triton X-100†	13.5
Polyoxyethylene sorbitan monostearate (Tween 60*)	14.9
Polyoxyethylene sorbitan monooleate (Tween 80*)	15.0
Polyoxyethylene sorbitan monolaurate (Tween 20*)	16.7
Pluronic F 68§	17.0
Sodium oleate	18.0
Potassium oleate	20.0
Sodium lauryl sulfate	40.0

* ICI Americas, Inc., Wilmington, DE
†Rohm and Haas, Philadelphia, PA
‡Amerchol Corporation, Edison, NJ
§BASF-Wyandotte Chemical Corporation, Parsippany, NJ

Table 13.3.   Activity and HLB Value of Surfactants

Activity	Assigned HLB
Antifoaming	1 to 3
Emulsifiers (w/o)	3 to 6
Wetting agents	7 to 9
Emulsifiers (o/w)	8 to 18
Solubilizers	15 to 20
Detergents	13 to 15

has an assigned HLB value of 4 if a w/o emulsion is desired and a value of 10.5 if an o/w emulsion is to be prepared. To prepare a stable emulsion, the emulsifying agent selected should have an HLB value similar to the one for mineral oil, depending on the type of emulsion desired. When needed, two or more emulsifiers may be combined to achieve the proper HLB value.

The accompanying Physical Pharmacy Capsule 13.3 summarizes the activities of surfactants and the calculations involved in determining the quantity of surfactant required to prepare a stable emulsion.

Methods of Emulsion Preparation

Emulsions may be prepared by several methods, depending upon the nature of the emulsion components and the equipment available for use. On a small scale, as in the laboratory or pharmacy, emulsions may be prepared using a dry Wedgewood or porcelain mortar and pestle, a mechanical blender or mixer such as a Waring blender or a milk-shake mixer, a hand homogenizer (Fig. 13.9), a bench-type homogenizer (Fig. 13.10), or sometimes a simple prescription bottle. On a large scale, large volume mixing tanks (Fig. 13.5) may be used to form the emulsion through the action of a highspeed impeller. As desired, the product may be rendered finer by passage through a colloid mill, in which the particles are sheared between the small gap separating a high speed rotor and the stator, or by passage through a large homogenizer, in which the liquid is forced under great pressure through a small valve opening. Industrial homogenizers have the capacity to handle as much as 100,000 liters of product per hour.

In the small-scale extemporaneous preparation of emulsions, three methods may be used. They are the *continental* or *dry gum method,* the *English* or *wet gum method,* and the *bottle* or the *Forbes bottle method.* In the first method, the emulsifying agent (usually acacia) is mixed with the oil before the addition of

Physical Pharmacy Capsule 13.3   **Blending of Surfactants**

Wetting agents are surfactants with HLB values of **7 to 9.** Wetting agents aid in attaining intimate contact between solid particles and liquids.

Emulsifying agents are surfactants with HLB values of **3 to 6 or 8 to 18.** Emulsifying agents reduce interfacial tension between oil and water, resulting in minimizing surface energy through the formation of globules.

Detergents are surfactants with HLB values of **13 to 16.** Detergents will reduce the surface tension and aid in wetting the surface and the dirt. The soil will be emulsified, and foaming generally occurs and a washing away of the dirt.

Solubilizing agents have HLB values of **16 to 18.**

HLB values are additive, and often surfactants are blended. For example if 20 mL of an HLB of 9.0 are required, then two surfactants (with HLB values of 8.0 and 12.0) can be blended in a 3:1 ratio. The following quantities of each will be required:

$$\frac{3}{4} \times 8.0 = 6.0$$
$$\frac{1}{4} \times 12.0 = 3.0$$
$$\text{Total HLB} = 9.0$$

water. In the second method, the emulsifying agent is added to the water (in which it is soluble) to form a mucilage, and then the oil is slowly incorporated to form the emulsion. The bottle method is reserved for volatile oils or less viscous oils and is a variation of the dry gum method.

Continental or Dry Gum Method

The method is also referred to as the "4:2:1" method because for every 4 parts (volumes) of oil, 2 parts of water and 1 part of gum are added in preparing the initial or *primary emulsion.* For instance, if 40 mL of oil are to be emulsified, 20 mL of water and 10 g of gum would be employed, with any additional water or other formulation ingredients being added afterward to the primary emulsion. In this method, the acacia or other o/w emulsifier is triturated with the oil in a perfectly dry Wedgewood or porcelain mortar until thoroughly mixed. A mortar with a rough rather than smooth inner surface must be used to ensure proper grinding action and the reduction of the globule size during the preparation of the emulsion. A glass mortar has too smooth a surface to produce the proper size reduction of the internal phase. After the oil and gum have been mixed, the two parts of water are then added all at once, and the mixture is triturated immediately, rapidly, and continuously until the primary emulsion that forms is creamy white and produces a crackling sound to the move-

ment of the pestle. Generally, about 3 minutes of mixing are required to produce such a primary emulsion. Other liquid formulative ingredients that are soluble in or miscible with the external phase may then be added to the primary emulsion with

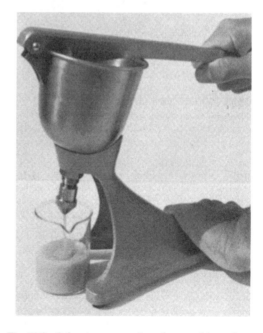

Fig. 13.9 *Laboratory preparation of an emulsion, using a hand homogenizer.*

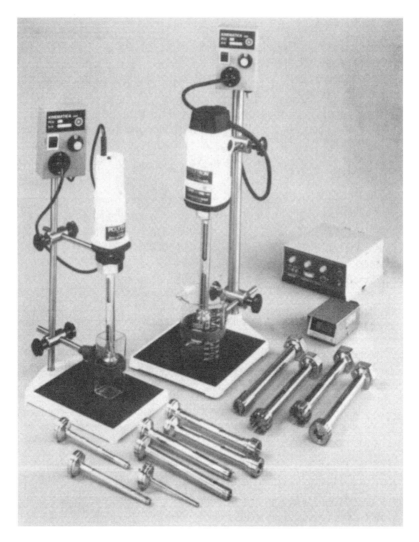

Fig. 13.10   *Brinkmann Homogenizer Models PT 10/35 and PT 45/80 with accessories. The equipment is used for the homogenization, dispersion and emulsification of solids or liquids. Volumes can be processed ranging from 0.5 mL to 25 liters. (Courtesy of Brinkmann Instruments Co., Division of Sybron Corporation.)*

mixing. Solid substances such as preservatives, stabilizers, colorants, and any flavoring material are usually dissolved in a suitable volume of water (assuming water is the external phase) and added as a solution to the primary emulsion. Any substances that might interfere with the stability of the emulsion or the emulsifying agent are added as near last as is practically possible. For instance, since alcohol has a precipitating action on gums such as acacia, alcohol or any solution containing alcohol should not be added directly to the primary emulsion, since the total alcoholic concentration of the mixture would be greater at that point than it would be

after other diluents had been previously added. When all necessary agents have been added, the emulsion is transferred to a graduate and made to volume with water previously swirled about in the mortar to remove the last portion of emulsion.

Provided the dispersion of the acacia in the oil is adequate, the dry gum method can almost be guaranteed to produce an acceptable emulsion. Sometimes, however, the amount of acacia needs to be adjusted upward to ensure an emulsion can be produced. For example, volatile oils, liquid petrolatum (mineral oil) and linseed oil usually require a "3:2:1 or 2:2:1" ratio for adequate preparation. Rather than use a mortar and pestle, the pharmacist can generally prepare an excellent emulsion using the dry gum method and an electric mixer or blender.

English or Wet Gum Method

By this method, the same proportions of oil, water, and gum are used as in the continental or dry gum method, but the order of mixing is different, and the proportion of ingredients may be varied during the preparation of the primary emulsion as is deemed necessary by the operator. Generally a mucilage of the gum is prepared by triturating granular acacia with twice its weight of water in a mortar. The oil is then added slowly in portions, and the mixture is triturated to emulsify the oil. Should the mixture become too thick during the process, additional water may be blended into the mixture before another successive portion of oil is added. After all of the oil has been added, the mixture is thoroughly mixed for several minutes to insure uniformity. Then, as with the continental or dry gum method, the other formulative materials are added, and the emulsion is transferred to a graduate and made to volume with water.

Bottle or Forbes Bottle Method

For the extemporaneous preparation of emulsions from volatile oils or oleaginous substances of low viscosities, the bottle method is useful. In this method, powdered acacia is placed in a dry bottle, two parts of oil are then added, and the mixture is thoroughly shaken in the capped container. A volume of water approximately equal to the oil is then added in portions, the mixture being thoroughly shaken after each addition. When all of the water has been added, the primary emulsion thus formed may be diluted to the proper volume with water or an aqueous solution of other formulative agents.

This method is not suited for viscous oils, because they cannot be thoroughly agitated in the bottle when mixed with the emulsifying agent. In instances in which the intended dispersed phase is a mixture of part fixed oil and part volatile oil, the dry gum method is generally employed for emulsification.

Auxiliary Methods

An emulsion prepared by either the wet gum or the dry gum methods can generally be increased in quality by passing it through a hand homogenizer. In this apparatus, the pumping action of the handle forces the emulsion through a very small orifice which reduces the globules of the internal phase to about 5 μm and sometimes less. The hand homogenizer is less efficient in reducing the particle size of very thick emulsions, and it should not be employed for emulsions containing a high proportion of solid matter because of possible damage to the valve.

In Situ Soap Method

The two types of soaps developed by this method are calcium soaps and soft soaps. Calcium soaps are water-in-oil emulsions which contain certain vegetable oils, e.g., oleic acid, in combination with lime water (syn: Calcium Hydroxide Solution USP), and are prepared simply by mixing equal volumes of the oil and lime water. The emulsifying agent in this instance is the calcium salt of the free fatty acid which is formed from the combination of the two entities. In the case of olive oil, the free fatty acid is oleic acid, and the resultant emulsifying agent formed is calcium oleate. A difficulty which sometimes arises when preparing this self-emulsifying product is that the amount of free fatty acids in the oil may be insufficient on a 1:1 basis with calcium hydroxide. Typically, to make up for this deficiency a little excess of the oil is needed to ensure a nice, homogeneous emulsion results. Otherwise, tiny droplets of water form on the surface of the preparation. Because the oil phase is the external phase, this formulation is ideal where occlusion and skin softening are desired, e.g., itchy, dry skin or sunburned skin. A typical example of this emulsion is calamine liniment:

Calamine ....
Zinc Oxide aa ....   80.0 g
Olive Oil ....
Calcium Hydroxide Sol'n aa qs ad .... 1000.0 mL

Microemulsions

Microemulsions are thermodynamically stable, optically transparent, isotropic mixtures of a biphasic oil-water system stabilized with surfactants. The diameter of droplets in a *micro*emulsion may be in the range of 100 Å (10 millimicrons) to 1000 Å whereas in a *micro*emulsion the droplets may be 5000 angstroms in diameter (6). Both o/w and w/o microemulsions may be formed spontaneously by agitating the oil and water phases with carefully selected surfactants. The type of emulsion produced depends upon the properties of the oil and surfactants utilized.

Physical Pharmacy Capsule 13.4   **Surface Area of Globules**

The following is an example calculation for determining the quantity of surfactant required to prepare a stable oil-in-water emulsion.

A surface-active agent will spread itself as a single layer when applied to the surface of still water. The dimensions of a molecule can be determined by their surface orientation. For example, if a micropipet is used to deliver 3 μL of a surfactant onto the clean, quiet surface of water, the area over which it spreads, determined experimentally using a film balance, is 12,000 cm². The actual thickness of the film can be calculated by dividing the volume of surfactant applied by the surface area, as follows:

$$\frac{0.003 \text{ cm}^3}{12,000 \text{ cm}^2} = 2.5 \times 10^{-7} \text{ cm}$$

The surfactant has a density of 0.910 g/cc and a molecular weight of 325 g/mole. To calculate the cross-sectional area occupied by each molecule, one can divide the area of the monomolecular film by the number of molecules present in the 3 μL of surfactant comprising the film, as follows:

1. The weight of the surfactant can be obtained by multiplying the volume by the density (0.003 mL × 0.910 g/cc = 0.00273 g).
2. To calculate the number of moles present, divide the weight of the surfactant by its molecular weight (0.00273 g/325 g/mole = 8.4 × 10⁻⁶ moles).
3. The number of molecules present is the number of moles times Avogadro's Number (8.4 × 10⁻⁶ × 6.02 × 10²³ = 5.0568 × 10¹⁸ molecules).
4. The cross-sectional area can now be calculated by dividing the surface area by the number of molecules (12,000 cm²/5.0568 × 10¹⁸ = 2.373 × 10⁻¹⁵ cm² = 23.73 × 10⁻¹⁶, or approximately 24 square angstroms.

The quantity of surfactant required to emulsify selected a quantity of oil for the preparation of an oil in water emulsion can be calculated as follows.

EXAMPLE
To emulsify 50 mL of oil to an average globular diameter of 1 micron, the volume of each globule is:

$$V_i = \frac{4}{3} \pi r^3 = \frac{4}{3} \pi (0.5 \times 10^{-4})^3 = 0.524 \times 10^{-12} \text{ mL}$$

To calculate the number of globules present per mL, divide 1 mL by the volume of each globule:

$$\frac{1 \text{ mL}}{0.524 \times 10^{-12} \text{ mL/globule}} = 1.91 \times 10^{12} \text{ globules per mL}$$

The surface area (S) of each individual globule will be:

$$S = 4\pi r^2 = 4\pi (0.5 \times 10^{-4})^2 = 3.14 \times 10^{-8} \text{ cm}^2$$

and the surface area of all the globules in 1 mL of oil is:

$$(1.91 \times 10^{12}) \times (3.14 \times 10^{-8}) = 6 \times 10^4 \text{ cm}^2$$

The number of surfactant molecules that will be adsorbed at the interface of the oil globules, and the dispersion medium from 1 cc of oil, is equal to the total surface area divided by the cross-sectional area of the surfactant:

$$\frac{6 \times 10^4 \text{ cm}^2}{2.373 \times 10^{-15} \text{ cm}^2/\text{molecule}} = 2.528 \times 10^{19} \text{ molecules}$$

Surface Area of Globules (Continued)

To calculate the number of moles of surfactant that will be required to emulsify 1 mL of oil is equal to the number of molecules adsorbed at the interface divided by Avogadro's number:

$$\frac{2.528 \times 10^{19} \text{ molecules}}{6.02 \times 10^{23} \text{ molecules/mole}} = 4.199 \times 10^{-5} \text{ moles}$$

and the quantity required for 50 mL will be:

$$50 \text{ mL} \times 4.199 \times 10^{-5} \text{ moles/mL} = 2.095 \times 10^{-3} \text{ moles}$$

$$2.095 \times 10^{-3} \text{ moles} \times 325 \text{ g/mole} = 0.681 \text{ g, or } 681 \text{ mg}$$

Therefore, 681 mg of surfactant will be required to emulsify 50 mL of the oil.

Hydrophilic surfactants may be used to produce "transparent" o/w emulsions of many oils, including flavor oils and vitamin oils such as A, D, and E. Surfactants in the HLB range of 15 to 18 have been used most extensively in the preparation of such emulsions. These emulsions are dispersions of oil, not true solutions; however, because of the appearance of the product, the surfactant is commonly said to "solubilize" the oil. Surfactants commonly used in the preparation of such oral liquid formulations are polysorbate 60 and polysorbate 80.

Among the advantages cited for the use of microemulsions in drug delivery are: more rapid and efficient oral absorption of drugs than through solid dosage forms; enhanced transdermal drug delivery through increased drug diffusion into the skin; and the unique potential application of microemulsions in the development of artificial red blood cells and in the targeting of cytotoxic drugs to cancer cells (6).

Stability of Emulsions

Generally speaking, an emulsion is considered to be physically unstable if: a) the internal or dispersed phase upon standing tends to form aggregates of globules, b) large globules or aggregates of globules rise to the top or fall to the bottom of the emulsion to form a concentrated layer of the internal phase, and c) if all or part of the liquid of the internal phase becomes "unemulsified" and forms a distinct layer on the top or bottom of the emulsion as a result of the coalescing of the globules of the internal phase. In addition, an emulsion may be adversely affected by microbial contamination and growth and by other chemical and physical alterations.

Aggregation and Coalescence

Aggregates of globules of the internal phase have a greater tendency than do individual particles to rise to the top of the emulsion or fall to the bottom. Such a preparation of the globules is termed the "creaming" of the emulsion, and provided coalescence is absent, it is a reversible process. The term is taken from the dairy industry and is analogous to the creaming or the rising to the top of cream in milk that is allowed to stand. The creamed portion of an emulsion may be redistributed rather homogeneously upon shaking, but if the aggregates are difficult to disassemble or if insufficient shaking is employed before each dose, improper dosage of the internal phase substance may result. Further, the creaming of a pharmaceutical emulsion is not esthetically acceptable to the pharmacist nor appealing to the consumer. More importantly, it increases the risk of the coalescing of the globules.

According to the Stokes' equation (See accompanying Physical Pharmacy Capsule), the rate of separation of the dispersed phase of an emulsion may be related to such factors as the particle size of the dispersed phase, the difference in the density between the phases, and the viscosity of the external phase. It is important to recall that the rate of separation is increased by increased particle size of the internal phase, a larger density difference between the two phases, and a decreased viscosity of the external phase. Therefore, to increase the stability of an emulsion, the globule or particle size should be reduced as fine as is practically possible, the density difference between the internal and external phases should be minimal, and the viscosity of the external phase should be reasonably high. Thickeners such as tragacanth and microcrystalline cellulose are frequently added to emulsions to increase the viscosity of the external phase. Upward creaming takes place in unstable emulsions of the o/w or w/o type in which the internal phase has a lesser density than the external phase. Downward creaming takes place in unstable emulsions in which the opposite is true.

Of greater destruction to an emulsion than creaming is the coalescence of the globules of the internal phase and the separation of that phase into a layer. The separation of the internal phase from the emulsion is called the "breaking" of the emulsion, and the emulsion is described as being "cracked" or "broken." This is irreversible, because the protective sheath about the globules of the internal phase no longer exists. Attempts to reestablish the emulsion by agitation of the two separate layers are generally unsuccessful. Additional emulsifying agent and reprocessing through appropriate machinery are usually necessary to reproduce an emulsion.

Generally, care must be taken to protect emulsions against the extremes of cold and heat. Freezing and thawing result in the coarsening of an emulsion and sometimes in its breaking. Excessive heat has the same effect. Because emulsion products may be transported to and used in various geographic locations having varying climates and conditions of extremely high and low temperature, pharmaceutical manufacturers must have predetermined knowledge of their emulsion stability before they may be shipped. For most emulsions, the industry performs tests of evaluation under experimental conditions of 5° C, 40° C, and 50° C to determine the product's stability. Stability at both 5° C and 40° C for 3 months is considered the minimal stability that an emulsion should possess. Shorter exposure periods at 50° C may be used as an alternate test.

Because other environmental conditions such as the presence of light, air, and contaminating microorganisms can adversely affect the stability of an emulsion, appropriate formulative and packaging steps are usually taken to minimize such possible hazards to product stability. For light-sensitive emulsions, light-resistant containers are used. For emulsions susceptible to oxidative decomposition, antioxidants may be included in the formulation and adequate label warning provided to ensure that the container is tightly closed to air after each use. Many molds, yeasts, and bacteria can bring about the decomposition of the emulsifying agent of an emulsion, thereby causing the disruption of the system. In cases in which the emulsifier is not affected by the microbes, the product can be rendered unsightly by their presence and growth and will of course not be efficacious from a pharmaceutical or therapeutic standpoint. Fungistatic preservatives are generally included in the aqueous phase of an o/w emulsion, since fungi (molds and yeasts) are more likely to contaminate emulsions than are bacteria. Combinations of methylparaben and propylparaben are frequently employed to serve this function. Alcohol in the amount of 12 to 15% based on the external phase volume is frequently added to orally used o/w emulsions for preservation.

Examples of Oral Emulsions

Mineral Oil Emulsion

This emulsion, also referred to as liquid petrolatum emulsion, is an oil-in-water emulsion prepared from the following formula:

Mineral Oil	500 mL
Acacia (finely powdered)	125 g
Syrup	100 mL
Vanillin	40 mg
Alcohol	60 mL
Purified Water, a sufficient quantity, to make	1000 mL

The emulsion is prepared by the dry gum method (4:2:1), mixing the oil with the acacia and adding 250 mL of purified water all at once to effect the primary emulsion. To this is slowly added with trituration the remainder of the ingredients, with the vanillin dissolved in the alcohol. A substitute flavorant for the vanillin, a substitute preservative for the alcohol, and a substitute emulsifying agent for the acacia and an alternative method of emulsification may be used as desired.

The emulsion is employed as a lubricating cathartic with a usual dose of 30 mL. The usual dose of the plain (unemulsified) mineral oil for the same purpose is 15 mL. The emulsion is much more palatable than is the unemulsified oil. Both are best taken at bedtime. There are a number of commercial preparations of emulsified oil, with many containing additional cathartic agents as phenolphthalein, milk of magnesia, agar, and others.

Castor Oil Emulsion

This emulsion is utilized as a laxative, for isolated bouts of constipation, and in preparation of the colon for x-ray and endoscopic examination. The castor oil present in the emulsion works directly on the small intestine to promote bowel movement. This, and other laxatives, should not be used regularly or excessively as they can lead to dependence for bowel movement. Castor oil may cause excessive loss of water and body electrolytes if used excessively which can have a debilitating effect. Laxatives should not be used when nausea, vomiting, or abdominal pain is present since these symptoms may indicate appendicitis, and use of a laxative in this instance could promote rupturing of the appendix.

The amount of castor oil in commercial castor oil emulsions varies from about 35 to 67%. The amount of oil present influences the dose of the emulsion required. Generally, for an emulsion containing about two-thirds oil, the adult dose would be 45 mL, about 3 tablespoonfuls. For children 2 to 6 years of age, 15 mL is usually sufficient and for children less than 2 years of age, 5 mL may be given. Castor oil is best taken on an empty stomach, followed with one full glass of water.

Simethicone Emulsion

Simethicone emulsion is a water-dispersible form of simethicone used as a defoaming agent for the relief of painful symptoms of excess gas in the gastrointestinal tract. Simethicone emulsion works in the stomach and intestines by changing the surface tension of gas bubbles enabling them to coalesce; thus, freeing the gas for easier elimination. The emulsion, in drop form, is useful for the relief of gas in infants due to colic, air swallowing, or lactose intolerance. The commercial product [Mylicon Drops (Johnson & Johnson Merck)] contains 40 mg of simethicone per 0.6 mL. Simethicone is also present in a number of antacid formulations [e.g., Mylanta (Johnson & Johnson Merck)] as a therapeutic adjunct to relieve the discomfort of gas.

Gels and Magmas

Gels are defined as semisolid systems consisting of dispersions made up of either small inorganic particles or large organic molecules enclosing and interpenetrated by a liquid.

Gels are also defined as semirigid systems in which the movement of the dispersing medium is restricted by an interlacing three-dimensional network of particles or solvated macromolecules of the dispersed phase. A high degree of physical or chemical cross-linking may be involved. The increased viscosity caused by the interlacing and consequential internal friction is responsible for the semisolid state. A gel may consist of twisted matted strands often wound together by stronger types of van der Waals forces to form crystalline and amorphous regions throughout the system., *e.g.* tragacanth and carboxymethylcellulose.

Some gel systems are as clear as water in appearance and others are turbid, since the ingredients involved may not be completely molecularly dispersed (soluble or insoluble) or they may form aggregates, which disperse light. The concentration of the gelling agents is mostly less than 10%, usually in 0.5 to 2.0% range, with some exceptions.

Gels in which the macromolecules are distributed throughout the liquid in such a manner that no apparent boundaries exist between them and the liquid are called *single-phase gels*. In instances in which the gel mass consists of floccules of small distinct particles, the gel is classified as a two-phase system and frequently called a *magma* or a *milk*. Gels and magmas are considered colloidal dispersions since they each contain particles of colloidal dimension.

Colloidal Dispersions

Many of the various types of colloidal dispersions have been given appropriate names. For instance, *sol* is a general term to designate a dispersion of a solid substance in either a liquid, a solid, or a gaseous dispersion medium. However, more often than not it is used to describe the solid-liquid dispersion system. To be more descriptive, a prefix such as *hydro-* for water (*hydrosol*) or *alco-* for alcohol (*alcosol*) may be employed to indicate the dispersion medium. The term *aerosol* has similarly been developed to indicate a dispersion of a solid or a liquid in a gaseous phase.

Although there is no precise point at which the size of a particle in a dispersion can be considered to be "colloidal," there is a generally accepted size range. A substance is said to be colloidal when its particles fall between 1 nm and 0.5 μm. Colloidal particles are usually larger than atoms, ions, or molecules and generally consist of aggregates of many molecules, although in certain proteins and organic polymers single, large molecules may be of colloidal dimension and form colloidal dispersions. One difference between colloidal dispersions and true solutions is the larger particle size of the disperse phase of the former type of preparation. Another difference is the optical properties of the two systems. True solutions do not scatter light and therefore appear clear, but colloidal dispersions contain opaque particles that do scatter light and thus appear turbid. This turbidity is easily seen, even with dilute preparations, when the dispersion is observed at right angles to a beam of light passed through the dispersion (Tyndall effect). Although reference is made here to dilute colloidal dispersions, most pharmaceutical preparations contain high concentrations of particles within the colloidal size range, and in these instances there is no difficulty in observing turbidity. In fact, certain preparations may be opaque, depending on the concentration of the disperse phase. Also, the particle size of the disperse phase in some pharmaceutical preparations may not be uniform, and a preparation may contain particles within and outside of the colloidal range, giving the preparation more of an opaque appearance than if all particles were uniformly colloidal.

Particle size is not the only important criterion for establishing the colloidal state. The nature of the dispersing phase with respect to the disperse phase is also of great importance. The attraction or lack of attraction between the disperse phase and the dispersion medium affects the ease of preparation of a colloidal dispersion as well as the character of the dispersion. Certain terminology has been developed to characterize the various degrees of attraction between the phases of a colloidal dispersion. If the disperse phase interacts appreciably with the dispersion medium, it is referred to as being *lyophilic*, meaning "solvent-loving." If the degree of attraction is small, the colloid is termed *lyophobic* or "solvent-hating." These terms are more suitably used when reference is made to the specific dispersion medium, for a single substance may be lyophobic with respect to one dispersion medium and lyophilic with respect to another. For instance, starch is lyophilic in water but lyophobic in alcohol. Terms such as *hydrophilic* and *hydrophobic*, which are more descriptive of the nature of the colloidal property, have therefore been developed to refer to the attraction or lack of attraction of the substance specifically to water. Generally speaking, because of the attraction to the solvent of lyophilic substances in contrast to the lack of attraction of lyophobic substances, lyophilic colloidal systems are usually easier to prepare and have the greater stability. A third type of colloidal sol, termed as *association* or *amphiphilic colloid*, is formed by the grouping or association of molecules that exhibit both lyophilic and lyophobic properties.

Lyophilic colloids are large organic molecules capable of being solvated or associated with the molecules of the dispersing phase. These substances disperse readily upon addition to the dispersion medium to form colloidal dispersions. As more molecules of the substance are added to the sol, the viscosity is characteristically increased and when the concentration of molecules is sufficiently high,

the liquid sol may become a semisolid or solid dispersion, termed a *gel*. Gels owe their rigidity to an intertwining network of the disperse phase which entraps and holds the dispersion medium. A change in the temperature can cause certain gels to resume the sol or liquid state. Also, some gels may become fluid after agitation only to resume their solid or semisolid state after remaining undisturbed for a period of time, a phenomenon known as *thixotrophy.*

Lyophobic colloids are generally composed of inorganic particles. When these are added to the dispersing phase, there is little if any interaction between the two phases. Unlike lyophilic colloids, lyophobic materials do not spontaneously disperse but must be encouraged to do so by special, individualized procedures. Their addition to the dispersion medium does not greatly affect the viscosity of the vehicle. Amphiphilic colloids form dispersions in both aqueous and nonaqueous media. Depending upon their individual character and the nature of the dispersion medium, they may or may not become greatly solvated. However, they generally cause an increase in the viscosity of the dispersion medium with an increase in concentration.

For the most part, the colloidal sols and gels used in pharmacy are aqueous preparations. The various preparations composed of colloidal dispersions are prepared, not according to any general method but according to the means best suited to the individual preparation. Some substances such as acacia are termed *natural colloids* because they are self-dispersing upon addition to the dispersing medium. Other materials that require special means for prompt dispersion are termed *artificial colloids.* They may require fine pulverization of coarse particles to colloidal size by a colloid mill or a micropulverizer, or colloidal size particles may be formed by chemical reaction under highly controlled conditions.

Terminology Related to Gels

A number of terms are commonly used in discussing some of the characteristics of gels, including imbibition, swelling, syneresis, thixotropy and xerogel. *Imbibition* is the taking up of a certain amount of liquid without a measurable increase in volume. *Swelling* is the taking up of a liquid by a gel with an increase in volume. Only those liquids that solvate a gel can cause swelling. The swelling of protein gels is influenced by pH and the presence of electrolytes. *Syneresis* is when the interaction between particles of the dispersed phase becomes so great that on standing, the dispersing medium is squeezed out in droplets and the gel shrinks. Syneresis is a form of instability in aqueous and nonaqueous gels. Separation of a solvent phase is thought to occur because of the elastic contraction of the polymeric molecules; in the swelling process during gel formation the macromolecules involved become stretched and the elastic forces increase as swelling proceeds. At equilibrium the restoring force of the macromolecules is balanced by the swelling forces, determined by the osmotic pressure. If the osmotic pressure decreases, *e.g.* on cooling, water may be squeezed out of the gel. The syneresis of an acidic gel from *Plantago albicans* seed gum may be decreased by the addition of electrolyte, glucose and sucrose, and by increasing the gum concentration. pH has a marked effect on the separation of water. At low pH marked syneresis occurs, possibly due to suppression of ionization of the carboxylic acid groups, loss of hydrating water, and the formation of intramolecular hydrogen bonds. This would reduce the attraction of the solvent for the macromolecule. *Thixotropy* is a reversible gel-sol formation with no change in volume or temperature-a type of non-Newtonian flow. A *xerogel* is formed when the liquid is removed from a gel and only the framework remains. Examples would include gelatin sheets, tragacanth ribbons and acacia tears.

Classification and Types of Gels

Table 13.4 is a general classification of gels, listing two classification schemes. The first scheme divides gels into "inorganic" and "organic." *Inorganic hydrogels* are usually two-phase systems such as Aluminum Hydroxide Gel and Bentonite Magma. Bentonite has also been used as an ointment base in about 10–25% concentrations. *Organic gels* are usually single-phase systems and may include such gelling agents as carbomer and tragacanth and those that contain an organic liquid, such as *Plastibase.*

The second classification scheme divides gels into hydrogels and organogels with some additional subcategories. *Hydrogels* include ingredients that are dispersible as colloidals or soluble in water and include organic hydrogels, natural and synthetic gums and inorganic hydrogels. Examples include hydrophilic colloids such as silica, bentonite, tragacanth, pectin, sodium alginate, methylcellulose, sodium carboxymethylcellulose and alumina, which in high concentration, form semisolid gels. Sodium alginate has been used to produce gels that can be employed as ointment bases. In concentrations greater than 2.5% and in the presence of soluble calcium salts, a firm gel, stable between pH 5 and 10, is formed. Methylcellulose, hydroxyethylcelluose and sodium carboxymethylcellulose are among the commercially available cellulose products that may be used in ointments. They are available in various viscosity types, usually high, medium and low. *Organogels* include the hydrocarbons, animal/vegetable fats, soap base greases and the hydrophilic organogels. Included in the hydrocarbon type is *Jelene,* or *Plastibase* a combination of mineral oils and heavy hydrocarbon waxes with a molecular weight of about 1300. Petrolatum is a semisolid gel consisting of a liquid component together with a "protosubstance"and a crystalline waxy fraction. The

Table 13.4. General Classification and Description of Gels

Class	Description	Examples
Inorganic	Usually are two-phase systems	Aluminum Hydroxide Gel Bentonite Magma
Organic	Usually are single-phase systems.	Carbopol Tragacanth
Hydrogels	Contain Water	Silica, bentonite, pectin, sodium alginate, methylcellulose, alumina
Organogels	Hydrocarbon type	Petrolatum, Mineral Oil/Polyethylene gel (Plastibase)
	Animal/Vegetable fats	Lard, Cocoa butter
	Soap base greases	Aluminum stearate with heavy mineral oil gel
	Hydrophilic Organogels Polar Nonionic	Carbowax bases (PEG Ointment)
Hydrogels	Organic Hydrogels Natural and synthetic gums Inorganic Hydrogels	Pectin paste, Tragacanth jelly Methylcellulose, sodium carboxymethylcellulose, Pluronic Bentonite gel (10–25%), Veegum

crystalline fraction provides rigidity to the structure, while the protosubstance or gel former stabilizes the system and thickens the gel. The hydrophilic organogels, or polar organogels include the polyethylene glycols of high molecular weight, the *Carbowaxes*. They are soluble to about 75% in water and are completely washable. The gels look and feel like petrolatum. They are nonionic and stable. *Jellies* are a class of gels in which the structural coherent matrix contains a high proportion of liquid, usually water. They usually are formed by adding a thickening agent such as tragacanth or carboxymethyl cellulose to an aqueous solution of a drug substance. The resultant product is usually clear and of a uniform semisolid consistency. Jellies are subject to bacterial contamination and growth and thus most are preserved with antimicrobials. Jellies should be stored with tight closures since water may evaporate, drying out the product.

Some substances, such as acacia, are termed natural colloids because they are self-dispersing in a dispersing medium. Other materials that require special treatment for prompt dispersion are called artificial colloids. The special treatment may involve fine pulverization to colloidal size with a colloid mill or a micropulverizer.

Preparation of Magmas and Gels

Some magmas and gels (inorganic) are prepared by freshly precipitating the disperse phase in order to achieve a fine degree of subdivision of the particles and a gelatinous character to those particles. The desired gelatinous precipitate results when solutions of inorganic agents react to form an insoluble chemical having a high attraction for water. As the microcrystalline particles of the precipitate develop, they strongly attract water to yield gelatinous particles, which combine to form the desired gelatinous precipitate. Other magmas and gels may be prepared by the direct hydration in water of the inorganic chemical, the hydrated form constituting the disperse phase of the dispersion. In addition to the water vehicle, other agents as propylene glycol, propylgallate and hydroxypropylcellulose may be used to enhance gel formation.

Because of the high degree of attraction between the disperse phase and the aqueous medium in both magmas and gels, these preparations remain fairly uniform on standing with little settling of the disperse phase. However, on long standing a supernatant layer of the dispersion medium develops, but the uniformity of the preparation is easily reestablished by moderate shaking. To ensure uniform dosage, magmas and gels should be shaken before use, and a statement to that effect must be included on the label of such preparations. The medicinal magmas and gels are used orally for the value of the disperse phase.

Examples of Gelling Agents

Examples of gelling agents include acacia, alginic acid, bentonite, carbomer, carboxymethylcellulose sodium, cetostearyl alcohol, colloidal silicon dioxide, ethylcellulose, gelatin, guar gum, hydroxyethylcellulose, hydroxypropyl cellulose, hydroxypropyl methylcellulose, magnesium aluminum silicate, maltodextrin, methylcellulose, polyvinyl alcohol, povidone, propylene carbonate, propylene glycol alginate, sodium alginate, sodium starch glycolate, starch, tragacanth and xanthan gum. A few of the more common ones will be discussed here.

Alginic acid is obtained from seaweed throughout the world and the prepared product is a tasteless, practically odorless, white to yellowish-white colored, fibrous powder. It is used in concentrations between 1 and 5% as a thickening agent in gels. It swells in water to about 200–300 times its own weight without dissolving. Crosslinking with increased viscosity occurs upon the addition of a calcium salt, such as calcium citrate. Alginic acid can be dispersed in water vigorously stirred for approximately 30 minutes. Premixing with another powder or with a water-miscible liquid aids in the dispersion process.

Bentonite is discussed later in the preparation of Bentonite Magma.

Carbomer (Carbopol) resins were first described in the literature in 1955 and are currently ingredients in a variety of pharmaceutical dosage systems, including controlled release tablets, oral suspensions and topical gels. Carbomer resins are high molecular weight, allylpentaerythritol-crosslinked, acrylic acid-based polymers, modified with C_{10}-C_{30} alkyl acrylates. They are fluffy, white, dry powders with large bulk densities. The pH of 0.5% and 1.0% aqueous dispersions are 2.7–3.5 and 2.5–3.0, respectively. There are many carbomer resins, with viscosity ranges from 0 to 80,000 cps. Carbomers 910, 934, 934P, 940 and 1342 are official in the USP 23/NF 18. Carbomer 910 is effective at very low concentrations when low viscosity is desired and is frequently used for producing stable suspensions. It is the least ion sensitive of these resins.

Carbomer 934 is highly effective in thick formulations such as viscous gels. Carbomer 934P is similar to 934 but is intended for oral and mucosal contact applications and is the most widely used in the pharmaceutical industry. In addition to thickening, suspending and emulsifying in both oral and topical formulations, the 934 polymer is also used to provide sustained-release properties in both the stomach and intestinal tract for commercial products. Carbomer 940 forms sparkling clear water or hydroalcoholic gels. It is the most efficient of all the Carbopol resins and has very good non-drip properties.

The addition of alcohol to prepared carbomer gels may decrease their viscosity and clarity. To overcome the loss of viscosity, an increase in the concentration of carbomer may be required. Also, gel viscosity is dependent upon the presence of electrolytes and the pH. Generally, a maximum of 3% electrolytes can be added before a rubbery mass forms. Overneutralization also will result in decreased viscosity that cannot be reversed by the addition of acid. Maximum viscosity and clarity occur at pH 7, but acceptable viscosity and clarity begins at pH 4.5 to 5.0 and extends to a pH of 11.

Preparation of aqueous dispersions of carbomer resins: Carbomer preparations are primarily used in aqueous systems, although other liquids can be used. In water, a single particle of carbomer will wet very rapidly but, like many other powders, carbomer polymers tend to form clumps of particles when haphazardly dispersed in polar solvents. As the surfaces of these clumps solvate, a layer is formed which prevents rapid wetting of the interior of the clumps. When this occurs, the slow diffusion of solvent through this solvated layer determines the mixing or hydration time. To achieve fastest dispersion of the carbomer, it is wise to take advantage of the very small particle size of the carbomer powder by adding it very slowly into the vortex of the liquid that is very rapidly stirred. Almost any device, like a simple sieve, that can sprinkle the powder on the rapidly stirred liquid is useful. The goal is to prevent clumping by slowly sprinkling the very small particle size powder over the rapidly agitated water.

A neutralizer is added to thicken the gel after the carbomer is dispersed. Sodium hydroxide or potassium hydroxide can be used in carbomer dispersions containing less than 20% alcohol. Triethanolamine will neutralize carbomer resins containing up to 50% ethanol. Other neutralizer agents include sodium carbonate, ammonia, and borax.

Carboxymethylcellulose in concentrations of 4 to 6% of the medium viscosity grades can be used to produce gels; glycerin may be added to prevent drying. Precipitation can occur at pH values less than 2, it is most stable at pH levels between 2 and 10, with maximum stability at pH 7 to 9. It is incompatible with ethanol.

Carboxymethylcellulose Sodium. Sodium carboxymethylcellulose is soluble in water at all temperatures. The sodium salt of CMC can be dispersed with high shear in cold water before the particles can hydrate and swell to sticky gel grains agglomerating into lumps. Once the powder is well dispersed, the solution is heated with moderate shear to about 60°C for fastest dissolution. These dispersions are sensitive to pH changes because of the carboxylate group. The viscosity of the product is decreased markedly below pH 5 or above pH 10.

Colloidal silicon dioxide can be used to prepare transparent gels when used with other ingredients of similar refractive index. Colloidal silicon dioxide adsorbs large quantities of water without liquefying. The viscosity is largely independent of temperature. Changes in pH may affect the viscosity: it is most effective at pH values up to about 7.5. Colloidal silicon dioxide (fumed silica) will form a gel when combined with 1-dodecanol and n-dodecane. These are prepared by adding the silica to the vehicle and sonicating for about one minute to obtain a uniform dispersion, sealing and storing at about 40°C overnight to complete gelation. This gel is more hydrophobic in nature than the others.

Gelatin. Gels are prepared from gelatin by dispersing the gelatin in hot water followed by cooling. As an alternative, moisten the gelatin with about 3 to 5 parts of an organic liquid that will not swell the polymer, such as ethyl alcohol or propylene glycol followed by the addition of the hot water and cooling.

Magnesium aluminum silicate, Veegum, in concentrations of about 10% form firm, thixotropic gels. The material is inert and has few incompatibilities but is best used above pH 3.5. It may bind to some drugs and limit their availability.

Methylcellulose is a long-chain substituted cellulose that can be used to form gels in concentrations up to about 5%. Since methylcellulose hydrates slowly in hot water, the powder is dispersed with high shear in about 1/3 of the required amount of water at 80–90° C. Once the powder is finely dispersed, the rest of the water is added cold or as ice with moderate stirring to cause prompt dissolution. Anhydrous alcohol or propylene glycol may be used to help prewet the powders. Maximum clarity, fullest hydration and highest viscosity will be obtained if the gel is cooled to 0–10°C for about an hour. A preservative should be added. A 2% solution of methylcellulose 4000 has a gel point about 50° C. High concentrations of electrolytes will salt out the macromolecules and increase their viscosity, ultimately precipitating the polymer.

Plastibase/Jelene is a 5% low-molecular-weight polyethylene/95% mineral oil mixture. The polymer is soluble in mineral oil above 90°C, close to its melting point. When cooled below 90°C, the polymer precipitates and causes gelation. The mineral oil is immobilized in the network of entangled and adhering insoluble polyethylene chains which probably even associate into small crystalline regions. This gel can be heated to about 60°C without substantial loss of consistency.

Poloxamer, or *Pluronic,* gels are made from selected forms of polyoxyethylene-polyoxypropylene copolymers in concentrations ranging from 15 to 50%. Poloxamers generally are white, waxy, free-flowing granules that are practically odorless and tasteless. Aqueous solutions of poloxamers are stable in the presence of acids, alkalis and metal ions. Commonly used poloxomers include the 124 (L-44 grade), 188 (F-68 grade), 237 (F-87 grade), 338 (F-108 grade) and 407 (F-127 grade) types, which are freely soluble in water. The "F" designation refers to the flake form of the product. The trade name "Pluronic" is used in the US by BASF Corp for pharmaceutical and industrial grade poloxamers. Pluronic F-127 has good solubilizing capacity and optical properties, low toxicity and is a good medium for topical drug delivery systems.

Polyvinyl alcohol (PVA) is used at concentrations of about 2.5% in the preparation of various jellies which dry rapidly when applied to the skin. Borax is a good agent that will gel PVA solutions. For best results, disperse PVA in cold water, followed by hot water. It is less soluble in the cold water.

Povidone, in the higher molecular weight forms, can be used to prepare gels in concentrations up to about 10%. It has the advantage of being compatible in solution with a wide range of inorganic salts, natural and synthetic resins and other chemicals. It has also been used to increase the solubility of a number of poorly soluble drugs.

Sodium alginate can be used to produce gels in concentrations up to 10%. Aqueous preparations are most stable between pH values of 4–10; below pH 3, alginic acid is precipitated. Sodium alginate gels for external use should be preserved, for example, with 0.1% chloroxylenol or the parabens. If the preparation is acidic, benzoic acid may be used. High concentrations will result in increased viscosity up to a point where the sodium alginate is salted out; occuring at about 4% with sodium chloride.

Tragacanth gum has been used to prepare gels that are most stable at pH 4–8. These gels must be preserved with either 0.1% benzoic acid or sodium benzoate or a combination of 0.17% methylparaben and 0.03% propylparaben. These gels may be sterilized by autoclaving. Since powdered tragacanth gum tends to form lumps when added to water, aqueous dispersions are prepared by adding the powder to vigorously stirred water. Also, the use of ethanol, glycerin or propylene glycol to pre-wet the tragancanth is very effective. If other powders are to be incorporated into the gel, they can be premixed with the tragacanth in the dry state.

Gel Formulation Considerations

In gel preparation, the powdered polymers, when added to water, may form temporary gels that slow the process of dissolution. As water diffuses into these loose clumps of powder, their exteriors frequently turn into clumps of solvated partcles encasing dry powder. The blobs of gel dissolve very slowly because of their high viscosity and low diffusion coefficient of the macromolecules.

As a hot, colloidal dispersion of gelatin cools, the gelatin macromolecules lose kinetic energy. With reduced kinetic energy, or thermal agitation, the gelatin macromolecules are associated through dipole-dipole interaction into elongated or thread-like aggregates. The size of these association chains increases to the extent that the dispersing medium is held in the interstices among the interlacing network of gelatin macromolecules, and the viscosity increases to that of a semisolid. Gums, such as agar, Irish moss, algin, pectin and tragacanth form gels by the same mechanism as gelatin.

Polymer solutions tend to cast gels because the solute consists of long, flexible chains of molecular thickness that tend to become entangled, attract each other by secondary valency forces, and even crystallize. Crosslinking of dissolved polymer molecules also causes these solutions to gel. The reactions produce permanent gels, held together by primary valence forces. Secondary valence forces are responsible for reversible gel formation. For example, gelatin will form a gel when lowered to about 30°C, the gel melting point, but aqueous methylcellulose solutions will gel when heated above about 50° C because the polymer is less soluble in hot water and precipitates. Lower temperatures, higher concentrations and higher molecular weights promote gelation and produce stronger gels. The reversible gelation of gelatin will occur at about 25°C for 10% solutions, 30°C for 20% solutions and about 32° C for 30% solutions. Gelation is rarely observed for gelatin above 34°C and, regardless of concentration, gelatin solutions do not gel at 37°C. The gelation temperature or gel point of gelatin is highest at the isoelectric point. Water soluble polymers have the property of thermal gelation, *i.e.,* they gel on heating, whereas natural gums gel on cooling. The thermal gelation is reversed on cooling.

Inorganic salts will compete with the water present in a gel and cause gelation to occur at lower concentrations. This is usually a reversible process and, upon the addition of water, the gels will reform. Alcohol may cause precipitation or gelation because alcohol is a nonsolvent or precipitant, lowering the dielectric constant of the medium and tending to dehydrate the hydrophilic solute. Alcohol lowers the concentrations at which electrolytes salt out hydrophilic colloids. Phase separation by adding alcohol may cause coacervation.

Aqueous polymer solutions, especially of cellulose derivatives, are stored for approximately 48 hours after dissolution to promote full hydration, maximum viscosity and clarity. If salts are to be added, they are done at this point rather than dissolving in water prior to adding polymer; otherwise the solutions may not reach their full viscosity and clarity.

Examples of Magmas and Gels

One official magma, Bentonite Magma, NF, is used as a suspending agent and finds application in the extemporaneous compounding of prescriptions calling for the suspension of medicinal agents. Sodium Fluoride and Phosphoric Acid Gel, USP, is applied topically to the teeth as a dental care prophylactic. Other official gels applied topically include Fluocinonide Gel, USP, an antiinflammatory corticosteroid, and Tretinoin Gel, USP, an irritant which stimulates epidermal cell turnover and causes peeling and is effective in the treatment of acne. Examples of such drugs and drug products are: erythromycin and benzoyl peroxide topical gel [(Benzamycin Topical Gel (Dermik Laboratories)]; clindamycin topical gel [Cleocin T Topical Gel (Pharmacia & Upjohn)], and benzoyl peroxide gel [Desquam-X 10 Gel (Westwood-Squibb)] used in the control and treatment of acne vulgaris; hydroquinone gel [Solaquin Forte Gel (ICN)], a bleach for hyperpigmented skin; salicylic acid gel [Compound W gel (Whitehall)], a keratolytic; and desoximetasone gel (Topicort Gel (Hoechst Marion Roussel)], an anti-inflammatory and antipruritic agent.

Other official magmas and gels are employed as antacids, namely: Aluminum Phosphate Gel, USP, Aluminum Hydroxide Gel, USP; Dihydroxya-luminum Aminoacetate Magma, USP, and Milk of Magnesia (Magnesia Magma), USP. Some of these preparations are discussed briefly below.

Bentonite Magma, NF

Bentonite magma is a preparation of 5% bentonite, a native, colloidal hydrated aluminum silicate, in purified water. It may be prepared mechanically in a blender with the bentonite added directly to the purified water while the machine is running, or it may be prepared by sprinkling the bentonite, in portions, upon hot purified water, allowing each portion to become thoroughly wetted without stirring before another portion is added. By the latter method, the mixture must be allowed to stand for 24 hours before it may be stirred. The standing period ensures the complete hydration and swelling of the bentonite. Bentonite, which is insoluble in water, swells to approximately twelve times its volume upon addition to water. The NF monograph for bentonite contains a test for "swelling power," in which 2 g of a bentonite sample is added in portions to 100 mL of water contained in a 100-mL glass-stoppered cylinder. At the end of a 2-hour period, the mass at the bottom of the cylinder is required to occupy an apparent volume of not less than 24 mL. Other required tests are for gel formation, fineness of powder, and pH, the latter being between 9.5 and 10.5. After bentonite magma has been allowed to stand undisturbed for some period of time, it sets to a gel. Upon agitation the sol form returns. The process may be repeated indefinitely. As mentioned earlier, this phenomenon is termed *thixotropy,* and bentonite magma is termed a *thixotropic gel.* The thixotropy occurs only when the bentonite concentration is somewhat above 4%.

Bentonite magma is employed as a suspending agent. Its alkaline pH must be considered, because this might be undesirable for certain drugs. Further, because the suspending capacity of the magma is drastically reduced if the pH is lowered to about pH 7, another suspending agent should be selected for drugs requiring a less alkaline medium rather than make bentonite magma more acidic.

Aluminum Hydroxide Gel, USP

Aluminum Hydroxide Gel, USP, is an aqueous suspension of a gelatinous precipitate composed of insoluble aluminum hydroxide and the hydrated aluminum oxide, equivalent to about 4% of aluminum oxide. The disperse phase of the gel is generally prepared by chemical reaction, using various reactants. Usually the aluminum source of the reaction is aluminum chloride or aluminum alum, which yields the insoluble aluminum oxide and aluminum hydroxide precipitate. To the gel, the USP permits the addition of peppermint oil, glycerin, sorbitol, sucrose, saccharin, or other flavorants and sweeteners as well as suitable antimicrobial agents.

This antacid preparation is a white, viscous suspension. It is effective in neutralizing a portion of the gastric hydrochloric acid and by virtue of its gelatinous, viscous, and insoluble character, coats the inflamed and perhaps ulcerated gastric surface and is useful in the treatment of hyperacidity and peptic ulcers. The main disadvantage to its use is its constipating effects. The usual dose is 10 mL, four or more times a day. Ten mL of the analogous commercial product (Amphojel, Wyeth-Ayerst) has the capacity to neutralize about 13 mEq of acid. The preparation should be stored in tight containers, and freezing should be avoided.

Because it possesses a trivalent cation, aluminum hydroxide has the capability to interfere with the bioavailability of tetracycline by chelating with the antibiotic in the gastrointestinal tract. Thus, when these two medicines are indicated for patient use, the doses of each should be staggered to ensure the patient receives the benefit of both drugs. Aluminum hydroxide gel has also been implicated at decreasing the bioavailability of other drugs as well by adsorption onto the gel. This is usually illustrated by a decrease in the area under the concentration time curve (AUC) for the concomitantly administered drug. Suffice to say that the clinical significance of the interaction might not be that great, but observation of the patient to insure the proper therapeutic outcome from the other drug is important. Thus, for example, if aluminum hydroxide gel is suspected of causing incomplete absorption of the second drug, then an upward alteration in the dose of the drug might be necessary provided the aluminum hydroxide gel administration remains the same.

Milk of Magnesia, USP

Milk of Magnesia, USP, is a preparation containing between 7 and 8.5% of magnesium hydroxide. Although there is no method of preparation indicated in the USP for this preparation, it may be prepared by a reaction between sodium hydroxide and magnesium sulfate (1), diluted solutions being used to ensure a fine, flocculent, gelatinous precipitate of magnesium hydroxide. The precipitate so produced is washed with purified water to remove the sodium

sulfate prior to its incorporation with additional purified water to prepare the required volume of product. Commercially, the product is more economically produced by the direct hydration of magnesium oxide.

1) $2NaOH + MgSO_4 \rightarrow Mg(OH)_2 + Na_2SO_4$
2) $MgO + H_2O \rightarrow Mg(OH)_2$

Irrespective of its method of preparation, milk of magnesia is a white, opaque, viscous preparation from which varying proportions of water separate on standing. For this reason it should be shaken before use. The preparation has a pH of about 10, which may bring about a reaction between the magma and the glass container imparting a bitter taste to the preparation. To minimize such an occurrence, 0.1% citric acid may be added to the preparation. Also, flavoring oils at a concentration not exceeding 0.05% may be added to enhance the palatability of the preparation.

Milk of Magnesia possesses reasonable acid-neutralizing ability and a dose of 5 mL will neutralize about 10 mEq of stomach acid. However, to neutralize more acid a higher dose, e.g., 15 mL is usually necessary, and this may predispose the patient to the development of diarrhea, a common side effect of this drug. Thus, to circumvent the problem of diarrhea from magnesium hydroxide and the constipating effects of aluminum hydroxide, frequently these two drugs are combined in an antacid preparation. The combination results in a more palatable product with optimum buffering of stomach contents between a pH of 4 to 5, and less of a chance for either diarrhea or constipation to occur. When a laxative effect is desired a bedtime dose of 30 to 60 mL of milk of magnesia will suffice very nicely by the next morning.

The preparation is best stored in tight containers preferably at a temperature above freezing and below 35°C. Freezing results in a coarsening of the disperse phase, and temperatures above 35°C decrease the gel structure.

Starch Glycerite

Starch	100 g
Benzoic Acid	2 g
Purified Water	200 g
Glycerin	700 g

The starch and benzoic acid are rubbed in the water to a smooth mixture. The glycerin is added and mixed. The mixture is heated to 140°C with constant, gentle agitation until a translucent mass forms. The heat ruptures the starch grains and permits the water to reach and hydrate the linear and branched starch molecules which trap the dispersion medium in the interstices to form a gel. Starch glycerinte has been used as a topical vehicle and protectant.

Lubricating Jelly Formula

Methylcellulose, 4000 cps	0.8%
Carbopol 934	0.24%
Propylene glycol	16.7%
Methylparaben	0.015%
Sodium hydroxide, qs ad	pH 7
Purified water, qs ad	100%

Disperse the methylcellulose in 40 mL of hot (80–90° C) water. Chill overnight in a refrigerator to effect solution. Disperse the Carbopol 934 in 20 mL water. Adjust the pH of the dispersion to 7.0 by adding sufficient 1% sodium hydroxide solution (about 12 mL is required) and bring the volume to 40 mL with purified water. Dissolve the methylparaben in the propylene glycol. Mix the methylcellulose, Carbopol 934 and propylene glycol fractions using caution to avoid incorporating air. Lubricating jellies are used to assist in medical procedures, to aid in insertion of various devices and drugs, including catheters and suppositories, and as vehicles for some drug products, especially in extemporaneous compounding.

Clear Aqueous Gel with Dimethicone

Water	59.8%
Carbomer 934	0.5%
Triethanolamine	1.2
Glycerin	34.2
Propylene Glycol	2.0
Dimethicone copolyol	2.3

Prepare the carbomer gel, add the other ingredients and mix well. Dimethicone copolyol is included to reduce the sticky feel associated with glycerin. These gels are commonly used as vehicles for drug products, especially for those that are extemporaneously compounded.

Poloxamer Gel Base

Pluronic F-127, NF	20 g–50 g
Purified Water/Buffer qs	100 mL

Poloxamer gel base is widely used as a vehicle for extemporaneously compounded products. In a combination with isopropyl palmitate and lecithin, it is an absorption enhancing topical vehicle.

Proper Administration and Use of Disperse Systems

The majority of dosage forms discussed thus far in this chapter are for oral use. As the oral solutions discussed in the the previous chapter, they can be measured by spoon, i.e., teaspoon, tablespoon, or administered dropwise depending upon the appropriate dosage. It is very important that the patient understand the proper quantity of product to use. For example, differences in dosage can occur between product category, e.g., OTC antidiarrheal suspensions [tablespoonfuls] *vs* OTC antacid suspensions [teaspoonfuls]. Differences in dosage can also occur within a category, most notably antacid suspensions. Some are recommended in teaspoon doses because of higher concentration whereas others are suggested in tablespoon quantities. It is important, therefore, that the pharmacist ensure that the patient knows how much to use, and then use a calibrated device to make sure the right amount is taken.

Reconstituted products, as mentioned earlier in the chapter frequently are suspensions. Several potential problems can emerge if the pharmacist is not careful to counsel the patient about them. Usually the patient or the guardian of the patient receives the product in an oversized bottle that allows for the proper shaking of the product prior to its use. To allay fears that all of the medicine may not be in the bottle, the pharmacist must make the patient or the guardian aware of this, and indicate this feature enhances the shakability before its administration. Further, some patients do not make the connection that the medicine should be administered by mouth. Oral antibiotic suspensions intended to treat a middle ear infection have been mistakenly administered directly into the ear by some patients or guardians. Thus, the pharmacist should review with the patient the proper administration. Lastly, because these are reconstituted with purified water stability problems with the drug usually dictate it be stored in the refrigerator until it is consumed. The patient has to be informed of this. Tiny labels on the container directing one to store the product in the refrigerator are sometimes overlooked by the consumer. Alternatively, not all suspensions need to be stored in the refrigerator, but because of prior experience with other liquid suspensions that necessitated refrigeration, a patient or guardian may assume this is necessary.

Certain suspensions by virtue of their active ingredients, e.g., aluminum hydroxide gel, cholestyramine, kaolin, have the ability to interfere with the absorption of other drugs that might be concurrently administered. For example, cholestyramine has been shown to interfere with and decrease the bioavailability of such drugs as warfarin, digitoxin and thyroid hormones. The pharmacist should be aware of this and make recommendations to help avoid this drug interaction whenever possible. The typical suggestion would be to stagger the administration of the liquid cholestyramine away from other drug administration by several hours, and in the case of warfarin, giving warfarin at least 6 hours after the cholestyramine reportedly avoids the impaired warfarin bioavailability (8). However, warfarin is a drug that undergoes enterohepatic recycling in the body, and if cholestyramine were present in the intestine because of earlier administration, it could bind it and decrease warfarin's subsequent reabsorption. In this instance, concomitant use of one of the two drugs should be discontinued by the physician. However, if concurrent use is necessary, the pharmacist should monitor the patient more frequently for the possibility of an altered anticoagulant response. This is important because if adjustments in warfarin dosage were made on the basis of cholestyramine interference and then the cholestyramine was discontinued, the warfarin dosage also would have to be decreased accordingly, i.e., based on the patient's prothrombin time.

Aerosols

Pharmaceutical aerosols are pressurized dosage forms containing one or more active ingredients which upon actuation emit a fine dispersion of liquid and/or solid materials in a gaseous medium. See Physical Pharmacy Capsule 13.5, Partial Pressure and Aerosol Formulation. Pharmaceutical aerosols are similar to other dosage forms in that they require the same types of considerations with respect to formulation, product stability, and therapeutic efficacy. However, they differ from most other dosage forms in their dependence upon the function of the container, its valve assembly, and an added component—the propellant—for the physical delivery of the medication in proper form.

The term *pressurized package* is commonly used when referring to the aerosol container or completed product. Pressure is applied to the aerosol system through the use of one or more liquefied or gaseous propellants. Upon activation of the valve assembly of the aerosol, it is the pressure exerted by the propellant which forces the contents of the package out through the opening of the valve. The physical form in which the contents are emitted is dependent upon the formulation of the product

and the type of valve employed. Aerosol products may be designed to expel their contents as a fine mist, a coarse, wet or a dry spray, a steady stream, or as a stable or a fast-breaking foam. The physical form selected for a given aerosol is based on the intended use of that product. For instance, an aerosol intended for inhalation therapy, as in the treatment of asthma or emphysema, must present particles in the form of a fine liquid mist or as finely divided solid particles if the product is to be efficacious. Particles less than 6 μm will reach the respiratory bronchioles, and those less than 2 microns will reach the alveolar ducts and alveoli (see Fig. 13.11). In contrast, the particle size for a dermatologic spray intended for deposition on the skin would be more coarse and generally less critical to the therapeutic efficacy of the product. Some dermatologic aerosols present the medication in the form of a powder, a wet spray, a stream of liquid (usually a local anesthetic), or an ointment-like product. Other pharmaceutical aerosols include vaginal and rectal foams.

Aerosols used to provide an airborne mist are termed *space sprays*. Room disinfectants, room deodorizers, and space insecticides characterize this group of aerosols. The particle size of the released product is generally quite small, usually below 50 μm, and must be carefully controlled so that the dispersed droplets or particles remain airborne for a prolonged period of time. A one-second burst from a typical aerosol space spray will produce 120 million particles, a substantial number of which will remain suspended in the air for an hour.

Aerosols intended to carry the active ingredient to a surface are termed *surface sprays* or *surface coatings*. The dermatologic aerosols can be placed in this group. Also included are a great many non-pharmaceutical aerosol products, as personal de-

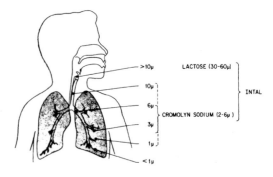

Fig. 13.11 *Relationship of INTAL (cromolyn sodium, Fisons) particle size to airway penetration. (Courtesy of Fisons Corporation.)*

Physical Pharmacy Capsule 13.5   **Partial Pressure and Aerosol Formulation**

Aerosols generally contain an active drug in a liquified gas propellant, in a mixture of solvents with a propellant, or in a mixture with other additives and a propellant. The gas propellants can be formulated to provide desired vapor pressures for enhancing the delivery of the medication through the valve and actuator, in accordance to the purpose of the medication. Aerosols are used as space sprays, surface sprays, aerated foams, and for oral inhalation.

Various propellants have properties including molecular weight, boiling point, vapor pressure, liquid density, and flash point that can be of importance. An example of a calculation to determine the vapor pressure of a certain mixture of hydrocarbon propellants follows.

EXAMPLE 1
What is the vapor pressure of a 60:40 mixture of propane and isobutane. Information on the two propellants is as follows:

Property	Propane	Isobutane
Molecular formula	C_3H_8	C_4H_{10}
Molecular weight	44.1	58.1
Boiling point (°F)	−43.7	10.9
Vapor pressure (psig @ 70°F)	110	30.4
Liquid density (g/mL @ 70°F)	0.50	0.56
Flash point (°F)	−156	−117

1. Assume an ideal solution.
2. For Raoult's Law, we need to determine the number of moles of each propellant:

$$n_{propane} = 60/44.1 = 1.36$$
$$n_{isobutane} = 40/58.1 = 0.69$$

3. From Raoult's Law, the partial pressure exerted by the propane is:

$$P_{propane} = [(n_{propane})/(n_{propane} + n_{isobutane})] \, P_{propane}$$
$$P_{propane} = [(1.36)/(1.36 + 0.69)] \, 110 = 72.98 \text{ psi}$$

4. The partial pressure exerted by the isobutane is:

$$P_{isobutane} = [(0.69)/(1.36 + 0.69)]30.4 = 10.23 \text{ psi}$$

5. The vapor pressure exerted by both gases, P_T, is:

$$P_T = 72.98 + 10.23 = 83.21 \text{ psi at } 70°F$$

The vapor pressure required for a specific application can be calculated in a similar manner and different ratios of propellants may be used to obtain that pressure.

odorant sprays, cosmetic hair lacquers and sprays, perfume and cologne sprays, shaving lathers, toothpaste, surface pesticide sprays, paint sprays, and various household products such as spray starch, waxes, polishes, cleaners, and lubricants. A number of veterinary and pet products have been put into aerosol form as have been such food products as dessert toppings and food spreads. Some of these products are sprays; others, foams; and a few, paste-like products.

Advantages of the Aerosol Dosage Form

Some features of pharmaceutical aerosols that may be considered advantages over other types of dosage forms are as follows:

1. A portion of medication may be easily withdrawn from the package without contamination or exposure to the remaining material.

2. By virtue of its hermetic character, the aerosol container protects medicinal agents adversely affected by atmospheric oxygen and moisture. Being opaque, the usual aerosol container also protects drugs adversely affected by light. This protection persists during the use and the shelf-life of the product. If the product is packaged under sterile conditions, sterility may also be maintained during the shelf-life of the product.

3. Topical medication may be applied in a uniform, thin layer to the skin, without touching the affected area. This method of application may reduce the irritation that sometimes accompanies the mechanical (fingertip) application of topical preparations. The rapid volatilization of the propellant also provides a cooling, refreshing effect.

4. By proper formulation and valve control, the physical form and the particle size of the emitted product may be controlled which may contribute to the efficacy of a drug; e.g., the fine controlled mist of an inhalant aerosol. Through the use of *metered valves,* dosage may be controlled.

5. Aerosol application is a "clean" process, requiring little or no "wash-up" by the user.

The Aerosol Principle

An aerosol formulation consists of two component parts, the *product concentrate* and the *propellant.* The product concentrate is the active ingredient of the aerosol combined with the required adjuncts, such as antioxidants, surface-active agents, and solvents, to prepare a stable and efficacious product. When the propellant is a liquefied gas or a mixture of liquefied gases, it frequently serves the dual role of propellant and solvent or vehicle for the product concentrate. In certain aerosol systems, nonliquefied compressed gases, as carbon dioxide, nitrogen, and nitrous oxide, are employed as the propellant.

For many years, the liquefied gas propellants most used in aerosol products were the chlorofluorocarbons (CFCs). However these propellants are being phased out and will be prohibited for nonessential use under federal regulations due to scientific recognition that they reduce the amount of ozone in the stratosphere, which results in an increase in the amount of ultraviolet radiation reaching the earth, an increase in the incidence of skin cancer, and other adverse environmental effects. Under the law, the FDA has the authority to exempt from the prohibition specific products under the agency's jurisdiction when there is sufficient evidence showing that: 1) there are no technically feasible alternatives to the use of a chlorofluorocarbon propellant in the product; 2) the product provides a substantial health or other public benefit unobtainable without the use of the chlorofluorocarbon; and 3) the use does not involve a significant release of chlorofluorocarbons into the atmosphere or, if it does, the release is warranted by the benefit conveyed. A number of metered-dose pharmaceutical products for oral inhalation have received such essential-use exemptions. Among the chlorofluorocarbons used as propellants in pharmaceuticals were dichlorodifluoromethane, dichlorotetrafluoroethane, and trichloromonofluoromethane (see Table 13.5).

Fluorinated hydrocarbons are gases at room temperature. They may be liquefied by cooling below their boiling point or by compressing the gas at room temperature. For example, dichlorodifluoromethane (Freon 12) gas will form a liquid when cooled to $-22°F$ or when compressed to 70 psig (pounds per square inch gauge) at 70°F. Both of these methods for liquefying gases are employed in aerosol packaging as will be discussed later in this section.

When a liquefied gas propellant or propellant mixture is sealed within an aerosol container with the product concentrate, an equilibrium is quickly established between that portion of propellant which remains liquefied and that which vaporizes and occupies the upper portion of the aerosol container (Fig. 13.12). The vapor phase exerts pressure in all directions—against the walls of the container, the valve assembly, and the surface of the liquid phase, which is composed of the liquefied gas and the product concentrate. It is this pressure which upon actuation of the aerosol valve forces the liquid phase up the dip tube and out of the orifice of the valve into the atmosphere. As the propellant meets the air, it immediately evaporates due to the drop in pressure, leaving the product concentrate as airborne liquid droplets or dry particles, depending upon the formulation. As the liquid phase is removed from the container, equilibrium between the propellant remaining liquefied and that in the vapor state is reestablished. Thus even during expulsion of the product from the aerosol package, the pressure within remains virtually constant, and the product may be continuously released at an even rate and with the same propulsion. However, when the liquid reservoir is depleted, the pressure may not be maintained, and the gas may be expelled from the container with diminishing pressure until it is exhausted.

Table 13.5. Physical Properties of Some Fluorinated Hydrocarbon Propellants

Chemical Name	Chemical Formula	Numerical Designation	Vapor Pressure (psia[b] 70°F)	Boiling Point (1 ATM) °F	Liquid Density (g/mL) 70°F
Trichloromonofluoromethane	CCl_3F	11	13.4	74.7	1.485
Dichlorodifluoromethane	CCl_2F_2	12	13.4	74.1	1.485
Dichlorotetrafluoroethane	$CClF_2CClF_2$	114	21.6	38.4	1.468
Chloropentafluoroethane	$CClF_2CF_3$	115	17.5	−37.7	1.29
Monochlorodifluoroethane	CH_3CClF_2	142[b]	43.8	15.1	1.119
Difluoroethane	CH_3CHF_2	152[a]	76.4	−11.2	0.911
Octafluorocyclobutane	$CF_2CF_2CF_2CFM_2$ 12	C318	40.1	21.1	1.513

[a]The numerical designations for fluorinated hydrocarbon propellants have been designed within the refrigeration industry to simplify communications when referring to these agents. The numerical designations are arrived at by the following method: (1) the digit at the extreme right refers to the number of fluorine atoms in the molecule; (2) the second digit from the right represents one *greater* than the number of hydrogen atoms in the molecule; (3) the third digit from the right is one *less* than the number of carbon atoms in the molecule; if this number is zero, it is omitted and a two-digit number is used; (4) a capital letter "C" is used before a number to indicate the cyclic nature of a compound; (5) the small letters following a number are used to indicate decreasing symmetry of isomeric compounds, with the "b" indicating less symmetry than the "a," and so forth. The number of chlorine atoms in a molecule may be determined by subtracting the total number of hydrogen and fluorine atoms from the total number of atoms which may be added to the carbon chain.

[b]psia is pounds per square inch absolute, which is equal to psig + 14.7.

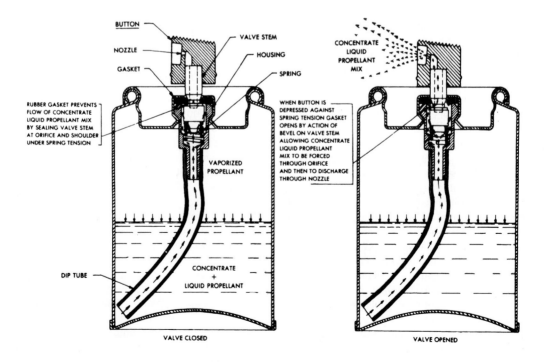

Fig. 13.12 *Cross section sketches of contents and operation of a typical two-phase aerosol system. (Courtesy of Armstrong Laboratories, Inc., Division of Aerosol Techniques, Inc.)*

Aerosol Systems

The pressure of an aerosol is critical to its performance. It can be controlled by 1) the type and amount of propellant and 2) the nature and amount of material comprising the product concentrate. Thus, each formulation is unique unto itself, and a specific amount of propellant to be employed in aerosol products cannot be firmly stated. However, some general statements may be made within the context of this discussion. Space sprays generally contain a greater proportion of propellant than do aerosols intended for surface coating, and thus they are released with greater pressure, and the resultant particles are projected more violently from the valve. Space aerosols usually operate at pressures between 30 and 40 psig at 70°F and may contain as much as 85% propellant. Surface aerosols commonly contain 30 to 70% propellant with pressures between 25 and 55 psig at 70°F. Foam aerosols usually operate between 35 and 55 psig at 70°F and may contain only 6 to 10% propellant.

Foam aerosols may be considered to be emulsions, in that the liquefied propellant is partially emulsified with the product concentrate rather than being dissolved in it. Because the fluorinated hydrocarbons are nonpolar organic solvents having no affinity for water, the liquefied propellant does not dissolve in the aqueous formulation. The utilization of surfactants or emulsifiers in the formulation encourages the mixing of the two components to enhance the emulsion. Shaking of the package prior to use further mixes the propellant throughout the product concentrate. When the aerosol valve is activated, the mixture is expelled to the atmosphere where the propellant globules vaporize rapidly, leaving the active ingredient in the form of a foam.

Blends of the various liquefied gas propellants are generally used in pharmaceutical aerosols to achieve the desired vapor pressure and to provide the proper solvent features for a given product. Some propellants are eliminated from use in certain products because of their reactivity with other formulative materials, or with the proposed container or valve components. For instance, trichloromonofluoromethane tends to form free hydrochloric acid when formulated with systems containing water or ethyl alcohol, the latter a commonly used cosolvent in aerosol systems. The free hydrochloric acid not only affects the efficacy of the product, but also exerts a corrosive action on some container components.

The physiologic effect of the propellant must also be considered in formulating an aerosol to assure safety of the product in its intended use. Even though an individual propellant or propellant blend and the active ingredient of a formulation are nontoxic when tested individually, the use of the combination in aerosol form may have undesirable features. For instance, when an active ingredient ordinarily used in a nasal or oral spray is placed in a fine aerosol mist, it may reach deeper into the respiratory tract than desired and may result in irritation. In other instances, as with new dermatologic, vaginal, and rectal aerosol products, the influence of the aerosol form of the drug on the recipient tissue membranes must be evaluated for irritating effects and changes in the absorption of the drug from the site of application. The absorption pattern of a drug may change due to an increased rate of solubility of the fine particles usually produced in aerosol products.

Although the fluorinated hydrocarbons have a relatively low order of toxicity and are generally nonirritating, certain individuals, who may be sensitive to the propellant agent and who utilize an inhalation aerosol, may exhibit cardiotoxic effects following rapid and repeated use of the aerosol product (9).

Two-phase Systems

As noted previously, the two-phase aerosol system is comprised of the liquid phase, containing the liquefied propellant and product concentrate, and the vapor phase.

Three-phase Systems

This system is comprised of a layer of water-immiscible liquid propellant, a layer of highly aqueous product concentrate, and the vapor phase. Because the liquefied propellant usually has a greater density than the aqueous layer, it generally resides at the bottom of the container with the aqueous phase floating above it. As with the two-phase system, upon activation of the valve, the pressure of the vapor phase causes the liquid phase to rise in the dip tube and be expelled from the container. To avoid expulsion of the reservoir of liquefied propellant, the dip tube must extend only within the aqueous phase (product concentrate) and not down into the layer of liquefied propellant. The aqueous product is broken up into a spray by the mechanical action of the valve. If the container is shaken immediately prior to use, some liquefied propellant may be mixed with the aqueous phase and be expelled through the valve to facilitate the dispersion of the exited product or the production of foam, depending upon the formulation. The vapor phase within the container is replenished from the liquid propellant phase.

Compressed Gas Systems

Compressed rather than liquefied, gases may be used to prepare aerosols. The pressure of the compressed gas contained in the headspace of the aerosol container forces the product concentrate up the dip tube and out of the valve. The use of gases that are insoluble in the product concentrate, as is nitrogen, will result in the emission of a product in essentially the same form as it was placed in the container. An advantage of nitrogen as a propellant is its inert behavior toward other formulative components and its protective influence on products subject to oxidation. Further, nitrogen is an odorless and tasteless gas and thus does not contribute adversely to the smell or taste of a product.

Other gases, such as carbon dioxide and nitrous oxide, which are slightly soluble in the liquid phase of aerosol products, may be employed in instances in which their expulsion with the product concentrate is desired to achieve spraying or foaming.

Unlike aerosols prepared with liquefied gas propellants, there is no reservoir of propellant in compressed gas filled aerosols. Thus higher gas pressures are required in these systems, and the pressure in these aerosols progressively diminishes as the product is used.

Aerosol Container and Valve Assembly

The effectiveness of a pharmaceutical aerosol depends on achieving the proper combination of formulation, container, and valve assembly. The formulation must not chemically interact with the container or valve components so as to interfere with the stability of the formulation or with the integrity and operation of the container and valve assembly. The container and valve must be capable of withstanding the pressure required by the product, it must be corrosive-resistant, and the valve must contribute to the form of the product to be emitted.

Containers

Various materials have been used in the manufacture of aerosol containers, including 1) glass, uncoated or plastic coated; 2) metal, including tin-plated steel, aluminum, and stainless steel; and 3) plastics. The selection of the container for an aerosol product is based on its adaptability to production

methods, compatibility with formulation components, ability to sustain the pressure intended for the product, the interest in design and aesthetic appeal on the part of the manufacturer, and cost.

Were it not for their brittleness and danger of breakage, glass containers would be preferred for most aerosols. Glass presents fewer problems with respect to chemical compatibility with the formula than do metal containers and is not subject to corrosion. Glass is also more adaptive to creativity in design. On the negative side, glass containers must be precisely engineered to provide the maximum in pressure safety and impact resistance. Plastic coatings are commonly applied to the outer surface of glass containers to render them more resistant to accidental breakage, and in the event of breaking, the plastic coating prevents the scattering of glass fragments. When the total pressure of an aerosol system is below 25 psig and no more than 50% propellant is used, glass containers are considered quite safe. When required, the inner surface of glass containers may be coated to render them more chemically resistant to formulation materials.

At the present time, tin-plated steel containers are the most widely used metal containers for aerosols. Because the starting material used is in the form of sheets, the completed aerosol cylinders are seamed and soldered to provide a sealed unit. When required, special protective coatings are employed within the container to prevent corrosion and interaction between the container and formulation. The containers must be carefully examined prior to filling to ensure that there are no flaws in the seam or in the protective coating that would render the container weak or subject to corrosion.

Most aluminum containers are manufactured by extrusion or by other methods that make them seamless. They have the advantage over the seam type of container in that there is greater safety against leakage, incompatibility, and corrosion. Stainless steel is employed to produce containers for certain small volume aerosols in which a great deal of chemical resistance is required. The main limitation of stainless steel containers is their high cost.

Plastic containers have met with varying success in the packaging of aerosols due to their inherent problem of being permeated by the vapor within the container. Also, certain drug-plastic interactions can occur which affect the release of drug from the container and reduce the efficacy of the product.

Valve Assembly

The function of the valve assembly is to permit the expulsion of the contents of the can in the desired form, at the desired rate, and, in the case of metered valves, in the proper amount or dose. The materials used in the manufacture of valves must be inert toward the formulations and must be approved by the Food and Drug Administration. Among the materials used in the manufacture of the various valve parts are plastic, rubber, aluminum, and stainless steel.

The usual aerosol valve assembly is composed of the following parts (Fig. 13.13):

1. *Actuator*—The actuator is the button which the user presses to activate the valve assembly for the emission of the product. The actuator permits the easy opening and closing of the valve. It is through the orifice in the actuator that the product is discharged. The design of the inner chamber and size of the emission orifice of the actuator contribute to the physical form (mist, coarse spray, solid stream, or foam) in which the product is discharged. The combination of the type and quantity of propellant used, and the actuator design and dimensions control the particle size of the emitted product. Larger orifices (and less propellant) are used for products to be emitted as foams and solid streams than for those intended to be sprays or mists.
2. *Stem*—The stem supports the actuator and delivers the formulation in the proper form to the chamber of the actuator.

3. *Gasket*—The gasket, placed snugly with the stem, serves to prevent leakage of the formulation when the valve is in the closed position.
4. *Spring*—The spring holds the gasket in place and also is the mechanism by which the actuator retracts when pressure is released, thereby returning the valve to the closed position.
5. *Mounting cup*—The mounting cup, which is attached to the aerosol can or container, serves to hold the valve in place. Because the underside of the mounting cup is exposed to the formulation, it must receive the same consideration as the inner part of the container, with respect to meeting criteria of compatibility. If necessary, it may be coated with an inert material (as an epoxy resin or vinyl) to prevent an undesired interaction.
6. *Housing*—The housing, located directly below the mounting cup, serves as the link between the dip tube and the stem and actuator. With the stem, its orifice helps to determine the delivery rate and the form in which the product is emitted.
7. *Dip tube*—The dip tube, which extends from the housing down into the product, serves to bring the formulation from the container to the valve. The viscosity of the product and its intended delivery rate dictate to a large extent the inner dimensions of the dip tube and housing for a particular product.

The actuator, stem, housing, and dip tube are generally made of plastic, the mounting cup and spring of metal, and the gasket of rubber or plastic predetermined to be resistant to the formulation.

Metered Dose Inhalers (MDIs)

Metering valves are employed when the formulation is a potent medication, as in inhalation therapy (Fig. 13.14). In these metered valve systems, the amount of material discharged is regulated by an auxiliary valve chamber by virtue of its capacity or dimensions. A single depression of the actuator causes the evacuation of this chamber and the delivery of its contents. The integrity of the chamber is controlled by a dual valving mechanism. When the actuator valve is in the closed position, a seal is effected between the chamber and the atmosphere. However, in this position the chamber is permitted to fill with the contents of the container to which it is open. Depression of the actuator causes a simultaneous reversal of positions sealed; the chamber becomes open to the atmosphere, releasing its con-

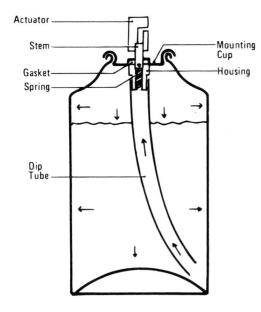

Fig. 13.13   *Sketch showing valve assembly components.*

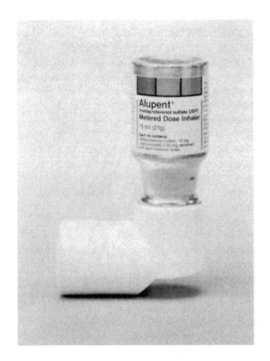

Fig. 13.14 *Example of metered dose inhaler. Each metered dose is delivered through the mouthpiece upon actuation of the aerosol unit's valve. (Courtesy of Boehringer Ingelheim.)*

tents, and at the same time becomes sealed from the contents of the container. Upon release of the actuator, the system is restored for the next dose. The USP contains a test to determine quantitatively the amount of medication from a metered valve.

As noted previously, the effectiveness in delivering medication to the lower reaches of the lungs for local or systemic effects depends in part on the particle size of the inhaled drug. Breathing patterns and the depth of respiration also play important roles in the deposition of inhaled aerosols into the lungs. Analysis of dose uniformity (10) particle size distribution patterns (11–13), and the "respirable" fractions of aerosol-delivered particles (14–15), are areas of current research interest in developing aerosol products for optimal oral inhalation therapy.

A unique translingual aerosol formulation of nitroglycerin has been developed (Nitrolingual Spray, (Rhône-Poulenc Rorer) that permits a patient to spray droplets of nitroglycerin onto or under the tongue for acute relief of an attack, or for prophylaxis, of angina pectoris due to coronary artery disease. The product is not to be inhaled. At the onset of an attack, two metered spray emissions, each containing 0.4 mg of nitroglycerin, are admin-

istered. The product contains 200 doses of nitroglycerin in a propellant mixture of dichlorodifluoromethane and dichlorotetrafluoroethane.

Filling Operations

As explained earlier, fluorinated hydrocarbon gases may be liquefied by cooling below their boiling points or by compressing the gas at room temperature. These two features are utilized in the filling of aerosol containers with propellant.

Cold Filling

In the cold method, both the product concentrate and the propellant must be cooled to temperatures of $-30°$ to $-40°F$. This temperature is necessary to liquefy the propellant gas. The cooling system may be a mixture of dry ice and acetone or a more elaborate refrigeration system. After the chilled product concentrate has been quantitatively metered into an equally cold aerosol container, the liquefied gas is added. The heavy vapors of the cold liquid propellant generally displace the air present in the container. However, in the process, some of the propellant vapors are also lost. When sufficient propellant has been added, the valve assembly is immediately inserted and crimped into place. Because of the low temperatures required, aqueous systems cannot be filled by this process, since the water turns to ice. For nonaqueous systems, some moisture usually appears in the final product due to the condensation of atmospheric moisture within the cold containers.

Pressure Filling

By the pressure method, the product concentrate is quantitatively placed in the aerosol container (Fig. 13.15), the valve assembly is inserted and crimped into place, and the liquefied gas, under pressure, is metered into the valve stem from a pressure burette (Fig. 13.16). The desired amount of propellant is allowed to enter the container under its own vapor pressure. When the pressure in the container equals that in the burette, the propellant stops flowing. Additional propellant may be added by increasing the pressure in the filling apparatus through the use of compressed air or nitrogen gas. The trapped air in the package may be ignored if it does not interfere with the quality or stability of the product, or it may be evacuated prior to filling or during filling, using special apparatus. After filling the container with sufficient propellant, the valve

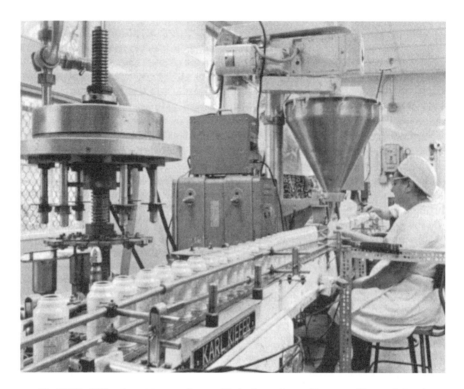

Fig. 13.15   *Filling the empty aerosol cans with the drug mixture. (Courtesy of Pennwalt Corp.)*

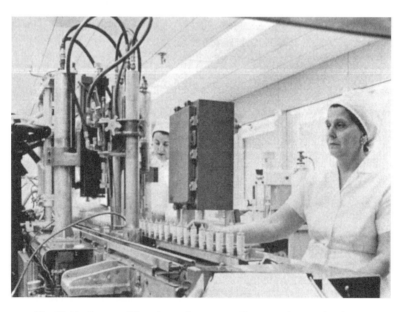

Fig. 13.16   *Pressure filling of aerosol containers. (Courtesy of Pennwalt Corp.)*

actuator is tested for proper function. This spray testing also rids the dip tube of pure propellant prior to consumer use.

Pressure filling is used for most pharmaceutical aerosols. It has the advantage over the cold filling method in that there is less danger of moisture contamination of the product, and also less propellant is lost in the process.

When compressed gases are employed as the propellant in aerosol systems, the gas is transferred from large steel cylinders into the aerosol containers. Prior to filling, the product concentrate is quantitatively placed in the container, the valve assembly is crimped into place, and the air is evacuated from the container by a vacuum pump. The compressed gas is then passed into the container through a pressure reducing valve attached to the gas cylinder; when the pressure within the aerosol container is equal to the predetermined and regulated delivery pressure, the gas flow stops, and the aerosol valve is restored to the closed position. For gases like carbon dioxide and nitrous oxide, which are slightly soluble in the product concentrate, the container is manually or mechanically shaken during the filling operation to achieve the desired pressure in the headspace of the aerosol container.

Testing the Filled Containers

After filling by either the cold method or the pressure method, the aerosol container is tested under various environmental conditions for leaks or weakness in the valve assembly or container.

Filled aerosol containers are also tested for the proper function of the valve. The *valve discharge rate* is determined by discharging a portion of the contents of a previously weighed aerosol during a given period of time, and calculating, by the difference in weight, the grams of contents discharged per unit of time. As is deemed desirable, aerosols may be tested for their spray patterns, for particle size distribution of the spray, and for accuracy and reproducibility of dosage when using metered valves.

Packaging, Labeling, and Storage

A unique aspect of pharmaceutical aerosols compared to other dosage forms is that the product is actually packaged as part of the manufacturing process. With most other dosage forms, the product is completely manufactured and then placed in the appropriate container.

Most aerosol products have a protective cap or cover that fits snugly over the valve and mounting cup. This protects the valve against contamination with dust and dirt. The cap, which is generally made of plastic or metal, also serves a decorative function.

Medicinal aerosols that are to be dispensed only upon prescription usually may be labeled by the manufacturer with plastic peel-away labels or easily removed paper labels so that the pharmacist may easily replace the manufacturer's label with his label containing the directions for use specified by the prescribing practitioner. Most other types of aerosols have the manufacturer's label printed directly on the container or on firmly affixed paper.

In addition to the usual labeling requirements for pharmaceutical products, aerosols have special requirements related to their use and storage. For example, for safety, labels must warn users not to puncture pressurized containers, not to use or store them near heat or an open flame, and not to incinerate. Exposure to temperatures above 120°F may cause an aerosol container to burst. Most medications in aerosol containers are intended for use at ambient room temperatures. When the canisters are cold, less than the usual spray may result. This may be particularly important to users of metered dose inhalation sprays. These products are generally recommended for storage between 15°C and 30°C (36°F and 86°F). Pharmaceutical aerosols are labeled with regard to shaking before use, holding at the proper angle and/or distance from the target; there are special detailed instructions for inhaler devices.

Aerosols should be maintained with the protective caps in place to prevent accidental activation of the valve assembly or its contamination by dust and other foreign materials. Examples of pharmaceutical aerosols are shown in Figure 13.17 and presented in Table 13.6.

Proper Administration and Use of Pharmaceutical Aerosols

The pharmacist should make every attempt to educate the patient about aerosol dosage forms, particularly for oral or nasal administration, because these are only effective when properly used. To complement verbal instructions the pharmacist should provide the patient with the written instructions found within the product package. It is difficult to predict what percentage of patients will read or even understand the printed instruction.

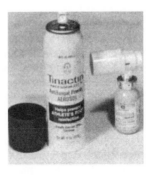

Fig. 13.17 *Examples of some pharmaceutical aerosols.*

Table 13.6.   Examples of Inhalation Aerosols

Aerosol	Some Representative Commercial Products	Category and Comments
Albuterol Inhalation Aerosol	Proventil Inhalation Aerosol (Schering) Ventolin Inhalation Aerosol (Glaxo Wellcome)	Beta-adrenergic agonist indicated for the prevention and relief of bronchospasm in patients with reversible obstructive airway disease and for the relief of exercise-induced bronchospasm.
Beclomethasone Dipropionate Inhalation Aerosol	Beclovent Inhalation Aerosol (Glaxo Wellcome) Vanceril Inhaler (Schering)	Adrenocortical steroid; aerosol for oral inhalation for control of bronchial asthma in patients requiring chronic treatment with corticosteroids with other therapy, e.g., xanthines, sympathomimetics.
	Beconase Nasal Inhaler (Alien & Hanburys) Vancenase Pockethaler Nasal Inhaler (Schering)	Adrenocortical steroid; aerosol for intranasal relief of symptoms of seasonal or perennial rhinitis in those cases poorly responsive to conventional treatment.
Cromolyn Sodium Inhalation Aerosol	Intal Inhaler (Rhône-Poulenc Rorer)	An antiasthmatic, antiallergic and mast cell stabilizer; metered-dose aerosol for oral administration for prevention of exercise-induced bronchospasm, and for prevention of acute bronchospasm induced by environmental pollutants and known allergens.
Ipratropium Bromide Inhalation Aerosol	Atrovent Inhalation Aerosol (Boehringer Ingelheim)	Anticholinergic (parasympatholytic) agent used as a bronchodilator in the treatment of bronchospasm.
Isoetharine Mesylate Inhalation Aerosol	Bronkometer (Sanofi)	Sympathomimetic for the temporary relief of bronchial asthma and other conditions of bronchospasm.
Metaproterenol Sulfate Inhalation Aerosol	Alupent Inhalation Aerosol (Boehringer Ingelheim)	Sympathomimetic for the relief of bronchospasm in patients with reversible obstructive airway disease.
Nedocromil Sodium Inhalation Aerosol	Tilade Inhaler (Rhone-Poulenc Rorer)	Maintenance therapy of patients with mild to moderate bronchial asthma.
Salmeterol Xinafoate Inhalation Aerosol	Serevent Inhalation Aerosol (Glaxo Wellcome)	Beta-adrenergic agonist used in the long-term maintenance treatment of asthma and prevention of bronchospasm in patients with reversible obstructive airway disease.
Terbutaline Sulfate Inhalation Aerosol	Brethaire (Novartis)	Beta-adrenergic agonist indicated for the relief of bronchospasm.
Triamcinolone Acetonide Oral Inhaler	Azmacort (Rhone-Poulenc Rorer)	Indicated in patients who require chronic treatment with corticosteroids for the control of symptoms of bronchial asthma.
Triamcinolone Acetonide Topical Aerosol	Kenalog Spray (Westwood-Squibb)	Anti-inflammatory; applied topically to the affected area.

Thus, the pharmacist must verbally transmit instruction for proper use. Using the oral, metered aerosols as a model, the pharmacist should demonstrate how the inhaler is assembled, stored and cleaned. The patient should be told whether the inhaler requires shaking before use and how to hold it between the index finger and thumb so that the aerosol canister is up side down. The patient should understand that coordination must be achieved between inhalation (after exhaling as completely as possible) and pressing down the inhaler to release one dose. The patient should be instructed to hold his breath for several seconds or as long as possible to gain the maximum benefit from the medication.

The patient is told to then remove the inhaler from the mouth and exhale slowly through pursed lips.

Some patients are unable to use metered-dose inhalers properly. Thus, after a new prescription is dispensed, it is advisable for the pharmacist to follow up with the patient to make sure the patient is capable of using the inhaler. If the patient confides an inability to use the inhaler, it is advisable for the pharmacist to recommend to the patient or the patient's physician the use of an extender device with the inhaler. Extender devices or "spacers" were originally developed for patients who could not learn to coordinate release of the medication with inhalation. These are now considered an important therapeutic aid because they can effectively assist the delivery of medication despite improper patient inhalation technique. By placing an extender device between the metered-dose inhaler's mouthpiece and the patient's mouth, the patient is permitted to separate activation of the aerosol from inhalation by up to 3 to 5 seconds (a valve in the spacer opens when the patient inhales). Another advantage of the extender device is that aerosol velocity is reduced, and droplet size is decreased because there is time for evaporation of the fluorohydrocarbon propellant. Thus, extender devices also cause less deposition of medication in the oropharynx. Extender devices are available that can be used with most pressurized canisters, e.g., Brethancer Inhaler (Geigy) and InspirEase (Schering).

To ensure continuity of therapy it is wise for the pharmacist to share with the patient ways to assess how much medication is left in the canister. This is important to ensure continuity of therapy, especially for those who suffer from respiratory illness and may need their medication on a moment's notice.

For topical administration of aerosol dosage forms, the patient should be told to first clean the affected area gently and to pat it dry. Holding the canister with the nozzle pointing toward the body area and about 6 to 8 inches away, the patient should press down the button to deliver enough medication to cover the area. The patient should allow the spray to dry and not cover the area with a bandage or dressing unless instructed to do so by the physician. The patient should avoid accidentally spraying the product into the eyes or mouth. If it is necessary to apply the product to a facial area, the patient should spray the product into the palm of the hand and apply it by this means.

As presented in Table 13.6, a number of drug substances are administered through pressure packaged *inhalation aerosols,* as the type shown in Figure 13.14. For the inhaled drug substance or solution to reach the bronchial tree, the inhaled particles must be just a few microns in size.

Topical Aerosols

Aerosol packages for topical use on the skin are convenient and include such drugs as some anti-infective agents: povidone-iodine, tolnaftate and thimerosal; the adrenocortical steroids: betamethasone dipropionate and valerate, dexamethasone, and triamcinolone acetonide; and the local anesthetic dibucaine hydrochloride.

The use of topical aerosols provides to the patient a means of applying the drug in a convenient

manner. The preparation may be applied to the desired surface area without the use of the fingertips, thus making the procedure less messy than with most other types of topical preparations. Among the disadvantages to the use of topical aerosols are the difficulty in applying the medication to a small area and the greater expense associated with the aerosol package.

Vaginal and Rectal Aerosols

Aerosol foams are commercially available containing estrogenic substances and contraceptive agents. The foams are used intravaginally in the same manner as that employed for creams. The aerosol package contains an inserter device which is filled with foam and the contents placed in the vagina through activation of the plunger. The foams are generally oil-in-water emulsions, resembling light creams. They are water-miscible and non-greasy.

Some available commercial preparations of rectal foams use rectal inserters for the presentation of the foam to the anal canal. One such product,

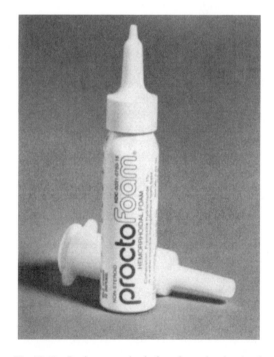

Fig. 13.18 *Product-example of a foam for anal and perianal use. To fill the applicator, the foam container is shaken vigorously, held upright, and the applicator tip placed on the container opening. With the plunger of the applicator drawn out all the way, pressure is exerted on the container cap and foam fills the applicator tube. (Courtesy of Reed & Carnrick.)*

ProctoFoam (Reed & Carnrick), contains pramoxine hydrochloride and is used to relieve inflammatory anorectal disorders (Fig. 13.18).

References

1. Heyd A, Dhabhar D. Particle shape effect on caking of coarse granulated antacid suspensions. Drug Cosmetic Industry 1979;125:42.
2. Oral Liquid Pharmaceuticals: Wilmington, DE: ICI Americas Inc., 1975.
3. Chang RK. Formulation approaches for sustained-release oral suspensions. Pharm Tech 1992;16:134–136.
4. Allen LV. Prednisone oral suspension. US Pharmacist 1989;14:84.
5. Allen LV. Ketoconazole oral suspension. US Pharmacist 1993;18:98.
6. Bhargava HN, Narurkar A, Lieb LM. Using microemulsions for drug delivery. Pharm Tech 1987;11:46.
7. Griffin WC. J Soc Cosmetics Chemists 1949;1:311; 1954;5:1.
8. Hansten PD, Horn JR. Drug Interactions. 6th Ed. Philadelphia: Lea & Febiger, 1989; 80.
9. Chiou WL. Aerosol propellants: Cardiac toxicity and long biological half-life. JAMA 1974;227:658.
10. Cyr TD, et al. Low first-spray drug content in albuterol metered-dose inhalers. Pharm Res 1991;8:658–660.
11. Miller NC, et al. Assessment of the twin impinger for size measurement of metered-dose inhaler sprays. Pharm Res 1992;9:1123–1127.
12. Ranucci JA, Chen FC. Phase Doppler anemometry: A technique for determining aerosol plume-particle size and velocity. Pharm Tech 1993;17:62–73.
13. Ranucci JA, Cooper D, Sethachutkul K. Effect of actuator design on metered-dose inhaler plume-particle size. Pharm Tech 1992;16:84–92.
14. Martonen TB, Katz IM. Deposition of aerosolized drugs within human lungs: Effects of ventilatory parameters. Pharm Res 1993;10:871–878.
15. Martonen TB, et al. Use of analytically defined estimates of aerosol respirable fraction to predict lung deposition patterns. Pharm Res 1992;9:1634–1639.

14

PARENTERALS

Chapter at a Glance

CONSIDERED IN this chapter are important pharmaceutical dosage forms that have the common characteristic of being prepared to be sterile; that is, free from contaminating microorganisms. Among these sterile dosage forms are the various small- and large-volume injectable preparations, irrigation fluids intended to bathe body wounds or surgical openings, and dialysis solutions. Biological preparations as vaccines, toxoids, and antitoxins are also among this group and discussed in Chapter 15. Sterility in these preparations is of utmost importance because they are placed in direct contact with the internal body fluids or tissues where infection can easily arise. Ophthalmic preparations, which are also prepared to be sterile, will be discussed separately in Chapter 16.

Injections

Injections are sterile, pyrogen-free preparations intended to be administered parenterally. The term *parenteral* refers to the injectable routes of administration. The term has its derivation from the Greek words *para* and *enteron*, meaning outside of the intestine, and denotes routes of administration other than the oral route. *Pyrogens* are fever-producing organic substances arising from microbial contamination and are responsible for many of the febrile reactions which occur in patients following intravenous injection. Pyrogens and the determination of their presence in parenteral preparations will be discussed later in this chapter. In general, the parenteral routes of administration are undertaken when rapid drug action is desired, as in emergency situations, when the patient is uncooperative, unconscious, or unable to accept or tolerate medication by the oral route, or when the drug itself is ineffective by other routes. With the exception of insulin injections, which are commonly *self*-administered by diabetic patients, most injections are administered by the physician, his/her assistant, or nurse in the course of medical treatment. Thus injections are employed mostly in the hospital, extended care facility, and clinic and less frequently in the home. An exception would be in *home health care* programs in which health professionals pay scheduled visits to patients in their homes, providing needed treatment, including intravenous medications. These programs enable patients who do not require or are unable to pay for more expensive hospitalization to remain in the familiar surroundings of their homes while receiving appropriate medical care. The pharmacist supplies injectable preparations to the physician and nurse, as required for their use in the institutional setting, clinic, office, or home health care program.

Perhaps the earliest injectable drug to receive official recognition was the hypodermic morphine solution, which appeared first in the 1874 addendum to the 1867 British Pharmacopeia, and later, in 1888 in the first edition of the National Formulary of the United States. Today, there are literally hundreds of drugs and drug products available for parenteral administration.

Parenteral Routes of Administration

Drugs may be injected into almost any organ or area of the body, including the joints *(intra-articular)*, a joint-fluid area *(intrasynovial)*, the spinal column *(intraspinal)*, into spinal fluid *(intrathecal)*, arteries *(intra-arterial)*, and in an emergency, even into the heart *(intracardiac)*. However, most commonly injections are performed into a vein *(intravenous, IV)*, into a muscle *(intramuscular, IM)*, into the skin *(Intradermal, ID, intracutaneous)*, or under the skin *(subcutaneous, SC, Sub-Q, SQ, hypodermic, Hypo)* (Fig. 14.1).

Intravenous Route

The intravenous injection of drugs had its scientific origin in 1656 in the experiments of Sir Christopher Wren, architect of St. Paul's Cathedral and amateur physiologist. Using a bladder and quill for a syringe and needle, he injected wine, ale, opium, and other substances into the veins of dogs and studied their effects. Intravenous medication was first given to humans by Johann Daniel Major of Kiel in 1662, but was abandoned for a period because of the occurrence of thrombosis and embolism in the patients so treated. The invention of the hypodermic syringe toward the middle of the 19th century created a new interest in intravenous techniques and toward the turn of the century, intravenous administration of solutions of sodium chloride and glucose became popular. Today, the intravenous administration of drugs is a routine occurrence in the hospital, although there are still recognized dangers associated with the practice. Thrombus and embolus formation may be induced by intravenous needles and catheters, and the possibility of particulate matter in parenteral solutions poses concern for those involved in the development, administration, and use of intravenous solutions.

Intravenously administered drugs provide rapid action compared with other routes of administration and because drug absorption is not a factor, optimum blood levels may be achieved with the accuracy and immediacy not possible by other routes. In emergency situations, the intravenous administration of a drug may be a life-saving procedure because of the placement of the drug directly into the circulation and the prompt action which ensues. On the negative side, once a drug is administered intravenously, it cannot be retrieved. In the case of an adverse reaction to the drug, for instance, the drug cannot be easily removed from the circulation as it could, for example, by the induction of vomiting after the oral administration of the same drug.

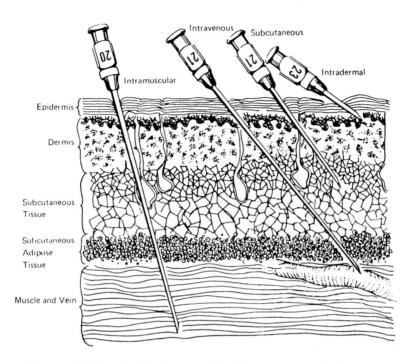

Fig. 14.1 *Routes of parenteral administration. Numbers on needles indicate size or gauge of needle based on outside diameter of needle shaft. (Reprinted with permission from Turco S, King RE. Sterile Dosage Forms: Their Preparation and Clinical Applications. 3rd Ed. Lea & Febiger, 1987.)*

Although most superficial veins are suitable for venipuncture, the veins of the antecubital area (situated in front of the elbow) are usually selected for direct intravenous injection. The veins in this location are large, superficial, and easy to see and enter. Most clinicians insert the needle with the bevel facing upward, at the most acute angle possible with the vein, to ensure that the direction of flow of the injectable is that of the flow of the blood. Strict aseptic precautions must be taken at all times to avoid risk of infection. Not only are the injectable solutions sterile, the syringes and needles used must also be sterilized and the point of entrance must be disinfected to reduce the chance of carrying bacteria from the skin into the blood via the needle. Before injection, administration personnel must withdraw the plunger of the syringe or squeeze a special bulb found on most IV sets to ensure that the needle has been properly located. In both instances, a "flashback" of blood into the administration set or the syringe indicates proper placement of the needle within the vein.

Both small and large volumes of drug solutions may be administered intravenously. The use of 1000-mL containers of solutions for intravenous infusion is commonplace in the hospital. These solutions containing such agents as nutrients, blood extenders, electrolytes, amino acids, and other therapeutic agents are administered through an indwelling needle or catheter by continuous infusion. The infusion or flow rates may be adjusted by the clinician according to the needs of the patient. Generally, flow rates for intravenous fluids are expressed in mL/hour, and range from 42 to 150 mL/hour. Lower rates are used for "keep open" lines. For intravenous infusion, the needle or catheter is placed in the prominent veins of the forearm or leg and taped firmly to the patient so that it will not slip from place during infusion. The main hazard of intravenous infusion is the possibility of thrombus formation induced by the touching of the wall of the vein by the catheter or needle. Thrombi are more likely to occur when the infusion solution is of an irritating nature to the biologic tissues. A *thrombus* is a blood clot formed within the blood vessel (or heart) due usually to a slowing of the circulation or to an alteration of the blood or vessel wall. Once such a clot circulates, it becomes an *embolus,* carried by the blood stream until it lodges in a blood vessel, obstructing it, and resulting in a blockage or occlusion referred to as an *embolism.* Such an obstruction may be a critical hazard to the patient, depending upon the site and severity of the obstruction.

Intravenously administered drugs ordinarily must be in aqueous solution; they must mix with the circulating blood and not precipitate from solution. Such an event could lead to pulmonary microcapillary occlusion and the subsequent blockage of blood passage. Intravenously delivered fat emulsions (e.g., Intralipid, 10%;20% [Clintec], Liposyn II, 10%;20% [Abbott], Liposyn III, 10%;20% [Abbott]) have gained acceptance for use as a source of calories and essential fatty acids for patients requiring parenteral nutrition for extended periods of time (usually for more than 5 days). The product contains up to 20% soybean oil emulsified with egg yolk phospholipids, in a vehicle of glycerin in water for injection. The emulsion is administered via a peripheral vein or by central venous infusion.

Naturally, the intravenous route is used in the administration of blood transfusions and it also serves as the point of exit in the removal of blood from patients for diagnostic work and for obtaining blood from donors.

In the late 1980s, automated intravenous delivery systems became commercially available for intermittent, self-administration of analgesics. Patient-controlled analgesia (PCA) has been used to control the pain associated with postoperative pain from a variety of surgical procedures, labor, sickle cell crisis, and chronic pain associated with cancer. For patients with chronic malignant pain, PCA allows a greater degree of ambulation and independence (1).

The typical PCA device includes a syringe or chamber that contains the analgesic drug and a programmable electomechanical unit. The unit, which might be compact enough to be worn on a belt or carried in a pocket (e.g., WalkMed™ PCA-Medex, Inc.), controls the delivery of drug by advancing a piston when the patient presses a button. The drug can be loaded into the device by a health care professional or dispensed from preloaded cartridges available through the manufacturer. The devices take advantage of intravenous bolus injections to produce rapid analgesia, along with slower infusion to produce steady-state opiate concentrations for sustained pain control.

The advantage of the PCA is its ability to provide constant and uniform analgesia. The typical intramuscular injection of an opioid into a depot muscular site may result in variable absorption, leading to unpredictable blood concentrations. Further, these injections are usually given when needed and are often inadequate to treat the pain. The PCA can prevent pharmacokinetic and pharmacodynamic differences between patients from interfering with the effectiveness of analgesia. Because opioid kinetics differ greatly among patients, the rates of infusion must be tailored (2).

The PCA also permits patients to medicate themselves when there is breakthrough pain. It eliminates the delay between the time of the patient's perception of pain and receiving the analgesic medication. Further, it saves nursing time. Otherwise, the nurse must check analgesic orders given by the physician, sign out the pain reliever from a controlled, locked location, and then administer the medication to the patient.

The PCA also provides better pain control with less side effects by minimizing the variations between suboptimal pain relief and overuse of narcotics. When the side effect profile of PCA patients is compared to patients maintained on IM narcotics, nausea, sedation, and respiratory depression occur less often in the PCA group. Lastly, patients accept the PCA as a favorable mode of relief, perhaps due to the sense of being in control and taking an active part in their pain relief.

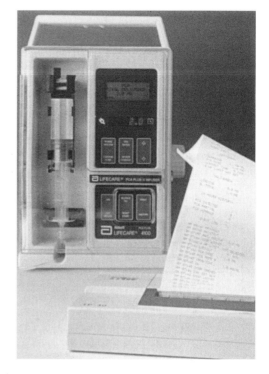

Fig. 14.2 *PCA Plus II (LifeCare 4100)-Patient-controlled analgesic infuser. (Courtesy of Abbott Hospital Products Division.)*

PCA devices can be used for intravenous, subcutaneous, or epidural administration. Usually, these devices are either *demand dosing* (i.e., a fixed dose of drug is injected intermittently) or *constant-rate infusion plus demand dosing* (2). Regardless of type utilized, the physician or nurse establishes the loading dose, the rate of background infusion, dose per demand, lockout interval (i.e., minimum time between demand doses), and maximum dosage over a specified time interval. Figure 14.2 demonstrates the PCA Plus II (Lifecare 4100) infuser. With this device, the patient pushes a button on a pendant to deliver a prescribed quantity of the analgesic.

Intramuscular Route

Intramuscular injections of drugs provide drug effects that are less rapid, but generally of greater duration than those obtained from intravenous administration (3). Aqueous or oleaginous solutions or suspensions of drug substances may be administered intramuscularly. Depending on the type of preparation employed, the absorption rates may vary widely. It would be expected that drugs in solution would be more rapidly absorbed than those in suspension and that drugs in aqueous preparations would be more rapidly absorbed than when in oleaginous preparations. The physical type of preparation employed is based on the properties of the drug itself and on the therapeutic goals desired.

Intramuscular injections are performed deep into the skeletal muscles. The point of injection should be as far as possible from major nerves and blood vessels. Injuries to patients from intramuscular injection usually are related to the point at which the needle entered and where the medication was deposited. Such injuries include paralysis resulting from neural damage, abscesses, cysts, embolism, hematoma, sloughing of the skin, and scar formation.

In adults, the upper outer quadrant of the gluteus maximus is the most frequently used site for intramuscular injection. In infants, the gluteal area is small and composed primarily of fat, not muscle. What muscle there is is poorly developed. An injection in this area might be presented dangerously close to the sciatic nerve, especially if the child is resisting the injection and squirming or fighting. Thus, in infants and young children, the deltoid muscles of the upper arm or the midlateral muscles of the thigh are preferred. An injection given in the upper or lower portion of the deltoid would be well away from the radial nerve. The deltoid may also be used in adults, but the pain is more noticeable here than in the gluteal area. If a series of injections are to be given, the injection site is usually varied. To be

certain that a blood vessel has not been entered, the clinician may aspirate slightly on the syringe following insertion of the needle to observe if blood enters the syringe. Usually, the volume of medication which may be conveniently administered by the intramuscular route is limited; generally a maximum of 5 mL is administered intramuscularly in the gluteal region and 2 mL in the deltoid of the arm.

The Z-Track Injection technique is useful for intramuscular injections of medications that stain upper tissue, e.g., iron dextran injection, or those that irritate tissue, e.g., Valium, by sealing these medications in the lower muscle. Because of its staining qualities, iron dextran injection, for example, must be injected only into the muscle mass of the upper outer quadrant of the buttock. The skin is displaced laterally prior to injection, then the needle is inserted and syringe aspirated, and the injection performed slowly and smoothly. The needle is then withdrawn and the skin released. This creates a "Z" pattern that blocks infiltration of medication into the subcutaneous tissue. The injection is 2 to 3 inches deep, and a 20 to 22 gauge needle is utilized. To further prevent any staining of upper tissue, usually one needle is used to withdraw the iron dextran from its ampul, and then replaced with another for the purposes of the injection.

Subcutaneous Route

The subcutaneous route may be utilized for the injection of small amounts of medication. The injection of a drug beneath the surface of the skin is usually made in the loose interstitial tissues of the outer surface of the upper arm, the anterior surface of the thigh, and the lower portion of the abdomen. The site of injection is usually rotated when injections are frequently given, e.g., daily insulin injections. Prior to injection, the skin at the injection site should be thoroughly cleansed. The maximum amount of medication that can be comfortably injected subcutaneously is about 1.3 mL and amounts greater than 2 mL will most likely cause painful pressure. Syringes with up to 3 mL capacities and utilizing needles with 24 to 26 gauges are used for subcutaneous injections. These needles will have cannula lengths that vary between 3/8 inch to 1 inch. Most typically, subcutaneous insulin needles are between 25 to 30 gauge with needle length between 5/16 to 5/8 inch. Upon insertion, if blood appears in the syringe, a new site should be selected.

Drugs that are irritating or those that are present in thick suspension form may produce induration, sloughing, or abscess formation and may be painful to the patient. Such preparations should be considered not suitable for subcutaneous injection.

Intradermal Route

A number of substances may be effectively injected into the corium, the more vascular layer of the skin just beneath the epidermis. These substances include various agents for diagnostic determinations, desensitization, or immunization. The usual site for intradermal injection is the anterior surface of the forearm. A short (3/8 in.) and narrow gauge (23- to 26-gauge) needle is usually employed. The needle is inserted horizontally into the skin with the bevel facing upward. The injection is made when the bevel just disappears into the corium. Usually only about 0.1 mL volumes may be administered in this manner.

Specialized Access

In those instances where it is necessary to administer repeated injections over a period of time, it might be more prudent to employ devices that provide continued access and help eliminate patient pain associated with administration. Thus, it is important to list a few at this juncture.

Several types of central venous catheters are used in institutions and on an outpatient basis. These are used for a variety of parenteral medications (e.g., cancer chemotherapy, long-term antibiotic therapy, total parenteral nutrition solutions), and their placement can remain for a few days to several months. When not in use, these require heparinization to maintain patency of the catheter lumen.

The use of plastic, indwelling catheters helps eliminate the need for multiple punctures during IV therapy. Composed of polyvinyl chloride, Teflon, and polyethylene, these should be radiopaque to ensure that they demonstrate visibility on x-ray films. Usually, these must be removed within 48 hours after insertion. The choice of catheter depends upon several factors (e.g., length of time of the infusion, purpose of the infusion, the condition/availability of the veins). Three types of catheters are available: plain plastic, catheter-over-needle or catheter-outside-needle, and catheter-inside-needle.

Implantable devices provide long-term venous access in various diseases. Broviac and Hickman catheters are notable examples. These do carry a risk of morbidity, including fracture of the catheters, entrance site infection, and catheter sepsis. These have been developed to overcome catheter complications and are designed to provide repeated access to the infusion site. The delivery catheter can be placed in a vein, cavity, artery, or CNS system. A Huber point needle allows system access through the skin into a self-sealing silicone plug positioned in the center of the portal.

Official Types of Injections

According to the USP, injections are separated into five general types, all of which are suitable for, and intended for, parenteral administration. These may contain buffers, preservatives, and other added substances.

1. [Drug] *Injection*—Liquid preparations that are drug substances or solutions thereof. (Ex: Insulin Injection, USP)
2. [Drug] *for Injection*—Dry solids that, upon the addition of suitable vehicles, yield solutions conforming in all respects to the requirements for Injections. (Ex: Cefamandole Sodium for Injection)
3. [Drug] *Injectable Emulsion*—Liquid preparations of drug substances dissolved or dispersed in a suitable emulsion medium. (Ex: Propofol)
4. [Drug] *Injectable Suspension*—Liquid preparations of solids suspended in a suitable liquid medium. (Ex: Methylprednisolone Acetate Suspension)
5. [Drug] for *Injectable Suspension*—Dry solids that, upon the addition of suitable vehicles, yield preparations conforming in all respects to the requirements for *Injectable Suspensions*. (Ex: Imipenem)

The form in which a given drug is prepared for parenteral use by the manufacturer depends upon the nature of the drug itself, with respect to its physical and chemical characteristics, and also upon certain therapeutic considerations. Generally, if a drug is unstable in solution, it may be prepared as a dry powder intended for reconstitution with the proper solvent at the time of its administration, or it may be prepared as a suspension of the drug particles in a vehicle in which the drug is insoluble. If the drug is unstable in the presence of water, that solvent may be replaced in part or totally by a solvent in which the drug is insoluble. If the drug is insoluble in water, an injection may be prepared as an aqueous suspension or as a solution of the drug in a suitable nonaqueous solvent, such as a vegetable oil. If an aqueous solution is desired, a water-soluble salt form of the insoluble drug is frequently prepared to satisfy the required solubility characteristics. Aqueous or blood-miscible solutions may be injected directly into the blood stream. Blood-immiscible liquids, e.g., oleaginous injections and suspensions, can interrupt the normal flow of blood within the circulatory system, and their use is generally restricted to other than intravenous administration. The onset and duration of action of a drug may be somewhat controlled by the chemical form of the drug used, the physical state of the injection (solution or suspension), and the vehicle employed. Drugs that are very soluble in body fluids generally have the most rapid absorption and onset of action. Thus, drugs in aqueous solution have a more rapid onset of action than do drugs in oleaginous solution. Drugs in aqueous suspension are also more rapid acting than drugs in oleaginous suspension due to the greater miscibility of the aqueous preparation with the body fluids after injection and the subsequent more rapid contact of the drug particles with the body fluids. Oftentimes more prolonged drug action is desired to reduce the necessity of frequently repeated injections. These long-acting types of injections are commonly referred to as repository or "depot" types of preparations.

The solutions and suspensions of drugs intended for injection are prepared in the same general manner as was discussed previously in this text for solutions (Chapter 12) and disperse systems (Chapter 13), with the following differences:

1. Solvents or vehicles used must meet special purity and other standards assuring their safety by injection.
2. The use of added substances, as buffers, stabilizers, and antimicrobial preservatives, fall under specific guidelines of use and are restricted in certain parenteral products. The use of coloring agents is strictly prohibited.
3. Parenteral products are always sterilized and meet sterility standards and must be pyrogen-free.
4. Parenteral solutions must meet compendial standards for particulate matter.
5. Parenteral products must be prepared in environmentally controlled areas, under strict sanitation standards, and by personnel specially trained and clothed to maintain the sanitation standards.
6. Parenteral products are packaged in special hermetic containers of specific and high quality. Special quality control procedures are utilized to ensure their hermetic seal and sterile condition.
7. Each container of an injection is filled to a volume in slight excess of the labeled "size" or volume to be withdrawn. This overfill permits the ease of withdrawal and administration of the labeled volumes.

8. There are restrictions over the volume of injection permitted in multiple-dose containers and also a limitation over the types of containers (single-dose or multiple-dose) which may be used for certain injections.
9. Specific labeling regulations apply to injections.
10. Sterile powders intended for solution or suspension immediately prior to injection are frequently packaged as *lyophilized* or freeze-dried powders to permit ease of solution or suspension upon the addition of the solvent or vehicle.

Solvents and Vehicles for Injections

The most frequently used solvent in the large-scale manufacturer of injections is *Water for Injection, USP.* This water is purified by distillation or by reverse osmosis and meets the same standards for the presence of total solids as does *Purified Water, USP,* not more than 1 mg per 100 mL Water for Injection, USP and may not contain added substances. Although water for injection is not required to be sterile, it must be pyrogen-free. The water is intended to be used in the manufacture of injectable products which are to be sterilized after their preparation. Water for injection should be stored in tight containers at temperatures below or above the range in which microbial growth occurs. Water for injection is intended to be used within 24 hours following its collection. Naturally, the water should be collected in sterile and pyrogen-free containers. The containers are usually glass or glass-lined.

Sterile Water for Injection, USP is water for injection which has been sterilized and packaged in single-dose containers of not greater than 1-liter size. As water for injection, it must be pyrogen-free and may not contain an antimicrobial agent or other added substance. This water may contain a slightly greater amount of total solids than water for injection due to the leaching of solids from the glass-lined tanks during the sterilization process. This water is intended to be used as a solvent, vehicle or diluent for already-sterilized and packaged injectable medications. The one-liter bottles cannot be administered intravenously because they have no tonicity. Thus, they are used for reconstitution of multiple antibiotics. In use, the water is aseptically added to the vial of medication to prepare the desired injection. For instance, a suitable injection may be prepared from the dry powder, Sterile Ampicillin Sodium, USP, by the aseptic addition of sterile water for injection.

Bacteriostatic Water for Injection, USP is sterile water for injection containing one or more suitable antimicrobial agents. It is packaged in pre-filled syringes or in vials containing not more than 30 mL of the water. The container label must state the name and proportion of the antimicrobial agent(s) present. The water is employed as a sterile vehicle in the preparation of small volumes of injectable preparations. Theoretically, presence of the bacteriostatic agent gives the flexibility for multiple-dose vials. If the first person to withdraw medication inadvertently contaminates the vial contents, the preservative will destroy the microorganism. Although, historically, there has been debate on how much protection the antimicrobial agent can provide in a multiple-dose vial (4). Because of the presence of antimicrobial agents the water must only be used in parenterals that are administered in small volumes. Its use in parenterals administered in large volume is restricted due to the excessive and perhaps toxic amounts of the antimicrobial agents which would be injected along with the medication. Generally, if volumes of greater than 5 mL of solvent are required, sterile water for injection rather than bacteriostatic water for injection is preferred. In using bacteriostatic water for injection, due regard must also be given to the chemical compatibility of the bacteriostatic agent(s) present with the particular medicinal agent being dissolved or suspended.

USP labeling requirements demand that the label state, "Not for Use in Newborns." This labeling statement was the result of problems encountered with neonates and the toxicity of the bacteriostat, i.e., benzyl alcohol. This toxicity results from the high cumulative amounts (mg/kg) of benzyl alcohol and the limited detoxification capacity of the neonate liver. This solution has not been reported to cause problems in older infants, children, or adults.

Benzyl alcohol poisoning is recognized as the "gasping syndrome." In one study, ten premature infants developed this clinical syndrome characterized by the development of multi-organ failure and eventually died (5). The typical clinical course included metabolic acidosis, respiratory distress requiring mechanical ventilation, central nervous system dysfunction, hyperactivity, hypotonia, depression of the sensorium, apnea, seizure, coma, intraventricular hemorrhage, hepatic and renal failure, and eventual cardiovascular collapse and death. In the study, the amount of benzyl alcohol received ranged from 99–234 mg/kg/day. Based on the concentration of 0.9% benzyl alcohol in the Bacteriostatic Water for Injection and Sodium Chloride Injection death resulted from as little as 11 mL/kg/day.

Following toxicity reports and the deaths of infants in the early 1980s, the FDA issued a very strong recommendation to stop the use of fluids preserved with benzyl alcohol for use in neonates as a flush solution or to reconstitute medications.

Sodium Chloride Injection, USP is a sterile isotonic solution of sodium chloride in Water for Injection. It contains no antimicrobial agents. The sodium and chloride ion contents of the injection are approximately 154 mEq of each per liter. The solution may be used as a sterile vehicle in preparing solutions or suspensions of drugs for parenteral administration.

Besides its use to reconstitute medications for injection, Sodium Chloride Injection is frequently used as a catheter or IV line flush to maintain patency. Catheters or IV lines are constantly used to infuse fluids and intravenous medications and draw blood for laboratory analysis, among others. Usually 2 mL is used to flush the line after each use or every 8 hours if the line is not used.

Bacteriostatic Sodium Chloride Injection, USP is a sterile isotonic solution of sodium chloride in Water for Injection. It contains one or more suitable antimicrobial agents which must be specified on the labeling. Sodium chloride is present at 0.9% concentration to render the solution isotonic. For the reasons noted previously for bacteriostatic water for injection, this solution may not be packaged in containers greater than 30 mL in size. When this solution is used as a vehicle, care must be exercised to assure the compatibility of the added medicinal agent with the preservative(s) present as well as with the sodium chloride.

Bacteriostatic Sodium Chloride Injection is also used to flush a catheter or IV line to maintain its patency. When used in only small quantities for flushing lines and reconstituting medications, the amount of benzyl alcohol is negligible and safe. But, in neonates, especially premature infants with very low birth weights, accumulation of benzoic acid and unmetabolized benzyl alcohol may occur due to the aforementioned liver immaturity. Because of their low physical weight, their need for more medications due to acute illness, and the frequent use of the umbilical catheter for various purposes, these patients may receive many more flush solutions relative to their body weight compared to adults. Thus, Bacteriostatic Sodium Chloride Injection also carries the warning, "Not for Use in Newborns."

Suffice to say, that benzyl alcohol may also be present in other parenteral medications and the pharmacist must be vigilant for its inappropriate use in neonates. Generally speaking, however, the amount of benzyl alcohol received through this means is negligible compared to the amount received from flush solutions. Preferably, the medication is available in a preservative-free formulation (i.e., single-use dose) and that should be utilized. However, if such a formulation is not available and there is no alternative, a medication preserved with benzyl alcohol might still be used based on the physician's clinical judgment and the risk-to-benefit ratio.

Ringer's Injection, USP is a sterile solution of sodium chloride, potassium chloride, and calcium chloride in water for injection. The three agents are present in concentrations similar to that found in physiologic fluids. The solution is employed as a vehicle for other drugs, or alone as an electrolyte replenisher and fluid extender. *Lactated Ringer's Injection, USP* has different quantities of the same three salts in Ringer's Injection and contains sodium lactate. This injection is a fluid and electrolyte replenisher and a systemic alkalizer.

Nonaqueous Vehicles

Although an aqueous vehicle is generally preferred for an injection, its use may be precluded in a formulation due to the limited water solubility of a medicinal substance or its susceptibility to hydrolysis. When such physical or chemical factors limit the use of a wholly aqueous vehicle, the pharmaceutical formulator must turn to one or more nonaqueous vehicles.

The selected vehicle must be nonirritating, nontoxic in the amounts administered, and nonsensitizing. Like water, it must not exert a pharmacologic activity of its own, nor may it adversely affect the activity of the medicinal agent. In addition, the physical and chemical properties of the solvent or vehicle must be considered, evaluated, and determined to be suitable for the task at hand before it may be employed. Among the many considerations are the solvent's physical and chemical stability at various pH levels, its viscosity, which must be such as to allow ease of injection (syringeability), its fluidity, which must be maintained over a fairly wide temperature range, its boiling point, which should be sufficiently high to permit heat sterilization, its miscibility with body fluids, its low vapor pressure to avoid problems during heat sterilization, and its constant purity or ease of purification and standardization. There is no single solvent that is free of limitations, and thus the cross-consideration and the assessment of each solvent's advantages and disadvantages help the formulator determine the most appropriate solvent for use in a given preparation. Among the nonaqueous solvents presently employed in parenteral products are fixed vegetable oils, glycerin, polyethylene glycols, propylene glycol, alcohol, and a number of lesser used agents as ethyl oleate, isopropyl myristate, and dimethylacetamide. These and other nonaqueous vehicles may be used provided they are safe in the amounts administered and do not interfere with the therapeutic efficacy of the preparation or with its response to prescribed assays and tests.

The USP specifies restrictions on the fixed vegetable oils which may be employed in parenteral products. For one thing, they must remain clear when cooled to 10°C to ensure the stability and clarity of the injectable product upon storage under refrigeration. The oils must not contain mineral oil or paraffin, as these materials are not absorbed by body tissues. The fluidity of a vegetable oil generally depends upon the proportion of unsaturated fatty acids, such as oleic acid, to saturated acids, such as stearic acid. Oils to be employed in injections must meet officially stated requirements of iodine number and saponification number.

Although the toxicities of vegetable oils are generally considered to be relatively low, some patients exhibit allergic reactions to specific oils. Thus, when vegetable oils are employed in parenteral products, the label must state the specific oil present. The most commonly used fixed oils in injections are corn oil, cottonseed oil, peanut oil, and sesame oil. Castor oil and olive oil have been used on occasion.

By the selective employment of solvent or vehicle, a pharmacist can prepare injectable preparations as solutions or suspensions of a medicinal substance in either an aqueous or nonaqueous vehicle. For the most part, oleaginous injections are administered intramuscularly. They must not be administered intravenously as the oil globules will occlude the pulmonary microcirculation. Some examples of official injections employing oil as the vehicle are presented in Table 14.1.

Added Substances

The USP permits the addition of suitable substances to the official preparations intended for injection for the purpose of increasing their stability or usefulness, provided the substances are not interdicted in the individual monographs and are harmless in the amounts administered and do not interfere with the therapeutic efficacy of the preparation or with specified assays and tests. Many of these added substances are antibacterial preservatives, buffers, solubilizers, antioxidants, and other

Table 14.1.   Examples of Some Injections in Oil

Injection	Oil	Category
Dimercaprol Injection	Peanut	Antidote to arsenic, gold and mercury poisoning
Estradiol Cypionate Injection	Cottonseed	Estrogen
Estradiol Valerate Injection	Sesame or Castor	Estrogen
Fluphenazine Decanoate Injection	Sesame	Antipsychotic
Fluphenazine Enanthate Injection	Sesame	Antipsychotic
Hydroxyprogesterone Caproate Injection	Castor	Progestin
Progesterone in Oil Injection	Sesame or Peanut	Progestin
Testosterone Cypionate Injection	Cottonseed	Androgen
Testosterone Cypionate and Estradiol Cypionate Injection	Cottonseed	Androgen and Estrogen
Testosterone Enanthate Injection	Sesame	Androgen
Testosterone Enanthate and Estradiol Valerate Injection	Sesame	Androgen and Estrogen

pharmaceutical adjuncts. Agents employed solely for their coloring effect are strictly prohibited in parenteral products.

The USP requires that one or more suitable substances be added to parenteral products that are packaged in multiple-dose containers, to prevent the growth of microorganisms regardless of the method of sterilization employed, unless otherwise directed in the individual monograph or unless the injection's active ingredients are themselves bacteriostatic. Such substances are used in concentrations that prevent the growth of or kill microorganisms in the preparations. Because many of the usual preservative agents are toxic when given in excessive amounts or irritating when parenterally administered, special care must be exercised in the selection of the appropriate preservative agents. For the following preservatives, the indicated maximum limits prevail for use in a parenteral product unless otherwise directed: for agents containing mercury and the cationic, surface-active compounds, 0.01%; for agents like chlorobutanol, cresol, and phenol, 0.5%; for sulfur dioxide as an antioxidant, or for an equivalent amount of the sulfite, bisulfite, or metabisulfite of potassium or sodium, 0.2%.

In addition to the stabilizing effect of the additives, the air within an injectable product is frequently replaced with an inert gas, such as nitrogen, to enhance the stability of the product by preventing chemical reaction between the oxygen in the air and the drug.

Methods of Sterilization

The term *sterilization,* as applied to pharmaceutical preparations, means the complete destruction of all living organisms and their spores or their complete removal from the preparation. Five general methods are used for the sterilization of pharmaceutical products:

1. Steam sterilization
2. Dry-heat sterilization
3. Sterilization by filtration
4. Gas sterilization
5. Sterilization by ionizing radiation

The method used in attaining sterility in a pharmaceutical preparation is determined largely by the nature of the preparation and its ingredients. However, regardless of the method used, the resulting product must pass a test for sterility as proof of the effectiveness of the method and the performance of the equipment and the personnel.

Steam Sterilization

Steam sterilization is conducted in an autoclave and employs steam under pressure. It is recognized as the method of choice in most cases where the product is capable of withstanding such treatment (Fig. 14.3).

Most pharmaceutical products are adversely affected by heat and cannot be heated safely to the temperature required for dry-heat sterilization (about 170°C). When moisture is present, bacteria are coagulated and destroyed at a considerably lower temperature than when a moisture is absent. In fact, bacterial cells with a large percentage of water are generally killed rather easily. Spores, which contain a relatively low percentage of water, are comparatively difficult to destroy. The mechanism of microbial destruction in moist heat is thought to

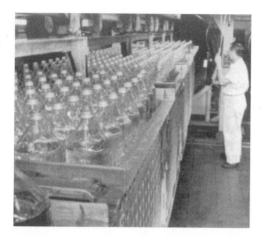

Fig. 14.3 *Autoclaving of intravenous electrolyte solutions. (Courtesy of Abbott Laboratories.)*

be by denaturation and coagulation of some of the organism's essential protein. It is the presence of the hot moisture within the microbial cell that permits destruction at relatively low temperature. Death by dry heat is thought to be by the dehydration of the microbial cell followed by a slow burning or oxidative process. Because it is not possible to raise the temperature of steam above 100°C under atmospheric conditions, pressure is employed to achieve higher temperatures. It should be recognized that the temperature, not the pressure, is destructive to the microorganisms and that the application of pressure is solely for the purpose of increasing the temperature of the system. Time is another important factor in the destruction of microorganisms by heat. Most modern autoclaves have gauges to indicate to the operator the internal conditions of temperature and pressure and a timing device to permit the desired exposure time for the load. The usual steam pressures, the temperatures obtainable under these pressures, and the approximate length of time required for sterilization after the system reaches the indicated temperatures are as follows:

10 pounds pressure (115.5°C), for 30 minutes
15 pounds pressure (121.5°C), for 20 minutes
20 pounds pressure (126.5°C), for 15 minutes.

As can be seen, the greater the pressure applied, the higher the temperature obtainable and the less the time required for sterilization.

The temperature at which most autoclaves are routinely operated is usually 121°C, as measured at the steam discharge line running from the auto-

clave. It should be understood that the temperature attained in the chamber of the autoclave must also be reached by the interior of the load being sterilized, and this temperature must be maintained for an adequate time. The penetration time of the moist heat into the load may vary with the nature of the load, and the exposure time must be adjusted to account for this latent period. For example, a solution packaged in a thin-walled 50-mL ampul may reach a temperature of 121°C in from 6 to 8 minutes after that temperature is registered in the steam discharge line, whereas 20 minutes or longer may be required to reach that temperature within a solution packaged in a completely filled thick-walled 1000-mL glass bottle. An estimate of these latent periods must be added to the total time in order to ensure adequate exposure times. Because this sterilization process depends upon the presence of moisture and an elevated temperature, air is removed from the chamber as the sterilization process is begun, because a combination of air and steam yields a lower temperature than does steam alone under the same condition of pressure. For instance, at 15 pounds pressure the temperature of saturated steam is 121.5°C, but a mixture of equal parts of air and steam will reach only about 112°C.

In general, this method of sterilization is applicable to pharmaceutical preparations and materials that can withstand the required temperatures and are penetrated by, but not adversely affected by, moisture. In sterilizing aqueous solutions by this method, the moisture is already present, and all that is required is the elevation of the temperature of the solution for the prescribed period of time. Thus solutions packaged in sealed containers, as ampuls, are readily sterilized by this method. The method is also applicable to bulk solutions, glassware, surgical dressings, and instruments. It is not useful in the sterilization of oils, fats, oleaginous preparations, and other preparations not penetrated by the moisture or the sterilization of exposed powders that may be damaged by the condensed moisture.

Dry-Heat Sterilization

Dry-heat sterilization is usually carried out in sterilizing ovens specifically designed for this purpose. The ovens may be heated either by gas or electricity and are generally thermostatically controlled.

Because dry heat is less effective in killing microorganisms than is moist heat, higher temperatures and longer periods of exposure are required. These must be determined individually for each product with consideration to the size and type of product and the container and its heat distribution characteristics. In general, individual units to be sterilized should be as small as possible, and the sterilizer should be loaded in such a manner as to permit free circulation of heated air throughout the chamber. Dry-heat sterilization is usually conducted at temperatures of 160° to 170°C for periods of not less than 2 hours. Higher temperatures permit shorter exposure times for a given article; conversely, lower temperatures require longer exposure times. For example, if a particular chemical agent melts or decomposes at 170°C, but is unaffected at 140°C, the lower temperature would be employed in its sterilization, and the exposure time would be increased over that required to sterilize another chemical that may be safely heated to 170°C.

Dry-heat sterilization is generally employed for substances that are not effectively sterilized by moist heat. Such substances include fixed oils, glycerin, various petroleum products such as petrolatum, liquid petrolatum (mineral oil), and paraffin and various heat-stable powders such as zinc oxide. Dry-heat sterilization is also an effective method for the sterilization of glassware and surgical instruments. Dry-heat sterilization is the method of choice when dry apparatus or dry containers are required, as in the handling of packaging of dry chemicals or nonaqueous solutions.

Sterilization by Filtration

Sterilization by filtration, which depends upon the physical removal of microorganisms by adsorption on the filter medium or by a sieving mechanism, is used for the sterilization of heat-sensitive solutions. Medicinal preparations sterilized by this method are required to undergo severe validation and monitoring since the effectiveness of the filtered product can be greatly influenced by the microbial load in the solution being filtered (Fig. 14.4).

Commercially available filters are produced with a variety of pore-size specifications. It would be well to mention briefly one type of these modern filters, the Millipore filters (Fig. 14.5). Millipore filters are thin plastic membranes of cellulosic esters with millions of pores per square inch of filter surface. The pores are made to be extremely uniform in size and occupy approximately 80% of the filter membrane's volume, the remaining 20% being the solid filter material. This high degree of porosity permits flow rates much in excess of other filters having the same particle-retention capability. Millipore filters are made from a variety of polymers to provide membrane characteristics required for the filtration of almost any liquid or gas system. Also, the filters are made of various pore sizes to meet the selective filtration requirements of the operator. They are available in pore sizes from 14 to 0.025 μm. For comparative purposes, the period that ended the last sentence is approximately 500 μm in size. The size of the smallest particle visible to the naked eye is about 40 μm, a red blood cell is about 6.5 μm, the smallest bacteria, about 0.2 μm, and a polio virus, about 0.025 μm.

Although the pore size of a bacterial filter is of prime importance in the removal of microorgan-

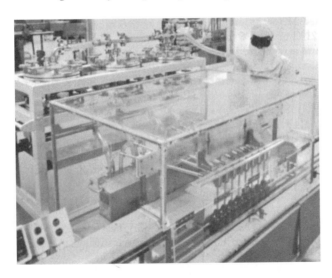

Fig. 14.4 *Sterilization by filtration. An eight-head bottle-filling machine using three large sterilizing filters for sterile filling of bottles in large scale pharmaceutical production. (Courtesy of Millipore Corporation.)*

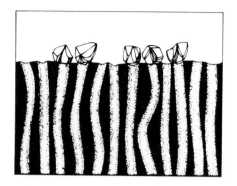

Fig. 14.5 *Membrane filters act as microporous screens that retain all particles and microorganisms larger than the rated pore size on their surface. (Courtesy of Millipore Corporation.)*

isms from a liquid, there are other factors such as the electrical charge on the filter and that of the microorganism, the pH of the solution, the temperature, and the pressure or vacuum applied to the system.

The major advantages of bacterial filtration include its speed in the filtration of small quantities of solution, its ability to sterilize effectively thermolabile materials, the relatively inexpensive equipment required, the development and proliferation of membrane filter technology, and the complete removal of living and dead microorganisms as well as other particulate matter from the solution.

The class of filter media lends itself to more effective standardization and quality control and also gives the user greater opportunity to confirm the characteristics or properties of the filter assembly before and after use. The fact that membrane filters are thin polymeric films offers many advantages but also some disadvantages when compared to depth filters such as porcelain or sintered material. Because much of the membrane surface is a void or open space, the properly assembled and sterilized filter offers the advantage of a high flow rate.

One disadvantage is that because the membrane is usually fragile, it is essential to determine that the assembly was properly made and that the membrane was not ruptured or flawed during assembly, sterilization, or use. The housing and filter assemblies that are chosen to be used should first be validated for compatibility and integrity by the user. This disadvantage is a circumstance not true of methods involving dry- or moist-heat sterilization in which the procedures are just about guaranteed to give effective sterilization. Also, filtration of large volumes of liquids would require more time, particularly if the liquid were viscous, than would, say,

steam sterilization. In essence, the bacterial filters are useful when heat cannot be used and also for small volumes of liquids.

Bacterial filters may be used conveniently and economically in the community pharmacy to filter extemporaneously prepared solutions (as ophthalmic solutions) that are required to be sterile (Figs. 14.6, 14.7). Further, the membrane filter method is the most commonly used sterilization method used by hospitals. Occasionally, hospitals may use the autoclave (i.e., moist heat method) to sterilize IV solutions, such as caffeine citrate IV injection.

To date, there has been limited information about drug adsorption to membrane filters. Several studies, however, have demonstrated that membrane filters have the capacity to remove drug from solution (6–9). For example, 0.22 micron filters reduce the in vitro antimicrobial activity of amphotericin B (a colloidal suspension), while filtration of the amphotericin B through 0.85 and 0.45 micron filters did not. Butler et al. demonstrated that the potency of drugs administered intravenously and in small doses could be significantly reduced during in-line filtration with a filter containing a cellulose ester membrane (10). The pharmaceutical literature indicates that drugs administered in low doses might present the problem of the drug's bonding to the filter. Many filters in clinical use are nitrate or acetate esters of cellulose. These compounds are polar and have residual hydroxyl groups that might become involved with drug adsorption interactions. Hydrophobic interactions between hydrocarbon portions of drug molecules being filtered and linear cellulose molecules of filters are also thought to be involved in drug adsorption.

In general, current information suggests that little or no adsorption takes place with membrane filters. However, it is recommended that minute dosages of drugs (i.e., <5 mg) should not be filtered until sufficient data are available to demonstrate

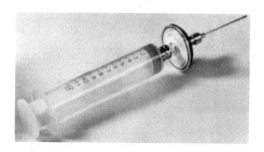

Fig. 14.6 *Luer-Lock syringe adapted with a MILLEX Filter Unit and hypodermic needle. (Courtesy of Millipore Corporation.)*

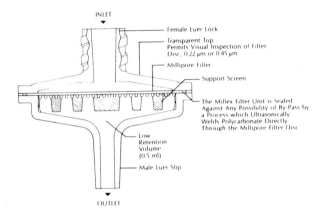

INLET

Female Luer Lock

Transparent Top
Permits Visual Inspection of Filter
Disc, 0.22 μm or 0.45 μm

Millipore Filter

Support Screen

The Millex Filter Unit is Sealed
Against Any Possibility of By-Pass by
a Process which Ultrasonically
Welds Polycarbonate Directly
Through the Millipore Filter Disc

Low
Retention
Volume
(0.5 ml)

Male Luer Slip

OUTLET

Fig. 14.7 *Cutaway showing composition of the MILLEX filter unit. (Courtesy of Millipore Corporation.)*

insignificant adsorption. With respect to amphotericin B, to assure the passage of the antibiotic colloidal dispersion, the filter's mean pore diameter should > 1 micron.

Membrane filter media which are now available include cellulose acetate, cellulose nitrate, fluorocarbonate, acrylic polymers, polycarbonate, polyester, polyvinyl chloride, vinyl, nylon, polytef, and even metal membranes, and they may be reinforced or supported by an internal fabric.

Gas Sterilization

Some heat-sensitive and moisture-sensitive materials can be sterilized much better by exposure to ethylene oxide or propylene oxide gas than by other means. These gases are highly flammable when mixed with air but can be employed safely when properly diluted with an inert gas such as carbon dioxide or a suitable fluorinated hydrocarbon. Such mixtures are commercially available.

Sterilization by this process requires specialized equipment resembling autoclaves, and many combination steam autoclaves-ethylene oxide sterilizers are commercially available. Greater precautions are required for this method of sterilization than for some of the others, because the variables—for instance, time, temperature, gas concentration, and humidity—are not as firmly quantitated as those of dry-heat and steam sterilization. In general, sterilization with gas is enhanced, and the exposure time required is reduced, by increasing the relative humidity of the system (to about 60%) and by increasing the exposure temperature (to between 50 and 60°C). If the material being sterilized cannot tolerate either the moisture or the elevated temperature, exposure time will have to be increased. Generally, sterilization with ethylene oxide gas requires from 4 to 16 hours of exposure. Ethylene oxide is thought to function as a sterilizing agent by

its interference with the metabolism of the bacterial cell.

The great penetrating qualities of ethylene oxide gas make it a useful sterilizing agent in certain special applications, as in the sterilization of medical and surgical supplies and appliances such as catheters, needles, and plastic disposable syringes in their final plastic packaging just prior to shipment. The gas is also used to sterilize certain heat-labile enzyme preparations, certain antibiotics, and other drugs, with tests being performed to assure of the absence of chemical reaction or other deleterious effects on the drug substance.

Sterilization by Ionizing Radiation

Techniques are available for the sterilization of some types of pharmaceuticals by gamma rays and by cathode rays, but the application of such techniques is limited because of the highly specialized equipment required and the effects of irradiation on products and their containers.

The exact mechanism by which irradiation sterilizes a drug or preparation is still subject to investigation. One of the proposed theories involves an alteration of the chemicals within or supporting the microorganism to form deleterious new chemicals capable of destroying the cell. Another theory proposes that vital structures of the cell, such as the chromosomal nucleoprotein, are disoriented or destroyed. It is probably a combination of irradiation effects that causes the cellular destruction, which is complete and irreversible.

Validation of Sterility

Regardless of the method of sterilization employed, pharmaceutical preparations required to be sterile must undergo sterility tests to confirm the absence of microorganisms. The USP contains monographs and standards for biologic indicators of a sterilization process. A *biologic indicator* is a characterized preparation of specific microorganisms resistant to a particular sterilization process. They may be utilized to monitor a sterilization cycle and/or to periodically revalidate the process. Biologic indicators are generally of two main forms. In one, spores are added to a carrier, as a strip of filter paper, packaged to maintain physical integrity while allowing the sterilization effect. In the other, the spores are added to representative units of the product being sterilized, with sterilization assessed based on these samples. In moist heat (i.e., steam) sterilization and ethylene oxide sterilization, spores of suitable strains of *Bacillus stearothermophilus* are commonly employed because of their resistance to this mode of sterilization. In dry heat sterilization, spores of *Bacillus subtilis* are commonly used. In sterilization by ionizing radiation, spores of suitable strains of *Bacillus pumilus, Bacillus stearothermophilus*, and *Bacillus subtilis* have been utilized.

The effectiveness of thermal sterilization procedures has been quantified through the determination and calculation of *F value* to express the time of thermal death. *Thermal death time* is defined as the time required to kill a particular organism under specified conditions. The F_0, at a particular temperature other than 121°C, is the time, in minutes, required to provide the lethality equivalent to that provided at 121° for a stated time.

Although heat distribution in an autoclave chamber is usually rapid with 121°C obtained nearly instantaneously throughout the autoclave, the product being sterilized may not achieve identical conditions due to a variety of factors of heat transfer, including the thermal conductivity of the packaging components, the viscosity and density of the product, container proximity, passage of steam around containers and other variables. F values may be computed from biologic data derived from the rate of destruction of known numbers of microorganisms, as shown in the following equation:

$$F_0 = D_{121}(\text{Log } A - \text{Log } B)$$

where D_{121} = the time required for a one-log reduction in the microbial population exposed to a temperature of 121°C
A = the initial microbial population
B = the number of microorganisms that survive after a defined heating time (11).

Pyrogens and Pyrogen Testing

As indicated earlier, *pyrogens* are fever-producing organic substances arising from microbial contam-

ination and responsible for many of the febrile reactions which occur in patients following injection. The causative material is thought to be a lipopolysaccharide from the outer cell wall of the bacteria and endotoxins. Because the material is thermostable, it may remain in water even after sterilization by autoclaving or by bacterial filtration.

Manufacturers of water for injection may employ any suitable method for the removal of pyrogens from their product. Because pyrogens are organic substances, one of the more common means of facilitating their removal is by oxidizing them to easily eliminated gases or to nonvolatile solids, both of which are easily separated from water by fractional distillation. Potassium permanganate is usually employed as the oxidizing agent, with its efficiency being increased by the addition of a small amount of barium hydroxide serving to impart alkalinity to the solution and to make nonvolatile barium salts of any acidic compounds that may be present. These two reagents are added to water that has previously been distilled several times, and the distillation process is repeated with the chemical-free distillate being collected under strict aseptic conditions. When properly conducted, this method results in a highly purified, sterile, and pyrogen-free water. However, in each instance the official pyrogen test must be performed for assurance of the absence of these fever-producing materials.

PYROGEN TEST. The USP Pyrogen Test utilizes healthy rabbits that have been properly maintained in terms of environment and diet prior to performance of the test. Normal, or "control" temperatures are taken for each animal to be used in the test. These temperatures are used as the base for the determination of any temperature increase resulting from the injection of a test solution. In a given test, rabbits are used whose temperatures do not differ by more than one degree from each other and whose body temperatures are considered to be unelevated. A synopsis of the procedure of the test is as follows.

Render the syringes, needles, and glassware free from pyrogens by heating at 250°C for not less than 30 minutes or by other suitable method. Warm the product to be tested to 37°C ± 2°C.

Inject into an ear vein of each of three rabbits 10 mL of the product per kg of body weight, completing each injection within 10 minutes after the start of administration. Record the temperature at 30-minute intervals between 1 and 3 hours subsequent to the injection.

If no rabbit shows an individual rise in temperature of 0.5° or more above its respective control temperature, the product meets the requirements for the absence of pyrogens. If any rabbit shows an individual temperature rise of 0.5° or more, continue the test using five other rabbits. If not more than three of the eight rabbits show individual rises in temperature of 0.5° or more and if the sum of the eight individual maximum temperature rises does not exceed 3.3°, the material under examination meets the requirements for the absence of pyrogens.

In recent years, it has been shown that an extract from the blood cells of the horseshoe crab (*Limulus polyphemus*) contains an enzyme and protein system that coagulates in the presence of low levels of lipopolysaccharides. This discovery has led to the development of the *Limulus* amebocyte lysate (LAL) test for the presence of bacterial endotoxins. The USP Bacterial Endotoxins Test utilizes LAL and is considered generally more sensitive to endotoxin than the rabbit test. The FDA has endorsed the test as a replacement for the rabbit test and it is used for a number of parenteral products.

Some parenteral products, however, cannot be tested with the LAL test because the active ingredient interferes with the test outcome. Such products include meperidine HCl and promethazine HCl, oxacillin sodium, sulfisoxazole, and vancomycin HCl, among others. These then, must be tested with the aforementioned USP Pyrogen Test.

Because the LAL test is so sensitive for the presence of bacterial endotoxins, in some cases, where the active ingredient of the small volume parenteral can interfere with the test, a strategy to overcome this interference is to dilute the product more than one twofold dilution. Such products include diphenhydramine HCl, ephedrine HCl, meperidine HCl, promethazine HCl, and thiamine HCl, among others, are thus tested in this manner.

The Industrial Preparation of Parenteral Products

Once the formulation for a particular parenteral product is determined, including the selection of the proper solvents or vehicles and additives, the production pharmacist must follow rigid aseptic procedures in preparing the injectable products. In most manufacturing plants the area in which parenteral products are made is maintained bacteria-free through the use of ultraviolet lights, a filtered air supply, sterile manufacturing equipment, such as flasks, connecting tubes, and filters, and sterilized work clothing worn by the personnel in the area (Fig. 14.8).

In the preparation of parenteral solutions, the required ingredients are dissolved according to good pharmaceutical practice either in water for injection, in one of the alternate solvents, or in a combination of solvents. The solutions are then usually filtered until sparkling clear through a membrane-type filter. After filtration, the solution is transferred as rapidly as possible and with the least possible exposure into the final containers. The product is then sterilized, preferably by autoclaving, and samples of the finished product are tested for sterility and pyrogens. In instances in which sterilization by autoclaving is impractical due to the nature of the ingredients, the individual components of the preparation that are heat or moisture labile may be sterilized by other appropriate means and added aseptically to the sterilized solvent or to a sterile solution of all of the other components sterilizable by autoclaving.

Suspensions of drugs intended for parenteral use may be prepared by reducing the drug to a very fine powder with a ball mill, micronizer, colloid mill, or other appropriate equipment and then suspending the material in a liquid in which it is insoluble. It is frequently necessary to sterilize separately the individual components of a suspension before combining them, as frequently the integrity of a suspension is destroyed by autoclaving. Autoclaving of a parenteral suspension may alter the viscosity of the product, thereby affecting the suspending ability of the vehicle, or change the particle size of the suspended particles, thereby altering both the pharmaceutic and the therapeutic characteristics of the preparation. If a suspension remains unaltered by autoclaving, this method is generally employed to sterilize the final product. Because parenterally administered emulsions, which are dispersions or suspensions of a liquid throughout another liquid, are generally destroyed by autoclaving, an alternate method of sterilization must be employed for this type of injectable.

Some injections are packaged as dry solids rather than in conjunction with a solvent or vehicle due to the instability of the therapeutic agent in the presence of the liquid component. These dry powdered drugs are packaged as the sterilized powder in the final containers to be reconstituted with the proper liquid prior to use, generally to form a solution or less frequently a suspension. The method of sterilization of the powder may be dry heat or another method that is appropriate for the particular drug

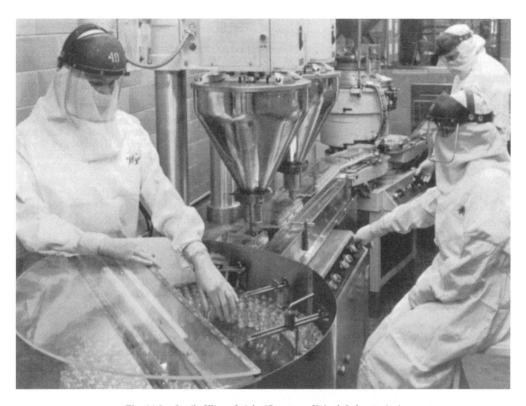

Fig. 14.8   *Sterile filling of vials. (Courtesy of Wyeth Laboratories.)*

involved. Examples of sterile drugs prepared and packaged *without* the presence of pharmaceutical additives as buffers, preservatives, stabilizers, tonicity agents, and other substances include:

Sterile Ampicillin Sodium
Sterile Ceftizoxime Sodium
Sterile Ceftazidime Sodium
Sterile Cefuroxime Sodium
Sterile Kanamycin Sulfate
Sterile Nafcillin Sodium
Sterile Penicillin G Benzathine
Sterile Streptomycin Sulfate
Sterile Tobramycin Sulfate

Antibiotics are prepared industrially in large fermentation tanks (Fig. 14.9).

Those sterile drugs formulated *with* pharmaceutical additives and intended to be reconstituted prior to injection include the following:

Cephradine for Injection
Cyclophosphamide for Injection
Dactinomycin for Injection
Erythromycin Lactobionate for Injection

Hyaluronidase for Injection
Hydrocortisone Sodium Succinate for Injection
Mitomycin for Injection
Nafcillin Sodium for Injection
Oxytetracycline Hydrochloride for Injection
Penicillin G Potassium for Injection
Vinblastine Sulfate for Injection

In certain instances, a liquid is packaged along with the dry powder for use at the time of reconstitution (Fig. 14.10). This liquid is sterile and may contain some of the desired pharmaceutical additives as the buffering agents. More frequently, the solvent or vehicle is not provided along with the dry product, but the labeling on the injection generally lists suitable solvents. Sodium chloride injection or sterile water for injection are perhaps the most frequently employed solvents used to reconstitute dry-packaged injections. The dry powders are packaged in containers large enough to permit proper shaking with the liquid component when the latter is aseptically injected through the container's rubber closure during its reconstitution. To facilitate the dissolving process, the dry powder is prevented from caking upon standing by the appropriate means including

Physical Pharmacy Capsule 14.1   **Colligative Properties of Drugs**

Drug molecules have properties that are often divided into additive, constitutive, or colligative.

Additive properties depend on the total contribution of the atoms in the molecule, or upon the sum of the properties of the constituents of the solution. An example is molecular weight.

Constitutive properties depend on the arrangement and, to a lesser extent, the number and kind of atoms in a molecule. Examples of this are the refraction of light, electrical properties, and surface and interfacial properties.

Colligative properties depend primarily on the number of particles in solution. Example properties include changes in vapor pressure, boiling point, freezing point and osmotic pressure. These values should be approximately equal for equimolar concentrations of drugs.

LOWERING OF VAPOR PRESSURE
A vapor, when in equilibrium with its pure liquid at a constant temperature, will exert a certain pressure known as the *vapor pressure*. When a solute is added to the pure liquid, it will alter the tendency of the molecules to escape the original liquid. In an ideal solution, or one that is very dilute, the partial vapor pressure of one component (p_1) is proportional to the mole fraction of molecules (N_1) of that component in the mixture:

$$p_1 = N_1 p_1^\circ$$

where p_1° is the vapor pressure of the pure component.

EXAMPLE 1
What is the partial vapor pressure of a solution containing 50 g dextrose in 1000 mL of water (the vapor pressure of water is given as 23.76 mm Hg).

1. (50 g dextrose)/(MW of 180) = 0.28 moles of dextrose
2. (1000 g water)/MW of 18) = 55.56 moles of water
3. 0.28 + 55.56 = 55.84 total moles
4. (55.56)/(55.84) = 0.995 mole fraction of water
5. p_1 = (0.995)(23.76 mm Hg) = 23.64 mm Hg

The vapor pressure of the solution is 23.64 mm Hg. The decrease in vapor pressure by the addition of the 50 g dextrose is 23.76 - 23.64 = 0.12 mm Hg.

INCREASE IN BOILING POINT
The *boiling point* of a liquid is that temperature when the vapor pressure of the liquid comes into equilibrium with the atmospheric pressure. The vapor pressure is reduced when a nonvolatile solute is added to a solvent, so the solution must be heated to a higher temperature to reestablish the equilibrium—hence, an increase in the boiling point. This is described in the following equation:

$$\Delta T_b = k_b m$$

where ΔT_b is the change in boiling point; k_b is the molar elevation constant of water, and m is the molality of the solute.

EXAMPLE 2
What is the boiling point elevation of a solution containing 50 g dextrose in 1000 mL of water (the molal elevation constant of water is 0.51).

1. (50 g dextrose)/(MW of 180) = 0.28 moles of dextrose in 1000 mL of water or 0.28 molal solution.
2. ΔT_b = (0.51) (0.28) = 0.143°C.

DECREASE IN FREEZING POINT
The *freezing point* of a pure liquid is the temperature at which the solid and liquid phases are in equilibrium at 1 atmosphere pressure. The freezing point of a solution is that temperature at which the solid phase of pure solvent and the liquid phase of solution are in equilibrium at 1 atmosphere pressure. When

Physical Pharmacy Capsule 14.1	**Colligative Properties of Drugs (Continued)**

a solute is added to a solvent, the decrease in freezing point is proportional to the concentration of the solute. The relationship is described by the following equation:

$$\Delta T_f = k_f m$$

where ΔT_f is the change in freezing point;
 k_f is the molal freezing point depression constant of water; and
 m is the molality of the solute.

EXAMPLE 3

What is the decrease in freezing point of a solution containing 50 g dextrose in 1000 mL of water (the molal elevation constant of water is $-1.86°C$).

1. (50 g dextrose)/(MW of 180) = 0.28 moles of dextrose in 1000 mL of water or 0.28 molal solution.
2. $\Delta T_f = (-1.86)(0.28) = -0.52°C$.

OSMOTIC PRESSURE

The pressure that must be applied to a more concentrated solution just to prevent the flow of pure solvent into the solution separated by a semipermeable membrane is called the *osmotic pressure*. This relationship can be expressed as follows:

$$PV = nRT$$

where P is the pressure (atm);
 V is the volume (L);
 n is number of moles of solute;
 R is the gas constant (0.082 L-atm/mole deg), and
 T is the absolute temperature in °C.

EXAMPLE 4

What is the osmotic pressure of 50 g dextrose in 1000 mL of water at room temperature (25°C)?

1. (50 g dextrose)/(MW of 180) = 0.28 moles of dextrose
2. 273°C + 25°C = 298°C
3. Volume will be 1 L
4. $P = [(0.28)(0.082)(298)]/(1) = 6.84$ atm

Deviations from reality in the above ideal examples of colligative properties are explained by the use of the Van't Hoff term, i. This "i" term considers that electrolytes exert more pressure than nonelectrolytes and is related to the number of ionic species present. These deviations may be caused by ionic interaction, degree of dissociation of weak electrolytes, or associations of nonelectrolytes.

MILLIEQUIVALENTS

An *equivalent weight* is the atomic weight, in grams, of a material divided by its valence, or charge. MilliEquivalents are related to equivalents, which are also considered measures of combining power, chemical activity, or chemical reactivity. Equivalency, or milliEquivalency, takes into consideration the total number of ionic charges in solution and the valence of the ions. Normally, plasma contains about 155 milliEquivalents of cations and anions in solution. The number of cations is always matched by the number of anions.

A *milliEquivalent* is the quantity, in mg, of a solute equal to 1/1000 of its gram-equivalent weight. Consider the following example.

EXAMPLE 1

What is the milliEquivalent weight of sodium?

1. The atomic weight of sodium is 23.
2. The valence of sodium is +1.

Physical Pharmacy Capsule 14.1   **Colligative Properties of Drugs (Continued)**

3. The equivalent weight of sodium is (23 g)/(1) = 23 g.
4. The milliEquivalent weight of sodium is (23 g)/1000 = 0.023 g, or 23 mg.
5. Therefore, one milliEquivalent of sodium weighs 23 mg.

MilliEquivalent calculations are commonly required in pharmacy practice today. The following are some examples.

EXAMPLE 2
How many milliEquivalents of potassium chloride are in a solution containing 74.5 mg/mL?

1. The atomic weight of potassium is 39 and chloride is 35.5. The combined molecular weight is 74.5.
2. Since the valence is 1 for both potassium and chloride, the equivalent weight for potassium chloride is 74.5 g and the milliEquivalent weight is 74.5 mg.
3. The solution contains 74.5 mg/mL, and the milliEquivalent weight is 74.5 mg; therefore, there is 1 mEq/mL of potassium chloride in the solution.

EXAMPLE 3
How many milliEquivalents of calcium are in 10 mL of 10% calcium chloride ($CaCl_2.2\ H_2O$) solution?

1. The formula weight for calcium chloride dihydrate is 147.
2. The equivalent weight is 147/2 = 73.5, since calcium is divalent.
3. Therefore, 1 milliEquivalent of calcium chloride weighs 73.5 mg.
4. (10 mL) (10%) = 1 g, or 1000 mg) of calcium chloride dihydrate.
5. (1000 mg)/(73.5 mg) = 13.6 mEq of calcium chloride dihydrate, which also is 13.6 mEq of calcium.

EXAMPLE 4
How many milliEquivalents of sodium are contained in a 1 liter bag of 0.9% sodium chloride solution?

1. (1000 mL) (0.009) = 9 g, or 9000 mg.
2. The formula weight for sodium chloride is 23 + 35.5 = 58.5.
3. The milliEquivalent weight for sodium chloride is 58.5 mg.
4. (9000)/(58.5) = 153.8 mEq, or 154 mEq.

In these cases, since sodium chloride is monovalent, there are 154 mEq of sodium, 154 mEq of chloride, or 154 mEq of sodium chloride.

OSMOLALITY AND TONICITY
Biologic systems are compatible with solutions having similar osmotic pressures, i.e., an equivalent number of dissolved species. For example, red blood cells, blood plasma, and 0.9% sodium chloride solution contain approximately the same number of solute particles per unit volume and are termed iso-osmotic and isotonic.

If solutions do not contain the same number of dissolved species i.e., they contain more (hypertonic) or less (hypotonic), then it may be necessary to alter the composition of the solution to bring them into an acceptable range.

An osmol (Osm) is related to a mole (gram molecular weight) of the molecules or ions in solution. One mole of glucose (180 g) dissolved in 1000 g of water has an osmolality of 1 Osm, or 1000 mOsm per kg of water. One mole of sodium chloride (23 + 35.5 = 58.5 g) dissolved in 1000 g of water has an osmolality of almost 2000 mOsm, since sodium chloride dissociates into almost two particles per molecule. In other words, a 1 molal solution of sodium chloride is equivalent to a 2 molal solution of dextrose.

Normal serum osmolality values are in the vicinity of 285 mOsm/kg (often expressed as 285 mOsm/L). Ranges may include values from about 275 to 300 mOsm/L). Pharmaceuticals should be close to this value to minimize discomfort on application to the eyes or nose, or when injected.

Physical Pharmacy Capsule 14.1   **Colligative Properties of Drugs (Continued)**

Some solutions may be iso-osmotic but not isotonic. This is because the physiology of the cell membranes must be considered. For example, the cell membrane of the red blood cell is not semi-permeable to all drugs. It allows ammonium chloride, alcohol, boric acid, glycerin, propylene glycol, and urea to diffuse freely. In the eye, the cell membrane is semi-permeable to boric acid, and a 1.9% solution of boric acid is an isotonic ophthalmic solution. But even though a 1.9% solution of boric acid is isotonic with the eye and is iso-osmotic, it is not isotonic with blood—since boric acid can freely diffuse through the red blood cells—and it may cause hemolysis.

Pharmacists are often called upon to calculate the quantity of solute that must be added to adjust a hypotonic solution of a drug to isotonic. This can be done using several methods, including the "L," sodium chloride equivalent, and cryoscopic methods.

One of the most frequently used methods for calculating the quantity of sodium chloride necessary to prepare an isotonic solution is the *sodium chloride equivalent method*. A "sodium chloride equivalent" is defined as the amount of sodium chloride that is osmotically equivalent to 1 g of the drug. For example, the sodium chloride equivalent of ephedrine sulfate is 0.23 (i.e., 1 g of ephedrine sulfate would be equivalent to 0.23 g of sodium chloride).

EXAMPLE 1

How much sodium chloride is required to make the following prescription isotonic?

Rx Ephedrine sulfate 2%
Sterile water, qs30 mL
M. isoton with sodium chloride.

1. (30 mL) (0.009) = 0.270 g sodium chloride would be required if only sodium chloride was present in the 30 mL of solution.
2. (30 mL) (0.02) = 0.6 g ephedrine sulfate is to be present.
3. (0.6 g) (0.23) = 0.138 g is the quantity of sodium chloride "represented" by the ephedrine sulfate present.
4. Since 0.270 g sodium chloride would be required if only sodium chloride is used, and the quantity of sodium chloride that is equivalent to 0.6 g of ephedrine sulfate is 0.138 g, then 0.270 − 0.138 g = 0.132 g of sodium chloride would be required to render the solution isotonic.
5. Therefore, to prepare the solution would require 0.6 grams of ephedrine sulfate, 0.132 grams of sodium chloride, and sufficient sterile water to make 30 mL.

its preparation by lyophilization (Fig. 14.11). Powders so treated form a honeycomb, lattice structure that is rapidly penetrated by the liquid, and solution is rapidly effected because of the large surface area of powder exposed.

Upjohn-Pharmacia has a newer Mix-O-Vial that incorporates the cover as part of the plunger. Once mixed, the small circle of plastic that covers the injection site is removed. This reduces the touch contamination potential.

The Abbott ADD-Vantage System IVPH is another example of a ready-to-mix sterile IV product designed for intermittent IV administration of potent drugs that do not have long-term stability in solution. With this system, antibiotics and other

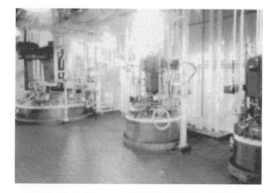

Fig. 14.9 *Fermentation tank in the preparation of antibiotics. (Courtesy of Schering-Plough.)*

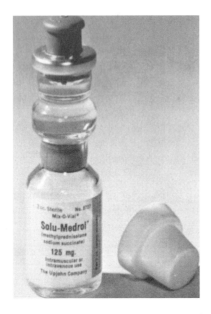

Fig. 14.10   *The Mix-O-Vial shown above is a combination vial containing dry ingredients in the bottom compartment and a liquid diluent in the top compartment, separated by a specially formulated center seal. The bottom compartment can either be liquid filled, frozen and dried to make a lyophilized product, or it may be powder filled. The top diluent contains a preservative and may or may not contain one or more active ingredients. To use the vial, the dust cover is removed (as shown above), pressure is applied with the thumb to the top plunger which dislodges the center seal and the vial is shaken until the solution is effected. The top of the plunger is then swabbed with a disinfectant; the syringe needle inserted through the target circle on the plunger and the contents of the vial withdrawn into the syringe. The Mix-O-Vial offers stability of product (until it is activated), convenience, fast operation and safety as regards the right drug with the proper diluent in the correct proportions. (Courtesy of The Upjohn Company.)*

drugs do not have to be mixed until just prior to administration.

ADD-Vantage consists of two components (Fig. 14.12): a flexible plastic IV container partially filled with diluent and a glass vial of powdered or liquid drug. The vials containing the medication and the piggybacks (i.e., 50–250 mL of Dextrose 5% in Water Injection [D_5W] or Normal Saline Solution [NSS]) are specially designed to be used together. The vial locks into a chamber inside the plastic container, and the drug is released by removing the stopper on the vial, allowing the two components to mix. This simple process is performed by external manipulation of the container, thereby preserving the closed, sterile system.

The ADD-Vantage unit may be assembled in a number of locations. Microbiological tests and sterility tests have been conducted at various intervals following assembly of the units under a laminar flow hood, in a pharmacy on a countertop and in a patient's hospital room. The final admixtures were sterile, demonstrating that the ADD-Vantage unit can be aseptically assembled under the conditions tested. However, whenever possible, this system should be assembled under a laminar flow hood.

The assembled, but not activated ADD-Vantage System can be used within 30 days from the date that the diluent container was removed from the overwrap. ADD-Vantage enables hospitals to reduce drug waste, often caused by cancelled or changed prescriptions, and helps the pharmacy conserve labor and reduce material costs.

The Monovial Safety Guard (Becton Dickinson Pharmaceutical Systems) is a new IV infusion sys-

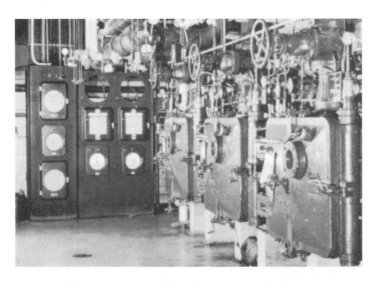

Fig. 14.11   *Antibiotic lyophilizers. (Courtesy of Abbott Laboratories.)*

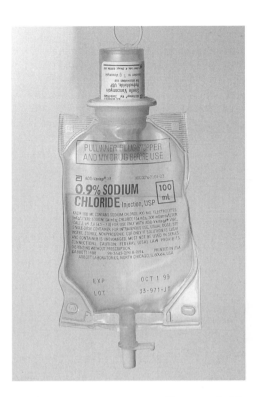

Fig. 14.12 *ADD-Vantage system. (Courtesy of Abbott Laboratories.)*

tem for use in preparing extemporaneous small-volume infusions utilizing plastic minibags (Fig. 14.13). When compared to the two traditional methods of preparing small-volume infusions, i.e., the transfer needle and vial (TFN) method, the syringe and vial (SYR) method, the Monovial system performed quite favorably by saving time, used fewer materials, and was less costly (12).

This system is an integrated device (i.e., drug, transfer mechanism) with a protective shield surrounding the attached transfer needle. The reconstitution and transfer of the drug into an infusion bag is accomplished safely, quickly, and necessitates fewer materials. The needle is inserted into the port of the infusion bag and then the transfer set is pushed down toward the vial until a "click" is heard. With the Monovial upright, the infusion bag is squeezed several times to transfer fluid into the Monovial. The Monovial is then shaken a few times to reconstitute the drug. It is then inverted and then the minibag is squeezed and released to transfer the drug back into the infusion bag. This process is repeated until the vial is empty. Presently, diltiazem HCl (i.e.,

Cardizem) for injection is available with the Monovial Safety Guard.

Several manufacturers now ship to the hospital pharmacy reconstituted intravenous antibiotic solutions, e.g., cefazolin sodium, in the frozen state. When thawed these nonpyrogenic solutions are stable for a finite amount of time, e.g., reconstituted cefazolin is stable for 48 hours at room temperature and for 10 days refrigerated (5°C). The product is packaged in a small plastic bag for piggy-back use in intravenous administration to the patient.

Packaging, Labeling, and Storage of Injections

Containers for injections, including the closures, must not interact physically or chemically with the preparation so as to alter its strength or efficacy (Fig. 14.14). If the container is made of glass, it must be clear and colorless or of a light amber color to permit the inspection of its contents. The type of glass suitable and preferred for each parenteral preparation is usually stated in the individual monograph. Injections are placed either in single-dose containers or in multiple-dose containers (Figs. 14.15 through 14.17). By definition:

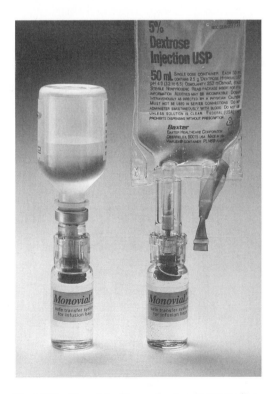

Fig. 14.13 *Monovial safety guard system. (Courtesy of Becton-Dickinson.)*

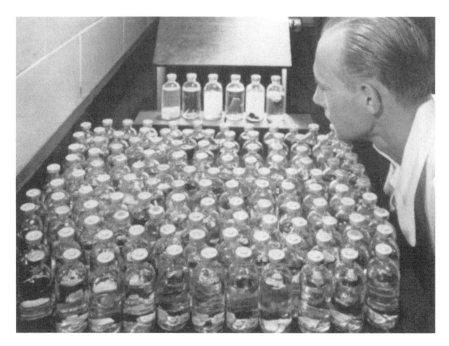

Fig. 14.14   *Testing compatibility of rubber closures with the solution with which they are in contact. (Courtesy of Abbott Laboratories.)*

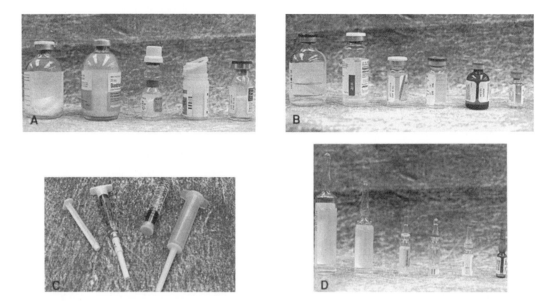

Fig. 14.15   *Examples of packaging of injectable products. A, Multiple-dose vials of suspensions and dry powders. B,Vials for solutions, including one with light-protective glass. C, Unit dose, disposable syringes. D,Various sizes of ampuls. (Courtesy of William B. French, PhD.)*

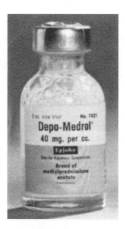

Fig. 14.16 *A typical vial used for sterile injectable products. It is made from Type I (borosilicate) glass. The rubber closure has been specially selected as regards compatibility with the product, desirable physical characteristics, etc. The overseal holds the closure in place and provides a means for ready access to the contents of the vial. (Courtesy of the Upjohn Company.)*

Single-dose container—A single-dose container is a hermetic container holding a quantity of sterile drug intended for parenteral administration as a single dose, and which when opened cannot be re-sealed with assurance that sterility has been maintained.

Multiple-dose container—A multiple-dose container is a hermetic container that permits withdrawal of successive portions of the contents without changing the strength, quality, or purity of the remaining portion.

Single-dose containers may be ampuls or single-dose vials. Ampuls (Fig. 14.18) are sealed by fusion of the glass container under aseptic conditions (Figs. 14.19, 14.20). The glass container is made so as to have a neck portion that may be easily separated from the body of the container without fragmentation of the glass. After opening, the contents of the ampul should be withdrawn into a syringe with a 5-μm filter needle/straw apparatus. The filter needle or straw is then replaced with a regular needle. The filter needle or straw is used to trap any glass particles that have entered the sterile solution when the neck of the ampul was broken. Otherwise, if a filter needle is not available, the withdrawal of glass can be minimized by holding the ampul in the upright position, tilted slightly, when inserting the needle, and avoiding the outer surface of the neck of the ampul. The needle should not be lowered to the bottom of the ampul, but held slightly above, to avoid drawing glass particulate matter into the syringe.

Once opened, the ampul cannot be resealed, and any unused portion may not be retained and used at a later time, since the contents would have questionable sterility. Some injectable products are packaged in pre-filled syringes, with or without special administration devices (Figs. 14.21 to 14.23). The types of glass for parenteral product containers have already been pointed out in Chapter 5, and the student should recall that Types I, II, and III are suitable for parenteral products, with Type I being the most resistant to chemical deterioration. The type of glass to be used as the container for a particular injection is indicated in the individual monograph for that preparation.

One of the prime requisites of solutions for parenteral administration is clarity. They should be sparkling clear and free of all particulate matter, that is, all of the mobile, undissolved substances which are unintentionally present. Included are such contaminants as dust, cloth fibers, glass fragments, material leached from the glass or plastic containers or seals, and any other material which may find its way into the product during its manufacture or administration, or develop during storage.

To prevent the entrance of unwanted particles into parenteral products, a number of precautions

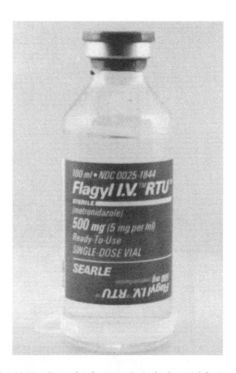

Fig. 14.17 *Example of a 100 mL single-dose vial for intravenous infusion in ready-to-use (RTU) form. (Courtesy of Searle Pharmaceuticals, Inc.)*

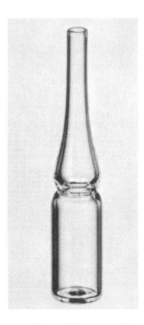

Fig. 14.18 *Ampul, before filling and sealing. (Courtesy of Owens Illinois.)*

must be taken during the manufacture, storage, and use of the products. During manufacture, for instance, the parenteral solution is usually final filtered before being placed into the parenteral containers. The containers are carefully selected to be chemically resistant to the solution being added

and of the highest available quality to minimize the chances of container components being leached into the solution. It has been recognized for some time, that some of the particulate matter found in parenteral products is generated from leached material from the glass or plastic containers. Once the container is selected for use, it must be carefully cleaned to be free of all extraneous matter (Fig. 14.24). During container-filling, extreme care must be exercised to prevent the entrance of air-borne dust, lint or other contaminants into the container. The provision of filtered and directed air flow in production areas is useful in reducing the likelihood of contamination. Laminar flow hoods have been developed which allow for the draft-free flow of clean, filtered air over the work area. These hoods are commonly found in the hospital setting for both the manufacture and the incorporation of additives into parenteral and ophthalmic products (Fig. 14.25). The personnel involved in the manufacture of parenterals must be made acutely aware of the importance of cleanliness and aseptic techniques. They are provided uniforms made of monofilament fabrics that do not shed lint. They wear face hoods, caps, gloves, and disposable shoe covers to prevent contamination (Fig. 14.26).

After the containers are filled and hermetically sealed, they are visually (Fig. 14.27) or automatically (Fig. 14.28) inspected for particulate matter. Usually an inspector passes the filled container

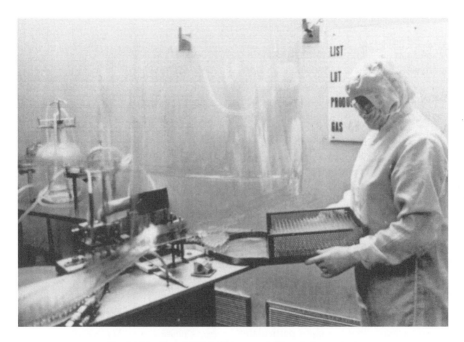

Fig. 14.19 *Ampul filling. (Courtesy of Abbott Laboratories.)*

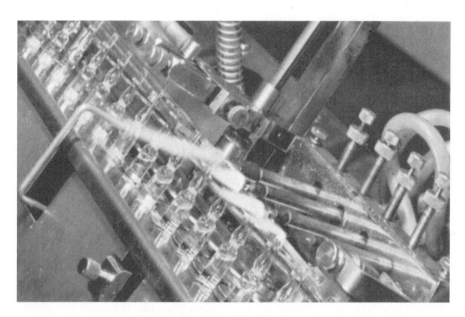

Fig. 14.20   *Ampul sealing. (Courtesy of Abbott Laboratories.)*

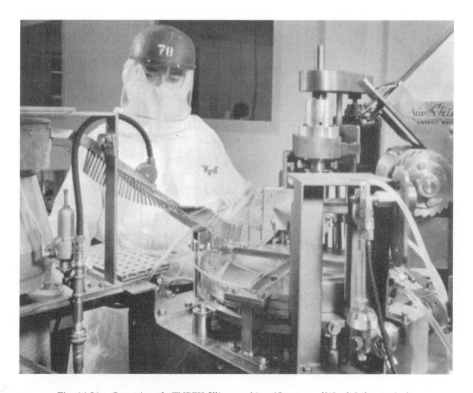

Fig. 14.21   *Operation of a TUBEX filling machine. (Courtesy of Wyeth Laboratories.)*

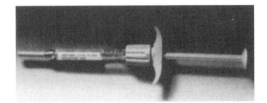

Fig. 14.22 *Tubex Injector. The ribbed collar and plunger rod securely hold a glass sterile cartridge-needle unit. Each prefilled unit contains a dose of medication with an attached sterile needle. After administration, the cartridge-needle unit is discarded; the Injector is reusable. (Courtesy of Wyeth-Ayerst Laboratories.)*

past a light source with a black background to observe for mobile particles. Particles of approximately 50 μm in size may be detected in this manner. Reflective particles, such as fragments of glass, may be visualized in smaller size, about 25 μm in size. Other methods are used to detect particulate matter smaller than that which may be detected by the unaided eye including microscopic examinations as well as the use of sophisticated equipment as the Coulter Counter which electronically counts particles present in a sample presented to it. Once past the inspection following production the product may be labeled. Prior to its use, however, the pharmacist should inspect each parenteral solution dispensed for evidence of particulate matter.

Although the total significance of injecting or infusing parenteral solutions containing particulate matter into a patient has not been ascertained, it is apparent that particulate matter has the potential of inducing thrombi and vessel blockage and depending upon the chemical composition of the particles the additional potential for introducing

into the patient chemical agents which are undesired and possibly toxic.

In formulating a single-dose parenteral product, the pharmacist must consider not only the physicochemical aspects of the drug, but also the intended therapeutic use of the product itself. Some single-dose preparations are prepared to be administered rapidly in small volumes, but other preparations are allowed to infuse slowly into the circulatory system over a period of hours. Most small-volume parenterals are formulated so that a convenient amount of solution, say 0.5 to 2 mL, contains the usual dose of the drug although larger volumes of more diluted solutions are frequently administered intravenously and intramuscularly. Generally, several strengths of injections of a given drug are marketed to permit a wider dosage selection by the physician without being wasteful of the drug as would be the case if only part of a given single-dose parenteral solution was administered. The large-volume, single-dose preparations generally are those solutions used to expand the blood volume or to replenish nutrients or electrolytes and are given by slow intravenous infusion. However, in no instance may a single-dose parenteral container permit the withdrawal and administration of greater than 1000 mL. In addition, preparations intended for intraspinal, intracisternal, or peridural administration must be packaged only in single-dose containers as a precaution against contamination.

Frequently in the hospital, a physician may order an additional agent to be placed in a large-volume parenteral solution for infusion. In these instances, the person filling such an order must be certain that aseptic conditions are employed and that the additive is compatible with the contents of the original large volume parenteral solution (13). Care must also be exercised not to introduce particulate matter into

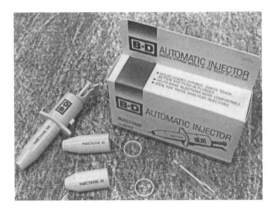

Fig. 14.23 *Inject-Ease automatically inserts the needle of an insulin syringe into the skin when activated. (Courtesy of William B. French, PhD.)*

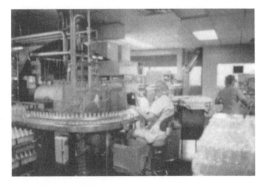

Fig. 14.24 *Production line in the preparation of vials for sterilization and filling. (Courtesy of Schering-Plough.)*

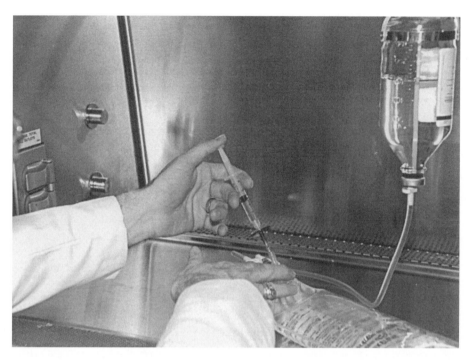

Fig. 14.25   *Hyperalimentation being prepared in a vertical laminae flow hood using millipore sterilization. (Courtesy of William B. French, PhD.)*

the solution. Many pharmaceutical companies have developed special devices for the aseptic transfer of pharmaceutical additives to large volume parenterals. An ordinary sterile needle and syringe, preferably affixed with a filtering device, may be effectively employed to transfer solutions from one parenteral product to another (Fig. 14.29). Many hospital pharmacies have established well controlled *IV additive* or *admixture* programs to assure additive-solution compatibility, safety and efficacy (14).

Multiple-dose containers are affixed with rubber closures to permit the penetration of a hypodermic needle without the removal or destruction of the closure. Upon withdrawing the needle from the container, the closure reseals and protects the contents from airborne contamination. The needle may be inserted to withdraw a portion of the prepared liquid injection, or it may be used to introduce a solvent or vehicle to a dry powder intended for injection. In either instance, the sterility of the injection may be maintained so long as the needle itself is sterile at the time of entry into the container. It

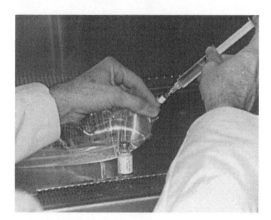

Fig. 14.26   *Pharmacist preparing a parenteral admixture in a laminar flow hood. (Courtesy of William B. French, PhD.)*

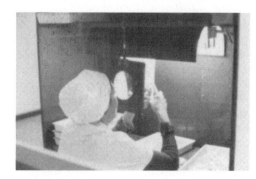

Fig. 14.27   *Industrial inspection of parenteral fluid for particulate matter. (Courtesy of Schering-Plough.)*

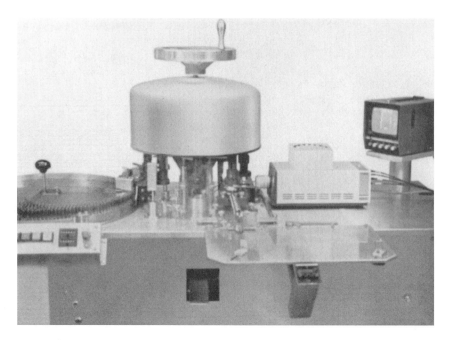

Fig. 14.28 *The AUTOSKAN industrial automatic inspection machine which detects the presence of particulate matter in injectables with a television camera and electronics, and automatically rejects them from the production line. (Courtesy of Lakso Company, Inc.)*

should be recalled that unless otherwise indicated in the monograph, multiple-dose injectables are required to contain added antibacterial preservatives. Also, unless otherwise specified, multiple-dose containers are not permitted to allow the withdrawal of greater than 30 mL in order to limit the number of penetrations made into the closure and thus protect against loss of sterility. The limited volume also guards against an excessive amount of antibacterial preservative being inadvertently co-administered with the drug when unusually large doses of an injection are required, in which case a non-preserved single-dose preparation is advisable. The usual multiple-dose container contains about ten usual doses of the injection, but quantity may vary greatly with the individual preparation and manufacturer.

Because it is impossible in practice to transfer the entire volume of a single-dose container or the last dose in a multiple-dose container into a hypodermic syringe, a slight excess in volume of the contents of ampuls and vials over the labeled "size" or volume of the package is permitted. Table 14.2 presents the recommended "overages" permitted by the USP to allow the withdrawal and administration of the labeled volumes.

For labeling purposes, a revised injectable product nomenclature process became official in the *United States Pharmacopeia* 23 (USP 23) on January

1, 1995. The main points of the revised process were as follows:

1. The term "Sterile" was eliminated from the titles of injectable products with the exception of appropriate monograph titles for WATER that are intended for parenteral use, e.g., Sterile Water for Injection.
2. For established names of injectable products, all

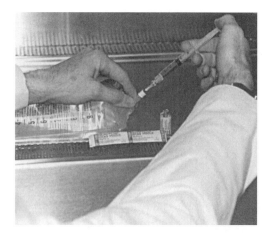

Fig. 14.29 *Utilization of a filter syringe for the aseptic addition of an additive to a large-volume parenteral solution. (Courtesy of William B. French, PhD.)*

Table 14.2. Recommended Overages for Official Parenteral Products

Labeled Size, mL	Excess Volume for Mobile Liquids, mL	Excess Volume for Viscous Liquids, mL
0.5	0.10	0.12
1.0	0.10	0.15
2.0	0.15	0.25
5.0	0.30	0.50
10.0	0.50	0.70
20.0	0.60	0.90
30.0	0.80	1.20
50.0 or more	2%	3%

of which are suitable for, and intended for parenteral administration, USP established the following criteria in determining the product's title:

a. Liquids

    1) *[Drug] Injection*—Title for liquid preparations that are drug substances or solutions thereof.

    2) *[Drug] Injectable Suspension*—Title for liquid preparations of solids suspended in a suitable liquid medium.

    3) *[Drug] Injectable Emulsion*—Title for liquid preparations of drug substances dissolved or dispersed in suitable emulsion medium.

b. Solids

    1) *[Drug] for Injection*—Title for dry solids that, upon the addition of suitable vehicles, yield solutions conforming in all respects to the requirements for *Injections*.

    2) *[Drug] for Injectable Suspension*—Title for dry solids that, upon the addition of suitable vehicles, yield preparations conforming in all respects to the requirements for *Injectable Suspensions*.

To facilitate this transition to a new nomenclature, the Center for Drug Evaluation and Research encouraged parenteral drug manufacturers to place a "flag" or reminder statement on the labels of the product for a six month period alerting practitioners to the changes. The intent was to facilitate practitioners becoming familiar with the revised rules. An example of a "flag" would be: "FORMERLY STERILE [Drug Name]."

In addition, the labels on containers of parenteral products must state: 1) the name of the preparation; 2) for a liquid preparation, the percentage content of drug or the amount of drug present in a specified volume, or for a dry preparation, the amount of active ingredient present and the volume of liquid to be added to the dry preparation to prepare a solution or suspension; 3) the route of administration; 4) a statement of storage conditions and an expiration date; 5) the name of the manufacturer and distributor; 6) an identifying lot number, which is capable of yielding the complete manufacturing history of the specific package, including all manufacturing, filling, sterilizing, and labeling operations. Injections for veterinary use are labeled to that effect. Preparations intended to be used as dialysis, hemofiltration or irrigation solutions should meet the requirements for injections, except those relating to volume present in the containers, and should bear a statement indicating that the solution is not intended for use by intravenous infusion. All containers appropriately labeled should allow a sufficient area of the container to remain free of label for its full length or circumference to permit inspection of the contents. Any injection which upon visual inspection reveals particulate matter other than normally suspended material should be discarded.

Each individual monograph for the official injection states the type of container (single-dose and/or multiple-dose) permitted for the injection, the type of glass preferred for the container, exemptions, if any, to usual package-size limitations, and any special storage instructions. Most injections prepared from chemically pure medicinal agents are stable at room temperature and may be stored without special concern or conditions. However, most biological products—insulin injection and the various vaccines, toxoids, toxins, and related products—are usually stored under refrigeration. Reference should be made to the individual monograph to find the proper storage temperature for a particular injection.

Quality Assurance for Pharmacy-Prepared Sterile Products

The American Society of Health System Pharmacists (formerly, the American Society of Hospital Pharmacists) publishes annually a technical assistance bulletin (TAB) on quality assurance for pharmacy-prepared sterile products (15). The TAB was developed to help pharmacists establish quality assurance procedures for the component of practice that encompasses the preparation of sterile products. The recommendations of the TAB are appropriate to all practice settings in which pharmacists directly serve patients (e.g., hospitals, community pharmacies, nursing homes, home health care). Note that these are not intended to apply to the manufacturing of sterile pharmaceuticals as defined in state and federal laws and regulations. Nor are they to apply the preparation of medications (i.e., by pharmacists, nurses, physicians) intended for immediate administration (i.e., minimal delay between preparation and administration) to patients.

The term *sterile products* used within the TAB refers to sterile or nutritional substances that are prepared (e.g., compounded or repackaged) by pharmacy personnel, using aseptic technique and other quality assurance procedures.

The objectives of these recommendations are to enable pharmacists to provide:

1. Information to pharmacists on quality assurance and quality control activities that may be applied to the preparation of sterile products in pharmacies, and
2. A scheme to match quality assurance and qual-

ity control activities with the potential risks to patients posed by various types of products.

The TAB defines the purpose of these recommendations and encourages pharmacists to participate in quality improvement, risk management, and infection control programs within their organizations. In doing so, pharmacists would be expected to report findings about quality assurance in sterile products to appropriate staffs or committees, and to cooperate with managers of quality improvement, risk management, and infection control to develop optimal sterile product procedures.

Originally, in February 1992, the then American Society of Hospital Pharmacists had proposed guidelines that formed the basis of TAB (16). This original document distinguished between quality control (QC) and quality assurance (QA). By definition, *quality control* is the acceptance or rejection of raw materials and packaging components, in-process test materials, and inspections (17). *Quality assurance* is a systematic method to identify problems in patient care that are resolved via administrative, clinical, or educational actions to ensure that final products and outcomes meet applicable specifications (17).

The TAB classifies sterile products into three levels based on risk to the patient. The risk levels range

Table 14.3.   ASHP Risk Level Classification of Pharmacy-Prepared Sterile Products[15]

Risk Level 1

1. Products
   A. Stored at room temperature and completely administered within 28 hours of preparation; or
   B. Stored under refrigeration for 7 days or less before complete administration to a patient over a period not to exceed 24 hours; or
   C. Frozen for 30 days or less before complete administration to a patient over a period not to exceed 24 hours.
2. Unpreserved sterile products prepared for administration to one patient, or batch-prepared products containing suitable preservatives prepared for administration to more than one patient.
3. Products prepared by closed-system aseptic transfer of sterile, nonpyrogenic, finished pharmaceuticals obtained from licensed manufacturers into sterile final containers (e.g., syringe, minibag, portable infusion-device cassette) obtained from licensed manufacturers.

Risk Level 2

1. Products stored beyond 7 days under refrigeration, or stored beyond 30 days frozen, or administered beyond 28 hours after preparation and storage at room temperature.
2. Batch-prepared products without preservatives that are intended for use by more than one patient. (*Note:* Batch-prepared products without preservatives that will be administered to multiple patients carry a greater risk to the patients than products prepared for a single patient because of the potential effect of product contamination on the health and well-being of a larger patient group.)
3. Products compounded by combining multiple sterile ingredients, obtained from licensed manufacturers, in a sterile reservoir, obtained from a licensed manufacturer, by using closed-system aseptic transfer before subdivision into multiple units to be dispensed to patients.

Risk Level 3 Products Exhibit Either Characteristic 1 or 2

1. Products compounded from nonsterile ingredients or compounded with nonsterile components, containers, or equipment, or
2. Products prepared by combining multiple ingredients—sterile or nonsterile—by using an open-system transfer or open reservoir before terminal sterilization or subdivision into multiple units to be dispensed.

from the least potential risk (level 1) to the greatest potential risk (level 3). The classification system is designed only to assist the pharmacist in selecting sterile preparation procedures. Pharmacists must exercise professional judgment in deciding which risk level applies to a specific sterile product or situation. Factors that increase risk (e.g., multiple system breaks, compounding complexities, high-risk administration sites, immunocompromised patients, microbial growth potential of the product, storage conditions) must be weighed by the pharmacist.

There will be situations when the pharmacist must make risk vs. benefit decisions to prepare these products outside of the guidelines (e.g., the preparation of a sterile investigational drug in a compassionate-use protocol for a lifesaving effort). The risk assignments listed in Table 14.3 provide a logical template within which the pharmacist can evaluate risk. These do not, however, preclude the possibility of alternative, logical arrangements that could be based upon scientific information and professional judgment.

Risk level 1 represents the minimum QA guidelines. In risk levels 2 and 3, products must meet or exceed each of the risk level 1 guidelines. In those instances where the risk level assignment might be nebulous, guidelines for the higher risk level should be followed.

The TAB delineates the quality assurance components for each risk level. These include: policies and procedures; personnel education, training, and evaluation; process validation; storage and handling; facilities and equipment; garb; aseptic technique and product preparation; process evaluation; expiration dating; labeling; end-product evaluation; and documentation. Specific recommendations germane to each of these components at each risk level are made in the TAB; the reader may refer to them for additional information.

Available Injections

There are hundreds of injections on the market of various medicinal agents. Tables 14.4 through 14.7 present some examples of those packaged in small-volume and large-volume containers, the latter for intravenous infusion.

Small Volume Parenterals

Table 14.4 presents some commonly employed injections given in small volume. Some of these injections are solutions and others suspensions.

Premixed intravenous delivery systems have simplified the delivery process for small-volume parenterals in particular. A distinct advantage of these ready-to-use systems is that they require little or no manipulation to make them patient specific, and thus a viable alternative to the traditional labor-intensive method of compounding parenteral medications from partial-fill (i.e., individual dose/multiple doses of IV medications) vials and an appropriate parenteral solution. Since the introduction of the first ready-to-use systems in the late 1970s, the availability and variety of systems has increased (e.g., Baxter Healthcare Corporation, Kendall McGaw Laboratories, Abbott Laboratories) (refer to Table 14.5).

The traditional method for preparing small-volume parenteral therapy for patient-specific use from a partial-fill drug vial into a minibag can be labor-intensive and costly (e.g., labor supply and inventory costs for materials such as syringes and needles). The savings accrued through ready-to-use systems can be significant and have been documented (18). Another key advantage of these systems is extended stability dating and reduced wastage. Doses can be put together (but not activated) in cycles, then activated just prior to patient use and delivered to the nursing station by the pharmacy personnel (18).

The down side of these ready-to-use small parenteral products is that they do not offer flexibility in changing the volume or concentration of the product. This may then pose a problem to the fluid-restricted patient (18). But, the introduction of minibags in volumes of 100 mL, 50 mL, and 25 mL, have helped this problem somewhat. Another disadvantage of the ready-to-use products is that some manufacturers' premixed products require thawing. Microwave use for quick thawing poses stability problems for some of these products (e.g., cefazolin, cephalothin). For example, the high energy source of the microwave oven could cause a structural alteration of the cephalothin molecule. Another possibility is that of leaching of substance from the rubber stopper when frozen ampuls of Neutral Keflin are thawed using the microwave.

General precautions (19) required with the use of microwave ovens for thawing frozen premixed products include:

1. Being aware that the possibility of radiation leakage does exist. However, manufacturers of microwave ovens are required by law to comply with federal standards.
2. Safeguarding pharmacy personnel who are exposed to these ovens, especially those with cardiac pacemakers.
3. The possible leaching of rubber stopper material when the rubber material on the container is exposed to microwave heating.

Table 14.4.   Examples of Some Injections Usually Packaged and Administered in Small Volume

Injection	Physical Form	Category and Comments
Butorphanol Tartrate Injection	solution	Narcotic Agonist-Antagonist Analgesic; administered IM or IV for relief of moderate to severe pain and as a preoperative or preanesthesia medication.
Chlorpromazine HCl Injection	solution	An antipsychotic drug with antiemetic (antidopaminergic) effects, this drug should not be administered sub-Q. It's injection should be IM slowly, deep into upper outer quadrant of the buttocks. Avoid injecting directly into the vein. The IV route is used ONLY for severe hiccoughs, surgery, or tetanus.
Cimetidine HCl Injection	solution	Histamine H_2 antagonist; administered IM or IV for patients with pathological GI hypersecretory conditions or intractable ulcers.
Dalteparin Sodium Injection	solution	A sterile, low molecular weight heparin which is indicated for prophylaxis against deep vein thrombosis (DVT) in patients undergoing abdominal surgery who are at risk. Available in a prefilled syringe, it is administered Sub-Q.
Dexamethasone Sodium Phosphate Injection	solution	Glucocorticoid; administered IM or IV for cerebral edema and unresponsive shock. Also used intra-articular, intralesional or soft tissue for joints, bursae, and ganglia.
Digoxin Injection	solution	Cardiotonic given IM (not preferred) or IV with highly individualized and monitored dosage.
Dihydroergotamine Mesylate Injection	solution	Alpha-adrenergic blocking agent specific in migraine, given IM or IV.
Diphenhydramine HCl Injection	solution	An ethanolamine, non-selective antihistamine administered intravenously or intramuscularly when oral administration is impractical and indicated for Type I (i.e., immediate) hypersensitivity reactions and active treatment of motion sickness.
Furosemide Injection	solution	Loop diuretic; administered IM or IV [slowly] for edema or acute pulmonary edema.
Granisetron HCl Injection	solution	5-HT_3 receptor antagonist indicated for the prevention of nausea and vomiting associated with initial and repeat courses of emetogenic cancer therapy, including high-dose cisplatin.
Heparin Sodium Injection	solution	Anticoagulant administered IV or SubQ, as indicated by activated partial prothrombin time (APTT) or actuated coagulation time (ACT).
Hydromorphone HCl Injection	solution	Narcotic analgesic used for the relief of moderate to severe pain; administered subcutaneously or IM or by slow IV injection.
Ibutilide Fumarate Injection	solution	An antiarrhythmic drug with predominantly class III (i.e., cardiac action potential prolongation) properties according to the Vaughn Williams Classification that is infused intravenously undiluted or diluted in 50 ml diluent.
Iron Dextran Injection	solution	A hematinic agent administered intravenously or intramuscularly for the treatment of patients with documented iron deficiency in whom oral administration is unsatisfactory or impossible.
Isoproterenol HCl Injection	solution	Adrenergic (bronchodilator) given IM, SubQ, or IV.
Ketorolac Tromethamine Injection	solution	Available in Tubex® syringes for IV/IM dosing, this NSAID is indicated for the short-term ($<$ 5 days) management of moderately severe, acute pain that requires analgesia at the opioid level, usually in a postoperative setting.
Lidocaine HCl Injection	solution	Cardiac depressant given IV as an antiarrhythmic; also as a local anesthetic, epidurally, by infiltration, and in peripheral nerve block.
Magnesium Sulfate Injection	solution	Anticonvulsant/electrolyte; administered by IM or direct IV injection, IV infusion, or in other IV infusions for management of convulsive toxemia of pregnancy, hyperalimentation therapy, mild magnesium deficiency, or severe hypomagnesemia.
Meperidine HCl Injection	solution	Narcotic analgesic given IM, SubQ, or slow continuous IV infusion.

continued

Table 14.4. Examples of Some Injections Usually Packaged and Administered in Small Volume

Injection	Physical Form	Category and Comments
Metoclopramide Monohydrochloride Injection	solution	Gastrointestinal stimulant; administered IM, direct IV, or slowly as an IV admixture for the prevention of chemotherapy-induced emesis.
Midazolam HCl Injection	solution	A short-acting benzodiazepine CNS depressant administered IV or IM and indicated for preoperative sedation, anxiolysis and amnesia.
Morphine Sulfate Injection	solution	Narcotic analgesic. IM, IV, PCA.
Nalbuphine HCl Injection	solution	Narcotic Agonist-Antagonist Analgesic; administered SC, IM or IV for relief of moderate to severe pain and for preoperative analgesia.
Naloxone HCl Injection	solution	A narcotic antagonist which prevents or reverses the effects of opioids including respiratory depression, sedation and hypotension; administered IV, IM, or subcutaneously.
Oxytocin Injection	solution	Oxytocic, given IM (erratic) or IV obstetrically for the therapeutic induction of labor.
Phenytoin Sodium Injection	solution	Anticonvulsant; administered IM [erratic absorption] as a prophylactic dosage for neurosurgery or IV [slowly] for status epilepticus.
Phytonadione Injection	dispersion	Vitamin K (prothrombogenic) employed in hemorrhagic situations. An aqueous dispersion of phytonadione, a viscous liquid.
Procaine Penicillin G Injection	suspension	Anti-infective; administered IM for moderately severe infections due to penicillin-G sensitive microorganisms.
Prochlorperazine Edisylate Injection	solution	Antidopaminergic; administered IM or IV for control of severe nausea and vomiting associated with adult surgery.
Propranolol HCl Injection	solution	A beta-adrenergic receptor blocking agent indicated in the management of hypertension. Oral dosage (tablets) is usual; intravenous administration is reserved for life-threatening arrhythmias or those occurring under anesthesia.
Sodium Bicarbonate Injection	solution	Electrolyte; administered IV, either undiluted or diluted in other IV fluids for cardiac arrest and in less urgent forms of metabolic acidosis.
Sumatriptan Succinate Injection	solution	A selective 5-hydroxytryptamine$_1$ receptor, subtype agonist, used for acute migraine attacks with or without aura. Self-administered SubQ from unit-of-use syringes and *SELFdose* unit.
Verapamil HCl Injection	solution	Calcium channel blocking agent; administered as a slow IV injection over at least 2 minutes for supraventricular tachyarrhythmias.

4. A possible explosion that may result from the increase in internal pressure as a result of placing a closed or sealed container into the microwave oven.
5. The possibility of unequal distribution of heat because microwave ovens do produce heterogeneous heat.
6. Developing protocols to ensure that the final solution temperature does not exceed room temperature.

Some manufacturers allow frozen premixed products to be warmed using a water bath, but warn not to submerge during the thawing process because there is a distinct possibility that water from the bath could enter and contaminate the contents of the dosage form. Forced clean air at 25° C flowing over the bags may help. In fact, using an old laminar flow hood for thawing has been used with some success. However, room temperature thawing is a lengthy process. Thus, appropriate planning is required so that large numbers of these products that are thawed in advance are used and recycled efficiently. Otherwise, these small-volume parenteral products potentially increase waste. Finally, getting a prescription label to adhere to a thawed minibag can be a problem.

The available ready-to-use systems have not demonstrated much impact in the pediatric and neonatal population. The unique dosing and fluid requirements of these patients make these systems inappropriate. In some institutions, the unique dosing and fluid requirements of pediatric and neonate

Table 14.5.   Representative Marketed Frozen, Premixed Products Illustrating Stability Data Frozen and After Thawing[a]

Drug	Diluent	Expiration Dating			
		Storage Stability	Frozen Stability	Refrigerated Stability	Room Temperature
Aztreonam 1g, 2g	Iso-osmotic in dextrose, 50 mL	Frozen	18 months	14 days	48 hours
Cefazolin sodium 500 mg, 1 g	Iso-osmotic in dextrose, 50 mL	Frozen	24 months	30 days	48 hours
Cefotaxime sodium, 1g, 2g	Iso-osmotic in dextrose, 50 mL	Frozen	15 months	10 days	24 hours
Cefoxitin sodium 1g, 2g	Iso-osmotic in dextrose, 50 mL	Frozen	18 months	21 days	24 hours
Ceftazidime sodium 1g, 2g	Iso-osmotic in dextrose, 50 mL	Frozen	9 months	7 days	24 hours
Ceftizoxime sodium 1g, 2g	Iso-osmotic in dextrose, 50 mL	Frozen	12 months	28 days	48 hours
Ceftriazone sodium 1g, 2g	Iso-osmotic in dextrose, 50 mL	Frozen	15 months	21 days	72 hours
Ticarcillin disodium and clavulanate potassium	Iso-osmotic in Water for Injection, 100 mL	Frozen	6 months	7 days	24 hours
Vancomycin HCl 500 mg	Iso-osmotic in dextrose, 100 mL	Frozen	12 months	30 days	72 hours

[a]Stability information provided by Baxter Healthcare Corporation.

patients are addressed by making dilutions of medications to standardized concentrations, filling and capping individual syringes, and administering these doses through a syringe pump.

Among the most used of the small volume injections are the various insulin preparations. Insulin, the active principle of the pancreas gland, is primarily concerned with the metabolism of carbohydrates, but also influences protein and fat metabolism. Insulin facilitates the cellular uptake of glucose and its metabolism in liver, muscle, and adipose tissue. It increases the uptake of amino acids and inhibits the breakdown of fats and the production of ketones. Insulin is administered to patients having abnormal or absent pancreatic beta cell function to restore glucose metabolism and maintain satisfactory carbohydrate, fat, and protein metabolism. It is used in the treatment of *diabetes mellitus,* in instances in which the condition cannot be controlled satisfactorily by dietary regulation alone or by oral hypoglycemic drugs. Insulin may also be used to improve the appetite and increase the weight in selected cases of nondiabetic malnutrition and is frequently added to intravenous infusions.

Insulin is administered by needle or jet injection (Figs. 14.30, 14.31, 14.32). A system for the

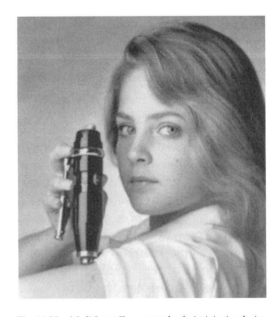

Fig. 14.30   *Medi-Jector II, an example of a jet injection device. The jet injection method utilizes pressure rather than a needle in providing the subcutaneous distribution of an injectable medication. The device shown can be used with U-100 insulin or a combination of insulins and can deliver 2 to 100 units in half-unit increments. (Courtesy of Derata Corporation.)*

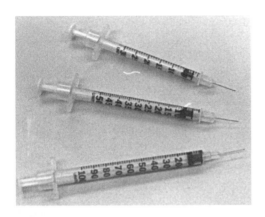

Fig. 14.31 *Examples of insulin syringes calibrated in units. (Courtesy of William B. French, PhD.)*

nasal administration of insulin is presently under study.

Since its introduction, U-100 insulin has been suggested as a replacement for the U-40 insulin strength, with the intention of making U-100 the single strength for in-home use by the patient. In December 1991, Eli Lilly announced that it would cease further production of U-40 insulins, and subsequently other insulin manufacturers also decided to cease production of this strength. The basis for this decision was a lack of patient demand (i.e., very low numbers of patient utilizing this strength). Recognizing, however, that lower strengths of insulin (i.e., under 100 U/mL) might still be needed (e.g., small children, veterinarian use), Lilly markets a diluting fluid for the Regular, NPH, and Lente insulins of U-100 strength. This fluid can be used to prepare any strength of insulin below 100 U/mL.

Age-associated sight difficulties and the vision deterioration associated with diabetes can interfere significantly with buying and using insulin products. Therefore, packaging of insulins must make allowances for the visual deficits of patients with diabetes. To facilitate identification of the proper medication at the site of purchase, the arrangement and size of the package lettering must make it easy for the insulin-dependent patient to recognize the insulin type and concentration of the product. In the case of Humulin insulins, an international symbol also appears on the cartons and bottles of all formulations. These symbols help assure that patients with diabetes secure the correct Humulin formulation anywhere in the world.

Insulin Injection (Regular)

Insulin Injection is a sterile aqueous solution of insulin. Commercially, the solution is prepared from beef or pork pancreas or both or through biosynthetic means (Human Insulin), discussed in the next section. The source must be stated on the labeling. In 1980, purified pork insulin [Iletin II, pork (Lilly)] became available for individuals allergic to or otherwise adversely affected by the mixed pork-beef product. The first insulin developed for clinical use was an amorphous insulin. This type has since been replaced by a more purified crystalline insulin composed of zinc-insulin crystals which produces a clear aqueous solution. Originally, insulin injection ("regular insulin") had been produced at a pH of 2.8 to 3.5. This was necessary, because particles formed in the vial when the pH was increased above the acid range. However, changes in the manufacturing methods resulting in the production of insulin of greater purity has allowed for the preparation of insulin injection having a neutral pH. The neutralized product has been shown to exhibit greater stability than the acidic product.

Insulin injection is prepared to contain 100 or 500 USP Insulin Units in each mL. The labeling must state the potency, in USP Insulin Units in each mL and the expiration date, which must not

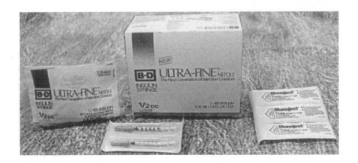

Fig. 14.32 *Example of packaging of disposable sterile insulin syringes and needles. (Courtesy of William B. French, PhD.)*

be later than 24 months after the date of distribution from the manufacturer's storage. As an added precaution against the inadvertent use of the incorrect strength of insulin by the patient during self-administration of the drug, the package colors vary, depending on the strength of the insulin. For instance, all insulins (of the various types) containing 100 units per mL have orange and the 500 units per mL preparation has brown with diagonal white stripes. U-500 insulin is indicated for patients with a marked insulin requirement (more than 200 units per day) because a large unit/dose may be administered subcutaneously in a small volume.

Insulin injection is a colorless to straw-colored solution, depending upon its concentration; that containing 500 Units per mL is straw-colored. It is substantially free from turbidity. A small amount of glycerin (1.4 to 1.8%) is added for stability and 0.1 to 0.25% of either phenol or cresol is added for preservation. Insulin remains stable if stored in a cold place, preferably the refrigerator. However, because the injection of cold insulin is somewhat uncomfortable, the patient may store the vial being used at room temperature (59–86°F or 15–30°C) for up to 1 month. Any insulin remaining in the vial after that time should be discarded. Freezing should be avoided, as this reduces potency.

The various insulin preparations differ as to their rapidity of action (onset of action) after injection, their peak of action, and their duration of action (Table 14.6). Insulin injection, being a solution, is categorized as a prompt-acting insulin preparation. Insulin preparations that are suspensions are slower acting. Only insulin injection may be administered intravenously; all others, as well as insulin injection, are normally given subcutaneously, usually 1/2 to 2 hours before a meal so that its physiological effects will parallel the absorption of glucose. The dosage is individually determined, with the usual dosage range being 5 to 100 USP Units. The insulin injection containing 500 units per mL is employed in cases of insulin resistance requiring very large doses.

It is important to emphasize at this point that the pharmacist plays a vital role in the education of the diabetic patient, particularly as it relates to the proper use of insulin. The insulin dosage should always be checked to ensure it is correct. Because it is a solution, Regular Insulin can be used in emergency situations, i.e., ketoacidosis, to effect a rapid decrease in blood glucose levels. However, with the exception of diabetic ketoacidosis, it is rare for a patient to ever require a dose of Regular Insulin greater than 25 units. Typically, diabetic patients combine Regular Insulin with a modified insulin, i.e., NPH, to provide daily coverage using two injections (morning, late-afternoon) or now use available pre-mixed preparations. So it is important that the patient understand how much of each to use and know in what order these should be mixed in the insulin syringe. The unmodified insulin, i.e., Regular Insulin, is drawn up first into the syringe.

In an institutional setting the pharmacist must make sure written insulin orders are correctly transcribed or transmitted. Errors in insulin dosage have occurred because of allied health professional error. Written orders for 6 U of insulin have been interpreted to mean 60 units, an order for 4 U has been read as 4 cc. Each of these occurred because

Table 14.6. Insulin Activity Profiles and Compatibility

	Insulin Preparations	Onset (hr)	Peak (hr)	Duration (hr)	Compatible mixed with
Rapid Acting	Insulin Injection (Regular)	0.5 to 1		8 to 12	All
	Prompt Insulin Zinc Suspension (Semilente)	1 to 1.5	5 to 10	12 to 16	Lente
	Lispro Insulin Solution	0.25	0.5 to 1.5	6 to 8	Ultralente, NPH
Intermediate Acting	Isophane Insulin Suspension (NPH)	1 to 1.5	4 to 12	24	Regular
	Insulin Zinc Suspension (Lente)	1 to 2.5	7 to 15	24	Regular, semilente
Long Acting	Protamine Zinc Insulin Suspension (PZI)	4 to 8	14 to 24	36	Regular
	Extended Insulin Zinc Suspension (Ultralente)	4 to 8	10 to 30	> 36	Regular, semilente
Premixed Insulins	Isophane Insulin Suspension 50% and Insulin Injection, 50%				
	Isophane Insulin Suspension 70% and Insulin Injection, 30%	0.5	2 to 12	18 to 24	Regular, NPH

the abbreviation "U" for units was read as a zero or a cc.

The patient should be instructed to rotate the site of insulin injections on a continual basis. Rotation of the site will help to avoid the development of lipohypertrophy, a buildup of fibrous tissue. Otherwise, if there is continual injection into one site, the tissue becomes spongy and avascular. The avascular nature of the site perpetuates the problem because the skin becomes anesthetized and the injection is not felt. This is a particular problem with children who continue to use the same site and do not realize that the absorption of insulin from this site becomes erratic and uncontrollable. Numerous brochures are available from manufacturers of diabetic supplies that demonstrate the appropriate rotation of insulin injection sites over the entire body.

Another encountered problem with insulin injection is the development of lipodystrophy. Generally, this problem appears within 2 months to 2 years following the beginning of insulin therapy and occurs predominantly in women and children. The etiology of the problem has been ascribed to the injection of refrigerated insulin (not giving enough time for it to warm up prior to injection), to a failure to rotate the injection site and to insulin impurities. The result is the formation of a subcutaneous indentation or "pothole" caused by a wasting or atrophy of the lipid tissue. It appears that the greater purity of current insulins significantly have decreased this problem, and a marked improvement in existing atrophic areas has been demonstrated by the injection of highly purified port or human insulin directly into or on the periphery of the atrophic areas.

Prior to use, the patient should be instructed to carefully inspect the insulin. Regular Insulin, a solution, should appear clear, while the other insulins which are suspensions should appear cloudy. With the insulins that are suspensions the patient should be instructed how to prepare the insulin, i.e., the vial is rotated slowly between the palms of the hands several times, prior to drawing the insulin into the syringe. This avoids frothing and bubble formation which would result in an inaccurate dose of insulin. The patient should not shake the insulin vial.

Proper storage should also be encouraged for insulins. These preparations should be stored in a cool place or a refrigerator. The patient should be warned to avoid having the insulin come into contact with extremes of temperature, i.e., freezing [overnight in the car during the wintertime], heat [glove compartment of a car, direct sunlight]. If this occurs, it is preferred that the patient discard the insulin and get a new bottle. Any bottle of insulin that appears "frosted" or "clumped" should be returned to the pharmacy where the purchase took place. Lastly, the patient should use the insulin in a timely fashion, but not beyond the expiration date indicated on the insulin vial.

Human Insulin

Biosynthetic human insulin was the first drug product developed through recombinant DNA techniques to receive approval by the federal Food and Drug Administration for marketing. This product, Humulin, Lilly, became available in 1983. It is produced by utilizing a special nondisease-forming laboratory strain of *Escherichia coli* and recombinant DNA technology. A recombined plasmid DNA coding for human insulin is introduced into the bacteria, and it is then cultured by fermentation to produce the A and B chains of human insulin. These A and B chains are freed and purified individually before they are linked by the specific disulfide bridges to form human insulin. The insulin produced is chemically, physically, and immunologically equivalent to insulin derived from the human pancreas. The biosynthetic insulin is free of contamination with *E. coli* peptides, and, is also free of the pancreatic peptides that are present as impurities in insulin preparations derived from animal pancreatic extraction. These latter impurities include proinsulin and proinsulin intermediates, glucagon, somatostatin, pancreatic polypeptide, and vasoactive intestinal peptide.

Pharmacokinetic studies in some normal subjects and clinical observations in patients indicate that formulations of human insulin have a slightly faster onset of action and a slightly shorter duration of action than their purified pork insulin counterparts. Two formulations of human insulin were initially marketed: Neutral Regular Human Insulin (Humulin R, Lilly) and NPH Human Insulin (Humulin N, Lilly). Neutral Regular human insulin consists of zinc-insulin crystals in solution. It has a rapid onset-of-action and a relatively short duration-of-action (6 to 8 hours). NPH human insulin is a turbid preparation that is intermediate-acting, with a slower onset-of-action and longer duration-of-action (slightly less than 24 hours) than regular human insulin.

Human insulins should be stored as other insulins, in a cold place, preferably a refrigerator. Freezing should be avoided.

Lispro Insulin Solution

Lispro insulin solution consists of zinc-insulin lispro crystals dissolved in a clear aqueous fluid. It is created when the amino acids at positions 28 and 29 on the insulin B-chain are reversed.

Lispro insulin solution is rapidly absorbed after subcutaneous administration and demonstrates no significant differences in absorption from abdominal, deltoid, and femoral sites of injection. Its bioavailability mimics that of regular insulin. Compared to regular insulin, however, peak serum levels of lispro insulin occur earlier, i.e., within 0.5 to 1.5 hours, are higher, and are shorter acting, i.e., 6–8 hours. Peak hypoglycemic effects are more pronounced with lispro insulin solution. Thus, hypoglycemia is the primary complication associated with its use. Comparative studies have demonstrated, however, that hypoglycemic episodes have been less frequent with lispro insulin than with regular insulin.

Lispro insulin solution administered fifteen minutes before meals has decreased the risk of hypoglycemic episodes and improved postprandial glucose excursions when compared to conventional regular insulin therapy. Some studies have demonstrated a greater impact on the quality of life with lispro insulin solution, and it has been shown to be more effective than regular insulin in reducing exercise-induced hypoglycemia when exercise is performed three hours after a meal. Thus, as a new insulin, it offers more flexibility for the diabetes patient and should be added to formularies as an alternative to regular insulin.

Lispro insulin solution should be stored in a refrigerator, but not in the freezer. If accidently frozen, it should not be used. If absolutely necessary, it may be stored at room temperature for up to 28 days. In this instance, storage temperature should be as cool as possible. The vial or cartridge containing this insulin should be kept away from direct light and heat. At the end of 28 days, any unused portion of the Lispro insulin solution should be discarded.

Isophane Insulin Suspension (NPH Insulin)

Isophane Insulin Suspension is a sterile suspension, in an aqueous vehicle buffered with dibasic sodium phosphate to between pH 7.1 and 7.4, of insulin prepared from zinc-insulin crystals modified by the addition of protamine so that the solid phase of the suspension consists of crystals composed of insulin, zinc, and protamine. Protamine is prepared from the sperm or the mature testes of fish belonging to the genus *Oncorhynchus* and others. As mentioned earlier during the discussion of the aqueous insulin solutions, suspensions of insulin with a pH on the alkaline side are inherently of a longer duration of action than those preparations that are solutions. Insulin is most insoluble at pH 7.2.

The rod-shaped crystals of isophane insulin suspension should be approximately 30 micrometers in length and the suspension free from large aggregates of crystals following moderate agitation. This is necessary for the insulin suspension to pass freely within the needle used in injection and for the absorption of the drug from the site of injection to be consistent from one manufactured batch of injection to another. When a portion of the suspension is examined microscopically, the suspended matter is largely crystalline with only traces of amorphous material. The official injection is required to contain glycerin and phenol for stability and preservation. The specified expiration date occurring in the labeling is 24 months after the immediate container was filled by the manufacturer. The suspension is packaged in multiple-dose containers having not less than 10 mL of injection. Each mL of the injection contains 100 units of insulin per mL of suspension. The suspension is best stored in a refrigerator, but freezing must be avoided.

As indicated earlier, isophane insulin suspension is an intermediate-acting insulin preparation administered as required mainly as hormonal replacement in diabetes mellitus. The usual dosage range subcutaneously is 10 to 80 USP Units.

The "NPH" used in some product names stands for "Neutral Protamine Hagedorn," since the preparation is about neutral (pH about 7.2), contains protamine, and was developed by Hagedorn. The term "isophane" is based on the Greek: *iso* and *phane,* meaning "equal" and "appearance" and refers to the equivalent balance between the protamine and insulin.

Isophane Insulin Suspension and Insulin Injection

In years past, patients needing a more rapid onset of insulin and the intermediate duration of activity approximately one day, would routinely mix isophane insulin suspension, an intermediate-acting insulin, with insulin injection, a rapid-acting insulin. Unexpected patient responses (e.g., hypoglycemic episodes) were encountered. It was not uncommon for the patient inadvertently to contaminate one of the vials during the mixing process. Subsequently, a premixed formulation of isophane insulin suspension and insulin injection became available. Currently there are two formulations, a 70/30 combination that consists of 70% isophane insulin suspension and 30% insulin injection, and a 50/50 combination that consists of 50% isophane insulin suspension and 50% insulin injection.

Humulin 50/50, for example, achieves a higher insulin concentration (C_{max}) and higher maximum glucose infusion rates with more rapid elimination than Humulin 70/30. However, as expected, the cumulative amounts of insulin absorbed (AUC) and the cumulative effects over 24 hours following injection are identical. Thus, the 70/30 combination provides an initial insulin response tempered with a more prolonged release of insulin. The 50/50 mixture would be useful in those situations where a greater initial response is required, and in those patients who have been using extemporaneously compounded insulin mixtures in a 50/50 ratio.

The Humulin 70/30 and 50/50 premixed insulins are cloudy suspensions with a zinc content of 0.01–0.04 mg/100 units. These insulins are neutral in pH and phosphate buffered. m-Cresol and phenol are the preservatives employed for both combinations. Protamine sulfate is used as the modifying protein salt.

Patients should not attempt to change the ratio of these products with the addition of NPH or regular insulin. If Humulin N and Humulin R mixtures are prescribed in a different proportion, the individual insulin products should be mixed in the amounts recommended by the physician.

Insulin Zinc Suspension

Insulin for Insulin Zinc Suspension is modified by the addition of zinc chloride so that the suspended particles consist of a mixture of crystalline and amorphous insulin in a ratio of approximately 7 parts of crystals to 3 parts of amorphous material. The sterile suspension is in an aqueous vehicle buffered to pH 7.2 to 7.5 with sodium acetate. In treating insulin with zinc chloride, it is possible to obtain both crystalline and amorphous zinc insulin. The amorphous form has the most prompt hypoglycemic effect, since the particles are the smallest and are absorbed into the system more rapidly after subcutaneous injection than are the zinc insulin crystals. Also, the larger the crystals the less prompt and the longer-acting will be the insulin suspen-

sion. By combining the crystalline and amorphous forms into one preparation, an intermediate-acting suspension is obtained. As noted in Table 14.6 the time-activity of insulin zinc suspension is only slightly different than that for isophane insulin suspension. The advantage of the former is that no additional foreign protein (other than the insulin) is present, such as protamine, which may produce local sensitivity reactions. Also, it may be combined as desired with either of the following two suspensions to produce an insulin preparation having the time-activity characteristics that most closely meet the desires and requirements of the individual patient. Suspensions available contain 100 USP Insulin Units per mL packaged in 10-mL vials. The individual crystalline and amorphous particles may be seen microscopically, with the crystals being predominantly between 10 to 40 μm in maximum dimension and the amorphous particles no greater than 2 μm in maximum dimension.

In addition to the sodium acetate as a buffer, the suspension contains about 0.7% sodium chloride for tonicity and 0.10% methylparaben for preservation. The expiration date of the suspension is 24 months after the immediate container was filled. The suspension must be stored in a refrigerator with freezing being avoided. As with all such preparations, the dose depends upon the individual needs of the patient, but generally ranges between 10 and 80 USP Units.

Extended Insulin Zinc Suspension

Extended insulin zinc suspension is a sterile suspension of zinc insulin crystals in an aqueous medium buffered to between pH 7.2 and 7.5 with sodium acetate. Present also are 0.7% sodium chloride for tonicity and 0.1% methylparaben for preservation. Because the suspended matter is composed solely of zinc insulin crystals, which are slowly absorbed, this preparation is classified as a long-acting insulin preparation. Because of the compatibility between the preparations, this suspension may be mixed with either insulin zinc suspension or prompt insulin zinc suspension to achieve the proper time-activity requirements of an individual patient. The usual dosage range is 10 to 80 USP Units. The suspension is commercially available in 10-mL vials providing 100 USP Insulin Units per mL. The suspension must be stored in a refrigerator with freezing being avoided. Under proper storage conditions, the expiration date of the injection is not later than 24 months after the immediate container was filled.

Prompt Insulin Zinc Suspension

The sterile suspension of insulin in Prompt Insulin Zinc Suspension is modified by the addition of zinc chloride so that the solid phase of the suspension is amorphous. The maximum dimension of the shapeless particles of zinc insulin must not exceed 2 micrometers. The suspension is available in 100 USP Insulin Units per mL in vials of 10 mL. This preparation has the same pH and additives as extended insulin zinc suspension, and they may be mixed as desired to achieve a preparation having the desired time-activity characteristics. This is a rapid-acting insulin preparation. It must be stored in a refrigerator and not permitted to freeze. Its expiration date is not greater than 24 months after the immediate container was filled.

Insulin Infusion Pumps

Insulin infusion pumps allow patients to achieve and maintain blood glucose at near-normal levels on a *constant basis.* Continuous infusion of insulin through use of these pumps eliminates the need for the patient to self-administer daily injections of insulin. This provides patient convenience, better patient compliance, and control over the disease. The main objective of pump therapy is the strict control of the blood glucose level between 70 to 140 mg/dL. This is the primary way to avoid complications in diabetic patients, such as gangrene and diabetic retinopathy.

Early insulin infusion pumps were large bedside units, used mainly in hospitals. Today, portable, battery-operated, and programmable units are available. These systems utilize microcomputers to regulate the flow of insulin from a syringe attached to a catheter (usually 18 gauge) connected to a 27- to 28-gauge needle inserted in the patient. The insulin may be delivered subcutaneously, intravenously, or intraperitoneally.

Patients who use infusion pumps for the continuous subcutaneous administration of insulin may develop hard nodules at the site of injection. Some patients may demonstrate nodules that are tender, develop a rock-hard consistency, and take several months to subside. Although the cause of this nodule formation is unknown, a change in insulin may be beneficial. Speculation as to the cause centers around the development of local trauma or hematoma formation with a subsequent local inflammatory response, stimulation of fibroblast replacement, or dystrophic calcification. The need to rotate sites of injection on a several day basis cannot be overemphasized. For additional information on infusion pumps, the reader is directed to the footnote reference at the end of this chapter (20).

Large Volume Parenterals (LVPs)

Common examples of large volume parenterals in use today were presented in Table 14.7. These solutions are usually administered by intravenous infusion to replenish body fluids, electrolytes, or to provide nutrition. They are usually administered in volumes of 100 mL to liter amounts and more per

Table 14.7.   Examples of Some Injections Administered in Large Volume by Intravenous Infusion That May Be Administered in Volumes of 1 Liter or More, Alone, or With Other Drugs Added

Injection	*Usual Contents*	*Category and Comments*
Amino Acid Injection	3.5, 5, 5.5, 7, 8.5, 10% crystalline amino acids with or without varying concentrations of electrolytes or glycerin	Fluid and nutrient replenisher.
Dextrose Injection, USP	2.5, 5.0, 10, 20% dextrose, and other strengths	Fluid and nutrient replenisher.
Dextrose and Sodium Chloride Injection, USP	Dextrose varying from 2.5 to 10% and sodium chloride from 0.11 (19 mEq sodium) to 0.9% (154 mEq sodium)	Fluid, nutrient, and electrolyte replenisher.
Mannitol Injection, USP	5, 10, 15, 20 and 25% mannitol	Diagnostic aid in renal function determinations; diuretic. Fluid and nutrient replenisher
Ringer's Injection, USP	147 mEq sodium, 4 mEq potassium, 4.5 mEq calcium, and 156 mEq chloride per liter	Fluid and electrolyte replenisher.
Lactated Ringer's Injection, USP	2.7 mEq calcium, 4 mEq potassium, 130 mEq sodium and 28 mEq lactate per liter	Systemic alkalinizer; fluid and electrolyte replenisher.
Sodium Chloride Injection, USP	0.9% sodium chloride	Fluid and electrolyte replenisher; isotonic vehicle.

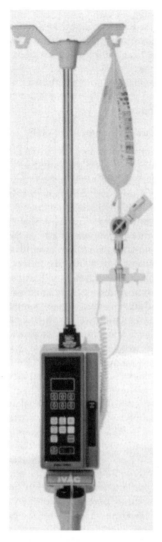

Fig. 14.33 *Accurate delivery of intravenous fluids and medications by use of a controlled rate infusion system (CRIS) for the drug vial and a volumetric infusion pump for the intravenous fluids. (Courtesy of Eli Lilly and Company.)*

day by slow intravenous infusion with or without controlled-rate infusion systems (Fig. 14.33). Because of the large volumes administered, these solutions must not contain bacteriostatic agents or other pharmaceutical additives. They are packaged in large single-dose containers (Figs. 14.34, 14.35).

As indicated previously, therapeutic additives as electrolytes, vitamins, and antineoplastics are frequently incorporated into large volume parenterals for coadministration to the patient. It is the responsibility of the pharmacist to be knowledgeable of the physical and chemical compatibility of the

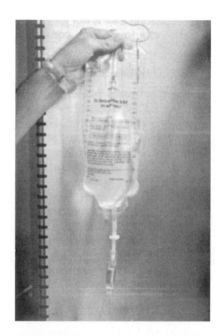

Fig. 14.34 *Intravenous solution packaged in pliable plastic.*

additive in the solution in which it is placed. Obviously, an incompatible combination which results in the formation of insoluble material or which affects the efficacy or potency of the therapeutic agent of the vehicle is not acceptable.

It is also important for the pharmacist to be vigilant of possible incompatibilities associated with multiple infusions that may be co-administered to a patient. A typical nursing question may involve,"can the dopamine infusion ('drip') be run in with the heparin infusion ('drip')?"To answer these questions, the pharmacist should become knowledgeable about parenteral therapy and be aware of incompatibilities through the literature. Numerous references (e.g., *Handbook of Injectable Drugs,* King's *Guide to Parenteral Admixtures* [Cutter Laboratories]) are available for sources listing and discussing par-

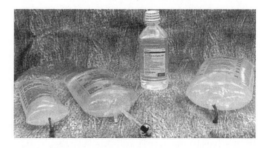

Fig. 14.35 *Examples of peritoneal dialysis and irrigation fluids. (Courtesy of William B. French, PhD.)*

enteral incompatibilities. However, the pharmacist should only use the most current editions of each of these references. Whenever possible, the pharmacist should attempt to answer these important questions and explain the incompatibilities that come to his/her attention as part of the daily routine. Further, the pharmacist should create a file of available data and add it from one's experience and the literature.

While it is impossible to chart every possible admixture incompatibility, principles can be learned and applied. For example, certain drugs are inactivated or precipitate at either high or low pH values, some drugs (e.g., sympathomimetics) encounter problems when added to IV fluids, and certain therapeutic large-volume solutions (e.g., sodium bicarbonate, urea, mannitol) should never contain additives.

Large volume parenteral solutions are employed in *maintenance therapy* for the patient entering or recovering from surgery, or for the patient who is unconscious and unable to obtain fluids, electrolytes, and nutrition orally. The solutions may also be utilized in *replacement therapy* in patients who have suffered a heavy loss of fluid and electrolytes.

Maintenance Therapy

When a patient is being maintained on parenteral fluids for only several days, simple solutions providing adequate amounts of water, dextrose, and small amounts of sodium and potassium generally suffice. When patients are unable to take oral nutrition or fluids for slightly longer periods, say 3 to 6 days, solutions of higher caloric content may be used. In instances in which oral feeding must be deferred for periods of weeks or longer, total parenteral nutrition must be implemented to provide all of the essential nutrients to minimize tissue break-down and to maintain normalcy within the body. Total nutrient admixtures (i.e., TNA, three-in-one) include all substrates necessary for nutritional support, e.g., carbohydrates, protein, fat, electrolytes, trace elements, that are usually mixed in a single plastic intravenous bag for more convenient administration.

These admixtures are very useful for patients undergoing chemotherapy, and for gastrointestinal patients, and anorexic patients. The use of three-in-one admixtures in pediatric patients, especially neonates is controversial. The concentration of calcium, phosphorus, and necessary warm administration conditions for pediatric TPNs do not lend themselves to stable preparations. As a result, many pediatric institutions will not compound three-in-one admixtures for their patients, but administer each component separately.

When using TNA, the pharmacist must consider the order of substrate mixing, differentiate between various brands of substrate and their physical-chemical properties, determine the type of plastic bag system that is most appropriate to use, determine whether (and by what mode) the TNA should be filtered prior to infusion, determine how the product should be stored, and assess any potential complications that might arise with the use of this method of administering nutritional products. For example, the use of "standard" total parenteral nutrition plastic bags may result in the leaching out of plasticizer into the solution, and be potentially injurious to the patient.

In April, 1994, the FDA issued a Safety Alert regarding the hazards of precipitation associated with parenteral nutrition (21). This was in response to two deaths and at least two other patient cases of respiratory distress associated with the use of three-in-one admixtures. Patient autopsies revealed diffuse microvascular pulmonary emboli linked to the presence of a calcium phosphate precipitate in the admixture. Consequently, the FDA Safety Alert recommends that a filter be used when infusing either central or peripheral parenteral nutrition admixtures. A 0.22-μm filter, containing both a bacterial-retentive and an air-eliminating filter, has been recommended for use with nonlipid (i.e., two-in-one) containing parenteral nutrient solutions.

Lipid emulsions and three-in-one admixture parenteral nutrient solutions can be safely filtered through filters with a pore size of ≥ 1.2 μm. A problem with the lipid emulsion in a three-in-one admixture is that it obscures the presence of any precipitate. Thus, if a lipid emulsion is needed, a preferable alternative is to employ a two-in-one admixture with a lipid infused separately via a Y-site.

Replacement Therapy

In instances in which there is a heavy loss of water and electrolytes, as in severe diarrhea or vomiting, greater than usual amounts of these materials may be initially administered and then maintenance therapy provided. Patients with Crohn's disease, AIDS, burn patients, or those experiencing trauma are candidates for replacement therapy.

Water Requirement

In normal individuals, the daily water requirement is that amount needed to replace normal and expected losses. Water is lost daily in the urine, feces, skin and from respiration. The normal daily requirement of water for adults is about 25 to 40 mL/kg of body weight, or an average of about 2,000 mL per square meter of body surface area (22). Nomograms for the determination of body surface area from body height and weight are presented in Chapter 2, Figure 2.8. Children and small adults need more water per pound of body weight than do larger adults; water requirements correlate more closely with body surface area than with weight and an employed guideline to estimate normal daily requirement for water in these patients is as follows:

1. <10 kg: 100 mL/kg/day
2. 10–20 kg: 1000 mL plus 50 mL/kg/day for weight over 10 kg.
3. >20 kg to maximum of 80 kg: 1500 mL plus 20 mL/kg/day for weight over 20 kg.

However, in the newborn, the volume administered in the first week or two should be about half that calculated from body surface area.

In water replacement therapy for adults, 70 mL of water per kg per day may be required in addition to the maintenance water requirements; a badly dehydrated infant may require even a greater proportion (22). Thus, a 50-kg patient may require 3500 mL for replacement plus 2400 mL for maintenance. In order to avoid the consequences of fluid overload, especially in elderly patients, and those with renal or cardiovascular disorders, monitoring of blood pressure is desirable.

Because water administered intravenously as such may cause the osmotic hemolysis of red blood cells, and, since a patient who requires water generally requires nutrition and/or electrolytes, the parenteral administration of water is generally as a solution with dextrose or electrolytes in which the solution has sufficient tonicity (sodium chloride equivalency) to protect the red blood cells from hemolyzing.

Electrolyte Requirement

Potassium, the primary intracellular cation, is particularly important for normal cardiac and skeletal muscle function. The usual daily intake of potassium is about 100 mEq and the usual daily loss is about 40 mEq. Thus, any replacement therapy should include a minimum of 40 mEq plus the amount needed to replace additional losses. Potassium can be lost through excessive perspiration, repeated enemas, trauma (such as severe burns), uncontrolled diabetes, diseases of the intestinal tract, surgical operations, and the use of such medications as thiazide and loop diuretics. People who suffer from poor nutrition, those using very low-calorie diet products, and victims of anorexia nervosa or acute alcoholism

also may have low potassium levels, i.e., hypokalemia, because they are not taking in enough of the mineral. Symptoms of potassium loss include a weak pulse, faint heart sounds, falling blood pressure, and generalized weakness. Severe loss of potassium can lead to death. Too much potassium is not a good thing, either. An excess may cause diarrhea, irritability, muscle cramps, and pain. Hyperkalemia can be caused by kidney failure or consuming excess amounts of potassium-rich foods. Prescribed potassium supplements, potassium-sparing diuretic therapy, angiotensin converting enzyme inhibitors (e.g., lisinopril) and the indiscriminate use of over-the-counter salt-substitute products have also been implicated to induce hyperkalemia.

In cases of severe potassium deficiency, electrolyte replacement through the intravenous administration of potassium is usually employed. The pharmacist who receives a prescription for intravenous potassium chloride must be careful and check the amount of potassium chloride in the prescription and the infusion rate at which the drug is to be administered to the patient. Potassium preparations must be diluted with a suitable large volume parenteral solution, mixed well, and given by slow IV infusion. They are not to be administered undiluted.

The most commonly used concentration of potassium chloride for continuous infusion, IV maintenance therapy is between 20–40 mEq/L. With a peripheral line, that concentration may increase to 60 mEq/L, and with a central line, the maximum concentration can be up to 80 mEq/L.

For intermittent potassium replacement therapy in patients suffering from hypokalemia, the usual infusion rate is 10 mEq/hr (maximum recommended rate is 20 mEq/hr). Because of potassium chloride's ability to effect ECG changes (e.g., progressive increase in height and peaking of T waves, lowering of the R wave, decreased amplitude and ultimate disappearance of the P waves), most hospitals establish a maximum infusion rate of 10 mEq/hr if the patient is not monitored by EKG. For patients monitored by EKG, the usual infusion rate is 20 mEq/hr with a maximum infusion rate of 40 mEq/hr depending upon the clinical condition of the patient.

For patients in need of aggressive potassium replacement, the potassium serum level should be assessed every 6 hours during the early intensive phase of therapy and once daily thereafter when normal potassium serum levels are achieved. For patients whose serum potassium is >2.5 mEq/L, the potassium level should be measured after the first 60 mEq are administered. For patients whose serum potassium is <2.5 mEq/L, the potassium level should be measured after the first 80 mEq are administered.

Sodium, the principal extracellular cation, is vital to maintain normal extracellular fluids. Average daily intake of sodium is 135 to 170 mEq (8 to 10 g of sodium chloride). The body is able to conserve sodium when this ion is lost or removed from the diet. When there is sodium loss or a deficit, the daily administration of 3 to 5 g of sodium chloride (51 to 85 mEq of sodium) should prevent a negative sodium balance. A low sodium level in the body may result from excessive sweating, the use of certain diuretics, or diarrhea. Fatigue, muscle weakness, apprehension, and convulsions are among the symptoms of excessive sodium loss. Sodium concentrations can increase when a person does not drink enough water, especially in hot weather, or if kidney function is impaired. Dry, sticky mucous membranes, flushed skin, elevated body temperature, lack of tears, and thirst are among the symptoms of sodium excess. In about 20% of individuals who suffer from high blood pressure, sodium has been implicated as a causative factor. Chloride, the principal anion of the extracellular fluid is usually paired with sodium. Chloride is also important for muscle contraction, balancing the fluid levels inside and outside the cells, and maintaining the acid-base balance of the extracellular fluid. An adequate supply of chloride is necessary to prevent bicarbonate, the second most prevalent anion, from tipping the acid-base balance to the alkaline side. (In 1979, a lack of chloride in a brand of infant formula caused metabolic alkalosis in babies who had been exclusively fed that formula. As a result of this episode, Congress passed the Infant Formula Act of 1980, which spells out the nutrients that must be in formulas and establishes quality control procedures for the manufacture of these infant foods.) Although other electrolytes and minerals as calcium, magnesium, and iron are lost from the body, they generally are not required during short-term parenteral therapy.

Caloric Requirements

Generally patients requiring parenteral fluids are given 5% dextrose to reduce the caloric deficit that usually occurs in patients undergoing maintenance or replacement therapy. The use of dextrose also minimizes ketosis and the breakdown of protein. Basic caloric requirements may be estimated by body weight; in the fasting state, the average daily loss of body protein is approximately 80 g/day for a 70 kg man. Daily ingestion of at least 100 g of glucose reduces this loss by half.

Parenteral Hyperalimentation

This is the infusion of large amounts of basic nutrients sufficient to achieve active tissue synthesis and growth. It is employed in the long-term intravenous feeding of protein solutions containing high concentrations of dextrose (approximately 20%), electrolytes, vitamins, and in some instances insulin. Among the components utilized in parenteral nutrition solutions are the following, listed in quantities commonly provided per liter of fluid. The individual components and amounts administered to a patient would vary depending on the patient's needs.

Electrolytes:

Sodium	25 mEq
Potassium	20 mEq
Magnesium	5 mEq
Calcium	5 mEq
Chloride	30 mEq
Acetate	25 mEq
Phosphate	18 mM

Vitamins:

Vitamin A	3300 I.U.
Vitamin D	200 I.U.
Vitamin E	10 I.U.
Vitamin C	100 mg
Niacin	40 mg
Vitamin B_2	3.6–4.93 mg
Vitamin B_1	3–3.35 mg
Vitamin B_6	4–4.86 mg
Pantothenic Acid	15 mg
Folic Acid	400 mcg
Vitamin B_{12}	5 mcg
Biotin	60 mcg

Amino Acids: Essential Amino Acids

L-Isoleucine	590 mg
L-Leucine	770 mg
L-Lysine acetate	870 mg
(free base	620 mg)
L-Methionine	450 mg
L-Phenylalanine	480 mg
L-Threonine	340 mg
L-Tryptophan	130 mg
L-Valine	560 mg

Nonessential Amino Acids

L-Alanine	600 mg
L-Arginine	810 mg
L-Histidine	240 mg
L-Proline	950 mg
L-Serine	500 mg
Aminoacetic Acid	1.19 g

The large proportion of dextrose increases the caloric value of the solution, while keeping the volume required to be administered to a minimum. The solutions are administered slowly through a large vein, such as the superior vena cava. The superior vena cava is accessed through the subclavian vein, which is located immediately beneath the clavicle and near to the heart. This permits the rapid dilution of the concentrated hyperalimentation fluid and minimizes the risk of tissue or cellular damage due to the hypertonicity of the solution. Generally, final concentrations of dextrose (≤10%) can be given peripherally. Solutions containing dextrose (>10%) should be given via the central route, i.e., the superior vena cava.

Calcium (usually as calcium gluconate) and phosphate (usually as potassium or sodium phosphate) are frequently present in parenteral admixtures. A significant problem associated with their use is the formation of calcium phosphate, an insoluble precipitate. As mentioned earlier in this chapter, the formation of this and its resultant deposition of calcium phosphate crystals in lung tissue led to the 1994 FDA Safety Alert (21).

Many factors have been implicated in the formation of the insoluble precipitate. Among these are the concentration of the individual ions, the salt form of the calcium, the concentration and type of amino acids, the concentration of the dextrose, the temperature and pH of the TPN, the presence of other additives (e.g., cysteine), and the order of mixing. The potential of calcium phosphate precipitation is especially challenging for compounding neonate/pediatric TPN admixtures because of the small volume they are able to tolerate and the need for aggressive replacement therapy. Thus, pharmacists must be alert to recognize and to avoid this potential serious compatibility problem.

Figure 14.36 demonstrates a Nutrimix Macro TPN Compounder. This device can pump four nutritional solutions (i.e., dextrose, water, amino acids, fat) simultaneously to compound nutritional admixtures by gravimetric means. The user programs the volume and specific gravity of the fluid to be pumped and the device calculates the weight of the solution that has to be transferred from the source station to the patient bag. The fifth load cell serves as a confirmation of the weights programmed vs. weights delivered.

With the increasing use of parenteral solutions in the pediatric population, including parenteral nutrition solutions, pharmacists are frequently confronted with inquiries concerning the appropriate method of parenteral drug delivery (20). A dilemma with pediatric patients is that they often have a limited fluid capacity caused by disease (e.g., congestive heart failure, renal insufficiency) and limited vascu-

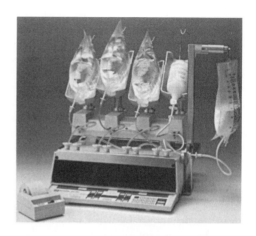

Fig. 14.36 *Nutrimix Macro TPN Compounder. (Courtesy of Abbott Hospital Products Division.)*

lar access. As a consequence, pharmacists are asked whether a medication can be administered along with a parenteral nutrition solution. Although this practice is to be discouraged, in the pediatric population it may be the only way to ensure that the patient is receiving adequate nutrition as well as appropriate drug therapy. Further, by administering the medication with the PN solution, rather than interrupting the PN to administer medication, rebound hypoglycemia is less likely to develop in the patient. The pharmacist must remember that the practice of administering medication through a central venous line intended for PN solutions is not without risks. Catheter sepsis and occlusion can result.

Formerly, TPNs were prepared one liter at a time. However, to conserve pharmacist and nursing time, a 24-hour supply is much more efficient and now the norm. Indeed, if a patient encounters a problem necessitating a bag to be remade, the cost difference between one or two liters and a 2000 mL bag is not that significant. Waste should not be a consideration because the attending physician should not use the TPN to minutely adjust for a patient's need. Typically, electrolyte requirements exceed the physical compatibilities of the TPN components (e.g., calcium/phosphate compatibilities in lipid containing TPNs), and when this occurs the pharmacist should encourage the physician to write for a separate infusion to make up the deficiency.

The following abbreviations may be used in the hospital in describing the desired order for parenteral nutrition:

CVTPN (Central Vein TPN)
TPN (Total Parenteral Nutrition)
PPN (Peripheral Parenteral Nutrition)

Enteral Nutrition

As appropriate, hospitalized and home care patients may be provided their nutritional needs through *enteral* rather than *parenteral* means. Enteral nutrition products may be administered orally, via nasogastric tube, via feeding gastrostomy, or via needle-catheter jejunostomy. These products are formulated to contain a variety of vitamins, minerals, carbohydrates, proteins, fats and caloric requirements to meet the specific needs of patients. While parenteral feeding is appropriate for short-term use in a hospital or long-term care facility, or when the gastrointestinal tract is unable to absorb nutrients, enteral feeding is preferable whenever possible. It is just as effective as a source of nutrients, less expensive than parenteral feeding, and has a low potential to cause serious complications.

The defined formula diets may be monomeric or oligomeric (i.e., amino acids or short peptides and simple carbohydrates) or polymeric (more complex protein and carbohydrate sources). Modular supplements are used for individual supplementation of protein (ProMod powder, Propac powder), carbohydrate (Moducal powder), or fat (Lipomul liquid) when formulas do not offer sufficient flexibility. For example, a physician may order a powder reconstituted one-quarter strength, half-strength, or full strength for a particular patient and then have this administered via a nasogastric tube, a feeding gastrostomy, or a needle-catheter jejunostomy.

There is no single classification system for these products, and there are different criteria for evaluating and categorizing them. Caloric density (generally in the range of 1, 1.5, or 2 kcal/mL) influences the density of other nutrients. Protein content is also a major determinant in these products. For those patients who experience diarrhea and cramping, high osmolality formulas may present difficulty. Low-fat-content products should be suggested for patients with significant malabsorption, hyperlipidemia, or severe exocrine pancreatic insufficiency. Medium chain triglycerides (MCT), while providing a useful source of energy in patients with malabsorption, do not provide essential fatty acids.

Originally, enteral feedings contained lactose and presented problems in lactase-deficient individuals. This ingredient has been eliminated from many of the nutritionally complete enteral formulas. For those patients with hepatic or renal disease, the sodium and potassium content of the formulations must be considered. For patients maintained on warfarin therapy, consideration should be focused on the content of Vitamin K in the formulation. Although many products now have less Vitamin K than before, caution is still warranted to avoid hypoprothrombinemic alterations in warfarin therapy.

Specific enteral products are selected according to the patient type they serve. For example, a requirement for less than 2000 calories per day, or increased protein typically involves an elderly, bedfast patient who is not physically active. This level of support is also advocated for postsurgical patients, and those who suffer from infection or fractured bones. While requiring fewer calories, these individuals still need normal nutrients, including protein. Such products as Ensure HN, Sustacal, and Osmolite HN are appropriate in this circumstance. Alternatively, most persons fall within the 2000 to 3000 calorie per day category, inclusive of patients with poor appetite or those suffering from cancer. The last category of patients are those with daily caloric needs which exceed 3000 calories. These individuals usually have high protein losses from severe trauma, e.g., burns, sepsis, multiple trauma. As in the first example there are numerous products for the latter two patient categories.

The pharmacist can be helpful in the selection of these products because these do differ in the amount of their carbohydrate, fat, and protein content, and in fiber. Further, these products differ in taste and consumer acceptability criteria, e.g., "mouth feel," cost. Pharmacists may encounter consumers who wish to self-administer an enteral product. If the intent is to supplement calories or protein in an otherwise healthy individual who simply wishes to assure a balanced dietary intake, a complete formula can be recommended. However, if it is intended to help a person regain weight which has been lost unexpectedly, the individual should be instead referred to a doctor. Sudden weight loss may indicate a serious pathologic problem requiring medical attention.

Pharmacists can also be helpful in cost management associated with these products. Composition (oligomeric or polymeric) and form (ready-to-use vs. powder) of the product influence cost. Generally, the polymeric products are less expensive than the oligomeric products. While powder forms may be less expensive compared to ready-to-use formulations, there is an indirect cost of labor required in the powder preparation.

Intravenous Infusion Devices

Since the early 1970s, the use of the intravenous route to administer drugs has become increasingly popular. In 1989, it was estimated that about 40% of all drugs and fluid administered in the hospital setting are done through intravenous administration (22). This increase has affected the development and use of mechanical infusion devices. Advances in infusion technology and computer technology have resulted in devices with extremely sophisticated drug-delivery capabilities (e.g., multiple-rate programming, pump or controller operation) (23). As a result, these cost-efficient devices provide greater accuracy and reliability of drug delivery than the traditional gravity-flow infusion methods. They also help reduce the fluid volume attributable to the medication infusion and decrease the need for monitoring fluid input (thus, decreased nursing time). Further, multiple-drug dosages can be administered, and incompatible drugs can be administered separately (22).

There are disadvantages associated with these mechanical devices, however, including the initial capital investment and extensive in-service education. Further, the influence of infusion pump devices on the delivery of a drug has not been fully recognized by clinicians. For example, intrinsic factors (operating mechanisms, flow accuracy, flow continuity, occlusion detection) and an extrinsic factor (backpressure) may alter the rate of drug delivery and the corresponding therapeutic response of the patient.

Pumps are classified by their *mechanism of operation* (peristaltic, piston, diaphragm), *frequency or type of drug delivery* (continuous or intermittent, bolus dosing, single-solution or multiple-solution), or *therapeutic application* (patient-controlled analgesia [PCA]) (24). Current research focuses upon the influence of drug delivery by these devices and the creation of new technologies (e.g., implantable pumps, pumps with chronobiological applications, osmotic-pressure devices, and open- or closed-loop systems) (24). Table 14.8 demonstrates several infusion devices which are used in parenteral nutrition support, including features associated with each.

Special Considerations Associated with Parenteral Therapy

Adsorption of Drugs

Numerous studies have demonstrated that some drugs are adsorbed onto the inner lining of IV containers and tubing or administration sets. Some of the drugs that have been implicated in this phenomenon and lost from aqueous solutions during infusion through plastic IV delivery systems include:

- Chlorpromazine HCl
- Diazepam
- Insulin
- Promazine HCl

- Promethazine HCl
- Thiopental sodium
- Thioridazine HCl
- Trifluoperazine HCl
- Warfarin sodium

Thus, pharmacists must be cognizant of this and take appropriate steps to prevent their occurrence. The significance of the loss is magnified with drugs that are used in lower quantities because a small amount lost to adsorption results in a higher percentage loss of the drug being delivered to the patient. One method to minimize this, is to administer infusions through short lengths of small-diameter tubing made of inert plastics.

Nitroglycerin, for example, should always be prepared in glass containers, and is adsorbed (40–80% of total dose) to polyvinylchloride (PVC), a plastic commonly used in administration components and some infusion containers. Thus, nitroglycerin for IV use is packaged with special non-PVC tubing by some manufacturers to avoid loss (<5%) of the drug into the tubing during administration. The amount of the adsorption depends upon such factors as concentration, flow rate, surface area of the tubing, and contact time with the tubing.

Intravenous nitroglycerin should be regulated by automatic infusion equipment (i.e., pumps, controllers) to enhance consistent dose administration. However, a problem may occur in that infusion pumps may fail to occlude the non-PVC infusion sets completely because the non-PVC (i.e., polyethylene) tubing is less pliable (i.e., more stiff) than standard PVC tubing. Excessive flow at low infusion rate settings may occur, causing alarms or unregulated gravity flow when the infusion pump is stopped. This could lead to overinfusion of nitroglycerin.

Some practitioners have responded by using the PVC containing tubing with the nitroglycerin and working around the problem. This is justified by some in that even though a great amount of drug is lost, the amount of drug the patient receives is based on hemodynamic functions. But, when the previous set is replaced, retitration of the drug is necessary. To allay this problem, several manufacturers have made available non-PVC containing pump administration sets.

The adsorption of insulin onto glassware and tubing depends upon several factors (i.e., concentration of insulin, contact time of insulin with glass and tubing, flow rate of the insulin infusion, presence of negatively charged proteins [human serum albumin]). Plastic IV infusion sets have reportedly removed up to 80% of a dose, but 20% to 30% is more common. The percent adsorbed is inversely

Table 14.8.　Selected Infusion Devices Used in Parenteral Nutrition Support[1]

Pump	Manufacturer	Cost ($)	Alarms, Features
Volumetric infusion pumps			
AVI 2000 #200	AVI, 3M HealthCare Group	2800	Safety alarms; variable occlusion pressure limits; automatic KVO rate switch when volume limit reached.
Flo-Gard 8100	Baxter Healthcare	2800	Visual/audible alarms for flow rate error, improperly loaded cassette or drop sensor, infusion complete, low battery, occlusion; disposable cassette, gravity control plunger eliminates "run-aways" and allows for use on pump or by gravity, adjustable differential occlusion detection.
IMED	IMED	2600	Alarms for air in line, door open, low battery, malfunction, occlusion; automatic priming, dual-rate sequential piggybacking, syringe-use, selectable tamper-proof modes.
Multiple-rate programmable pumps			
CADD-TPN	Sims Deltec	3500	Alarms for infusion period completed, low reservoir volume, invalid rate, high pressure, system error; ambulatory system, may be stored and operated in backpack, programmable taper features.
Volumetric infusion pumps			
Provider One	Pancretec	2995	Alarms for air in line, computer error, end of infusion, low battery, low reservoir, occlusion, programming error; ability to taper up, down, or both, ability to adjust flow rate automatically, convenient carry case.
Quest 521 Intelligent	McGaw	2895	Alarms for air in line, check set, door open, low battery, repair, set volume; selectable variable pressure limits, 9 programmable cycles of time and rate.
Multiple-solution programmable pumps			
Gemini PC-2	IMED	4250	Alarms for check i.v. set, open-close door, air in line, occlusion inpatient or fluid side; 2 channels allowing delivery of 2 fluids at independent rates, can be operated as pump, controller, or both.
LifeCare 5000 Plum	Abbott	3500	Alarms for high or low flow, distal and proximal air in line or occlusion, dose end, low battery; history bank with last 15 alarms, variable pressure limits, tubing conversion to gravity flow, allows delivery of 2 fluids at independent rates, can be operated as pump, controller, or both.
Omni-Flow 4000	Abbott	4995	Alarms for air in line, cassette unlocked, empty container, low battery, occlusions in patient lines or upstream; automatic air elimination, can deliver up to 4 fluids simultaneously in continuous or intermittent modes.

[1]Copyright permission, American College of Clinical Pharmacy

proportional to the insulin concentration and will take place within 30 to 60 minutes. Because this phenomenon cannot be easily and accurately predicted, patient monitoring is essential.

Handling/Disposal of Chemotherapeutic Agents for Cancer

In the 1980s awareness developed among health care personnel about environmental cont-amination that was possible after handling cytotoxic agents. Mutagenic and allergic case reports began to emerge in the literature, and in response in 1985, the then American Society of Hospital Pharmacists (now the American Society of Health-System Pharmacists) published a technical assistance bulletin on handling cytotoxic and hazardous drugs. This bulletin has been updated through the years and is now found in the *Practice Standards of ASHP* (25).

In theory, "correct and perfect preparation and handling techniques will prevent drug particles or droplets from escaping from their containers while they are being manipulated" (25). However, near perfect technique is uncommon and quite impossible. Thus, there must be structured training and quality-assurance programs in place within institutions that use these hazardous drugs, and the pharmacist must play a vital role in creating and executing these.

At potential risk for harm are those personnel who handle cytotoxic drugs, and steps should be taken to minimize unnecessary exposure by implementing basic steps and following common sense (26). These basic steps include:

1. Utilizing vertical laminar flow hoods (or bacteriological glove boxes) for the preparation and reconstitution of cytotoxic drugs.
2. Wearing protective gloves and mask during product preparation.
3. Handling and disposing of cytotoxic drugs centrally utilizing specially designed waste containers and incineration.
4. Periodic monitoring of personnel involved with handling admixtures of cytotoxic drugs (e.g., CBC, blood chemistry screen, differential cell count).
5. Informing personnel handling cytotoxic drugs that a potential risk to their health exists.
6. Instituting specialized labeling of containers to ensure proper handling and disposal of the cytotoxic agent.

Other Injectable Products— Pellets or Implants

Historically, pellets or implants were sterile, small, usually cylindrical-shaped solid objects about 3.2 mm in diameter and 8 mm in length, prepared by compression and intended to be implanted subcutaneously for the purpose of providing the continuous release of medication over a prolonged period of time. The pellets, which are implanted under the skin (usually of the thigh or abdomen) with a special injector or by surgical incision, are used for potent hormones. Their implantation provides the patient with an economical means of obtaining long-lasting effects (up to many months after a single implantation) and obviates the need for frequent parenteral or oral hormone therapy. The implanted pellet, which might contain 100 times the amount of drug (e.g., desoxycorticosterone, estradiol,

testosterone) given by other routes of administration, release the drug slowly into the general circulation.

Pellets were formulated with no binders, diluents, or excipients, to permit total dissolution and absorption of the pellet from the site of implantation. Recently, a levonorgestrel implant contraceptive system was developed. Rather than dissolve entirely, the surgically implanted capsules are intended to be removed subsequently by surgery after an appropriate amount of time (up to 5 years).

Levonorgestrel Implants

These are a set of six flexible, closed capsules of a dimethylsiloxane/methylvinylsiloxane copolymer, each containing 36 mg of the progestin levonorgestrel (27). These are found in an insertion kit to facilitate surgical subdermal implantation through a 2 mm incision in the mid-portion of the upper arm about eight to ten cm above the elbow crease. These are implanted in a fan-like pattern, about 15° apart, for a total of 75°. Appropriate insertion facilitates removal by the end of the fifth year. This system provides long-term (up to 5 years) reversible contraception.

Diffusion of the levonorgestrel through the wall of each capsule provides a continuous low dose of progestin. Initially, the dose of levonorgestrel is about 85 mcg/day, followed by a decline to about 50 mcg/day by 9 months, and to about 35 mcg/day by 18 months, with a further decline thereafter to about 30 mcg/day. The resulting blood levels are substantially below those generally observed among users of combination oral contraceptives containing the progestins norgestrel or levonorgestrel. Because of the range of variability in blood levels and variation in individual response, blood levels alone are not predictive of the risk of pregnancy in an individual woman (27).

Irrigation and Dialysis Solutions

Solutions for irrigation of body tissues and for dialysis resemble parenteral solutions in that they are subject to the same stringent standards. The difference is in their use. These solutions are not injected into the vein, but employed outside of the circulatory system. Since they are generally used in large volumes, they are packaged in large volume containers, generally of the screw-cap type which permits the rapid pouring of the solution.

Table 14.9.   Examples of Irrigation Solutions

Solution	Description
Acetic Acid Irrigation, USP	This solution is employed topically to the bladder as a 0.25% solution for irrigation. It has a pH of between 2.8 and 3.4 and a calculated osmolarity of 42 mOsm/L, and is employed during urologic procedures. It is administered to wash blood and surgical debris away while maintaining suitable conditions for the tissue and permitting the surgeon an unobstructed view.
Neomycin and Polymyxin B Sulfates Solution for Irrigation, USP	This sterile urogenital solution contains 57 mg neomycin sulfate (40 mg of neomycin) and Polymyxin B Sulfate 200,000 Units (of polymyxin B) per ml and is employed as a topical antibacterial in the continuous irrigation of the bladder. It has a pH between 4.5 to 6.0. One ml of this solution is added to 1 L of 0.9% sodium chloride solution and administered via a 3-way catheter at the rate of 1 L every 24 hours (i.e., approximately 40 mL/hr).
Ringer's Irrigation, USP	This solution contains sodium chloride (8.6 g/L), potassium chloride (0.3 g/L), and calcium chloride (0.33 g/L) in purified water, in the same proportions, as is present in Ringer's Injection. The solution is sterile and pyrogen-free. It is used topically as an irrigation and must be labeled "not for injection." It has a pH between 5.0 and 7.5 and a calculated osmolarity of 309 mOsm/L.
Sodium Chloride Irrigation, USP	This sterile solution of sodium chloride in water for injection contains 77 or 154 mEq/L each of sodium and chloride in the 0.45 and 0.9% solution, respectively. Sodium chloride irrigation has a pH of approximately 5.3, and the 0.45 and 0.9% solutions have a calculated osmolarity of 154 and 308 mOsm/L, respectively. The solution is employed topically to wash wounds and into body cavities where absorption into the blood is not likely. The solution may also be employed rectally as an enema; for simple evacuation, 150 mL is usually employed and for colonic flush, 1500 mL may be used.
Sterile Water for Irrigation, USP	This is water for injection that has been sterilized and suitably packaged. The label designations "for irrigation only" and "not for injection" must appear prominently on the label. The water must not contain any antimicrobial or other added agent.

Irrigation Solutions

Irrigation solutions are intended to bathe or wash wounds, surgical incisions, or body tissues. Examples are presented in Table 14.9.

Dialysis Solutions

Dialysis may be defined as a process whereby substances may be separated from one another in solution by taking advantage of their differing diffusibility through membranes. *Peritoneal dialysis* solutions, allowed to flow into the peritoneal cavity, are used to remove toxic substances normally excreted by the kidney. In cases of poisoning or kidney failure, or in patients awaiting renal transplants, dialysis is an emergency life-saving procedure. Solutions are commercially available containing dextrose as a major source of calories, vitamins, minerals, electrolytes, and amino acids or peptides as a source of nitrogen. The solutions are made to be hypertonic (with dextrose) to plasma to avoid absorption of water from the dialysis solution into the circulation.

Peritoneal dialysis involves the principles of osmosis and diffusion across the semipermeable peritoneal membrane and includes the osmotic and chemical equilibration of the fluid within the peritoneal cavity with that of the extracellular compartment. The semipermeable peritoneal membrane restricts the movement of formed elements (e.g., erythrocytes) and large molecules (e.g., protein) but allows the movement of smaller molecules (e.g., electrolytes, urea, water) in both directions across the membrane according to the concentration on each side of the membrane, with net movement occurring in the direction of the concentration gradient. Instillation of dialysis solutions containing physiologic concentrations of electrolytes intraperitoneally allows for the movement of water, toxic substances and/or metabolites across the membrane in the direction of the concentration gradient, resulting in removal of these substances from the body following drainage of the solution from the peritoneal cavity (i.e., outflow).

Hemodialysis is employed to remove toxins from the blood. In this method, the arterial blood is shunted through a polyethylene catheter through an artificial dialyzing membrane bathed in an electrolyte solution. Following the dialysis, the blood is returned to the body circulation through a vein.

Various dialysis solutions are available commercially and the pharmacist may be called upon to provide them or to make adjustments in their composition.

References

1. Rapp RP, Bivins BA, Littrell RA, Foster, TS. Patient-controlled analgesia: A review of effectiveness of therapy and an evaluation of currently available devices. DICP, Ann Pharmacother 1989;23:899–904.
2. Kwan JW. Use of infusion devices for epidural or intrathecal administration of spinal opioids. Am J Hosp Pharm 1990;47 (Suppl 1):S18-S23.
3. Erstad BL, Meeks ML. Influence of injection site and route on medication absorption. Hosp Pharm 1993; 28:853–856; 858–860; 863–864, 867–868; 871–874; 877–878.
4. Highsmith AK, Greenhood GP, Allen JR. Growth of nosocomial pathogens in multiple-dose parenteral medication vials. J Clin Microbiol 1982;15:1024–1028.
5. Gershanik J, Boecler B, Ensley H, McCloskey S, George W. The gasping syndrome and benzyl alcohol poisoning. N Engl J Med 1982;307:1384–1388.
6. Nema S, Avis KE. Loss of LDH activity during membrane filtration. J Parenter Sci Technol 1993;47:16–21.
7. Sarry C, Sucker H. Adsorption of proteins on microporous membrane filters: Part I. Pharm Technol 1992; 16(Oct):72–82.
8. Sarry C, Sucker H. Adsorption of proteins on microporous membrane filters: Part II. Pharm Technol 1993;17(Jan):60–70.
9. McKinnon BT, Avis KE. Membrane filtration of pharmaceutical solutions. Am J Hosp Pharm 1993;50: 1921–1936.
10. Butler LD, Munson JM, DeLuca PP. Effect of inline filtration on the potency of low-dose drugs. Am J Hosp Pharm 1980;37:935–941.
11. Akers MJ, Attia IA, Avis KE: Understanding and Utilizing F_0 Values. Pharm Tech 1987;11:44–48.
12. Wall DS, Noe LI, Abel SR, Hardwick LI, Plesek SR. A resource use comparison of Monovial® with traditional methods of preparing extemporaneous small-volume intravenous infusions. Hosp Pharm 1997;32: 1647–1656.
13. Turco S, Miele WH, Barnoski D. Evaluation of an aseptic technique testing and challenge kit (Attack). Hosp Pharm 1993; 28:11–16.
14. Crawford SY, Narducci WA, Augustine SC. National survey of quality assurance activities for pharmacy-prepared sterile products in hospitals. Am J Hosp Pharm 1991;48:2398–2413.
15. ASHP Technical Assistance Bulletin on Quality Assurance for Pharmacy-Prepared Sterile Products. *Practice Standards of ASHP,* 1997–1998. American Society of Health-System Pharmacists, Bethesda, MD, 1997: 171–172.
16. ASHP. Draft guidelines on quality assurance for pharmacy-prepared sterile products. Am J Hosp Pharm 1992;49:407–417.
17. Erskine CR, Herzog KA. Quality assurance and control. In Gennaro AR, ed. Remington: The Science and Practice of Pharmacy. 19th ed. Easton: Mack Publishing, 1995, 648–652.
18. Maliekal J, Bertch KE, Witte KW. An update on ready-to-use intravenous delivery system. Hosp Pharm 1993; 28:970–971, 975–977.
19. Turco S. Parenteral admixtures and incompatibilities. In: Sterile Dosage Forms. Philadelphia: Lea & Febiger, 1994;11:263.
20. Munzenberger PJ, Levin S. Home parenteral antibiotic therapy for patients with cystic fibrosis. Hosp Pharm 1993;28:20–28.
21. McKinnon BT. FDA Safety Alert: Hazards of precipitation associated with parenteral nutrition. Nutr Clin Pract 1996;11:59–65.
22. Kwan JW. High-technology IV infusion devices. Am J Hosp Pharm 1989;46:320–335.
23. KITS: Kit for Infusion Technology Self-Instruction. Marketing Department, Electronic Drug Delivery Systems, Abbott Laboratories, Abbott Park, IL.
24. Keefner KR. Parenteral pumps and controlled-delivery devices. US Pharmacist 1992;17(8):H-3-H.16.
25. ASHP Technical Assistance Bulletin on Handling Cytotoxic and Hazardous Drugs. *Practice Standards of ASHP,* 1997–1998. American Society of Health-System Pharmacists, Bethesda, MD, 1997:136–152.
26. *op. cit.* ref 19, 267.
27. Fung S, Ferrill M. Contraceptive update: Subdermal implants. California Pharmacist 1992;40:35–41.

15

BIOLOGICALS

Chapter at a Glance

THE FOOD and Drug Administration refers to immunizing agents as *biologics* (e.g., biologicals, biological products). In an encompassing manner, a biological refers to a substance produced by a living source and includes antibiotics, hormones, and vitamins, among others. Alternatively, the Advisory Committee on Immunization Practices (i.e., ACIP) refers to immunizing agents as *immunobiologics*.

According to the *Code of Federal Regulations (CFR)*, a biological product is any virus, therapeutic serum, toxin, antitoxin or analogous product which is employed for the prevention, treatment, or cure of diseases in humans. The underlying objective of these products is to help develop a type of immunity in the person receiving them or are concerned with aspects of immunity. Immunity is defined as the natural or acquired resistance to disease.

The provision of gaining immunity through the use of a biological is referred to as immunization. More commonly, vaccination is a term used, and refers to the use of a biological product (i.e., a vaccine) to develop active immunity in the patient.

Types of Immunity

Before discussing specific biologicals, it is important to have an understanding of the different types of immunity. There are two main categories of immunity, natural and acquired.

Natural Immunity

Natural, innate, or native immunity depends on factors that are inborn and can be classified as species immunity, racial immunity, and individual immunity.

Species Immunity

In general, cold-blooded animals are not susceptible to diseases common to warm-blooded animals. Humans are not all susceptible to certain diseases of lower animals, such as chicken cholera. There are, however, a number of infections, which occur primarily in animals that can be transmitted to humans. Among the most important are anthrax (from cattle, sheep, horses), plague (rodents) and rabies (cats, dogs, bats). Correspondingly, many human diseases do not naturally occur in animals. Examples include gonorrhea, typhoid fever, influenza, measles, mumps, and poliomyelitis.

Racial Immunity

Among human races there are differences in susceptibility to common infections (e.g., yellow fever, pneumonia, tuberculosis). Factors that determine racial immunity are elusive and not well known. Racial immunity should not be used synonymously or confused with environmental immunity. Environmental immunity may be the result of resistance to infection among individuals within a community due to the degree of acquired immunity and to other factors (e.g., nutrition, genetic constitution, fatigue). For example, tuberculosis and smallpox wreaked havoc among the Eskimos and American Indians when these groups were first exposed to them. However, with the course of time, the disease tends to become less severe, and it may eventually reach the same level of incidence and severity as it has among other races with whom the disease has been endemic for long periods of time.

Individual Immunity

Apart from any specific immunity toward a particular infectious agent that they may happen to possess, individuals vary in their abilities to resist common microbiological diseases. Some individuals demonstrate decreased capacity to resist skin disorders, the common cold, and other familiar diseases. The natural resistance of the same individual may vary from time to time.

General good health is demonstrated by healthy body tissues, skin, and mucous membranes, leukocytes in plentiful supply, an active and positive (i.e., little or no smoking, drinking alcohol, social drug use) lifestyle provide adequate barriers to bacteria infiltration. Resident bacterial flora within the gastrointestinal tract and in the upper respiratory tract, for example, provide resistance to infection. These play a vital role in resisting invasion by other species of microorganisms capable of producing infection. Also, stomach acid is bacteriocidal to a degree and capable of destroying bacteria that are ingested during eating and drinking. Intestinal enzymes are also known to provide secondary defense mechanisms.

Acquired Immunity

This is a specific immunity that may be actively acquired (active immunity) or passively acquired

(passive immunity). *T lymphocytes* regulate cell-mediated immunity and are responsible for controlling certain bacterial and viral infections. These lymphocytes are responsible for mediating graft *vs* host disease, allograft rejection, and delayed hypersensitivity reactions.

T lymphocytes augment the activity of *B lymphocytes* that are primarily involved with humoral immunity and antibody production. Once an antigen is introduced into the body, *B lymphocytes* differentiate into plasma cells that are capable of producing antibodies specific to the invading antigen. These antibodies, known synonymously as immunoglobulins (i.e., Igs), attach to the invading antigen and cause its destruction by phagocytes and the complement system.

Once exposed to an antigen, the *T* and *B lymphocytes* demonstrate "memory" which will allow them to recognize and respond to a specific antigen when re-exposed again. The second response is far greater in magnitude to the first immunological response. This "memory" of an antigen by the immune system allows sensitized individuals to resist infections following subsequent exposure.

Active Immunity

This type develops within an individual in response to the introduction of antigenic substances into his/her body. This may occur by natural means, as by infection, in which case it is termed *naturally acquired active immunity,* or it may be developed in response to the administration of a specific vaccine or toxoid, in which case it is termed *artificially acquired active immunity.* In either case, the body builds up its own defenses in response to the antigen.

Vaccines are administered primarily for prophylactic action in the development of active immunity (acquired). Vaccines may contain living, attenuated (weakened), or killed microorganisms, or fractions of these microorganisms. Toxoids are bacterial toxins modified and detoxified by the use of moderate heat and chemical treatment so that the antigenic properties remain while the substance is rendered nontoxic. Although toxoids do not cause disease, exposure of immunocompetent patients may result in antibody production that will protect the patient against disease caused by the naturally occurring toxin. A problem with toxoids is that they produce inadequate immunological responses when administered alone. Thus, they are often combined with adjuvants (e.g., alum, aluminum phosphate, aluminum hydroxide) that enhance their antigenicity. These agents do so through their insoluble nature that acts to keep the immunogens in tissue for longer periods and thus, causes a prolonged immune response.

A vaccine composed of killed whole bacteria or viruses or substructures of these is known as an inactivated vaccine. Those vaccines that contain live, but significantly weakened, microorganisms are known as attenuated vaccines. Both of these types of vaccines are capable of producing immunity. However, the attenuated vaccines typically have more antigenicity, and thus, more likely to confer permanent immunity. To maintain adequate antibody titers, inactivated vaccines must be readministered over time.

Caution must be exercised when vaccinating patients who are immunocompromised. This group of patients includes those with HIV infection, thymic abnormalities, lymphoma, leukemia, generalized malignancy, advanced debilitating diseases, receiving therapy with corticosteroids, alkylating agents, antimetabolites, or radiation chemotherapy. These patients are unable to mount immune responses against even weakened microorganisms in the attenuated vaccines. The result could be a disseminated bacterial or viral infection. Thus, inactivated vaccines should be employed for these special patient types.

Immunization during pregnancy is another concern. Live, attenuated vaccines should be avoided for use in pregnant patients because of the danger of bacterial/viral transmission to the fetus.

Passive acquired immunity occurs by the introduction of the immunoglobulins produced in another individual (i.e., human or lower animal) into the host who is not involved in their production. In similar fashion to active acquired immunity, passive acquired immunity can be classified as natural or artificial.

Naturally acquired passive immunity occurs by placental transmission of immunoglobulin G (i.e., IgG) from the mother to the fetus. Because of the transfer of these immunoglobulins, the infant may have passive immunity to diphtheria, tetanus, measles, mumps and other infections for the first 4 to 6 months of life.

Several biological products containing immunoglobulins provide passive immunity. These are limited to the provision of temporary prophylaxis to susceptible individuals, for example, during an epidemic, and to supplying immediate immunoglobulins for the treatment of infections and toxicities. Notable in this category are the antivenins used for the treatment of bites from poisonous snakes (e.g., North American Coral Snake Antivenin) and spiders (e.g., Black Widow Spider Antivenin).

The acquired passive immunity provided by immunoglobulins is not long lasting. Usually, the time frame for immunity ranges from one to two weeks. The important feature, however, of their use is that they offer the susceptible patient protection during a critical period of exposure (e.g., the patient exposed to diphtheria). Immunoglobulins do not last long because their function is to bind to the pathogen as needed. Remaining immunoglobulin is metabolized by the body if not needed for immunological purposes.

Production of Biologicals

Biologicals are produced by manufacturers licensed to do so in accordance with the terms of the federal Public Health Service Act (58 Stat. 682) approved July 1, 1944, and each product must meet the specified standards as administered by the Center for Biologics Evaluation and Research of the federal Food and Drug Administration (1). Each lot of a licensed biological is approved for distribution when it has been determined that the lot meets the specific control requirements for that product set forth by the Center. Licensing includes approval of a specific series of production steps and in-process control tests as well as end-product specifications that must be met on a lot-by-lot basis.

Generally, each lot of a biological product must pass rigid control requirements before it may be distributed for general use. Provisions generally applicable to biological products include tests for potency, general safety, sterility, purity, water (residual moisture), pyrogens, identity, and constituent materials. Constituent materials include ingredients: preservatives, diluents, and adjuvants (which generally should meet compendial standards), extraneous protein in cell-culture produced vaccines (which, if other than serum-originating, is excluded) and antibiotics other than penicillin added to the production substrate of viral vaccines for which compendial monographs on antibiotics and antibiotic substances are available. Additional safety tests are also required to be performed on live vaccines and certain other items.

Biologicals intended to be administered by injection are packaged and labeled in the same manner as other injections. In addition, however, the label of a biological product must include the title or proper name (the name under which the product is licensed under the Public Health Service Act); the name, address, and license number of the manufacturer; the lot number; the expiration date; and the recommended individual dose for multiple-dose containers. The package label includes all of the above, with the addition of: the preservative used and its amount; the number of containers, if more than one; the amount of product in the container; the recommended storage temperature; a statement, if necessary, that freezing is to be avoided; and such other information as the Food and Drug regulations may require to ensure the safe and effective use of the product (1).

With few exceptions, most biologicals are stored in a refrigerator (between 2°C and 8°C), and freezing is avoided. In many instances it is not the biological substance that is harmed by freezing, but rather the container which may be broken through the freezing and expansion of an aqueous vehicle so that some of the product is lost. Diluents packaged with biologicals should not be frozen. Some products are to be maintained during shipment at specified temperatures.

The expiration date for biological products varies with the product and the storage temperatures employed. Generally, most biological products have an expiration date of a year or longer after the date of manufacture or issue. For biological products the stated date on each lot determines the dating period, which begins on the date of manufacture and beyond which the product cannot be expected beyond reasonable doubt to yield its specific result and to retain the required safety, purity, and potency. The dating period may comprise an in-house storage period during which the lot is permitted to be held under prescribed conditions in the manufacturer's storage facilities followed by a period after issue. The individual monographs for biologicals usually indicate both, the after issue time frame for use and (in parentheses) the permissible in-house storage period (1).

Storage, Handling, and Shipping of Biologicals

Biologicals are sensitive to extreme temperatures, and exposure to heat or freezing can decrease their potency and dramatically reduce their effectiveness. Not providing adequate storage, handling, and shipping conditions for these products not only wastes the intrinsic value of the products, but wastes money as well. Biologicals are very expensive products and can add significantly to one's inventory. An inventory of vaccines and other immunological products can amount to tens of thousands of dollars or more.

A real danger is that if damaged products are administered to a patient, that patient might get little of the intent of the product whether it be prophylaxis or therapeutic benefit. This patient might not be able to build up his/her immunity and get the infection. Or, the patient might get the disease that the biological was intended to protect the patient.

The overriding theme for the pharmacist in the storage, handling, and shipping of the biological product is to maintain the "cold chain" (2). This implies a continuity from the manufacturer's refrigerator at the manufacturing facilities through to one's pharmacy, clinic, office, etc., to ultimate patient administration. If the "cold chain" is maintained, the pharmacist can be assured that the quality of the product will not be diminished.

In the pharmacy, there should be a clear understanding of primary and alternative individuals who are responsible to receive, handle, and ship these products. A key ingredient also is good equipment to store these products. Whenever possible, separate commercial refrigerators and freezers should be used for these products. For small volume biologicals, a standard refrigerator-freezer should be used. Frost-free freezers should be utilized because ice buildup interferes with the freezer's ability to maintain very low temperatures. Also, defrosting requires that product be removed from the freezer during thawing to temporary storage.

Refrigerators and freezers cool by convection. Thus, cool air must have room to circulate around the products (or boxes of product) to cool them. If one packs the refrigerator too tightly, this can lead to small, incremental elevations in the temperature of the product.

A separate refrigerator dedicated to biologicals is preferable to minimize the times the refrigerator door is opened on a routine basis. The World Health Organization recommends that the door not be opened more frequently than four times per day. Also, doors should be closed as quickly as possible after securing the product. Further, pharmacists should avoid using the inside of the refrigerator door to store product to avoid unacceptable temperature variations. The door shelving can be used to store diluents or bottles of water. This then helps provide insulation and a thermal reserve (2).

If out of necessity, a vaccine must be kept outside of the refrigerator for a few minutes after its removal from the refrigerator, it is advisable to insulate the product within an insulated container with coolant packs (syn. thermal packs, blue-ice packs, chemical packs) taken from the freezer. Coolant packs should be kept in the freezer and ready for use in shipping. An additional advantage of freezer packs is that their presence in the freezer provides extra insulation and cooling power in the case of an interruption of electric power or outage.

Coolant packs that contain water have about as much cooling capacity as ethylene glycol packs. An easy way to create a coolant pack is to fill a plastic bottle with water and then freeze it for use. It is important, however, that the product not come in direct contact with these coolant packs because the vial contents may freeze and be damaged. An easy method to separate the product from the coolant pack is to use a towel or sheet of cardboard to separate the two (2).

Periodically, it is advisable for the pharmacist to test the refrigerator and freezer to determine their ability to maintain the desired temperature range. Refrigerator temperatures should range between 2°C and 8°C, and freezers should maintain their temperatures well below 0°C. Usually, an optimal temperature is -15°C (5°F).

With respect to personnel, pharmacists should educate and train every person who will handle biologicals in good storage and handling procedures. These individuals should understand the importance of reporting any encountered problems or interruption associated with proper handling and storage guidelines. It is far more important to report a breach in handling and storage than to discount and overlook it intentionally. The subsequent use of a useless, inactivated biological could have devastating consequences on the patient who receives it.

When storing biological products, store containers of the same vaccine together. To help avoid selecting the wrong product or something that has similar packaging separate the products. A good example of this occurs with pediatric and adult dosage forms (e.g., tetanus-diphtheria toxoids) which could be confused. Keep them separate. Look-alike packaging can easily confuse any conscientious practitioner.

Biologicals for Active Immunity

Bacterial Vaccines

A vaccine is a suspension of attenuated (i.e., live) or inactivated (i.e., killed) microorganisms or fractions thereof that are administered to induce immunity and subsequently prevent disease. Originally, the organism is grown in a suitable broth medium under a controlled environment of temperature, pH, and oxygen tension. To reduce the potential of hypersensitivity reactions of the finished product, the medium, whenever possible, should consist of chemically defined ingredients.

Following a suitable amount of time for bacterial growth, the culture is then processed in two steps. If the vaccine is to be inactivated microorganisms,

the organisms are treated with phenol or formaldehyde. Heat and phenol or heat and acetone are employed for the typhoid fever vaccine. Next, the organisms are separated from the medium through centrifugation and resuspended in sterile water or 0.9% sodium chloride for injection. Beyond this step, if necessary, the preparation may be further purified by several methods including dialysis and/or additional centrifugation.

A live, attenuated vaccine can also be produced through biotechnological technique by genetically altering the pathogenic organism. This allows the organism to survive and multiply, but not produce the disease. Usually, several base pairs of DNA within a key region of the gene structure are eliminated or altered. Thus, the organism is incapable of reverting to its more pathogenic form.

Another mode to create a vaccine is to employ purified antigen subunits which are produced through recombinant DNA technology. Known as a subunit vaccine, the genes that code for the desired antigen in the immunization process are introduced into the nonpathogenic organisms. There is no potential to cause harm to the patient because there is no possibility that a pathogenic organism can be created from only a limited number of components from the original organism. Also, the subunit vaccine would be expected to have a lower incidence of side effects associated with its use.

To date, subunit vaccines have had limited clinical utility because of an inability to effect a sufficient specific immune response. However, alternative biotechnological strategies have been employed to produce subunit vaccine immunogens and adjuvant-active compounds that can be added to enhance the immune response.

The final vaccine product may contain one single immunogen (i.e., monovalent) or it may contain multiple immunogens (i.e., polyvalent, trivalent) to promote immunity against the same disease state. Further, the final product may be a mixed vaccine. For example, the measles, mumps, and rubella vaccine (MMR) is a single product with three different viral immunogens for three different viral disease states. A mixed biological may contain a vaccine and a toxoid in the same product, e.g., DTP.

The strength of a vaccine may be expressed as total organisms, total protective units per mL or dose, or micrograms of immunogen in each mL or in each dose of vaccine.

Viral Vaccines

Viruses cannot be grown on inanimate media employed to grow bacteria and thus are propagated on one of several types of animate media. Examples of animate media include embryonic egg, cell cultures of chick embryo, human diploid cell culture, monkey cell culture, skin of living calves, and intact mice.

In similar fashion to vaccine preparation, following growth various techniques are employed to separate the virus from the host cell. Purification steps are then employed to reduce the incidence of hypersensitivity reactions due to animate media or host cells, most notably embryonic egg. The final viral product may contain a single immunogen (i.e., monovalent) or it may contain multiple immunogens (i.e., polyvalent) to elicit immunity against the same disease.

The vaccine may remain as the whole virion or be further chemically processed to split the virion into a subvirion vaccine, as is the case with the influenzavirus vaccine. This virus is prepared yearly, with three virus strains (usually two Type A and one Type B) chosen on the basis of information provided by a worldwide surveillance network. The information identifies strains most likely to circulate widely during the upcoming season. Strains to be included in the influenza vaccine usually are selected during the preceding January through February because of scheduling requirements for production, quality control, packaging, distribution, and vaccine administration before the onset of the next influenza season.

For 1998–1999, the FDA's Vaccines and Related Biologic Products Advisory Committee (VRBPAC) recommended that the trivalent vaccine for the United States contain A/Sydney/5/97-like(H3N2), A/Beijing/262/95-like(H1N1), and B/Beijing/184/93-like viruses (3). When there is a good match between the strains included in the vaccine and those circulating in the community, inactivated vaccine is 70 to 90 percent effective in preventing the disease in people under 65 years of age (4).

To prolong stimulation of antibodies, the virion may be adsorbed onto aluminum phosphate (as is the case with Rabies vaccine [adsorbed]). Typically, viral vaccines are available as lyophilized (i.e., freeze-dried) products that require reconstitution prior to administration with the provided diluent. Some inactivated vaccines are available in suspensions for injection, whereas living polio vaccine is in a liquid form for oral use.

Belshe et al. reported the effectiveness of a live attenuated, cold-adapted, trivalent influenza-virus vaccine that was administered intranasally to over 1000 healthy school-aged children (5). This placebo-controlled trial demonstrated that those children re-

ceiving the active vaccine had fewer febrile illnesses, including 30 percent fewer episodes of febrile otitis media when compared to the placebo group. This was one significant outcome of the study because otitis media is a recognized complication of influenza in children, and the influenzavirus has been isolated from middle-ear fluid in children with influenza and middle-ear effusion. The incidence of otitis media increases in the 14 day period after influenzavirus infection. Further, administration of inactivated influenzavirus vaccine has been shown to reduce outbreaks of otitis media in day care centers (6). Thus, if efforts are employed to immunize more day care children, this might ultimately result in lower incidence of otitis media and less need for prescribed antibiotics.

The introduction of a nasally administered vaccine has much implication to help overcome barriers associated with people becoming immunized (e.g., fear of side effects, the need for yearly immunizations, perception of low vaccine effectiveness). Widespread use of the nasal vaccine in high-risk children may therefore be more easily achievable than has been the case with injected vaccines and would be a very effective way to reduce the incidence of influenza in this population.

The strength of viral vaccines can be provided in Tissue Culture Infectious Doses (i.e., $TCID_{50}$), which is the quantity of virus estimated to infect 50% of inoculated cultures. Also, microgram, μg, of immunogen present, international units, D-antigen units, and plaque-forming units (PFUs) for yellow fever vaccine are employed for these products.

Cancer Vaccines

For over a century, the role of the immune system and its relationship to cancer has been researched. It has been only in recent years, however, that the immune response is becoming clinically explored as a mode to prevent and treat cancer. Those cancer vaccines in development are intended to increase the recognition of the cancer cells by the immune system.

This approach to cancer treatment is exciting as it offers another modality to complement surgery, radiation therapy, and chemotherapy. Another cause for guarded optimism is that the development of these vaccines may play a role in preventing cancer in patients who run a high risk because of familial diseases to develop cancer.

For the immune system to recognize and kill a tumor cell, immune cells must recognize antigens on the tumor cell as foreign to the body and receive co-stimulatory signals. Otherwise, tumor cells go undetected by the immune system and proliferate. Thus, a goal of cancer vaccine development is to increase antigen awareness to the immune cells or increase co-stimulatory signals that induce an immune response.

T cells, lymphokine-activated killer (LAK) cells, and *natural killer (NK) cells* within the body's immune system have antitumor activity. Thus, tumor vaccine development is to stimulate these immune cells instead of antibody producing cells [which is the operational model used to protect one from an infection]. The aforementioned tumor killing cells recognize antigens (syn. tumor associated antigens [TAAs]) on the surface of the tumor cells. These antigens demonstrate peptide fragments that appear on the cell surface either by the cancer cell or taken up by a phagocytic cell.

Tumor-associated antigens fall into one of three categories. These are patient-specific, tumor-specific, and shared. Those antigens unique to a specific patient are termed patient-specific. An example might be an antigen expressed on the surface of a B-cell malignancy. A tumor-specific TAA is unique to a particular tumor. Most notable as an example would be the prostate specific antigen (PSA) found in prostate tumors. Shared TAAs are created by tumor cells that have a common histology. A notable example of this is the carcinoembryonic antigen located on adenocarcinoma cells found in colon, ovarian, and lung tumors.

Four different types of cancer vaccines are under investigation and a thorough explanation of each is beyond the scope of this presentation. Nonetheless these types are important to mention. They are autologous, allogeneic, anti-idiotypic, and gene-therapy derived vaccines.

Autologous tumor vaccines are developed from antigenic material procured from the tumor of the patient. Tumor cells are isolated from tissue procured during biopsy or surgery. These cells are then killed or attenuated and then reinfused into the patient. Typically, to enhance immunogenicity, they are combined with an adjuvant (e.g., BCG, c parvum). A major problem with this approach is the work and cost associated with the production of the vaccine for the individual patient. Also, some tumors escape the immune system because their antigens are not expressed on the tumor surface.

Allogeneic tumor vaccines use the concept of shared or tumor-specific antigens. These vaccines are produced from cell lines that express tumor-specific or shared TAAs. To induce an immune response, either the fragment of the allogeneic tumor cell or the whole cell is injected. The beneficial aspect of this vaccine is that it can be used in a wide population of patients.

Anti-idiotypic vaccines are three dimensional, immunogenic regions on the antibody that bind antigen. Those antibodies that bind TAAs are isolated and injected into mice. The resulting antibodies are then harvested and used to vaccinate another mouse. The resulting antibodies have a three dimensional binding site that mimics the original structure of the TAA. These antibodies are then combined with an adjuvant and given as a vaccine. Because the produced anti-idiotypic antibody closely resembles the antigen, these can be used to induce immune responses (i.e., cellular, antibody-antigen) to a given antigen.

Gene therapy allows a DNA template to be placed within a cell, to be transcribed into messenger RNA, and then expressed as a co-stimulatory protein. One can then induce a cell to synthesize this protein as part of its normal cellular function. A gene that encodes for interleukins or other co-stimulatory proteins can then be placed in cells expressing TAAs. This then produces stimulation of the immune response.

Clinical trials are now being undertaken for cancer vaccines developed for melanoma, colorectal cancer, renal cell carcinoma, breast and ovarian cancers, lung cancer, and cervical cancer. These are being studied also as a combination modality with chemotherapy, surgery, and radiation therapy.

Toxoids

In similar fashion to bacterial vaccines, bacteria are propagated, and after the required growth is achieved, the culture is filtered through a sterilizing membrane filter. The filtrate that contains the toxin (exotoxin) is then processed. Processing then involves the addition of a concentrated salt solution to precipitate the toxin from the filtrate. After the precipitated toxin is washed and dialyzed to purify it, the toxin is detoxified with formaldehyde.

The detoxified toxin (*syn* toxoid) may be plain or contain an adjuvant (e.g., alum, aluminum hydroxide, aluminum sulfate). Further, the product may contain single (e.g., Tetanus Toxoid), multiple or mixed immunogens (e.g., Tetanus and Diphtheria Toxoids Adsorbed for Adult Use). The latter example contains two toxoids in a single preparation for active immunization against different toxicities. A mixed biological such as Diphtheria and Tetanus Toxoids and Pertussis Vaccine Adsorbed for pediatric use has two toxoids and a vaccine in a single dosage form for active immunization against different toxicities and infection. The advantage to their use is the broad immunization coverage and minimum number of injections.

These mixtures or types of biologicals differ from polyvalent products which are used for different strains of the same toxicity or infection (e.g., Influenza Virus Vaccine, Pneumococcal Vaccine Polyvalent).

The strength of a toxoid is in flocculating (Lf) units (e.g., Tetanus toxoid, 4 to 5 Lf Units/0.5 ml dose). A flocculating unit is the smallest amount of toxin which flocculates most rapidly one unit of standard antitoxin in a series of mixtures containing fixed amounts of antitoxin and varying amounts of toxin.

Biologicals for Passive Immunity

Human Immune Sera and Globulins (Homologous Sera)

Human immune sera or homologous sera include immune globulin and hyperimmune sera for specific diseases. These are sera containing the specific antibodies obtained from the blood of humans and produced as a result of having had the specific disease or having been immunized against it with a specific biological product. The source of homologous sera is the pooled plasma of adult donors either from the general population (for immune globulin) or from hyperimmunized donors (for immune globulins for specific diseases). Thus, these products confer passive immunity.

The pooled plasma from adult donors must be free of hepatitis B antigen and antibodies to human immunodeficiency virus (i.e., HIV). Processing steps include fractional precipitation (e.g., with cold ethanol) maintaining rigorous control of pH and ionic strength. Further purification takes place with a finished biological product that contains not less than 15% and not more than 18% protein. There are of course exceptions (e.g., Varicella-zoster immune globulins contain not less than 10% protein).

These preparations are for intramuscular injection and should not be intravenously administered. However, two immune globulins (i.e., immune globulin intravenous [3 to 12% protein], cytomegalovirus immune globulin) are intravenously administered.

Sera are of the greatest value for the treatment of acute disease, although they are also useful in some instances for the prevention of illness when immediate protection is needed. Immunity resulting from the injection of an immune serum is of brief duration (i.e., a few weeks) because the foreign serum along with the antibodies that it produces are eliminated from the body within a few weeks.

Animal Immune Sera (Heterologous Sera)

Most of the commonly employed immune sera are prepared through the immunization of horses which have been immunized against the specific immunogen (e.g., toxin, venom). After the plasma has been harvested, it is separated into two components which are immunologically active (i.e., immunoglobulins) and immunologically inactive (i.e., albumins, clotting factors) by fractional precipitation. The immunologically active component is then treated with pepsin to remove the complement-activating component of the molecules and render it less immunogenic. Subsequently, the active component is recovered through dialysis and fractional precipitation or centrifugation.

This category of pharmaceuticals includes antitoxins and antivenins. Antitoxins are produced by inoculating horses with increasing doses of the respective toxoids and exotoxins. After several injections spread out over a period of weeks or months, the animal is bled with adequate safeguards to avoid contamination and the plasma harvested. Antivenins are produced similarly by inoculating horses with the venoms of selected species of snakes (e.g., crotalids [pit vipers]) or the black widow spider and then harvesting the plasma.

Before using these products, precaution must be taken to ensure the safety of the patient who may be sensitive to horse protein. Appropriate measures, including a sensitivity test with suitable controls, should be taken to detect the presence of dangerous hypersensitivity.

Table 15.1 demonstrates representative biologicals according to category (i.e., vaccines, toxoids, antitoxins, immune sera, miscellaneous diagnostic antigen products). Although the scope of this book does not permit a thorough description of each according to its intended use, adverse effects, etc., nonetheless the listing demonstrates the wide applicability of these products to effect active or passive immunity, provide prophylaxis, or serve as a diagnostic tool.

Administration and Toxicity Associated with Biological Products

Biologicals must be dispensed in their original containers to avoid contamination and deterioration. They are sterile when packaged and are injected by aseptic techniques. A few are administered by mouth.

Traditional vaccines, for example, often constituted by inactivated whole cells can cause unwanted side effects. Those developed from selected antigens

Table 15.1   Examples of Official Biologic Products

Biologic Product	Nature of Contents	Route of Administration*	Use
Vaccines and Vaccine Combinations			
BCG Vaccine	Attenuated, living culture of the bacillus Calmette-Guerin strain of *Mycobacterium bovis.*	Percutaneous via a multiple-puncture disc	Active immunizing agent
Cholera Vaccine	Suspension of inactivated cholera vibrios (*Vibrio Cholerae*).	Intramuscular or subcutaneous	Active immunizing agent
Hepatitis B Vaccine	Originally, biochemically and biophysically inactivated human hepatitis B surface antigen (HBsAg) particles, obtained by plasmapheresis from plasma of screened chronic HBsAG carriers. Currently, only recombinant vaccines derived from HBsAg produced in yeast cells are available in the U.S.	Intramuscular	Active immunizing agent
Influenza Virus Vaccine	Aqueous suspension of inactivated influenza virus prepared from allantoic fluid of influenza virus-infected chick embryo in a phosphate-buffered isotonic sodium chloride injection.	Intramuscular or subcutaneous	Active immunizing agent
Measles Virus Vaccine Live	Live, attenuated Enders' line measles virus derived from attenuated Edmonston strain in chick embryo cell cultures.	Subcutaneous	Active immunizing agent
Measles, Mumps, and Rubella Virus Vaccine Live	Combination of viruses propagated in chick embryo tissue (measles and mumps) and in human diploid cell cultures (rubella).	Subcutaneous	Active immunizing agent
Measles and Rubella Virus Vaccine Live	Live viral vaccine with the measles virus grown on chicken embryo tissue and the rubella virus on duck embryo tissue.	Subcutaneous	Active immunizing agent
Mumps Virus Vaccine Live	Live, attenuated organisms of the Jeryl Lynn (B level) strain of mumps virus propagated in chick embryo tissue cultures.	Subcutaneous	Active immunizing agent
Plague Vaccine	Suspension of inactivated 195/P strain of plague bacilli (*Yersinia pestis*) in 0.9% sodium chloride injection.	Intramuscular	Active immunizing agent
Pneumococcal Vaccine, Polyvalent	A sterile solution containing antigenic capsular polysaccharides extracted from *Streptococcus pneumoniae.* This vaccine contains 23 capsular polysaccharide types. Each 0.5 ml dose of the vaccine contains 25 μg of each type of capsule polysaccharide dissolved in 0.9% sodium chloride injection. The vaccine also contains phenol or thimerosal as a preservative.	Subcutaneous or intramuscular	Active immunizing agent
Poliovirus Vaccine Live Oral	A preparation of one or a combination of the three types of live, attenuated polioviruses, grown separately in primary cultures of monkey kidney tissue.	Oral	Active immunizing agent
Rabies Vaccine	A preparation of inactivated rabies virus harvested from human (HDCV) or rhesus diploid-cell (RDCV) cultures.	HDCV—intramuscular or intradermal; RDCV—intramuscular only	Active immunizing agent
Rubella Virus Vaccine Live	Live rubella (German measles) virus propagated in human diploid (WI-38) cell culture.	Subcutaneous	Active immunizing agent

continued

Table 15.1 Examples of Official Biologic Products

Biologic Product	Nature of Contents	Route of Administration*	Use
Rubella and Mumps Viral Vaccine Live	Combination of rubella virus propagated in human diploid cell culture and mumps virus grown on chicken embryo tissue.	Subcutaneous	Active immunizing agent
Smallpox Vaccine	A dried form of living virus of vaccinia that has been grown in the skin of a vaccinated bovine calf.	Intradermal	Active immunizing agent
Typhoid Vaccine	Parenteral acetone-killed and dried or heat/phenol-inactivated *Salmonella typhi* of Ty2 strain or oral form, as enteric-coated capsules, lyophilized, live *S. typhi* of the attenuated Ty21a strain.	Subcutaneous or intradermal; oral	Active immunizing agent
Varicella Virus Vaccine Live	Live, attenuated varicella-zoster virus of the Oka/Merck strain. Attenuated by multiple passages through human embryonic lung cell cultures, embryonic guinea pig cell cultures, the WI-38 strain of human diploid cell cultures, and the MRC-5 strain of human diploid cell cultures.	Subcutaneous	Active immunizing agent
Yellow Fever Vaccine	Dried, frozen, attenuated strain of living yellow fever virus prepared by culturing the virus in the living chick embryo prepared, processed, freeze-dried, and sealed under nitrogen.	Subcutaneous	Active immunizing agent
Toxoids			
Diphtheria and Tetanus Toxoids Adsorbed	Suspension prepared by mixing purified diphtheria toxoid and tetanus toxoid alum precipitated or adsorbed onto aluminum phosphate.	Deep intramuscular	Active immunizing agent
Tetanus Toxoid	Suspension of formaldehyde-treated products of growth of the tetanus bacillus (*Clostridium tetani*).	Intramuscular or subcutaneous	Active immunizing agent
Tetanus Toxoid Adsorbed	Suspension of tetanus toxoid alum precipitated or adsorbed onto aluminum phosphate.	Deep intramuscular	Active immunizing agent
Tetanus and Diphtheria Toxoids Adsorbed for Adult Use	Suspension of tetanus toxoid and diphtheria toxoid alum precipitated or adsorbed onto aluminum phosphate.	Intramuscular	Active immunizing agent
Antitoxins			
Botulism Antitoxin	Solution of refined and concentrated proteins, chiefly globulins, containing antitoxin obtained from the blood serum or plasma of healthy horses immunized against the toxins produced by type A, B, and E strains of *Clostridium botulinum*.	Intramuscular or intravenous	Passive immunizing agent
Tetanus Antitoxin	Solution of the refined and concentrated proteins, chiefly globulins, containing antitoxic antibodies obtained from the blood serum or plasma of a healthy animal, usually the horse, that has been immunized against tetanus toxoid or toxin.	Intramuscular or subcutaneous (prophylactic) or intravenous (therapeutic)	Passive immunizing agent

continued

Table 15.1   Examples of Official Biologic Products

Biologic Product	Nature of Contents	Route of Administration*	Use
Immune Serums			
Cytomegalovirus Immune Globulin Intravenous, Human	IgG anitbodies from a lare number of healthy persons who contributed to plasma pools.	Intravenous	Passive for kidney transplant recipients who are seronegative for CMV and who receive a kidney from a CMV seropositive donor.
Immune Globulin IM (IGIM)	Nonpyrogenic solution of globulins containing many antibodies normally present in adult human blood prepared by cold alcohol fractionation of pooled plasma from venous blood of at least 1000 individuals.	Intramuscular	Passive immunity to hepatitis A and B infections, measles, varicella zoster, primary immunodeficiency diseases.
Immune Globulin IV (IGIV)	Nonpyrogenic solution of globulins containing many antibodies normally present in adult human blood prepared by cold alcohol fractionation of pooled plasma from venous blood of at least 1000 individuals.	Intravenous	Primary immunodeficiency diseases, HIV infections, idiopathic thrombocytopenia purpura, bone marrow transplantation, and beta-cell chronic lymphocytic leukemia.
Rh_o (D) Globulin	Prepared from plasma or serum of adults with a high titer of anti-Rh_o antibody to the red blood cell antigen Rh_o (D). It contains 10–18% protein, of which not less than 90% is immunoglobin G (gamma globulin, IgG). Commerically available solutions contain glycine as a stabilizing agent and thimerosal as a preservative; pH is adjusted with sodium carbonate or sodium chloride.	Intramuscular	Passive immunizing agent
Tetanus Immune Globulin	Solution of globulins derived from the blood plasma of adult human donors who have been hyperimmunized with tetanus toxoid.	Intramuscular	Passive immunizing agent
Miscellaneous Biologic Products			
Antivenin (Crotalidae) Polyvalent	A preparation derived by drying frozen solution of specific venom-neutralizing globulins obtained from the serum of healthy horses immunized against venoms of four species of pit vipers, *Crotalus atrox, C. adamanteus, C. durissus terrificus,* and *Bothrops atrox.*	Intramuscular or intravenous	To neutralize the toxic effects of venoms of crotalids native to North, Central and South America
Candida albicans Skin Test Antigen	Prepared from the culture filtrate and cells of two strains of *Candida albicans.*	Intradermal	To detect reduced cellular (or delayed-type) hypersensitivity (DTH) and assess diminished cellular immunity in persons infected with HIV.

continued

Table 15.1   Examples of Official Biologic Products

Biologic Product	Nature of Contents	Route of Administration*	Use
Histoplasmin, USP	Standardized culture filtrates of the fungus *Histoplasma capsulatum* grown on a liquid synthetic medium.	Intradermal	Diagnostic aid (histoplasmosis)
Plasma Protein Fraction, USP	Solution of selected proteins derived from the blood plasma of adult human donors. It contains about 5% of protein, about 85% of which is albumin, the remainder alpha and beta globulins.	Intravenous	Blood-volume expansion
Tuberculin, USP	Solution of the concentrated, soluble products of growth of the tubercle bacillus, *Mycobacterium tuberculosis.* Old Tuberculin or, a soluble partially purified product of growth of the tubercle bacillus prepared in a special liquid medium free from protein (Purified Protein Derivative, PPD).	Intradermal	Diagnostic aid (tuberuclosis)

*The doses to be administered and the schedule of doses vary widely, depending upon the patient's age, exposure, previous record of immunizations, etc.

have demonstrated fewer systemic side effects. Liposomal delivery has decreased side effects while helping to enhance the vaccine's effectiveness.

Itching, erythema, pain, and tenderness around the injection site occur with subcutaneous, intramuscular, and intradermal administration. Using vaccines as an example, those that contain adjuvants (e.g., BCG) can cause the aforementioned in addition to induration and ulceration at the site. Low-grade fever, myalgia, and arthralgia have occurred in patients who have received a BCG-containing biological product.

These adverse effects are controlled with the use of OTC analgesic agents. However, before these are used, a patient drug history should be obtained to ensure that the use of an analgesic is permissible given a patient's health status and other drug therapy.

The foremost adverse effect of concern with immunization is hypersenstivity type reactions, most notably anaphylaxis (i.e., ranging from pruritis/urticaria to bronchospasm, respiratory distress, laryngeal edema, circulatory collapse and death). Life threatening anaphylaxis is a rarity, but still very possible. The risk of an anaphylactic reaction occurring is in the magnitude of one for every 600,000 to 6.4 million doses of vaccine distributed (7).

The immunopathologic classification of allergic drug reactions places anaphylactic reactions in Type I. In this situation, initial exposure to an antigen results in production of specific IgE antibodies. Upon re-exposure, antigen reacts with antibodies bound to the surface of mast cells or basophils causing the release of histamine and other mediators. A period of several weeks is required after initial exposure to antigen and sensitization before an anaphylactic reaction can occur. Once sensitized, however, the patient can demonstrate an attack within minutes upon re-exposure to small amounts of the drug administered by any route.

Because of the rare nature of anaphylactic reactions, it is difficult to determine if the patient is allergic to the proteins that make up the active antigenic portion of the vaccine or to the excipients (e.g., thimerosal, neomycin, gelatin, aluminum gels) which constitute the formulation. Several viruses that constitute vaccines are grown in animate media including embryonic egg and cell cultures of chick embryo. Even though purification techniques decrease dramatically the amount of egg protein (e.g., ovalbumin) in the final product, still even small amounts (e.g., picograms, nanograms) can elicit a response.

Before a vaccination is administered, it is important that a complete and thorough history of previous allergic reactions be taken. This includes the names of the offending agents and the type of reaction that was elicited by the allergen. Also, one should determine how long ago that the reaction took place. Not only should one inquire about drugs (e.g., neomycin, gelatin), but also foods (e.g., severe allergy to egg products). It may be necessary for an allergist to perform skin testing to determine if a patient may be suspected to demonstrate an immediate, Type I, hypersensitivity reaction to a vaccine.

Even though anaphylactic reactions after immunizations are rare, these still can occur. Thus, at the time of immunization adequate safeguards must be in place (e.g., proper emergency supplies and adequately trained personnel) to handle such an emergency.

Administration of Biologicals by Health Care Providers

According to the National Childhood Vaccine Injury Act of 1986, health care-providers who administer certain vaccines and toxoids are required to record permanently and to report adverse effects resulting from the use of one of the biological products. Becoming effective on March 21, 1988, the Act has three primary objectives:

- To avoid future "crises" that could interrupt the National Immunization Program,
- To achieve optimal prevention of adverse reactions to these preparations, and
- To provide financial compensation for those patients who suffer vaccine-related injuries.

The Act requires that certain specified adverse reaction events be reported in detail to the US DHHS Vaccine Adverse Event Reporting System (VAERS) to expand knowledge of such reactions. Those adverse events that occur within 7 days after administration (e.g., encephalopathy with DPT vaccine) or within such other time period as specified for certain vaccines (e.g., paralytic poliomyelitis from OPV within 30 days of administration) and/or toxoid are to be reported. This is very important as such an event may be a rarity and one that should be known. For more information about reporting requirements or completion of the reporting forms, health-care providers can contact VAERS at 1-800-822-7967. The Act also requires that a surcharge be placed on biological products to establish a fund to compensate victims.

The Act requires that health-care providers who administer any vaccine containing measles, mumps, rubella, poliomyelitis, diphtheria, tetanus or pertussis antigens maintain permanent vaccination records. These records include: the type of biological administered; date of administration; manufacturer and lot number; name, address and title of the person administering the vaccine; and the patient's occupation, lifestyle and history of vaccine-preventable illnesses. Further, information on other vaccines and toxoids administered should be a part of the permanent record. Pharmacists can work with allied health practitioners (e.g., physicians, nurses) to immunize patients, and in 22 states (i.e., Alabama, Alaska, Arkansas, California, Georgia, Illinois, Indiana, Iowa, Kansas, Kentucky, Michigan, Mississippi, Missouri, Nebraska, New Mexico, Oklahoma, South Carolina, South Dakota, Tennessee, Texas, Virginia, Washington), pharmacists are permitted to give vaccinations.

The Public Health Service Act (42 U.S.C.§ 300aa–26), Section 2126, effective October 1, 1994, mandated that all health care providers who administer any vaccine containing diphtheria, tetanus, pertussis, measles, mumps, rubella or polio vaccine shall, prior to administration of the vaccine, provide a copy of relevant vaccine information materials contained in this notice:

- To any adult to whom the provider intends to administer the vaccine; and
- To the legal representative (i.e., parent, other individual qualified under state law to consent to the immunization of a minor) of any child to whom the vaccine will be administered (8).

Also, the materials are to be supplemented with visual presentation or oral explanations. There is no requirement that the health care provider obtain the signature or initials of the patient or legal representative affirming that the vaccine information materials were provided. Instead, the health care provider is to make a notation in the patient's permanent medical record indicating that these materials were provided at the time of vaccination (8).

In addition to complying with the mandatory requirements of the Act, the American Academy of Pediatrics strongly urges health-care providers to complete an official immunization record and provide it to the recipient's legal representative. This record should be accorded the status of a birth certificate or passport and retained with other vital documents for subsequent referral. The health care provider should encourage the legal representative to preserve this important record and present it for record keeping with each immunization. This facilitates accurate record keeping and immunization evaluation, particularly for those who move often. This record also serves a vital purpose for needed documentation of immunization history for school admission.

Childhood Immunization Schedule

Childhood immunization has been shown to be effective and inexpensive. The U.S. Public Health Service's *Healthy People 2000: National Health*

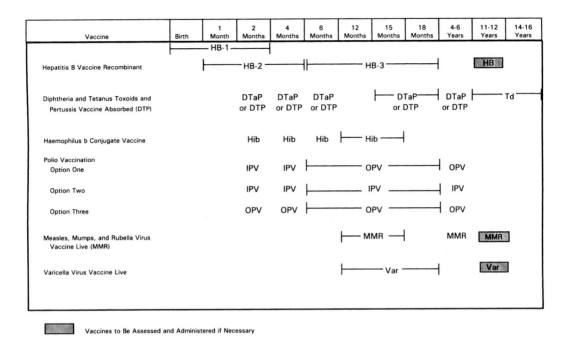

Fig. 15.1   *Recommended childhood immunization schedule—United States, January-December, 1998.*

Promotion and Disease Prevention Objectives established a goal of completely immunizing 90% of infants in the United States by 24 months of age (9). Yet, regrettably, only 40 to 50% of 2-year old children in the United States are completely immunized. It is estimated that four million children are at risk to develop serious, preventable diseases.

Residents of rural or large urban areas have particularly low immunization rates. Further, various ethnic minorities (e.g., Native Americans, Hispanics, African Americans) also demonstrate low rates of immunization. It is believed that this low immunization rate in children has been responsible for increased incidence of measles and pertussis.

In 1995, the CDC's Advisory Committee on Immunization Practices (ACIP), the American Academy of Pediatrics (AAP), and the American Academy of Family Physicians (AAFP) announced a unified version of a recommended immunization schedule for children. Subsequently, in January, 1997, and January, 1998 updated versions of the recommended childhood schedule were issued. Figure 15.1 demonstrates this recommended childhood immunization schedule as of January, 1998 (10). The intervals demonstrated in Figure 15.1 indicate the range of acceptable ages for vaccination, including catch-up vaccination.

Infants born to hepatitis B surface antigen (HB-sAg)-negative mothers should receive 2.5 μg of Merck vaccine (i.e., Recombivax HB) or 10 μg of SmithKline Beecham (SB) vaccine (i.e., Engerix-B). The second dose should be administered at least 1 month after the first dose. The third dose should be administered at least 2 months after the second, but not before 6 months of age.

Those infants born to HBsAg-positive mothers should receive 0.5 mL hepatitis B immune globulin (HBIG) within 12 hours of birth, and either 5 μg of Merck vaccine (i.e., Recombivax HB) or 10 μg of SB vaccine (i.e., Engerix-B) at a separate site. The second dose is recommended at age 1–2 months and the third dose at age 6 months.

Infants born to women whose HBsAg status is unknown should receive either 5 μg of Merck vaccine (i.e., Recombivax HB) or 10 μg of SB (i.e., Engerix-B) within 12 hours of birth. The second dose of the vaccine is recommended at age 1 month and the third dose at 6 months of age.

Blood should be drawn at the time of delivery to determine the mother's HBsAg status. If it is positive, the infant should receive HBIG as soon as possible, and no later than 1 week of age. The dosage and timing of subsequent vaccine doses should be based on the mother's HBsAg status.

Children and adolescents who have not been vaccinated against hepatitis B in infancy may begin the series during any visit. Those who have not previously received three doses of hepatitis B vaccine should initiate or complete the series during the routine visit to a health-care provider at age 11–12 years. An unvaccinated older adolescent should be vaccinated whenever possible. The second dose should be administered at least one month after the first dose, and the third dose should be administered at least four months after the first dose and at least two months after the second dose.

Diphtheria and tetanus toxoids and acellular pertussis vaccine (DTaP) is the preferred vaccine for all doses in this vaccination series, including completion of the series in children who have received one or more doses of whole-cell diphtheria and tetanus toxoids and pertussis vaccine (i.e., DTP). Whole-cell DTP is an acceptable alternative for DTaP.

The fourth dose of DPT may be administered as early as 12 months of age, provided that at least six months have elapsed since the third dose of DPT, and if the child is unlikely to return at age 15 to 18 months. Tetanus and diphtheria toxoids, adsorbed, for adult use (Td), is recommended at age 11–12 years if at least five years have elapsed since the last dose of DTP, DTaP, or diphtheria and tetanus toxoids, adsorbed, for pediatric use (DT). Subsequent routine Td boosters are recommended every ten years.

Three *H. influenza* type b (Hib) conjugate vaccines are licensed for infant use. These are: Hib oligosaccharide conjugate vaccine (diphtheria protein conjugate) [HbOC]; Hib polyribosylribitol phosphate-tetanus toxoid conjugate (tetanus toxoid conjugate) vaccine [PRP-T]; and *Haemophilus b* conjugate vaccine (meningococcal protein conjugate) vaccine [PRP-OMP].

These three products are now considered interchangeable for primary as well as booster vaccination (10). Excellent immune responses have been achieved when vaccines from different manufacturers have been used interchangeably in the primary series. Children who received the *Haemophilus b* conjugate vaccine (i.e., meningococcal protein conjugate [PRP-OMP], PedvaxHIB) at two and four months of age do not require a dose at six months of age. If PRP-OMP is administered in a series with one of the other two products licensed for infant use, the recommended number of doses to complete the series is determined by the other product (and not by PRP-OMP). For example, if PRP-OMP is administered for the first dose at 2 months of age, and another vaccine utilized at 4 months of age, a third dose of any of the three licensed Hib vaccines is recommended at age 6 months to complete the primary series.

Two poliovirus vaccines (i.e., Inactivated poliovirus vaccine [IPV], oral poliovirus vaccine [OPV]) are licensed and distributed within the U.S. There are three schedules acceptable to the ACIP, AAP, and AAFP. Parents and providers may elect any of the following three options. These are: two doses of IPV followed by two doses of OPV; four doses of IPV; or four doses of OPV. ACIP recommends the first option, i.e., two doses of IPV at ages two and four months followed by a dose of OPV at age 12–18 months and at age four to six years. IPV is the only poliovirus vaccine recommended for immunocompromised persons and their household contacts.

Routinely, the second dose of MMR vaccine is recommended between 4 to 6 years of age. It can, however, be administered during any visit, provided at least 1 month has elapsed since receipt of the first dose and that both doses are administered beginning at or after age 12 months. Those who have not previously received the second dose should complete the schedule no later than the routine visit to a health-care provider at age 11–12 years.

Varicella virus vaccine live (VAR) can be administered at any time after 12 months of age. Those children who are without a reliable history of chickenpox and who have not previously received VAR should be vaccinated between 11 to 12 years of age. Susceptible children aged ≥13 years should receive two doses at least 1 month apart.

Influenza continues to be a major cause of morbidity and mortality within the United States. In spite of efforts to vaccinate persons at high risk, the annual rate of influenza may reach as high as 40 percent in children, far above that (i.e., 10 to 20%) encountered in the general population. So, a question that occurs with the availability of an effective intranasal influenzavirus vaccine (11) is whether it is now more reasonable to vaccinate healthy children, especially those prone to otitis media and those with a high exposure rate to influenza. There will be much appeal to do so because the administration technique is not as invasive and the likelihood of less adverse effects. Certainly the potential health and economic benefit must be balanced with the challenge to develop and implement such a program and the unpredictable nature of the influenzavirus.

In late 1998, the FDA approved the first vaccine to prevent rotavirus gastroenteritis in children. Rotavirus gastroenteritis is the most common cause of severe and sometimes fatal diarrhea in children. Infants and children between the ages of 6 months and about 3 years are most vulnerable to rotavirus infection. The infection causes dehydration and an estimated one million deaths occur from it on a worldwide basis. In the United States, this virus causes about 50 deaths a year while it is estimated to infect about 3.5 million children.

The Rotavirus vaccine, RotaShield (Wyeth-Lederle), contains four live viruses: a rhesus rotavirus and three rhesus-human reassortant viruses. The vaccine provides protection against the four rotavirus serotypes that are responsible for a majority of rotavirus disease in infants and young children within the United States. The vaccine is administered orally (i.e., 2.5 ml per dose) to infants at 2, 4, and 6 months of age. The first dose may be administered as early as 6 weeks of age, but giving the dose after the sixth month of life is not recommended because of the increased risk of fever. The vaccine is available in a single-dose vial that must be reconstituted with a citrate-bicarbonate diluent. The vaccine is for oral administration and should not be administered by injection.

The Rotavirus will not protect 100% of the patients immunized or protect against diarrhea caused by other strains of rotavirus. Because it contains four live viruses, it is contraindicated for use in patients with compromised immune systems, and those being treated with systemic corticosteroids, alkylating agents, antimetabolites, radiation, or other immunosuppressive therapies. Additionally, this vaccine should not be administered to patients who have ongoing diarrhea and/or vomiting. An important precaution is to keep the vaccinated infant away from immunocompromised patients because the live virus vaccine could be transmitted to them.

Demonstrated adverse reactions in clinical trials involving this new vaccine included fever, decreased appetite, irritability, and decreased activity. Because the vaccine packaging contains dry natural rubber, the vaccine should be administered with extreme caution to patients with a history of latex sensitivity.

Adult Immunization Schedule

Between 50 to 70,000 adults die each year from vaccine-preventable diseases and their complications (12). At least 100 times as many adults as children succumb from these illnesses. Many adults do not recognize the need for immunization throughout their lifetime (12).

Figure 15.2 demonstrates an adult immunization schedule (12). Hepatitis A and B vaccines are recommended for persons who are or will be at increased risk of infection with Hepatitis A and B. These higher risk groups include health-care personnel, dialysis patients, morticians, embalmers, immigrants from areas of high Hepatitis A or B endemicity, homosexually active males, users of illicit injectable drugs, prisoners and clients in institutions for mentally retarded patients. Also included in this group would be health professional students who partake in the experiential component of their respective curricula in health care environments.

The influenzavirus vaccine is recommended for everyone ≥ 65 years and for those under this age who are at special risk to develop complications associated with influenza. Research demonstrates that the immunization of high risk patients is cost effective and reduces complications. However, data demonstrates that this vaccine is actually underutilized in high-risk adults and children (4). In 1994, for example, vaccination coverage in people ≥ 65 years of age only reached 55 percent, and was only 30 percent among high risk adults ≤ 65 years of age (4).

Groups at greatest risk include adults and children with chronic pulmonary and/or cardiovascular diseases that require routine medical examination or hospitalization during the preceding year, including children with asthma. Adults and children who have required regular medical follow up or hospitalizations during the preceding year because of chronic metabolic diseases (including diabetes mellitus), renal dysfunction, hemoglobinopathies, or immunosuppression (including immunosuppression caused by medications).

Other groups at high risk to develop influenza-related complications include persons ≥65 years of age and residents of nursing homes, extended care facilities, retirement villages, and other chronic care facilities housing patients of any age with chronic medical conditions should be vaccinated. Also, children and teenagers (age 6 months to 18 years) who are receiving long-term aspirin therapy and therefore might be at risk to develop Reye Syndrome after influenza. Lastly, women who will be in their second or third trimester of pregnancy during the influenza season should consider vaccination.

Those high risk individuals who should also be immunized with the influenzavirus vaccine include health-care workers (e.g., physicians, pharmacists, nurses), employees of nursing homes and chronic care facilities, providers of home care to persons at high risk (e.g., visiting nurses, volunteer workers) and individuals (e.g., family members) in close contact with high risk individuals. These individuals can become clinically or subclinically infected and transmit the virus to persons at high risk that they care for or live with. Some persons (e.g., the elderly, transplant recipients, persons with AIDS) can have a low antibody response to the influenza vaccine, and efforts to protect these patients must be

VACCINE	TIMING OF IMMUNIZATIONS			
Hepatitis A (Hep A) for those at risk	Two doses are needed to ensure long-term protection. Travelers to countries where the disease is common should get the first dose at least 4 weeks prior to departure.			
	first dose		second dose 6 to 12 months later	
Hepatitis B (Hep B) for those at risk	first dose	second dose 1 month later	third dose 5 months after second dose	
Influenza (Flu)	Given yearly in the fall to people age 65 or older. Also recommended for people younger than 65 who have medical problems such as heart disease, lung disease, diabetes, and other chronic conditions, and for others who work or live with high-risk individuals.			
Measles, Mumps, Rubella (MMR)	Two doses one month apart are recommended for adults born in 1957 or later if immunity cannot be proved.			
Pneumococcal	Usually given once at age 65 or older. Also recommended for people younger than 65 who have chronic illnesses such as those listed for influenza, and also those with kidney disorders and sickle cell anemia. A repeat dose 5 years later may be given to those at highest risk. Can be given at any time during the year.			
Tetanus, Diphtheria(Td) if initial series not given during childhood	first dose	second dose 4 to 8 weeks after first dose	third dose 6 to 12 months after second dose	booster shot every 10 years
Chickenpox (Varicella)	Two doses are recommended for persons 13 and older who have not had chickenpox.			
	first dose		second dose 1 to 2 months later	

Fig. 15.2   *Adult immunization schedule. Copyright 1997 by the American Pharmaceutical Association. Originally published in the* Pharmacy Today, *September 1997, Vol. 3, No. 9, page 9.* (American Pharmacy). *Reprinted with permission.*

made to reduce the likelihood they will contract influenza from their caregivers.

The Measles, Mumps, and Rubella (MMR) vaccine should not be given to a pregnant woman or those considering pregnancy within three months of vaccination. It is not known whether measles virus can cause fetal harm or can affect reproductive capacity. In addition, although mumps virus can infect the placenta and fetus, there is no good evidence that it causes congenital malformations in humans. Attenuated mumps vaccine virus can in-

fect the placenta, but the virus has not been isolated from fetal tissues of susceptible women who were vaccinated and underwent elective abortions. Further, there is evidence suggesting that transmission of attenuated rubella virus to the fetus occurs, although the vaccine is not known to cause fetal harm when administered during pregnancy. Suffice to say, it is prudent not to administered MMR to pregnant females. If postpubertal females are vaccinated, these women should be counseled to avoid pregnancy for three months after vaccination. Generally, most IgG passage across the placenta occurs during the third trimester.

The Tetanus and Diphtheria (Td) Toxoids are preferred for immunizing adults and children after the seventh year of age. All persons should maintain tetanus immunity by means of booster doses throughout their lifetime because tetanus spores are all over. Tetanus immunity is especially important for military personnel, farm and utility workers, those working with horses, firemen and all individuals whose occupation or vocation renders them prone to even minor lacerations and abrasions. Similarly, those traveling to developing nations should maintain active tetanus immunization to obviate the need for therapy with equine tetanus antitoxin and avoid its associated complications.

The Varicella Virus Vaccine in adults is intended to cover those that have not had chickenpox earlier in life. Studies demonstrate that the vaccine is quite effective at blunting breakthrough chickenpox following household exposure. And, when chickenpox does occur, reported body lesions are usually far less than that normally encountered during a chickenpox attack (i.e., 300 to 500 maculopapular or vesicular lesions accompanied by fever).

Those immunized with the chickenpox vaccine may potentially be capable of transmitting the vaccine virus to close contacts. Therefore, vaccine recipients should avoid close association with susceptible high-risk individuals (e.g., newborns, pregnant women, immunocompromised persons). Vaccinated persons should also be informed to avoid the use of salicylates for six weeks after vaccination with the varicella vaccine as Reye's Syndrome has been reported following the use of salicylates during natural varicella infections.

Because it is not known whether varicella vaccine can cause fetal harm or affect reproductive ability when administered during pregnancy it is prudent to avoid vaccination during pregnancy. Natural varicella, however, has sometimes caused fetal harm. In similar fashion to vaccination with MMR, females contemplating pregnancy should be counseled to avoid pregnancy within one month of vaccination with the chickenpox vaccine.

Vaccination Advocacy from Pharmacists

Perhaps one of the greatest achievements of medical science has been the ability to shield individuals from once-common, life threatening diseases through the process of providing immunity through the administration of vaccines or antibody-containing solutions. Indeed the practice of widespread childhood immunizations has reduced dramatically the morbidity and mortality of several infectious diseases and their sequelae. The best examples are the worldwide elimination of smallpox and the virtual elimination of polio from developed countries.

Preschool immunization programs against measles, mumps, pertussis and tetanus have resulted in >95% reductions in these diseases. In addition, to the vast human savings, there is also a health care cost benefit that accrues. It has been estimated that for every dollar spent on immunizing children against measles, mumps, and rubella, $14 in health care cost savings is achieved. Unfortunately, however, as mentioned earlier, between 50,000 to 70,000 adults die each year from vaccine-preventable diseases and their complications (12). This is at least 100 times greater than the number of children who die from similar afflictions. Adult deaths from hepatitis B and influenza demonstrate that more information must reach adults, among these being that pediatric immunization does not necessarily confer lifetime immunization.

Pharmacists can encourage immunization through 1) formulary management; 2) administrative measures, such as participation on infection committees and policy and procedures development; 3) patient history and screening; 4) counseling and documentation; and 5) public administration/advocacy (13). Depending upon the pharmacist's practice environment, all of these might not be possible. However, the key is involvement and advocacy regardless of one's practice setting.

For example, pharmacists should attempt to screen adult patients to determine those who may be susceptible to the development of preventable infectious diseases. Certain patients should be advised to receive influenza (e.g., >65 y.o. living in a nursing home) immunization, pneumococcal (e.g., alcoholics or coexisting diseases including diabetes and functional impairment of cardiorespiratory, hepatic, or renal systems), or hepatitis (e.g., dialysis patients, homosexually active persons) vaccination.

Compliance with established immunization guidelines can also be improved through the use of patient profile systems. Pharmacist incorporation of immunization histories into the patient's pharmacy profile can serve as a reminder when "booster" immunizations are needed. This is especially important with new patients (e.g., newborns, patients who migrate/move into the neighborhood).

The profession of pharmacy is in an optimal position to become part of a local community immunization effort. Because pharmacists are in residential neighborhoods, people do not have to travel far to reach them, and the convenience of when the pharmacy is open during the day and weekends make it an optimal site for immunization awareness and immunization programs. Further, as mentioned previously, the pharmacist has a legal right in 22 states to administer immunizations.

Professional organizations (e.g., American Pharmaceutical Association) have resources available to assist pharmacists in this endeavor of patient immunization. The APhA program, for example, is directed toward pharmacist preparation to develop immunization clinics for children and adults in their pharmacies. The program includes recommended immunization schedules, vaccination administration, techniques, and storage, and valuable marketing guidance (14).

Diagnostic Skin Antigens

Clinically, it may be necessary to utilize antigens *in vivo* as diagnostic tools. Typically, these are injected intradermally into the skin and are based on the patient's development of a hypersensitivity reaction. A positive reaction is determined by the extent of induration (in mms) and degree of reaction (i.e., from slight induration to vesiculation and necrosis) and demonstrates patient sensitivity to the antigen and the presence of antibodies due to either the present or past infection with the particular organism.

The number of available diagnostic skin biologicals is relatively small. In the late 1970s, many were removed from the market as a result of the recommendations of the FDA Panel on Review of Skin Antigens (15). Specifically, the Panel questioned the reliability of skin test antigens for trichinosis, lymphogranuloma venereum, and mumps and recommended that these be withdrawn from the market and not licensed.

Several diagnostic skin antigens are featured in Table 15.1. One of the newer *in vivo* diagnostic biologicals, *Candida albicans* Skin Test Antigen, is useful in the assessment of diminished cellular immunity in persons infected with HIV. Because HIV infection can modify the delayed-type hypersensitivity (DTH) response to tuberculin, it is advisable to skin test HIV-infected patients at high risk of tuberculosis with antigens in addition to tuberculin, to assess their competency to react to tuberculin. Responses to DTH antigens also have prognostic value in patients with cancer.

The Multiple Skin Test Antigens (Multitest CMI [Merieux]) is a skin test for multiple antigens and consists of a disposable applicator with eight sterile heads preloaded with seven delayed hypersensitivity skin test antigens and a glycerin negative control for percutaneous administration. The seven antigens are as follows: Tetanus Toxoid Antigen, Diphtheria Toxoid Antigen, Streptococcus Antigen, Old Tuberculin, Candida Antigen, Trichophyton Antigen, and Proteus Antigen. The intent of this multiple test is to detect anergy (i.e., nonresponsiveness to antigens) through delayed hypersensitivity skin testing.

References

1. Biologics. USP 23, The United States Pharmacopeial Convention, Inc., 12601 Twinbrook Parkway, Rockville MD 20852, 1994, p 1849.
2. Grabenstein JD, Kendal AP, Snyder RH. Storing, handling, and shipping immunologic drugs. Hosp Pharm 1996;31:936–948.
3. CDC. Update: Influenza activity—United States and worldwide, 1997–98 season, and composition of the 1998–99 influenza vaccine. MMWR 1998;47(14): 280–284
4. CDC. Prevention and control of influenza: Recommendations of the Advisory Committee on Immunization Practices (ACIP). MMWR 1997;46 [RR-9]:1–25.
5. Belshe RB, Mendelman PM, Treanor J, et al. The efficacy of live attenuated, cold-adapted, trivalent, intranasal Influenzavirus vaccine in children. N Engl J Med 1998;338(20):1405–1412.
6. Clements DA, Langdon L, Bland C, Walter E. Influenza A vaccine decreases the incidence of otitis media in 6- to 30-month old children in day care. Arch Pediatr Adolesc Med 1995;149:1113–7.
7. Grabenstein JD. Clinical management of hypersensitivities to vaccine components. Hosp Pharm 1997;32 (1):77–84.
8. Vaccine Information Materials. Federal Register 1994;59(117):31889-31892.
9. CDC. Reported vaccine-preventable diseases—United States, 1993, and the Childhood Immunization Initiative. MMWR 1994;43:57–60
10. CDC. Recommended childhood immunization schedule—United States, 1998. MMWR 1998;47(1): 8–12.
11. Barnett ED. Editorial: Influenza immunization for children. N Engl J Med 1998;338(20):1459–1461.
12. Williams CM. Operation immunization focuses on vaccinating adults. Pharmacy Today 1997;3(9):1,9.
13. ASHP technical assistance bulletin on the pharmacist's role in immunizations. Am J Hosp Pharm 1993; 50:501–505.
14. Hoeben BJ, Dennis MS, Bachman RL, et al. Role of the Pharmacist in Childhood Immunizations. JAPhA 1997;NS37(#5):557–562.
15. FDA skin test panel report. FDA Drug Bulletin 1978; 8(#2):15–16.

16

OPHTHALMIC SOLUTIONS AND SUSPENSIONS

Chapter at a Glance

PHARMACEUTICAL DOSAGE forms and drug delivery systems applied topically to the eye include solutions, suspensions, gels, ointments and drug-impregnated inserts. Ophthalmic inserts (Chapter 8) and ophthalmic ointments and gels (Chapter 9) previously have been discussed. The purpose of the present chapter is to build on the general considerations of solutions and suspensions presented in Chapters 12 and 13 by describing additional requirements of these dosage forms when designed specifically for ophthalmic use.

Ophthalmic Drug Delivery

Pharmaceutical preparations are applied topically to the eye to treat surface or intraocular conditions, including: infections of the eye or eyelids due to bacterial, fungal and viral pathogens; allergic or infectious conjunctivitis or inflammation; elevated intraocular pressure and glaucoma; and, dry-eye due to an inadequate production of fluids bathing the eye. In treating certain ophthalmic conditions, as glaucoma, both systemic drug use and topical treatments may be employed.

The normal volume of tear fluid retained in the cul-de-sac of the human eye is about 7–8 μL (1–3). An eye that is maintained in a nonblinking state can accommodate a maximum of about 30 μL of fluid but when blinked can retain only about 10 μL (2). Because the capacity of the eye to retain liquid and semisolid preparations is limited, topical applications are administered in small amounts; liquids drop-wise and ointments as a thin ribbon applied to the margin of the eyelid. Larger volumes of liquid preparations may be used to flush or bathe the eye.

Excessive liquids, both normally produced and externally delivered, are rapidly drained from the eye. A single drop of an ophthalmic solution/suspension measures about 50 μL (based on 20 drops/mL) and thus, much of an administered drop may be lost. The optimal volume to administer, based on eye capacity, would be 5 to 10 μL (1). Since microliter-dosing eye droppers are not generally available for self-use, loss of instilled medication using standard eye droppers is a common occurrence.

Due to the dynamics of the lacrimal system, the retention time of an ophthalmic solution on the eye surface is short, and the amount of drug absorbed is usually only a small fraction of the quantity administered. For example, following the administration of pilocarpine ophthalmic solution, the solution is flushed from the precorneal area within 1 to 2 minutes, resulting in the ocular absorption of less than 1 percent of the administered dose (4–5). This necessitates repeated administration of the solution. Decreased frequency of dosing, increased ocular retention time and greater bioavailability are achieved by formulations which extend corneal contact time, as gel systems, liposomes, polymeric drug carriers and ophthalmic suspensions and ointments (6–7).

Pharmacologic Categories of Ophthalmic Drugs

The major categories of drugs applied topically to the eye are:

Anesthetics. Topical anesthetics as tetracaine, cocaine and proparacaine are employed to provide pain relief preoperatively, postoperatively, for ophthalmic trauma, and during ophthalmic examination.

Antibiotic/Antimicrobial Agents. Used systemically and locally to combat ophthalmic infection. Among the agents used topically are gentamicin, sulfacetamide, tetracycline, ciprofloxacin, ofloxacin, chloramphenicol, polymyxin B-bacitracin, and tobramycin.

Antifungal Agents. Among the agents used topically against fungal endophthalmitis and fungal keratitis are amphotericin B, natamycin, and flucytosine.

Anti-inflammatory Agents. Used to treat inflammation of the eye, as allergic conjunctivitis. Among the topical anti-inflammatory steroidal agents used are fluorometholone, prednisolone, and dexamethasone salts.

Nonsteroidal anti-inflammatory agents include diclofenac, flurbiprofen, ketorolac, and suprofen.

Antiviral Agents. Used against viral infections, as that caused by herpes simplex virus. Among the antiviral agents used topically are trifluridine, idoxuridine, and vidarabine.

Astringents. Used in the treatment of conjunctivitis. Zinc sulfate is a commonly used astringent in ophthalmic solutions.

Beta-Adrenergic Blocking Agents. Agents as betaxolol hydrochloride and timolol maleate are used topically in the treatment of intraocular pressure and chronic open-angle glaucoma.

Miotics and other Glaucoma Agents. Miotics are used in the treatment of glaucoma, accommodative esotropia, convergent strabismus, and for the local treatment of myasthenia gravis. Among the miotics are pilocarpine, echothiophate iodide, and demecarium bromide. In addition to the miotics, several other types of agents are used in the treatment of glaucoma, including: carbonic anhydrase inhibitors, as acetazolamide (oral), beta-blockers, as timolol, and an ester prodrug analogue of prostaglandin F2a (latanoprost).

Mydriatics and Cycloplegics. Mydriatics allow examination of the fundus through the dilation of the pupil. Mydriatics having a long duration of action are termed *cycloplegics.* Among the mydriatics and cycloplegics are atropine, scopolamine, homatropine, cyclopentolate, phenylephrine, hydroxyamphetamine, and tropicamide.

Protectants/Artificial Tears. Solutions employed as artificial tears or as a contact lens fluids to lubricate the surface of the eye contain agents as carboxymethyl cellulose, methylcellulose, hydroxypropyl methylcellulose, and polyvinyl alcohol.

Vasoconstrictors/Ocular Decongestants. Vasoconstrictors, when applied topically to the mucous membranes of the eye cause transient constriction of the conjunctival blood vessels. They are intended to soothe, refresh, and remove redness due to minor eye irritation. Among the vasoconstrictors used topically are naphazoline, oxymetazoline, and tetrahydrozoline hydrochlorides. Antihistamines, as pheniramine maleate, are included in some products to provide relief of itching due to pollen, ragweed, and animal dander.

Pharmaceutic Requirements

The preparation of solutions and suspensions for ophthalmic use requires special consideration with regard to sterility, preservation, isotonicity, buffering, viscosity, ocular bioavailability and packaging.

Sterility and Preservation

Ophthalmic solutions/suspensions must be sterilized for safe patient-use. Although it is preferable to sterilize ophthalmics in their final containers by autoclaving at 121°C for 15 minutes, this method sometimes is precluded by the thermal instability of the formulation's components. As an alternative, bacterial filters may be used. Although bacterial filters work with a high degree of efficiency, they are not as reliable in achieving sterility as the autoclave. However, since final product testing is used to validate the absence of microbes, sterility may be assured by either method employed. One advantage of filtration is the retention of *all* particulate matter (microbial, dust, fiber), the removal of which is of substantial importance in the manufacture and use of ophthalmic solutions. Figures 16.1 and 16.2 show bacterial filtration equipment which may be used in the extemporaneous preparation of ophthalmic solutions.

To maintain sterility during patient use, antimicrobial preservatives generally are included in ophthalmic formulations; an exception being for preparations intended to be used during surgery or in the treatment of traumatized eyes because of the capacity of some preservatives to cause eye irritation. These non-preserved preparations are packaged in single-use containers.

During pre-formulation studies, antimicrobial preservatives must demonstrate stability, chemical/physical compatibility with other formulation and packaging components, and effectiveness at the concentration employed. Among the antimicrobial preservatives used in ophthalmic solutions/suspensions and their effective concentrations are: benzalkonium chloride, 0.004–0.01%; benzethonium chloride, 0.01%; chlorobutanol, 0.5%; phenylmercuric acetate, 0.004%; phenylmercuric nitrite, 0.004%; and, thimerosal, 0.005–0.01%. Certain preservatives have limitations to use, as chlorobutanol which cannot be autoclaved because it decomposes even under moderate conditions of heat with the formation of hydrochloric acid. This preservative degradation not only renders a product susceptible to microbial growth but could alter its pH and thereby affect the stability and/or physiologic activity of the therapeutic ingredient.

In concentrations tolerated by the eye, all of the aforementioned preservative agents are *in*effective against some strains of *Pseudomonas aeruginosa,*

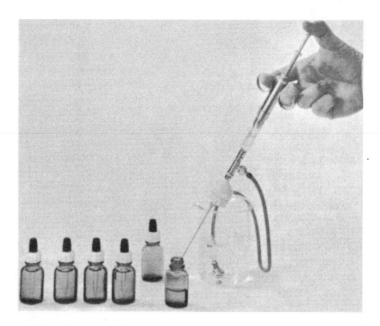

Fig. 16.1 *Sterilization by filtration. The preparation of a sterile solution by passage through a syringe affixed with a microbial filter. (Courtesy of Millipore Corporation.)*

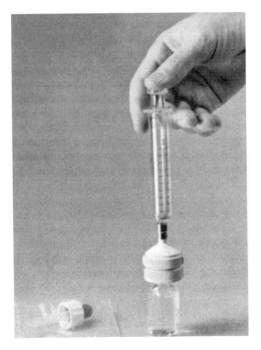

Fig. 16.2   *The preparation of a sterile ophthalmic solution by filtration. (Courtesy of Millipore Corporation.)*

an organism that can invade an abraded cornea and cause ulceration and even blindness. However, preservative mixtures of benzalkonium chloride (0.01%) and either polymyxin B sulfate (1000 USP Units/mL) or disodium ethylenediaminetetraacetate (0.01 to 0.1%) *are* effective against most strains of *Pseudomonas*. The latter agent, which is commonly employed as a chelating agent for metals, renders strains of *Pseudomonas aeruginosa* more sensitive to benzalkonium chloride.

Isotonicity Value

If a solution is placed behind a membrane that is permeable only to solvent molecules and not to solute molecules (a *semipermeable membrane*), a phenomenon called *osmosis* occurs as the molecules of solvent traverse the membrane. If a solution-filled membrane is placed in a solution of a higher solute concentration than its own, the solvent, which has free passage in either direction, passes into the more concentrated solution until an equilibrium is established on both sides of the membrane and an equal concentration of solute exists on the two sides. The pressure responsible for this movement is termed *osmotic pressure.*

The concentration of a solution with respect to osmotic pressure is concerned with the number of "particles" of solute in solution. That is, if the solute is a nonelectrolyte (as sucrose), the concentration of the solution will depend solely on the number of molecules present. However, if the solute is an electrolyte (as sodium chloride), the number of particles that it contributes to the solution will depend not only upon the concentration of the molecules present, but also on their degree of ionization. A chemical that is highly ionized will contribute a greater number of particles to the solution than will the same amount of a poorly ionized substance. The effect is that a solution with a greater number of particles, whether they be molecules or ions, has a greater osmotic pressure than does a solution having fewer particles.

Body fluids, including blood and lacrimal fluid, have an osmotic pressure corresponding to that of a 0.9% solution of sodium chloride. Thus, a 0.9% sodium chloride solution is said to be *isosmotic,* or having an equal osmotic pressure as physiologic fluids. The term *isotonic,* meaning equal tone, is commonly used interchangeably with isosmotic although it is correctly used only with reference to a specific body fluid whereas isosmotic is a physical chemical term which compares the osmotic pressure of two liquids which may or may not be physiologic fluids. Solutions with a lower osmotic pressure than body fluids or a 0.9% sodium chloride solution are commonly referred to as *hypotonic,* whereas solutions having a greater osmotic pressure are termed *hypertonic.*

Theoretically, a hypertonic solution added to the body's system will have a tendency to draw water from the body tissues toward the solution in an effort to dilute and establish a concentration equilibrium. In the blood stream, a hypertonic injection could cause the *crenation* (shrinking) of blood cells; in the eye, the solution could cause the drawing of water toward the site of the topical application. Conversely, a hypotonic solution might induce the hemolysis of red blood cells, or the passage of water from the site of an ophthalmic application through the tissues of the eye.

In practice, the isotonicity limits of an ophthalmic solution in terms of sodium chloride, or its osmotic equivalent, may range from 0.6 to 2.0% without marked discomfort to the eye. Sodium chloride itself does not have to be used to establish a solution's osmotic pressure. Boric acid in a concentration of 1.9% produces the same osmotic pressure as does 0.9% sodium chloride. All of an ophthalmic solution's solutes, including the active and inactive ingredients, contribute to the osmotic pressure of a solution.

The calculations involved in preparing isosmotic

solutions may be made in terms of data relating to the colligative properties of solutions (8). Like osmotic pressure, the other colligative properties of solutions, namely, vapor pressure, boiling point, and freezing point, depend upon the number of particles in solution. These properties, therefore, are related, and a change in any one of them will be accompanied by corresponding changes in the others. Although any one of these properties may be used to determine isosmoticity, a comparison of freezing points between the solutions in question, is most used.

When 1 g molecular weight of a non-electrolyte, such as boric acid, is dissolved in 1000 g of water, the freezing point of the solution is about 1.86°C below the freezing point of pure water. By simple proportion, therefore, the weight may be calculated for any non-electrolyte that should be dissolved in each 1000 g of water to prepare a solution isosmotic with lachrymal fluid and blood serum, which have freezing points of −0.52°C.

Boric acid, for example, has a molecular weight of 61.8, and thus 61.8 g in 1000 g of water should produce a freezing point of −1.86°C. Therefore:

$$\frac{1.86(\text{°C})}{0.52(\text{°C})} = \frac{61.8\ (\text{g})}{\times\ (\text{g})}$$

$$\times = 17.3\ \text{g}$$

Hence, 17.3 g of boric acid in 1000 g of water theoretically should produce a solution isosmotic with tears and blood.

The calculation employed to prepare a solution isosmotic (with tears of blood) when using electrolytes is different than when the calculation is made for a non-electrolyte. Since osmotic pressure depends upon the number of particles, substances that dissociate have an effect that increases with the degree of dissociation; the greater the dissociation, the smaller the quantity required to produce a given osmotic pressure. If we assume that sodium chloride in weak solutions is about 80% dissociated, then each 100 molecules yield 180 particles, or 1.8 times as many particles as are yielded by 100 molecules of a non-electrolyte. This dissociation factor, commonly symbolized by the letter i, must be included in the proportion when we seek to determine the strength of an isosmotic solution of sodium chloride (molecular weight, 58.5):

$$\frac{1.86\ (\text{°C}) \times 1.8}{0.52\ (\text{°C})} = \frac{58.5\ (\text{g})}{\times\ (\text{g})}$$

$$\times = 9.09\ \text{g}$$

Therefore, 9.09 g of sodium chloride in 1000 g of water should make a solution isosmotic with blood

or lachrymal fluid. As indicated previously, a 0.90% (w/v) sodium chloride solution is taken to be isosmotic (and isotonic) with the body fluids.

Simple isosmotic solutions, then, may be calculated by this general formula:

$$\frac{0.52 \times \text{molecular weight}}{1.86 \times \text{dissociation } (i)} = \begin{array}{l}\text{g of solute per} \\ \text{1000 g of water}\end{array}$$

Although the i value has not been determined for every medicinal agent that might be named, the following values may be (generally) used:

Non-electrolytes and substances
  of slight dissociation 1.0
Substances that dissociate into 2 ions:............. 1.8
Substances that dissociate into 3 ions:............. 2.6
Substances that dissociate into 4 ions:............. 3.4
Substances that dissociate into 5 ions:............. 4.2

Since 0.9% sodium chloride solution is considered to be isosmotic (and isotonic) with lacrimal fluid, other medicinal substances are compared with regard to their "sodium chloride equivalency." An often used rule states (8):

quantities of two substances that are tonicic equivalents are proportional to the molecular weights of each multiplied by the i value of the other.

Using the drug atropine sulfate as an example:

Molecular weight of sodium chloride = 58.5;
$i = 1.8$

Molecular weight of atropine sulfate = 695;
$i = 2.6$

$$\frac{695 \times 1.8}{58.5 \times 2.6} = \frac{1\ (\text{g})}{\times\ (\text{g})}$$

$$x = 0.12\ \text{g of sodium chloride}$$

represented by 1 g of atropine sulfate

Thus, the *sodium chloride equivalent* for atropine sulfate is 0.12 g. To put it one way, 1.0 g of atropine sulfate equals the "tonic effect" of 0.12 g of sodium chloride. To put it another way, atropine sulfate is 12% as effective as an equal weight of sodium chloride in contributing toward tonicity. When a combination of drugs is used in a prescription or formulation to be rendered isotonic, each agent's contribution to tonicity must be taken into consideration. For instance, consider the following prescription:

Atropine Sulfate 1%
Sodium Chloride .... q.s. to isotonicity
Sterile Purified Water, ad............ 30.0 mL

To make the 30 mL isotonic with sodium chloride; 30 mL x 0.9% = 0.27 g or 270 mg of sodium chloride would be required. However, since 300 mg of atropine sulfate is to be present, its contribution to tonicity needs to be taken into consideration. Since the sodium chloride equivalent for atropine sulfate is 0.12, its contribution is calculated as follows:

$$0.12 \times 300 \text{ mg} = 36 \text{ mg}$$

Thus, 270 mg − 36 mg = 234 mg of sodium chloride would actually be required.

Table 16.1 presents an abbreviated list of sodium chloride equivalents. A more complete list may be found in pharmaceutical calculations or physical pharmacy textbooks.

As a convenience, the USP XXI listed precalculated amounts of some common ophthalmic drugs which may be used to prepare isotonic solutions. Some of the drugs and the related values are presented in Table 16.2. The data shown are utilized in the following manner. One gram of each of the drugs listed, when added to purified water, will prepare the corresponding volume of an isotonic solution. For instance, 1 g of atropine sulfate will prepare 14.3 mL of isotonic solution. This solution may then be diluted with an isotonic vehicle to maintain the isotonicity while changing the strength of the active constituent in the solution to any desired level. For instance, if a 1% isotonic solution of atropine sulfate is desired, the 14.3 mL of isotonic solution containing 1 g of atropine sulfate should be diluted to 100 mL (1 g atropine sulfate in 100 mL = 1% w/v solution) with an isotonic vehicle. By utilizing sterile drug, sterile purified water, a sterile isotonic vehicle, and aseptic techniques, a sterile product may be prepared. In addition to being sterile and isotonic, the diluting vehicles generally used are also buffered and contain suitable preservative to maintain the stability and sterility of the product.

Buffering

The pH of an ophthalmic preparation may be adjusted and buffered for one or more of the following purposes (9): 1) for greater comfort to the eye; 2) to render the formulation more stable; 3) to enhance the aqueous solubility of the drug; and, 4) to enhance the drug's bioavailability (i.e., by favoring unionized molecular species); and 5) to maximize preservative efficacy.

The pH of normal tears is considered to be about 7.4, but varies among patients (e.g., more acidic in contact lens wearers) (9). Tears have some buffer capacity. The introduction of a medicated solution into the eye stimulates the flow of tears, which attempts to neutralize any excess hydrogen or hydroxyl ions introduced with the solution. Most drugs used ophthalmically are weakly acidic and have only weak buffer capacity. Normally, the buffering action of the tears is capable of neutralizing the ophthalmic solution and is thereby able to prevent marked discomfort. The eye apparently can tolerate

Table 16.1   Some Sodium Chloride Equivalents

Substance	Molecular Weight	Ions	i	Sodium Chloride Equivalent
Atropine Sulfate·H_2O	695	3	2.6	0.12
Benzalkonium Chloride	360	2	1.8	0.16
Benzyl Alcohol	108	1	1.0	0.30
Boric Acid	61.8	1	1.0	0.52
Chlorobutanol	177	1	1.0	0.18
Cocaine Hydrochloride	340	2	1.8	0.17
Ephedrine Sulfate	429	3	2.6	0.20
Epinephrine Bitartrate	333	2	1.8	0.18
Ethylmorphine Hydrochloride·$2H_2O$	386	2	1.8	0.15
Naphazoline Hydrochloride	247	2	1.8	0.27
Physostigmine Salicylate	413	2	1.8	0.14
Pilocarpine Hydrochloride	245	2	1.8	0.24
Procaine Hydrochloride	273	2	1.8	0.21
Scopolamine Hydrobromide·$3H_2O$	438	2	1.8	0.13
Tetracycline Hydrochloride	481	2	1.8	0.12
Zinc Sulfate·$7H_2O$	288	2	1.4	0.16

Table 16.2   Isotonic Solutions Prepared from Common Ophthalmic Drugs*

Drug (1.0 g)	Volume of Isotonic Solution Yielded (mL)
Atropine Sulfate	14.3
Boric Acid	55.7
Chlorobutanol (hydrous)	26.7
Cocaine Hydrochloride	17.7
Colistimethate Sodium	16.7
Dibucaine Hydrochloride	14.3
Ephedrine Sulfate	25.7
Epinephrine Bitartrate	20.0
Eucatropine Hydrochloride	20.0
Fluorescein Sodium	34.3
Homatropine Hydrobromide	19.0
Neomycin Sulfate	12.3
Penicillin G Potassium	20.0
Phenylephrine Hydrochloride	35.7
Physostigmine Salicylate	17.7
Physostigmine Sulfate	14.3
Pilocarpine Hydrochloride	26.7
Pilocarpine Nitrate	25.7
Polymyxin B Sulfate	10.0
Procaine Hydrochloride	23.3
Proparacaine Hydrochloride	16.7
Scopolamine Hydrobromide	13.3
Silver Nitrate	36.7
Sodium Bicarbonate	72.3
Sodium Biphosphate	44.3
Sodium Borate	46.7
Sodium Phosphate (dibasic, heptahydrate)	32.3
Streptomycin Sulfate	7.7
Sulfacetamide Sodium	25.7
Sulfadiazine Sodium	26.7
Tetracaine Hydrochloride	20.0
Tetracycline Hydrochloride	15.7
Zinc Sulfate	16.7

*Adapted from USP XXI, p. 1339.

a greater deviation from physiologic pH toward alkalinity (and less discomfort) than toward the acidic range (9). For maximum comfort, an ophthalmic solution should have the same pH as the lacrimal fluid. However, this is not pharmaceutically possible, since at pH 7.4, many drugs are insoluble in water. A few drugs—notably pilocarpine hydrochloride and epinephrine bitartrate—are quite acid and overtax the buffer capacity of the lacrimal fluid.

Most drugs, including many used in ophthalmic solutions, are most active therapeutically at pH levels which favor the undissociated molecule. However, the pH that permits greatest activity may also be the pH at which the drug is least stable. For this reason, a compromise pH is generally selected for a solution and maintained by buffers to permit the greatest activity while maintaining stability.

An isotonic phosphate vehicle, prepared at the desired pH (Table 16.3) and adjusted for tonicity, may be employed in the extemporaneous compounding of solutions. The desired solution is prepared through the use of two stock solutions, one containing 8.00 g of monobasic sodium phosphate (NaH_2PO_4) per liter, and the other containing 9.47 g of dibasic sodium phosphate (Na_2HPO_4) per liter, the weights being on an anhydrous basis.

The vehicles listed in Table 16.3 are satisfactory for many ophthalmic drugs with the exception of pilocarpine, eucatropine, scopolamine and homatropine salts which show instability in the vehicle. The vehicle is used effectively as the diluent for ophthalmic drugs already in isotonic solution, as those prepared according to the method presented in Table 16.2. When drug substances are added directly to the isotonic phosphate vehicle, the solution becomes slightly hypertonic. Generally, this provides no discomfort to the patient. However, if such a solution is not desired, the appropriate adjustment can be made through calculated dilution of the vehicle with purified water.

Viscosity and Thickening Agents

Viscosity is a property of liquids related to the resistance to flow. The reciprocal of viscosity is *fluidity*. Viscosity is defined in terms of the force required to move one plane surface past another under specified conditions when the space between is filled by the liquid in question. More simply, it can be considered as a relative property with

Table 16.3   Isotonic Phosphate Vehicle

Monobasic Sodium Phosphate Solution, mL	Dibasic Sodium Phosphate Solution, mL	Resulting Buffer Solution, pH	Sodium Chloride Required for Isotonicity, g/100 mL
90	10	5.9	0.52
80	20	6.2	0.51
70	30	6.5	0.50
60	40	6.6	0.49
50	50	6.8	0.48
40	60	7.0	0.46
30	70	7.2	0.45
20	80	7.4	0.44
10	90	7.7	0.43
5	95	8.0	0.42

Physical Pharmacy Capsule 16.1   **pH and Solubility**

pH is one of the most important factors involved in the formulation process. Two areas of critical importance are the effects of pH on solubility and stability. The effect of pH on solubility is critical in the formulation of liquid dosage forms, from oral and topical solutions to intravenous solutions and admixtures.

The solubility of a weak acid or base is often pH dependent. The total quantity of a monoprotic weak acid (HA) in solution at a specific pH is the sum of the concentrations of both the free acid and salt (A^{-2D}) forms. If excess drug is present, the quantity of free acid in solution is maximized and constant due to its saturation solubility. As the pH of the solution is increased, the quantity of drug in solution increases because the water-soluble ionizable salt is formed. The expression is:

$$HA \xrightleftharpoons{K_a} H^+ + A^-$$

where K_a is the dissociation constant.

There may be a certain pH level reached where the total solubility (S_T) of the drug solution is saturated with respect to both the salt and acid forms of the drug, i.e., the pH_{max}. The solution can be saturated with respect to the salt at pH values higher than this, but not with respect to the acid. Also, at pH values less than this, the solution can be saturated with respect to the acid, but not to the salt. This is illustrated in the accompanying figure.

To calculate the total quantity of drug that can be maintained in solution at a selected pH, two different equations can be used, depending upon whether the product is to be in a pH region above or below the pH_{max}. (See Figure on next page). The following equation is used when below the pH_{max}:

(Equation 1)

$$S_T = S_a \left(1 + \frac{K_a}{[H^+]}\right)$$

The next equation is used when above the pH_{max}:

(Equation 2)

$$S_T = S'a \left(\frac{1 + [H^+]}{K_a}\right)$$

where S_a is the saturation solubility of the free acid, and

$S'a$ is the saturation solubility of the salt form.

EXAMPLE

A pharmacist prepares a 3.0% solution of an antibiotic as an ophthalmic solution and dispenses it to a patient. A few days later the patient returns the eye drops to the pharmacist because the product contains a precipitate. The pharmacist, checking the pH of the solution and finding it to be 6.0, reasons that the problem might be pH-related. The physicochemical information of interest on the antibiotic includes the following:

Molecular weight	285 (salt) 263 (free acid)
3.0% solution of the drug is a	0.1053 molar solution
Acid form solubility (S_a)	3.1 mg/mL (0.0118 molar)
K_a	5.86×10^{-6}

Using Equation 1, the pharmacist calculates the quantity of the antibiotic that would be in solution at a pH of 6.0 (Note: pH of 6.0 = $[H^+]$ of 1×10^{-6})

$$S_T = 0.0118 \left(\frac{1 + 5.86 \times 10^{-6}}{1 \times 10^{-6}}\right) = 0.0809 \text{ molar}$$

Physical Pharmacy Capsule 16.1 **pH and Solubility (Continued)**

From this the pharmacist knows that, at a pH of 6.0, a 0.0809 molar solution could be prepared. However, the concentration that was to be prepared was a 0.1053 molar solution; consequently, the drug will not be in solution at that pH. What may have occurred was the pH was all right initially but shifted to a lower pH after a period of time, resulting in precipitation of the drug. The question is then asked, at what pH (hydrogen ion concentration) will the drug remain in solution? This can be calculated using the same equation and the information that is available. The S_T value is 0.1053 molar.

$$0.1053 = 0.0118 \left(\frac{1 + 5.86 \times 10^{-6}}{[H^+]} \right)$$

$[H^+] = 7.333 \times 10^{-7}$, or a pH of 6.135

The pharmacist then prepares a solution of the antibiotic, adjusting the pH to greater than about 6.2 using a suitable buffer system, and dispenses the solution to the patient—with positive results.

An interesting phenomenon can be discussed briefly concerning the close relationship of pH to solubility. At a pH of 6.0, only a 0.0809 molar solution could be prepared, but at a pH of 6.13 a 0.1053 molar solution could be prepared. In other words, a difference of 0.13 pH units resulted in:

$$\frac{0.1053 - 0.0809}{0.0809} = \begin{array}{l} 30.1\% \text{ more drug going into solution at} \\ \text{the higher pH compared to the lower pH} \end{array}$$

In other words, a very small change in pH resulted in about 30% more drug going into solution. According to the figure, the slope of the curve would be very steep for this example drug and a small change in pH (x-axis) results in a large change in solubility (y-axis). From this, it can be reasoned that if one observes the pH:solubility profile of a drug, it is possible to predict the magnitude of the pH change on its solubility.

In recent years, it has been interesting to note that more and more physicochemical information on drugs is being made available to pharmacists in routinely used reference books. This type of information is important for pharmacists in different types of practice, especially those involved in compounding and pharmacokinetic monitoring.

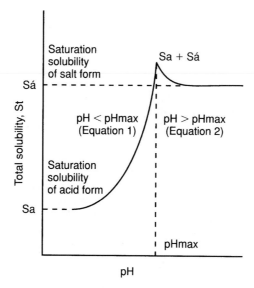

water as the reference material and all viscosities expressed in terms of the viscosity of pure water at 20°C. The viscosity of water is given as one centipoise (actually 1.0087 centipoise). A liquid material ten times as viscous as water at the same temperature has a viscosity of 10 centipoises. The centipoise, abbreviated cp. (*cps.* plural), is a more convenient term than the basic unit, the poise; one poise is equal to 100 centipoises.

Specifying the temperature is important because viscosity changes with temperature; generally, the viscosity of a liquid decreases with increasing temperature. The determination of viscosity in terms of poise or centipoise results in the calculation of *absolute* viscosity. It is sometimes more convenient to use the kinematic scale in which the units of viscosity are *stokes* and *centistokes* (1 stoke equals 100 centistokes). The kinematic viscosity is obtained from the absolute viscosity by dividing the latter by the density of the liquid at the same temperature:

$$\text{kinematic viscosity} = \frac{\text{absolute viscosity}}{\text{density}}$$

Using water as the standard, examples of some viscosities at 20°C are:

Ethyl alcohol	— 1.19	cps
Olive oil	— 100	cps
Glycerin	— 400	cps
Castor oil	— 1000	cps

Viscosity can be determined by any method that will measure the resistance to shear offered by the liquid. For ordinary Newtonian liquids, it is customary to determine the time required for a given sample of the liquid to flow at a regulated temperature through a small vertical capillary tube and to compare this time with that required to perform the same task by the reference liquid. Many capillary tube viscosimeters have been devised, and nearly all are modifications of the Ostwald type. With an apparatus such as this, the viscosity of a liquid may be determined by the following equation:

$$\frac{\eta_1}{\eta_2} = \frac{\rho_1 t_1}{\rho_2 t_2}$$

where η_1 is the unknown viscosity of the liquid, η_2 is the viscosity of the standard, ρ_1 and ρ_2 are the respective densities of the liquids, and t_1 and t_2 are the respective flow times in seconds.

In the preparation of ophthalmic solutions, a suitable grade of methylcellulose or other thickening agent is frequently added to increase the viscosity and thereby aid in maintaining the drug in contact with the tissues to enhance therapeutic effectiveness. Generally, methylcellulose of the 4000 cps viscosity type is used in concentrations of 0.25% and the 25 cps type at 1% concentration. Hydroxypropyl methylcellulose and polyvinyl alcohol are also used as thickeners in ophthalmic solutions. Occasionally a 1% solution of methylcellulose without medication is used as a tear replacement. Viscosity for ophthalmic solutions is considered optimal in the range of 15 to 25 cps.

Ocular Bioavailability

Ocular bioavailability is an important factor in the effectiveness of an applied medication. There are physiologic factors which can affect a drug's ocular bioavailability, including protein binding, drug metabolism, and lacrimal drainage. Protein-bound drugs are incapable of penetrating the corneal epithelium due to the size of the protein-drug complex (1). Because of the brief time in which an ophthalmic solution may remain in the eye (due to lacrimal drainage) the protein binding of a drug substance could quickly negate its therapeutic value by rendering it unavailable for absorption. Normally, tears contain between 0.6 and 2.0% of protein, including albumin and globulins, but disease states (as uveitis) can raise these protein levels (1). Although ocular protein binding is reversible, tear turnover results in the loss of both bound and unbound drug (2).

As in the case with other biological fluids, tears contain enzymes (such as lysozyme) capable of the metabolic degradation of drug substances. However, only a limited amount of research has been conducted on the ocular metabolism of pharmacologic agents and thus the full extent to which drug metabolism occurs and affects therapeutic effectiveness is undetermined at this time (10).

In addition to physiologic factors affecting ocular bioavailability, other factors, as the physicochemical characteristics of the drug substance and product formulation are important. Because the cornea is a membrane barrier containing both lipophilic and hydrophilic layers, it is permeated most effectively by drug substances having both lipophilic and hydrophilic characteristics (1).

As discussed previously, ophthalmic suspensions, gels, and ointments mix with lacrimal fluids less readily than do low-viscosity solutions, and thus, remain in the cul-de-sac for longer periods of time thereby enhancing the availability of the drug substance for its activity.

Additional Considerations

Ophthalmic solutions must be sparkling clear and free of all particulate matter for patient comfort and safety. The formulation of an ophthalmic suspension may be undertaken when it is desired to prepare a product with extended corneal contact time, or, it may be necessary when the medicinal agent is insoluble or unstable in an aqueous vehicle.

Drug particles in an ophthalmic suspension must be finely subdivided, usually micronized, to minimize eye irritation and/or scratching of the cornea. The suspended particles must not associate into larger particles upon storage and must be easily and uniformly redistributed by gentle shaking of the container prior to use.

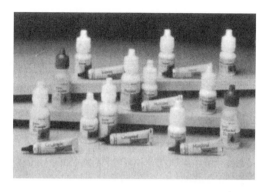

Fig. 16.4   *Examples of ophthalmic product packaging. Liquids are in 5-mL and 15-mL Drop-Tainer dispensers and ointments are in tubes containing 3.5 g of product. (Courtesy of Alcon.)*

Packaging Ophthalmic Solutions and Suspensions

Although a few commercial ophthalmic solutions/suspensions are packaged in small glass bottles with separate glass or plastic droppers, the vast majority are packaged in soft plastic containers having a fixed, built-in dropper (Figs. 16.3, 16.4). The latter type of packaging is preferred both to facilitate administration and to protect the product from external contamination. Ophthalmic solutions and suspensions are commonly packaged in containers holding 2, 2.5, 5, 10, 15, and 30 mL of product.

Patients must exercise care in protecting an ophthalmic solution/suspension from external contamination. Obviously, the fixed dropper containers are less likely to acquire airborne contaminants than the screw-type bottles which are fully opened when in use. However, each type is subject to contamination during use by airborne contaminants

and by the inadvertent touching of the tip of the dropper to the eye, eyelids or other surface.

Ophthalmic solutions used as eye washes are generally co-packaged with an eye cup which should be cleaned and dried thoroughly before and after each use.

Proper Administration of Ophthalmic Solutions and Suspensions

Prior to the administration of an ophthalmic solution or suspension, the patient or caregiver should be advised to wash his/her hands thoroughly. If the ophthalmic drops are supplied with a separate dropper, the patient should inspect the dropper to make sure it has no chips or cracks. Ophthalmic solutions should be inspected for color and clarity. Out of date or darkened solutions should be discarded. Ophthalmic suspensions should be shaken thoroughly prior to administration to evenly distribute the suspensoid.

The cap of an eye-drop container should be removed immediately prior to use and returned immediately after use. The combined dropper-container as shown in Figure 16.3 is used by holding it between the thumb and middle finger with the index finger on the bottom of the container. One or more drops are delivered by gently squeezing the container. A product packaged with a separate dropper is used by holding the dropper between the thumb and forefinger then drawing up and discharging the medication drop-wise in the usual and familiar manner.

To instill eye drops, the patient should tilt his/her head back and with the index finger of the free hand gently pull downward the lower eyelid of the

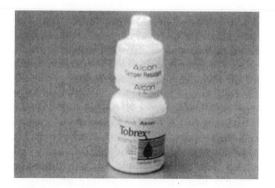

Fig. 16.3   *Commercial package of an ophthalmic solution in a plastic container with built-in dropper device. (Courtesy of Alcon.)*

affected eye to form a pocket or cup. While looking up, and without touching the dropper to the eye, the prescribed number of drops should be instilled into the formed pocket. The lower eyelid should be released and the eye closed to allow the medication to spread over the eye. The eye should be held closed preferably for a full minute without blinking, rubbing, or wiping. While the eye is closed, gentle pressure should be applied just under the inner corner of the eye by the nose to compress the nasolacrimal duct to prevent drainage and enhance corneal contact time. Then, any excess liquid may be wiped away with a tissue.

During handling and administration, care must be taken not to touch the dropper to the eye, eyelid or any other surface. If a separate dropper is used, it should be returned to the container and capped tightly. The dropper should not be rinsed or wiped off. If a combined dropper-container unit is used, the container-cap should be returned and tightly closed.

In every case, the patient should be advised about the correct number of drops to instill, the frequency of application, the duration of treatment, the proper storage of the medication and usual side effects specific to the product used. Among the side effects encountered with the use of ophthalmic medication are a transient stinging/burning, foreign body sensation, itching, tearing, decreased vision, margin crusting, and occasionally a bad (drug) taste.

Examples of some commercially available ophthalmic solutions and suspensions are presented in Table 16.4.

Contact Lenses and Care/Use Solutions

The number of persons wearing contact lenses grows each year. Their popularity and increased use has fostered the development of new types of lenses and lens care products. In order to counsel patients properly, it is important for pharmacists to be knowledgeable of the characteristics and features of the types of contact lenses and the products available for their care and use (11–14).

The three basic types of contact lenses are classified by their chemical composition and physical properties, i.e., hard, soft, and rigid gas permeable (RGP).

Hard contact lenses provide durability and clear, crisp vision for the patient. The lenses are termed *hard* because they are made of a rigid plastic resin, polymethylmethacrylate (PMMA). The lenses are 7–10 mm in diameter and are designed to cover

only part of the cornea. They float on the tear layer overlying the cornea. Hard lenses require an adaption period sometimes as long as a week for wearing comfort (15). Even then, because of their rigidity, some patients find them difficult to wear. PMMA lenses are practically impermeable to oxygen and moisture (they absorb only about 0.5% water), a disadvantage to corneal epithelial respiration and to patient comfort. Care must be exercised to prevent the hard lens from resting directly on the corneal surface and causing physical damage to epithelial tissue. To prevent direct contact, solutions are used that wet the surface of the lens and provide a cushioning layer between the corneal epithelium and the inner surface of the lens.

Soft contact lenses are more popular than hard lenses because of their greater comfort. They range from about 13 to 15 mm in diameter and cover the entire cornea. Because of their size and coverage, soft lenses are less likely than hard lenses to dislodge spontaneously. They also are less likely to permit irritating foreign particles (e.g., dust or pollen) to lodge beneath them. However for some patients, soft lenses do not provide the same high level of visual acuity as hard lenses. They are less durable than hard lenses and carry some risk of absorbing medication which may be concomitantly applied to the eye.

Soft contact lenses are made of a hydrophilic transparent plastic, hydroxyethylmethacrylate (HEMA), with small amounts of cross-linking agents that provide a hydrogel network (14). Soft lenses contain between 30 and 80% water which enables enhanced permeability to oxygen. There are two general types of soft contact lens: daily-wear and extended-wear. Whereas daily-wear lenses must be removed at night before the wearer goes to sleep, extended-wear lenses are designed to be worn for more than 24 hours with some approved for up to 30 days of continuous wear. However, it is advisable that lenses not be retained in the eye for longer than 4 to 7 days without removal for cleaning and disinfection. Else the wearer can be predisposed to eye infection.

Disposable soft lenses do not require cleaning and disinfection for the recommended period of use; they are simply discarded and replaced with a new pair. Patients should be advised to resist any temptation to wear the lenses for longer than recommended to avoid risk of eye infection. *Rigid gas permeable (RGP)* contact lenses take advantage of features of both soft and the hard lenses. They are constructed of material that is oxygen-permeable but hydrophobic. Thus, compared to hard lenses they permit greater movement of oxygen through

Table 16.4   Examples of Some Ophthalmic Agents by Category

Ophthalmic Agent	Corresponding Commerical Product	Concentration of Active Ingredient	Comments
Adrenergic			
Naphazoline HCI	Naphcon-A Ophthalmic Solution (Alcon)	0.025%	Used as a topical ocular vasoconstrictor.
Antiallergic			
Cromolyn Sodium	Opticrom Ophthalmic Solution (Fisons)	4%	For treatment of allergic ocular disorders as vernal conjunctivitis.
Antibacterial			
Chloramphenicol	Ophthochlor Ophthalmic Solution (Parke-Davis)	0.5%	
Ciprofloxacin Hydrochloride	Ciloxan Sterile Ophthalmic Solution (Alcon)	0.35%	
Gentamicin Sulfate	Garamycin Ophthalmic Solution (Schering)	0.3%	Used for superficial infections of the eye due to susceptible microorganisms.
Tetracycline Hydrochloride	Achromycin Ophthalmic Suspension (Lederle)	1%	
Tobramycin	Tobrex Ophthalmic Solution (Alcon)]	0.3%	
Sulfacetamide Sodium	Sodium Sulamyd Ophthalmic Solution (Schering)	10 and 30%	
Antiviral			
Trifluridine	Viroptic Ophthalmic Solution (Burroughs Wellcome)	1%	Indicated in the treatment of herpes simplex keratitis.
Artificial Tears			
Dextran 70, Hydroxypropyl Methylcellulose	Tears Naturale II (Alcon)	. . .	For relief of dry eyes.
Astringent			
Zinc Sulfate	Zincfrin Ophthalmic Solution (Alcon)	0.25%	Used for relief of discomfort and congestion caused by minor irritations to the eyes, such as dust, fatigue, and allergies.
Anti-inflammatory			
Dexamethasone Sodium Phosphate	Decadron Phosphate Sterile Ophthalmic Solution (Merck Sharpe & Dohme)	0.1%	Combats inflammation due to mechanical, chemical, or immunologic causes.
Antibacterial/Antiinflammatory Combinations			
Neomycin Sulfate and Dexamethasone Sodium Phosphate	NeoDecadron Ophthalmic Solution (Merck Sharpe & Dohme)	0.35% neomycin base equivalent and 0.1% dexamethasone	For steroid-responsive inflammatory ocular conditions where bacterial infection or a risk of bacterial ocular infection exists.
Oxytetracycline and Hydrocortisone Acetate	Terra-Cortril Ophthalmic Suspension (Roerig)	0.5% oxytetracycline equivalent and 1.5% hydrocortisone acetate	
Tobramycin and Dexamethasone	TobraDex Sterile Ophthalmic Suspension (Alcon)]	0.3% tobramycin and 0.1% dexamethasone	

continued

Table 16.4   Examples of Some Ophthalmic Agents by Category

Ophthalmic Agent	Corresponding Commerical Product	Concentration of Active Ingredient	Comments
Beta-Adrenergic Blocking Agents			
Betaxolol HCI	Betoptic Sterile Ophthalmic Solution (Alcon)	0.5%	Used for ocular hypertension and chronic open-angle glaucoma.
Timolol Maleate	Timoptic Sterile Ophthalmic Solution (Merck, Sharpe & Dohme)	0.25%, 0.5%	Used in patients with chronic open-angle glaucoma and aphakic patients with glaucoma.
Cholinergic			
Pilocarpine HCI	Isopto Carpine Ophthalmic Solution (Alcon)	0.25 to 10%	Used as a miotic in treating glaucoma, especially open-angle glaucoma. Also used to neutralize mydriasis following ophthalmoscopy or surgery.
Cholinesterase Inhibitor			
Demecarium Bromide	Humorsol Sterile Ophthalmic Solution (Merck & Co.)	0.125% and 0.25%	Produces intense miosis and ciliary muscle contractions due to inhibition of cholinesterase. Used in open-angle glaucoma when shorter-acting miotics have proved inadequate.

the lens while retaining the characteristic durability and ease of handling. RGP lenses provide greater wearing comfort than hard lenses. The basic-type lens is intended for daily wear; some of the newer "super-permeable" RGP lenses are suitable for extended-wear.

There are advantages and disadvantages associated with each type of contact lens. Hard contact lenses and RGP lenses provide strength, durability, and relatively easy care regimens. They are easy to handle during insertion and removal and are relatively resistant to the absorption of medications, lens-care products, or environmental contaminants. These lenses provide visual acuity superior to that provided by soft contact lenses. On the other hand, hard contact lenses and RGP lenses require a greater adjustment period for the wearer and are more easily dislodged in the eye. Soft contact lenses have a shorter adaption period and may be worn comfortably for longer periods time. They do not dislodge as easily nor fall out of the eye as readily as the hard lenses. However, they have a shorter life span than hard or RGP lenses and the wearer must ensure that the lenses remain hydrated and do not dry out.

Color Additives to Contact Lenses

Contact lens manufacturers produce clear as well as colored lenses. The use of color additives in med-

ical devices, including contact lenses, is regulated by the federal Food and Drug Administration through authority granted by the Medical Device Amendments of 1976. Color additives that come into direct contact with the body for a significant period of time must be demonstrated to be safe for consumer use. This includes the color additives used in contact lenses. The FDA permits the use of a specific color additive in contact lenses only after reviewing and approving a manufacturer's official *Color Additive Petition.* The petition must contain the requisite chemical, safety, manufacturing, packaging, and product labeling information for FDA review. Many colored contact lenses are prepared as a reaction product, formed by chemically bonding a dye [e.g., Color Index (C.I.) Reactive Red 180 (CibaVision)] to the vinyl alcohol/methyl methacrylate copolymeric lens material.

Care of Contact Lenses

It is important that contact lenses receive appropriate care to retain their shape and optical characteristics and for their safe use. Wearers should be instructed in the techniques for insertion and removal of the lenses as well as methods of cleaning, disinfecting and storage.

With the exception of disposable soft contact lenses, all soft lenses require a routine care program that includes 1) cleaning to loosen and remove lipid and protein deposits, 2) rinsing to remove the cleaning solution and material loosened by cleaning, and 3) disinfection to kill microorganisms. If these lenses are not maintained at proper intervals, they are prone to deposit build-up, discoloration, and microbial contamination. The moist, porous surface of the hydrophilic lens provides an attractive medium for the growth of bacteria, fungi and viruses. Thus, disinfection is essential to prevent eye infections and microbial damage to the lens material.

Hard contact lenses require a routine care program that includes 1) cleaning to remove debris and deposits from the lens, 2) soaking the lens in a storage/disinfecting solution while not in use, and 3) wetting the lenses to decrease their hydrophobic characteristics.

To achieve the care needs of contact lenses the following types of solutions are used: 1) cleaning solutions, 2) soaking solutions, 3) wetting solutions, and 4) combination purpose solutions.

Products for Soft Contact Lenses

Cleaners

Because of their porous composition, soft lenses tend to accumulate proteinaceous material which forms a film on the lens, decreasing clarity and serving as a potential medium for microbial growth. The two main categories of cleaners are *surfactants,* which emulsify accumulated oils, lipids and inorganic compounds, and *enzymatic cleaners,* which break down and remove protein deposits. Surfactant agents are utilized either within a mechanical washing device or by placing several drops of the solution on the lens surface and gently rubbing the lens back and forth with the thumb and forefinger or by placing the lens in the palm of the hand and rubbing gently with a fingertip (about a 20 to 30 second procedure). The ingredients in these cleaners usually include a nonionic detergent, wetting agent, chelating agent, buffers, and preservatives. Enzymatic cleaning is accomplished by soaking the lenses in a solution prepared from enzyme tablets. This procedure is recommended at least once per week or twice per month in conjunction with regular surfactant cleansing. The enzyme tablets contain either papain, pancreatin, or subtilisin, which causes the hydrolysis of protein to peptides and amino acids. Typically these are added to saline solution, but one solution can be prepared using 3% hydrogen peroxide, which combines enzymatic cleaning with disinfection. After the lenses have

been soaked for the recommended length of time they should be thoroughly rinsed.

Rinsing/Storage Solutions

Saline solutions for soft lenses should have a neutral pH and be isotonic with human tears, i.e., 0.9% sodium chloride. Besides rinsing the lenses, these solutions are used for storage because saline maintains their curvature, diameter, and optical characteristics. The solutions also facilitate lens hydration, preventing the lens from drying out and becoming brittle.

Because they are used for storage, some saline solutions contain preservatives which, while inhibiting bacterial growth, can induce sensitivity reactions or eye irritation. Thus some manufacturers make available preservative-free saline solutions and package them in aerosol containers or unit-of-use vials. The use of salt tablets to prepare a normal saline solution is discouraged because of the potential of contamination and risk of serious eye infections.

Disinfection and Neutralization

Disinfection can be accomplished by either of two methods, i.e., thermal (heat) or chemical (no heat). In the past both methods were equally used, however, with the introduction of hydrogen peroxide systems for chemical disinfection, chemical disinfection has become more popular.

For thermal disinfection, the lenses are placed into a specially designed heating unit with saline solution. The solution is heated sufficiently to kill microorganisms, e.g., for 10 minutes at a minimum of 80°C. It is important that after disinfection the lenses be stored in the unopened case until ready to be worn. Further, the wearer must ensure that the lenses have been thoroughly cleaned prior to using heat disinfection. Otherwise, heating can hasten lens deterioration.

In years past chemical disinfection was conducted with products that contained thimerosal in combination with either chlorhexidine or a quaternary ammonium compound. Unfortunately, many wearers encountered sensitivity reactions and these products and the chemical method of disinfection fell into disfavor. The subsequent introduction of hydrogen peroxide systems for chemical disinfection revitalized this method of disinfection. It is thought that the "free radicals" chemically released from the peroxide react with the cell wall of the microorganisms. Further, the bubbling action of the peroxide is thought to promote the removal of any remaining debris on the lens.

To prevent eye irritation from residual peroxide after disinfection, it is necessary that the lenses be exposed to one of three types of neutralizing agents:

the *catalytic type* (an enzyme catalase or a platinum disc), the *reactive type* (such as sodium pyruvate or sodium thiosulfate), or the *dilution-elution* type.

Chemical disinfection systems may come as two-solution systems, which use separate disinfecting and rinsing solutions, or one-solution systems, which use the same solution for rinsing and storage. It is important that the wearer realize that lenses must not be disinfected by heating when using these solutions.

Products for Hard Contact Lenses

Cleaners

Hard lenses should be cleaned immediately after their removal from the eye. Otherwise, oil deposits, proteins, salts, cosmetics, tobacco smoke and air-borne contaminants can build up, interfere with clear vision and possibly cause irritation upon reinsertion. A surfactant cleaner is used by applying the solution or gel onto both surfaces of the lens, and then rubbing the lens in the palm of the hand with the index finger for about 20 seconds. The wearer should realize that too vigorous rubbing can cause scratching or warping of the lens.

Soaking/Storage Solutions

Hard lenses are placed in a soaking solution once they are removed from the eye. Soaking solutions contain a sufficient concentration of disinfecting agent, usually 0.01% benzalkonium chloride and 0.01% edetate sodium, to kill surface bacteria. Overnight soaking is advantageous because it keeps the lenses wettable and the prolonged contact time helps to loosen deposits that remain after routine cleaning.

Wetting Solutions

These solutions contain surfactants to facilitate the hydration of the hydrophobic lens surface. Wetting solutions enable the tears of the eye to evenly spread across the lens surface by providing temporary hydrophilic qualities to the hydrophobic surface of the lens. These solutions also facilitate a cushion between the lens and the cornea and the eyelid. Typical ingredients include a viscosity-inducing agent, as hydroxyethylcellulose, a wetting agent, as polyvinyl alcohol, preservatives, as benzalkonium chloride or edetate disodium, and buffering agents/salts to adjust the pH and maintain tonicity.

Combination Solutions

These solutions provide combination effects as cleaning/soaking, wetting/soaking, or cleaning/soaking/wetting. While patient ease of use is im-

proved with their use, combination products may lower the effectiveness of the cleaning function if the concentration of cleaning solution is too low to adequately remove debris from the lens surface. These combination solutions should be reserved for those wearers who have a demonstrated need for simplification of the lens care process.

Products for Rigid Gas Permeable (RGP) Contact Lenses

Care of these lenses requires the same general regimen as for hard contact lenses except that RGP-specific solutions must be used. One of two cleaning methods may be used, i.e., hand washing or mechanical washing. In the first method, the lens may be cleaned by holding the concave side up in the palm of the hand. The lens should not be held between the fingers because the flexibility of the lens may inadvertently cause the lens to warp or turn inside out. Mechanical washing is advantageous because the possibility of the lens turning inside out or warping during cleaning is minimized.

After cleansing, the RGP lens should then be thoroughly rinsed and soaked in a wetting/soaking solution overnight. After soaking, the next morning the lens is rubbed with fresh wetting/soaking solution and then inserted into the eye. To facilitate removal of stubborn protein deposits, weekly cleaning with enzymatic cleaners is recommended.

Clinical Considerations in the Use of Contact Lenses

Although most medicated eyedrops may be used in conjunction with the wearing of contact lenses some caution should be exercised and drug-specific information utilized, particularly with soft contact lenses use because this type of lens has been shown to be capable of absorbing certain topically administered drugs and affecting bioavailability (12, 15).

Use of ophthalmic suspensions and ophthalmic ointments by contact lens wearers presents some difficulties. The drug particles in ophthalmic suspensions can build up between the corneal surface and the contact lens causing discomfort and undesired effects. Ophthalmic ointments not only cloud vision but are capable of discoloring the lens. Thus, an alternative dosage form, as an ophthalmic solution, may be prescribed or the wearing of contact lenses deferred until the therapy is completed.

Some drugs administered by various routes of administration for systemic effects can find their way to the lacrimal fluid and produce drug-contact lens interactions. This may result in lens discoloration (e.g., orange staining by rifampin), lens clouding (ribavirin), ocular inflammation (salicylates), and refractive changes (acetazolamide) (12). In addition, drugs which cause ocular side effects have the potential to interfere with contact lens use. For example, drugs with anticholinergic effects (e.g., antihistamines, tricyclic antidepressants) decrease tear secretion and may cause lens intolerance and damage. Isotretinoin, prescribed for severe, recalcitrant acne, can induce marked dryness of the eye and may interfere with the use of contact lenses while acne therapy is being conducted. Drugs that promote excessive lacrimation (e.g., reserpine) or ocular or eyelid edema (e.g., primidone, hydrochlorothiazide, chlorthalidone) also may interfere with lens wear.

Use of ophthalmic vasoconstrictors occasionally cause dilation of the pupil of the eye, especially in people who wear contact lenses or whose cornea is abraded. Although this effect lasts only 1 to 4 hours and is not clinically significant, some patients have expressed concern. To allay their concern, the FDA has recommended that patients be advised of this side-effect through product labeling stating: "Pupils may become dilated (enlarged)" (16).

The following guidelines to the use of contact lenses should be used by pharmacists in patient counseling. Contact lens wearers should wash their hands thoroughly with a nonabrasive, non-cosmetic soap before and after handling lenses. Wearers should not rub the eyes when the lens are in place, and if irritation develops, the lens should be removed until these symptoms subside.

Only contact lens care-products specifically recommended for the type of lens worn should be used. Also, to avoid differences between products of different manufacturers, it is preferable to use solutions made by a single manufacturer. Cleaning and storing lenses should be performed in the specific solution for that purpose. Lenses should not be stored in tap water, nor should saliva be used to help reinsert a lens into the eye. Saliva is not sterile and contains numerous microorganisms, including *Pseudomonas aeruginosa.*

As appropriate, contact lens users should be counseled with regard to cosmetic use. It is prudent to purchase makeup in the smallest container since once opened and the longer a container is used the greater the likelihood of bacterial contamination. Mascara and pearlized eye shadow should be avoided by women wearing hard lenses because particles of these products can get into the eye and cause irritation, with corneal damage a possibility. Aerosol hairsprays should be used before the lens is inserted and preferably applied in another room since airborne particles could attach to the lens during its insertion and cause irritation. Lenses should be inserted prior to makeup application because oily substances on the fingertips can smudge the lenses when they are handled. For similar reasons, lenses should be removed before removing makeup.

Wearers of contact lenses normally do not experience ocular pain. If pain is present it may be a sign of ill-fitting contact lenses, corneal abrasion, or other medical condition and the patient should be advised to consult his/her ophthalmologist (15). Lastly, hard or soft contact lenses may occasionally cause superficial corneal changes, which may be painless and not evident to the patient. Thus it is important that all contact lens wearers have their eyes examined regularly to make certain that no damage has occurred.

References

1. Akers HJ. Ocular bioavailability of topically applied ophthalmic drugs. Am Pharm 1983;NS23:33–36.
2. Reddy IK, Ganesan MG. Ocular therapeutics and drug delivery: an overview. In: Reddy IK, ed. Ocular therapeutics and drug delivery. Lancaster, PA: Technomic Publishing Co, 1996;3–29.
3. Reddy IK, Azia W, Sause RB. Artificial tear formulations, irrigating solutions and contact lens products. In: Reddy IK, ed. Ocular therapeutics and drug delivery. Lancaster, PA:Technomic Publishing Co., 1996; 171–211.
4. Lee VHL, Robinson JR. Mechanistic and quantitative evaluation of precorneal pilocarpine distribution in albino rabbits. J Pharm Sci 1979;68:673–684.
5. Shell JW. Pharmacokinetics of topically applied ophthalmic drugs. Surv Ophthalmol 1982;26:207–218.
6. Nadkarni SR, Yalkowski SH. Controlled delivery of pilocarpine 1: in vitro characterization of gelfoam matrices. Pharm Res 1993;10:109–112.
7. Davies NM, et al. Evaluation of mucoadhesive polymers in ocular delivery II: polymer-coated vesicles. Pharm Res 1992; 9:1137–1144.
8. Stoklosa MJ, Ansel HC. Pharmaceutical calculations, 10th ed. Baltimore, MD: Williams & Wilkins, 1996.
9. Gangrade NK, Gaddipati NB, Ganesan MG, Reddy IK. Topical ophthalmic formulations: basic considerations. In: Reddy IK, ed. Ocular therapeutics and drug delivery. Lancaster, PA:Technomics Publishing Co:1996; 377–403.
10. Kumar GN. Drug metabolizing enzyme systems in the eye. In: Reddy IK, ed. Ocular therapeutics and drug delivery. Lancaster, PA:Technomics Publishing Co:1996;149–167.
11. Hind HW, Zuccaro VS. Pharmacist's handbook of contact lenses and contact lens solutions. Sunnyvale, CA: Barnes-Hind, Inc., 1986.

12. Engle JP. Assessing and counseling contact lens wearers. Am Pharm 1993;NS33:39–45.

13. Engle JP. Contact lens solutions. Drug Topics 1988; 132:56–66.

14. Reddy IK, Aziz W, Sause RB. Artificial tear formulations, irrigating solutions and contact lens products. In: Reddy IK, ed. Ocular therapeutics and drug delivery. Lancaster, PA:Technomics Publishing Co:1996; 171–211.

15. Berkow R, ed. The Merck Manual: Rahway, NJ: Merck Sharp & Dohme Research Laboratories, 1987:15: 2242–2244.

16. 63 Federal Register 8888–8890 (1998).

RADIOPHARMACEUTICALS

Chapter at a Glance

BY DEFINITION, a radiopharmaceutical is a radio-active pharmaceutical agent or drug that is used for diagnostic or therapeutic procedures (1). For a product to be classified as a radiopharmaceutical agent safe for human use, the preparer must satisfy two branches of the federal government whose responsibilities in this category of drug/agent have overlapping jurisdictions (i.e., Food and Drug Administration [FDA], Nuclear Regulatory Commission [NRC]) and a state agency, the State Board of Pharmacy.

The extent of oversee by the local state board of pharmacy differs between states. Because of the stringent regulations of the NRC, some state boards defer and do not have specific rules for nuclear pharmacies. Alternatively, other state board of pharmacies will actually have rules within their pharmacy practice act that relate to the practice of nuclear pharmacy.

Over the past three decades, the discipline of nuclear pharmacy (syn. radiopharmacy) has become highly specialized and contributed positively to the practice of nuclear medicine. Nuclear pharmacy was the first specialty in pharmacy recognized (in 1978) by the Board of Pharmaceutical Specialties (BPS), and focuses on the safe and effective use of radioactive drugs (syn. radiopharmaceuticals).

The application of radiopharmaceuticals is divided into two major areas (i.e., diagnostic, therapeutics). The diagnostic side is well established, while the therapeutic side of nuclear medicine is in its infancy. For example, there are over 100 radiopharmaceutical products available, with a largest proportion of these having application in cardiology (e.g., myocardial perfusion), oncology (e.g., tumor imaging/localization), and neurology (e.g., cerebral perfusion). Diagnostically, these are also used for infection imaging and in nephrology. At present, nuclear medicine as a therapeutic modality is utilized in four main conditions: thyroid cancer, Graves Disease, hyperthyroidism, and bone pain palliation. However, current research demonstrates that ongoing investigative studies involving radiopharmaceuticals are being conducted for more than 35 other potential diseases. Thus, it is anticipated that many of these radiopharmaceuticals have the potential to become available clinically by 2005 (2).

A radiopharmaceutical consists of a drug component and a radioactive component. Most radioactive isotopes contain a component that emits *gamma* radiation. It should be recalled from general chemistry that substances that have the same number of protons but have varying numbers of neutrons are called *isotopes*. Isotopes may be stable or unstable; those that are unstable are radioactive because their nuclei undergo a rearrangement while changing to a stable state, and energy is given off.

An important distinction between radiopharmaceuticals and traditional drugs is a lack of pharmacological activity on their part. For intensive purposes, radiopharmaceuticals are used as tracers of physiological processes. The huge advantage of their use is that their radioactivity allows non-invasive external monitoring or targeted therapeutic irradiation while creating very little effect on the biological processes in the body. Indeed, radiopharmaceuticals have an excellent safety record and their incidence of adverse effects is extremely low (3).

Background Information

All of the atoms of an unstable isotope do not completely rearrange at the same instant. The time required for a radioisotope to decay to 50% of its original activity is termed its radioactive half-life. Isotopes range widely in their half-life; carbon-14 has a radioactive half-life of some 5730 years, whereas sodium-24 has only a 15 hour half life and krypton-81 has a 13 second half life.

The activity of radioactive material may be calculated by a decay equation that allows the clinician to predict the activity at any point in time, regardless if it is earlier or later than the specific assay. The specific decay equation is:

$$A_e = A_o\, e^{-\lambda t}$$

where, A_e is the specific activity at time t; A_o is the initial activity; λ is the decay constant calculated as *ln 2*/half life, and t is time.

Decay tables have been formulated for various isotopes by calculating the last portion of the decay equation (i.e., $e^{-\lambda t}$). Thus,

$$A_e = A_o\, (\text{decay factor})$$

The activity of a radioactive material is expressed as the number of nuclear transformations per unit time. Because of decay, all radioactivity decreases with time because fewer atoms remain as the atoms decay. The fraction of nuclei disintegrating with time is always constant, and progressively fewer atoms are left. The larger the decay constant, the faster the process of decay, and the shorter the half-life. Thus, as demonstrated by the following, the half-life is inversely proportional to the decay constant:

$$t_{1/2} = \frac{0.69315}{\lambda}$$

where λ is the transformation or decay constant, which has a characteristic value for each radionuclide.

The fundamental unit of radioactivity is the *curie* (Ci), defined as 3.700×10^{10} nuclear transformations per second or disintegrations per second (i.e., dps). By multiplying this unit by 60, the definition can be expressed as disintegrations per minute (dpm). Multiples and submultiples (e.g., *millicurie* [mCi], *microcurie* [μCi], and *nanocurie* [nCi]) of the curie unit can be expressed also in disintegrations per second or minute:

1 millicurie = 10^{-3} curie
1 microcurie = 10^{-6} curie
1 nanocurie = 10^{-9} curie

In July, 1974, at the meeting of the International Commission of Radiation Units and Measurements (i.e, ICRU), a recommendation was made that within a period of no less than 10 years, the curie would be replaced with a new Si (i.e., Systeme International d'Unites) unit, the reciprocal second (i.e., sec^{-1}) (4). The intent was that this new unit be used to express the unit of activity as a function of the rate of spontaneous nuclear transformations of radionuclides, as one per second (i.e., dps). Further, it was recommended that this new unit of activity be given the name *becquerel,* and bearing the symbol *Bq.* Thus, the intent was that the *becquerel* would be equivalent to 1 dps or approximately 2.703×10^{-11} Ci. For example, a 15 mCi dose of ^{99m}Tc would then be referred to as a 555 megabecquerel (555 MBq) dose. To date, the conversion to Si units within the United States has been slow.

The amount of radiation absorbed by body tissue in which a radioactive substance resides is called the "radiation dose." Traditionally, this is measured in units of rads (i.e., *radiation absorbed dose)*; 1 rad = 100 ergs of energy absorbed by 1 g of tissue. The Gray (Gy) is the international unit of absorbed dose and equal to 1 joule of energy absorbed in 1 kg of tissue (i.e., 1 Gy = 100 rads).

Radiopharmaceutical doses are dispensed to patients in units of activity, typically mCi or μCi. Traditional therapeutic agents are dispensed according to weight-based calculations to determine appropriate activity in mCi. But, the pharmacist remains responsible to ensure that the proper prescribed dose is prepared and dispensed for the patient. Due to the nature of radiopharmaceuticals, the amount of radioactivity in the unit dose at the time of preparation must be sufficient to allow for decay of radioactivity before the product is administered to the patient.

The three main types of radiation decay are alpha particles, beta particles, and gamma photons. Alpha particles have the largest mass and charge of the three types of radiation consisting of two protons and two neutrons, thus being identical with the helium nucleus. As an alpha particle loses energy, its velocity decreases. It then attracts electrons and becomes a helium atom. Most alpha particles are unable to pierce the outer layers of skin or penetrate a thin piece of paper. However, due to the large charge, it does cause a great deal of damage to the immediate area by breaking down DNA. Beta particles may be either electrons with negative charge, *negatrons*, or positive electrons, *positrons*. These two particles, β and β+, have a range of over 100 feet in air and up to about 1 mm in tissue. Beta particles are not as destructive as alpha particles, but can be used therapeutically. Nuclear medicine depends mostly on radiopharmaceuticals that decay by gamma γ emission. Gamma rays are electromagnetic vibrations comparable with light but of much shorter wavelength. Because of their short wavelength and high energy, they are very penetrating.

The optimum dosage of radiopharmaceuticals is that which allows the acquisition of the desired information with the least amount of radiation dose or exposure to the patient. Thus, the clinical utility of a radiopharmaceutical is determined mainly by the radionuclide's physical properties (e.g., radiation, energy, half-life). Therefore, the best diagnostic images at the lowest radiation dose are attained if the radionuclide has a short half-life and emits only gamma radiation. Technetium-99m is a prime example of a radionuclide with these properties. Its half-life is 6 hours and gamma emission is of the nature of 140 keV, efficiently detected by the gamma camera. For therapeutic use, however, radionuclides should emit particulate radiation (i.e., beta particles), which deposits the radiation within the target organ. Iodine-131 is a prime example and used for hyperthyroidism and eradication of metastatic disease of the thyroid gland. But because iodine-131 emits both beta and gamma radiation, it can be used diagnostically (gamma rays) and therapeutically (beta rays).

The majority of radiopharmaceuticals are produced by the process of nuclear activation in a nuclear reactor. In such a reactor, stable atoms are bombarded with excess neutrons present in the reactor. The resulting neutron additions to the stable atoms produce unstable atoms and radioactive isotopes. The facilities for the production, use, and storage of radioactive pharmaceuticals are subject to licensing by the Nuclear Regulatory Commission (NRC) or in certain instances to appropriate state agencies. As for all pharmaceuticals, the Federal Food and Drug Administration enforces strict adherence to good manufacturing practice and proper labeling and use of the products. The Federal Department of Transportation regulates the conditions of shipment of the radiopharmaceuticals, as do state and local agencies.

Radiopharmaceuticals are used to diagnose the presence of disease or evaluate the progression of disease following specific therapy intervention. Radiopharmaceuticals can also be used to evaluate drug-induced toxicity, and to a lesser extent have been used to treat diseased tissue with radiation.

The distribution pattern of radiopharmaceuticals can be used for imaging purposes to attain diagnostic information about organs or various body systems (5). Imaging procedures are classified either as *dynamic* or *static*. The dynamic study provides useful information through the rate of accumulation and removal of the radiopharmaceutical from a specific organ. A static study merely provides perfusion and morphological information, i.e., assessing adequacy of blood flow, organ size, shape, position, presence of space occupying lesions.

Diagnostic Imaging

Some radiopharmaceuticals are formulated with the intent to localize it within a target organ. Sodium iodide, I-131, is actively taken up by thyroid cells following its absorption into the bloodstream after oral administration from either a capsule or a solution dosage form. The extent of the uptake of the dose by the gland helps assess thyroid function, or an image of the gland can be obtained after administration to visualize, i.e., static imaging, thyroid morphology. Alternatively, if I-131 is labeled to orthoiodohippuric acid (i.e., ^{131}I-orthoiodohippurate [OIH]) and intravenously injected, kidney tubules will actively secrete this agent into urine. Measuring the time course of activity over the kidney with a gamma camera and plotting the rate of radioactivity accumulation and removal *versus* time, yields a measure of kidney function. Such a dynamic study is termed a *renogram,* a particularly useful procedure to assess renal function in patients with transplanted kidneys.

There are, however, limitations to the use of ^{131}I-orthoiodohippurate. Due to its β emissions, the dose must be reduced to 200–400 μCi. The required lower dose with the 364 KeV α and β emissions results in a lower quality of image in comparison to ^{99m}Tc-Mag-3 which has pure α emissions of 140 KeV and thereby allowing for a higher dose to enhance the image quality without increasing the total body radiation burden. MAG-3 undergoes both tubular secretion and glomerular filtration within the kidney and provides excellent renograms.

Radiopharmaceuticals also are useful to evaluate a patient's response to drug therapy and surgery. These agents can detect early changes in physiologic function which come before morphologic or biochemical endpoints. An example is perfusion lung imaging using Tc-99m macroaggregated albumin particles to detect pulmonary embolism. Once the embolism is confirmed and thrombolytic and/or anticoagulant therapy initiated, this lung perfusing agent can be re-administered to evaluate its resolution with drug therapy. Cardiac radionuclide ventriculograms utilizing Tc-99m labeled red blood cells are performed to assess left ventricular function (e.g., ejection fraction, regional wall motion) to evaluate the effect of surgery (e.g., coronary artery bypass graft, valve repair) or the response to drug therapy (e.g., beta-blocking agents, calcium channel blocking agents).

Radiopharmaceuticals also find utility to help monitor drug therapy inclusive of toxicity. For example, the ability of doxorubicin to cause irreversible drug-induced heart failure is well known and the cumulative dosage of this drug should not exceed 550 mg/m². Because there is much variability in the individual response to this drug, serial determinations of left ventricular ejection fraction using Tc-99m radiopharmaceuticals are useful to determine on an individual basis the risk of developing doxorubicin-induced heart failure. Also, a Tc-99m ejection fraction study can be performed to assess the benefits of heart medications, e.g., digoxin.

Therapeutic Use of Radiopharmaceuticals

To a limited degree, radiopharmaceuticals can be used therapeutically. Thyroid disease can be treated with sodium iodide, I-131, polycythemia vera can be treated with sodium phosphate, P-32, peritoneal ef-

fusions can be treated with chromic phosphate, P-32, and Sr-89 used palliatively for pain relief associated with metastatic bone lesions. The intent is to use the beta radiation of the radiopharmaceutical to selectively destroy diseased tissue in which it resides. Thus, a minimum, sufficient dosage must be administered. In the case of I-131, the therapeutic dosage is between 5 to 10,000 times greater than the diagnostic dosage used to assess organ function. The major indications for radioiodine therapy include hyperthyroidism (e.g., diffuse toxic goiter [Graves' disease], toxic multinodular goiter) and eradication of metastatic disease (i.e., thyroid cancer).

A number of new areas of nuclear medicine are emerging, including the use of radiolabeled monoclonal antibodies (MoAbs) in the imaging and treatment of targeted cancer cells. In 1996, the FDA granted licenses to three manufacturers to market four radiolabeled antibodies for diagnostic imaging. For example, CEA-Scan is a murine MoAB fragment linked to technetium-99m. It is reactive with carcinoembryonic antigen, a tumor marker for cancer of the colon and rectum. It is indicated with other standard diagnostic modalities for the detection of recurrent and/or metastatic colorectal cancer.

Cytogen Corporation developed a linker payload systems with the attachment of diagnostic (OncoScint Colorectal/Ovarian) or therapeutic substances (cancer-cell-killing yttrium in OncoRad Ovarian and OncoRad Prostate systems) on the carbohydrate region of MoABs. After injection, the MoABs bind to the targeted tumor antigen to facilitate diagnosis or treatment. Peptides are being investigated to succeed antibodies as delivery vehicles for linked diagnostic or therapeutic agents. Peptides would have the advantage over MoABs of being more rapidly cleared from the body with a potentially lower level of toxicity.

Radiolabeled peptides are a new class of radiotracer that have the ability to "target" a cell or tissue and deliver a diagnostic signal or therapeutic agent to the site of the disease. Peptides are naturally occurring or synthetic compounds that contain one or more amino acid sequences or groups. Hormones are among the most common and important of the naturally occurring peptides. In addition to the pharmacokinetic advantage of using smaller molecules for targeting, peptides offer the added advantage of being able to provide physiological evidence of the nature of the disease process or progress of treatment, and may even be able to influence the course of the disease directly.

An example of this new class of radiopharmaceuticals is octreotide, a synthetic analog of the peptide hormone, somatostatin. A variety of cells, including those of the central and peripheral nervous system, the gastrointestinal and respiratory tracts, the kidneys, and activated platelets, lymphocytes, and other white blood cells have receptors for somatostatin. Certain tumors, most notably breast cancer, lymphomas, and neuroendocrine tumors, also express somatostatin receptors. In most cases, these tumors express these receptors more so than normal tissue.

A radiolabeled analog of somatostatin, octreotide, has been radiolabeled with ^{111}In-labeled analog pentetreotide. The resulting product, OctreoScan became the first radiolabeled peptide approved by the FDA. This agent has made possible the detection of small primary and metastatic tumors (i.e., 0.5 to 1.0 cm), including those of the several brain tumor types, pancreatic islet tumors, neuroblastomas, carcinoids, thymomas, and melanomas, among others.

Radiopharmaceuticals

There are over 40 official radioactive pharmaceuticals listed in the USP 23/NF 18 (6). Examples of some radiopharmaceuticals are presented in Table 17.1 (7). The following describes some of those radiopharmaceuticals frequently used in daily practice. Several of these radiopharmaceuticals are being used for the delivery of MoABs, biotechnological drugs. Thus, for a more in-depth understanding of these biotechnological drugs, including terminology, the reader is referred to Chapter 18 (i.e., Products of Biotechnology).

Technetium-99m (Tc-99m) possesses a relatively short half life of six hours and this allows the administration of higher amounts of activity for faster and clearer images while exposing the patient to a low radiation dose. It offers an abundance of gamma photons for imaging without the hazardous effects of beta particles. Also, its chemistry profile is flexible which allows it to be used as a binding agent for several pharmaceuticals that are used for imaging purposes. Thus, kits are available for the preparation of various technetium Tc-99m compounds that assist in hepatobiliary imaging (i.e., mebrofenin) and ischemic heart disease (i.e., sestamibi, tetrofosmin).

Technetium has also begun to become popular as a radiolabel for MoABs. This is so because of its wide availability in nuclear pharmacies and thus, is

Table 17.1 Representative Radiopharmaceutical Drugs, Inclusive of Trade Names When Appropriate, and Primary Uses

Radiopharmaceutical	Trade Name	Primary Use(s)
IN-111 Oxyquinoline	Indium Oxine	Radiolabel autologous leukocytes and platelets
I-123 sodium iodide	—	Thyroid imaging and uptake
I-131 sodium iodide	—	Thyroid imaging, uptake, and therapy
Tc-99m exametazime (HMPAO)	Ceretec	Cerebral perfusion, radiolabeling autologous leukocytes
Tc-99m Macroaggregated Albumin (MAA)	Pulmonite, Macrotec	Pulmonary perfusion
Tc-99m Mebrofenin	Choletec	Hepatobiliary imaging
Tc-99m Medronate (MDP)	—	Bone imaging
Tc-99m Mertiatide	Technescan MAG3	Renal imaging
Tc-99m Oxidronate (HDP)	Osteoscan HDP	Bone imaging
Tc-99m Pentetate (DTPA)	Techneplex, Technescan DTPA	Renal imaging and function studies; radioaerosol ventilation imaging
Tc-99m Pertechnetate	—	Imaging of thyroid, salivary glands, ectopic gastric mucosa, parathyroid glands, dacryocystography, cystography
Tc-99m Red Blood Cells (RBCs)	Ultratag	Imaging of gastrointestinal bleeding cardiac chambers, and cardiac first pass and gated equilibrium imaging.
Tc-99m Sestamibi	Cardiolite, Miraluma	Myocardial perfusion imaging and breast tumor imaging
Tc-99m Sulfur Colloid (SC)	—	Imaging of the reticuloendothelial (RES-liver/spleen) system, bone marrow, gastric emptying, gastrointestinal bleeding, lymphoscintigraphy, and arthrograms.
Tc-99m Tetrofosmin	Myoview	Myocaridal perfusion imaging
Thallium-201	—	Myocardial perfusion imaging; parathyroid and tumor imaging
Xenon-133	—	Pulmonary ventilation imaging

relatively inexpensive and easy to obtain. It provides low radiation dosimetry and highly efficient detection of photons by planar scintigraphy. Unfortunately, widespread use of this isotope in immunoscintigraphy has been hindered by the lack of a simple, efficient, and stable method for attaching the Tc-99m to the antibody molecule.

Verluma is a MoAB Fab fragment linked to technetium -99m. Verluma identifies advanced-stage disease in patients with small-cell lung cancer (SCLC). The determination of disease stage has important prognostic and therapeutic implications. Clinical trials to date have demonstrated that Verluma can accurately determine if a disease process is extensive or limited to an impressive degree (i.e., 82% of the time it is used). This drug product was approved for clinical use by the FDA in August, 1996.

Strontium-89 Chloride (Sr-89), available as Metastron, is a sterile, non-pyrogenic, aqueous solution for intravenous use and containing no preservative. It decays by beta emission with a physical half life of 51 days. This beta emission is very harmful to skeletal tissue, and thus, its clinical indication is reserved for bone pain palliation associated with primary bone tumors and metastatic involvement (i.e, blastic lesions). An advantage of its use is that it is retained and accumulated in significantly greater concentration in metastatic bone lesions much longer than in normal bone.

Following its intravenous administration, strontium compounds demonstrate similar characteristics to calcium analogs. They clear rapidly from the blood stream and selectively localize in bone mineral. The uptake by bone of strontium occurs preferentially in sites of osteogenesis imperfecta (e.g., a condition characterized by the formation of brittle bones prone to fractures). Thus, as mentioned, it finds utility with primary bone tumors and metastatic bone lesions.

Prior to administration a risk-to-benefit ratio must be determined due to Sr-89's bone marrow toxicity. It should be used with caution in patients with platelet counts below 60,000 and white cell counts below 2,400. After administration of Sr-89, weekly blood tests should be performed and the patient's status monitored. Because the average hematological recovery time is six months of treatment, a period of at least 90 days is required prior to retreatment.

A small percentage of patients receiving Sr-89 may report a transient increase in bone pain within 36 to 72 hours after injection. This is usually mild and self-limiting and controllable with analgesic therapy. Pain relief from the administration of Sr-89 will typically evidence itself within 7–20 days post-injection and a key benefit of its use is a decreased dependence on narcotics.

Thallous Chloride (Tl-201) is available as a sterile, non-pyrogenic solution for intravenous administration. It demonstrates a physical half life of 73.1 hours and decays by electron capture to mercury, Hg (201). Tl-201 is a potassium analog which undergoes rapid active transport into the myocardium. Thus, it is an advantageous agent to diagnose and visualize a myocardial infarction or ischemic heart disease.

When utilized in conjunction with exercise stress testing to help differentiate between ischemic and infarcted tissue, Tl-201 should be administered at the inception of a period of maximum stress which is sustained for 30 seconds after injection of the agent. Imaging then commences within ten minutes after administration to obtain maximum target-to-background ratios. If, however, the patient is unable to undergo a treadmill stress exercise because of physical limitation (e.g., pulmonary problems, orthopedic problems), pharmaceutical agents (e.g., Adenoscan, Persantine) may be utilized to induce cardiac stress.

Tl-201 undergoes fast redistribution in normal myocardium. In ischemic cardiac tissue, the uptake and washout of Tl-201 is not quick and is delayed due to decreased blood flow. If the image demonstrates no uptake, the tissue is classified as infarcted tissue.

Gallium Citrate (Ga-67) is available as a sterile, pyrogen-free, aqueous solution, with no carrier added. Chemically, this drug behaves similar to ferric ion (i.e., Fe^{+3}) and demonstrates a half life of 78 hours.

Ga-67 can localize in certain viable primary and metastatic tumors as well as focal sites of infection. Investigational studies demonstrate that perhaps Ga-67 accumulates in lysosomes and is bound to a soluble intracellular protein. Presently, Ga-67 may be useful in demonstrating the presence and extent of malignancies associated with Hodgkin's disease, lymphomas, and bronchogenic carcinoma. It can also be useful for localization of focal inflammatory lesions (e.g., granulomatous diseases [sarcoidosis], abscesses, pyelonephritis). It finds utility in the diagnosis and monitoring of *Pneumocystis carinii* pneumonia which occurs in acquired immunodeficiency syndrome (i.e, AIDS) and can be used as a diagnostic screening test in cases of prolonged fever, when physical examination, laboratory tests, and other imaging studies have not disclosed the source of the fever.

Concurrent use of ferric ion can increase Ga-67 renal excretion from the body. Although not firm on the exact mechanism, it is thought that elevated serum iron levels may displace Ga-67 from plasma-protein binding sites and hasten its excretion resulting in decreased tumor and abscess localization.

The optimal tumor-to-background concentration ratios are often obtained 48 hours post injection and delayed imaging is necessary to allow for the ideal target to tissue ratio. However, considerable biological variability can occur in individuals, acceptable imaging may be performed in as little as six hours post administration to as late as 120 hours after injection. The optimal tumor-to-background ratios also depend upon the location of the area of interest. For example, a lower abdominal scan can be hindered by Ga-67 fecal excretion. Thus, the use of laxatives facilitate faster scanning of the patient.

Indium Chloride (In-111) has become a popular isotope as a label for MoABs. The advantages of using ^{111}In for immunoscintigraphy are that it possesses a long half life that allows multiple images to be taken up to ten to 14 days after administration. In addition, its dual photon peaks provide superior planar and tomographic images. Because it lacks β-emission it can be administered in rather high doses. Lastly, unlike radioiodine complexes, ^{111}In-MoAb complexes are relatively stable in the body.

Myoscint is a murine MoAB Fab fragment linked to indium-111, and approved for clinical use by the FDA in July, 1996. This product binds with high affinity and specificity to human cardia myosin, which is exposed following a loss of integrity of the myocyte cell membrane. It functions as a cardiac imaging agent indicated for detecting the presence and location of myocardial injury in patients with suspected myocardial infarction. It is anticipated that Myoscint will be utilized in situations where electrocardiography and cardiac enzymes are non-diagnostic. Myoscint was approved for clinical use in July, 1996.

ProstaScint is a MoAB imaging agent linked to Indium-111. This drug seeks out and attaches itself to prostate cancer and its metastases. ProstaScint images can aid in the patient management by helping identify when the cancer has disseminated or spread (i.e., metastasized) from the prostate bed to regional lymph nodes or to distant soft tissues. This product was approved for use by the FDA in late 1996.

Sodium Iodide (I-123) is available as an oral capsule and is generally more preferable to sodium iodide (I-131) because of its lower patient radiation doses and better imaging properties. It is used diagnostically to evaluate thyroid function and mor-

phology. Sodium Iodide I-123 emits only gamma rays. In the euthyroid patient, 5 to 30% of the administered dose is concentrated in the thyroid gland at 24 hours and has an effective half life of 13 hours. The remaining administered activity is distributed within the extracellular fluid and has an effective half life of 8 hours.

Although it is more expensive than Tc-99m, because of its higher target-to-background ratio, I-123 produces a superior image. Also, it gives a lower radiation dose.

There are concurrently administered drugs that can decrease the thyroid uptake of sodium iodide I-123 for a variety of reasons, and it is recommended that these medications be withheld for a period of time prior to the administration of I-123. For example, corticosteroids should be withheld one week prior to I-123 administration. Benzodiazepines should be withheld up to 4 weeks prior to I-123 administration. Vitamins, expectorants, antitussives, and topical medications (e.g., clioquinol, Betadine) should be withheld between 2–4 weeks prior to the administration of I-123.

Sodium Iodide I-131 is available as a volatile solution that can be purchased through a manufacturer or compounded by the nuclear pharmacist into an oral capsule or solution dosage form. In small amounts, it is used for thyroid function studies or thyroid uptake tests by determining the fraction of administered radioiodine activity taken up by the thyroid gland. The thyroid uptake test is used in the diagnosis and confirmation of suspected hyperthyroidism and in calculating the activity to be administered for radioactive iodine therapy.

Typically, the diagnostic dose of I-131 is between 2 mCi to 5 mCi. The therapeutic dose is higher and usually ranges from 5 mCi to 200 mCi. The upper limit can be calculated to determine just how much radiation a particular patient can withstand. However, more than a 200 mCi dose is usually not given.

Sodium iodide I-131 is also indicated for the evaluation of size, thyroid nodules, carcinoma, masses in the lingual region, neck and mediastinum, and in the localization of functioning metastatic thyroid tumors. It finds utility in the pre- and post-operative evaluation of patients with thyroid carcinoma, and can be used to assess the therapeutic effects on these patients.

The beta emissions from the I-131 kill thyroid tissue, and in small amounts can be used for diagnostic thyroid imaging. It is not recommended for this use because of its relatively long half life (i.e, 8 days) and beta emission. However, if cost is a consideration, I-131 is used in lieu of I-123.

The time to radioactivity visualization is generally between 18 to 24 hours. However, imaging of functional thyroid metastases is generally performed at 24 to 96 hours to allow maximal uptake and minimal blood-pool retention.

Positron Emission Tomography

Positron Emission Tomography (PET) has been employed since the early 1970s to study cerebral physiology (8). Since that time there has been increased interest in using this cross-sectional physiological imaging modality in clinical medicine (8). At present, there are over 50 PET centers within the United States.

Positron emission tomography allows the physician to secure a patient image that is essentially a low-resolution "autoradiograph" showing the regional concentration of a positron-emitting nuclide inside the living body (9). It is a method for quantitative imaging of regional function and chemical reactions within various organs of the living human body. Imaging applications of PET have shown great use, for instance, in mapping regional blood flow (i.e., perfusion), mapping of regional blood volume, mapping of the rates of use of metabolic substrates, and mapping receptor-specific tracer binding.

The nature of the tracers used in PET imaging is that of natural biochemicals labeled with radionuclides of carbon, nitrogen, oxygen, and fluorine. This allows analysis in terms of physiology and biochemistry at a level of sophistication beyond that encountered in traditional nuclear medicine procedures. No other technology can image body chemistry with such sensitivity, so that the moment-to-moment change in concentration of a tracer in the blood or tissue can be determined in absolute units. Other imaging modalities, such as x-ray computed tomography (CT) and magnetic resonance imaging (MRI), provide predominantly anatomic information. CT scanning is based on the portrayal of the distribution of attenuation of x-rays passing through the body. MRI exploits the variation in regional concentrations of hydrogen and nuclear relaxation parameters to generate image contrast and to provide information about free water content, relative blood flow and the concentration of contrast agents.

Chemical changes occur prior to anatomic changes in most disease states, and PET offers the advantage of being capable to detect functional abnormalities before anatomic changes have occurred. Historically, PET evolved with its main focus on studies of the brain and heart, and today, that is where it has its greatest impact. However, it is emerging as a valued diagnostic tool for the diagnosis and therapy monitoring of patients with lymphoma, as a means to assess estrogen receptors in primary and metastatic breast cancers, and better identify resectable colorectal tumor recurrence. In epilepsy, PET and surface electroencephalography (EEG) are used in concert with clinical assessment of symptoms and signs to try to localize areas of the brain that are the foci of epileptic seizures when surgical intervention is the only remaining method to prevent the seizures.

As an example, tumors have more intermediary metabolism than normal tissue, and PET use is advantageous because of its ability to qualitatively and quantitatively study metabolism. Several processes, including glycolysis, increased membrane glucose transfer capability, and RNA, DNA, and protein synthesis are demonstrated and/or accelerated in tumors. The radiopharmaceutical most widely used for evaluating tumors with PET imaging is [^{18}F]-fluorodeoxyglucose because it has been demonstrated useful for tracing glucose metabolism, for detecting malignant tissue, and for quantifying changes in tumor glycolysis during and after treatment. ^{18}F-FDG has a 110 minute half life which is much easier to work with instead of a two minute half life.

When a radionuclide within the body decays by emission of a positron (a positively charged electron), that particle travels a very short distance (i.e., 1–4 mm) in body tissues or water before expending its 511 KeV kinetic energy and combining with an electron. Their interaction results in the simultaneous emission of two photons, each having a specific energy and emitted at an angle of exactly 180° from each other. Thus, if two scintillation detectors are placed, one on either side of the tissue in which the isotope is located, and detectors connected to a coincident circuit which provides an output only when a certain level of gamma ray radiation can be simultaneously detected by both, the result is a low background detector, highly specific for the particular isotope used and also giving excellent resolution.

Radionuclides that decay by PET generally have very short half-lives (e.g., ^{15}O;t$_{1/2}$ = 2.04 minutes) which permits administration of large doses of activity without subjecting the patient to excessive radiation exposure. The high count rates which result facilitate collection of statistically significant images in a very short time interval and a dynamic study of physiological processes that produce a quick fluctuation in tissue concentrations of the tracer. The short half lives also allow repeat image studies within a brief time interval with no confounding background activity from the prior injection.

It is optimal to label radiopharmaceuticals using radionuclides with the shortest half-life that is compatible with the time-scale of the physiological process to be studied. However, a practical consequence of using short-lived ($t_{1/2} < 1$ hour) radionuclides in diagnostic medicine is the necessity for the radionuclide production and radiotracer synthesis to occur within the hospital where the imagining procedure will be conducted. The major production of radionuclides around which PET imaging has been developed (i.e., ^{11}C, ^{13}N, ^{15}O, ^{18}F) are generally produced through in-house biomedical cyclotrons. For those tracers that have demonstrated great utility in PET imaging studies, robotic technique and automated systems have been created for routine radiopharmaceutical synthesis. These systems cannot, however, reduce the personnel needed to supply PET radiopharmaceuticals, but the automated systems encourage frequent syntheses using large amounts of activity to be performed without exposing the personnel to unnecessary/excessive radiation exposure.

PET is conducted primarily in large medical centers. Another consideration is that PET radionuclides have short half-lives (e.g., 2 to 20 minutes) which makes their availability from commercial sources almost nonexistent. By the time the nuclear pharmacist would receive the nuclide it would already be gone. Out of necessity the production facility must be on site and after rapid synthesis, the pharmaceutical needs to be purified. Thus, research continues to focus upon noncyclotron, e.g., radionuclide generators, sources of PET radionuclides that would allow PET technology in community-based nuclear medicine/pharmacy environments.

Parent/daughter generator systems are now being investigated as a possible, alternative mode to produce PET radionuclides. Potentially, it would free PET imaging from its current dependence upon cyclotron generation within a hospital. Also, this could have economic benefit and make PET a viable clinical diagnosis tool away from the hospital or large medical center. To date, however, very few positron emitters can be created by these systems, and only two radionuclides (i.e., rubidium-82, gallium-68) have been extensively reported on in the nuclear medicine literature.

Studies of new drug entities in the future will include pharmacokinetic determination using PET technology. Further, PET will allow the manufacturer actually to quantify how much of the drug reaches a specific drug receptor. Thus, comparative PET studies will shed light on which drug, for example, within a therapeutic category attains the most optimal distribution and concentration at the intended receptor site. It is also conceivable that PET technology will open new vistas for the interpretation of drug interactions, particularly where there is competition by two drugs for one receptor site.

Longer-lived PET isotopes such as ^{89}Zr ($t_{1/2} = 78.1$ hr), ^{76}Br ($t_{1/2} = 61.1$ hr), ^{124}I ($t_{1/2} = 4.15$ days), and ^{64}Cu ($t_{1/2} = 12.8$ hr) are being investigated as radiolabels for MoAB-based PET imaging. Early clinical research has demonstrated that these might be useful for detecting small metastases (<1.5 cm). In addition to cancer diagnosis, radiolabeled MoABs have been used to evaluate cardiovascular disorders. Clinical use of ^{111}In-antimyosin include detection of acute myocardial infarct, perioperative myocardial damage assessment, detection of acute myocarditis, diagnosis of rejection and management of patients after heart transplantation, and diagnosis of active rheumatic carditis, among others.

There are 12 radiopharmaceuticals for positron imaging that have monographs in the United States Pharmacopeia. Table 17.2 demonstrates PET radiopharmaceuticals used in common imaging procedures and the following section highlights a few of the more frequently used PET radiopharmaceuticals.

Carbon-11 Radiopharmaceuticals

Carbon-11 has been incorporated into a number of organic molecules (e.g., carboxylic acids, alcohols, glucose) for use in diagnostic imaging despite its relatively long half life (i.e., 20 minutes). Palmitic acid is the carboxylic acid used the most to date in PET imaging and as a tracer has found useful in the study of myocardial metabolism.

Randomly labeled ^{11}C-labeled glucose has been produced photosynthetically for use in studies of cerebral glucose metabolism. The use of ^{11}C-glucose for cerebral glucose metabolism requires an imaging procedure of less than five minutes duration after injection.

Nitrogen-13 Radiopharmaceuticals

Nitrogen-13 ammonia has been used as a tracer for cerebral and myocardial blood flow and demonstrates a half life of 10 minutes. It undergoes a relatively long extraction into these organs and exhibits prolonged retention as a major fraction of extractor tracer is metabolically incorporated into amino acids. Nitrogen-13 gas is superior to the radioactive noble gases to study pulmonary ventilation because of its lower solubility in blood.

Table 17.2   Positron-Emitting Radiopharmaceuticals Used in Common PET Imaging Procedures

Radiopharmaceutical	Application	Typical Dose/Procedure*
[^{15}O]-oxygen (O$_2$)	Cerebral oxygen extraction and metabolism	50–100 mCi
[^{15}O]-carbon monoxide (CO)	Cerebral blood volume	50–100 mCi
	Myocardial blood volume	50–100 mCi
[^{15}O]-water (H$_2$O)	Cerebral blood flow	80 mCi
	Myocardial blood flow	150 mCi
[^{13}N]-ammonia (NH$_3$)	Myocardial blood flow	15–25 mCi
[^{11}C]-acetate	Myocardial metabolism	30 mCi
[^{11}C]-N-methylspiperone	Dopamine receptor binding	20 mCi
[^{18}F]-fluorodeoxyglucose	Cerebral glucose metabolism	5–10 mCi
	Myocardial glucose metabolism	
	Tumor glucose metabolism	
[^{82}Rb]-Rb$^+$	Myocardial blood flow	10–40 mCi

*Note that many PET studies combine multiple PET imaging procedures (e.g., measurements of both blood flow and metabolism); the doses given here are typical of those actually used in each procedure of the study. For a single imaging procedure, an allowable dose (i.e., a dose that does not lead to excessive radiation exposure) may be significantly higher than these values.

Oxygen-15 Radiopharmaceuticals

Oxygen-15 is the radionuclide of oxygen with the longest half-life (i.e., 2.04 minutes). Because very little time is available for tracer synthesis, PET imagining studies employing oxygen-15 are restricted to use of a few relatively simple molecules.

Four oxygen-15 radiopharmaceuticals are available for clinical use. These are ^{15}O-oxygen gas (^{15}OO), ^{15}O-carbon monoxide (C^{15}O), ^{15}O-carbon dioxide CO^{15}O), and ^{15}O-water (H$_2$^{15}O) have been used in hemodynamic studies that take advantage of their short half life to allow administration of large doses of activity (up to 100 mCi) in imaging studies that can be repeated within 8–10 minutes with no carryover effect.

Labeled oxygen gas, i.e., ^{15}O-oxygen gas (^{15}OO), for example, can be used directly in studies of oxygen metabolism or can be converted to carbon monoxide (CO), carbon dioxide (CO$_2$) or water. ^{15}O-carbon-monoxide can be safely administered via inhalation and serves as a tracer for RBC volume upon binding of the C^{15}O to hemoglobin.

Oxygen-15 labeled water can be used in equilibrium studies of tissue water content and finds its greatest use as a tracer for regional blood flow. Commonly used as a tracer in PET evaluation of cerebral and myocardial perfusion, its two minute half life outweighs its limitation of ability to freely diffuse across the blood-brain barrier at high flow rates.

Fluorine-18 Radiopharmaceuticals

Fluorine-18 demonstrates a prolonged half-life of 110 minutes. Compared to other, shorter half-life

radiopharmaceuticals this presents several distinct advantages for radiopharmaceutical synthesis and allows delivery of the radionuclide to imaging centers located a distance for the generating cyclotron.

Fluorine-18 also demonstrates specific activity that makes it attractive for use as a receptor-specific tracer binding. Its major use remains in imaging of cerebral, myocardial, and tumor metabolism with ^{18}F-2-fluorodeoxyglucose (FDG). In brain-imaging procedures, FDG maps normal brain metabolic activity. In cardiac studies, its use is to identify ischemic regions in which glucose metabolism increases as a consequence of decreased fatty acid metabolism. As mentioned earlier, glucose metabolism increases in tumor tissue, and FDG localization in that tissue is extremely helpful in the imaging study (10).

Gallium-68 Radiopharmaceuticals

Gallium-68 is rapidly bound by the iron-binding sites of transferrin following the intravenous injection of ^{68}Ga-citrate and is very useful in studies of regional plasma volume. When combined with a [^{15}O]-carbon monoxide measurement of regional blood cell volume, the ^{68}Ga-transferrin PET study allows calculation of the regional hematocrit. ^{68}Ga-transferrin has also been employed in pulmonary studies of vascular permeability.

Nonradioactive Pharmaceutical use in Nuclear Medicine

The advantage of radiopharmaceutical imaging is that it is a non-invasive modality in the diagnosis and work-up of a disease. Generally, radiopharmaceuticals used diagnostically help to monitor a physiological process without altering it. Sometimes, however, the information gained from the procedure is inadequate to address the clinical question(s). Thus, to overcome this deficiency, interventional pharmaceutical drugs are utilized to complement the administration of the radiopharmaceutical (11).

These interventional pharmaceutical drugs effect alterations within the physiological process being studied through the use of radiopharmaceuticals. And, when used in conjunction with the nuclear medicine procedure, the amount of information gained is greatly improved. This pharmacological intervention helps to facilitate increased information acquisition about the physiological process under study, and may increase the specificity and sensitivity of the procedure, or decrease the time frame of the imaging process.

Acetazolamide (i.e., Diamox), an agent used to treat glaucoma through its diuretic action has been shown to increase cerebral blood flow following its IV administration. On an average basis, it can increase cerebral blood flow $23\% \pm 8\%$ in normal vessels. Thus, its use in cerebral perfusion studies is to enhance the differentiation between normal vessels and diseased vessels which cannot easily dilate. Thus, it is indicated for use in patients with transient ischemic attack, carotid artery disease, or a cerebrovascular accident to help identify areas of the brain that are at risk for an infarct. The drug also is used in other neurological conditions (e.g., Alzheimer's disease, multi-infarct dementia) where cerebral perfusion is far from optimal.

Captopril (i.e., Capoten) intervention is used to help diagnose renovascular hypertension in hypertensive patients with abdominal bruits, declining renal function, and poorly controlled hypertension with drug therapy. As an angiotensin-converting enzyme (ACE) inhibitor, this drug blocks the conversion of angiotensin I to angiotensin II and prevents vasoconstriction of the efferent arterioles of the kidney. This results in a decreased glomerular filtration pressure in the affected kidney.

Within the pediatric population, Meckel's diverticulum, a congenital anomaly of the gastrointestinal tract presents itself in about a quarter of the cases as rectal bleeding and abdominal pain. This diverticulum is an abnormal remnant of the developing gastrointestinal tract which contains gastric mucosa that bleeds abnormally. This gastric mucosa concentrates ^{99m}Tc-pertechnetate as normal mucosa and cimetidine (i.e., Tagamet) demonstrates usefulness in Meckel's diverticulum imaging by virtue of its action as a histamine-H_2 receptor antagonist. Cimetidine

effects a reduction in the volume and concentration of stomach acid produced by the stomach, and following its administration in a Meckel's study, the cells of the gastric mucosa continue to accumulate ^{99m}Tc-pertechnetate, but their secretion of acid into the gastric lumen is reduced or prevented. This allows for continual ^{99m}Tc-pertechnetate accumulation in the gastric mucosa with little transit through the intestinal tract. This results in an enhanced ability to visualize the small area of ectopic gastric mucosa.

Dipyridamole (i.e, Persantine) is used as an alternative to a treadmill stress test prior to cardiac imaging. Typically, patients who are candidates to receive this intervention (i.e, pharmaceutical stress) as part of the imaging procedure rather than perform the stress test are those with cardiac, respiratory, and/or orthopedic problems, those maintained on beta-blocker or calcium-channel blocker medications, and/or those with poor motivation. Dipyridamole blocks adenosine deaminase, the enzyme responsible for the degradation of adenosine, a potent coronary vasodilator which is capable of increasing coronary blood flow up to four to five times that at rest. Blood flow through stenosed arteries will be less compared to normal.

Adenosine (i.e., Adenocard) is an ideal agent to use in combination with myocardial perfusion imaging agents. It possesses an ultrashort half-life (i.e., <10 seconds) while demonstrating potency as a coronary vasodilator. This drug can increase coronary blood flow four to five times that of rest and can be beneficial as a pharmaceutical stress agent to help diagnose and identify stenosed arteries.

In preparation for the use of adenosine or dipyridamole, theophylline- and caffeine-containing drugs, beverages, etc., must be discontinued and the patient is on *npo* status overnight. An advantage of adenosine use over dipyridamole is that adverse effects caused by adenosine (e.g., chest pain, pain in the throat, jaw, or arm, headache, flushing and dyspnea) generally disappear within one to two minutes after discontinuation of the infusion. Dipyridamole has a longer half life (i.e., 15–30 minutes) with a peak effect of 2–3 minutes after infusion. When this agent is used, chest pain, headache, and dizziness occur most often.

For adenosine and dipyridamole, aminophylline can be given intravenously to reverse their effects, if necessary. Nitroglycerin can be given to relieve the chest pain experienced after dipyridamole administration.

Furosemide (i.e., Lasix), a loop diuretic is administered to help confirm or rule out mechanical renal obstruction during renal scintigraphy when there is a significant retention of radioactivity noted in the renal pelvis. It inhibits the reabsorption of electrolytes, most notably sodium, in the ascending limb of the loop of Henle, as well as in the proximal and distal tubules. In an obstructed kidney, furosemide diuresis will have little effect on the clearance of the radioactivity retained in the kidney. A non-obstructed kidney will rapidly clear the radioactivity into the bladder following furosemide's administration, and the renograms produced over the test will show a rapid emptying with a steeply declining radioactivity curve.

The Schilling's Test is utilized to determine a patient's capability to absorb radioactive vitamin B-12 from the intestine. Normally, vitamin B-12 is released from food sources (e.g., meat, eggs, milk) and bound to intrinsic factor in the stomach. Ultimately, in the ileum this intrinsic factor-vitamin B-12 complex is absorbed and then stored in the liver. Once the storage capacity of the liver for this complex is exceeded, Vitamin B-12 is excreted in urine. In cases of Vitamin B-12 deficiency, it is crucial that the cause of the deficiency be determined, that is either a lack of a proper diet or due to inadequate absorption. For the procedure, one mg of nonradioactive vitamin B-12 is given IM two hours before the ^{57}Co-labeled vitamin B-12 is administered. This large dose is intended to saturate the storage sites and helps flush absorbed radiolabeled B-12 into the urine. Thus, the excreted radioactivity demonstrates the amount absorbed. If the excretion is ≤5%, this is diagnostic of B-12 malabsorption. Typically, urinary excretion of B-12 ranges between 15 to 40%.

Practice of Nuclear Pharmacy

There are several activities that typify the provision of nuclear pharmacy services. Determined by task analyses, these serve as the basic underpinning for the American Pharmaceutical Association's Nuclear Pharmacy Practice Guidelines (12). A listing of tasks with related knowledge statements for each activity aid to further delineate and interpret the practice of nuclear pharmacy.

Nuclear pharmacy is a patient-oriented service that embodies the scientific knowledge and professional judgment required to improve and promote health through the assurance of the safe and efficacious use of radioactive drugs for diagnosis and therapy. The pharmacist is expected to understand nuclear medicine procedures, their advantages and disadvantages, when used for diagnostic or therapeutic purposes (7, 13).

Typically, nuclear pharmacy practice occurs primarily in two settings, either within a clinic or within a commercial, centralized operation. With practice site differences, activities might not be all inclusive at each site. The nine general activities encompassing nuclear pharmacy practice are: procurement, compounding, quality assurance, dispensing, distribution, health and safety, provision of drug information and consultation, monitoring patient outcome, and research and development.

Procurement and Storage

Nuclear pharmacists are responsible to secure radiopharmaceuticals, other appropriate drugs, supplies, and materials necessary to effect appropriate outcomes. For example, the effectiveness of some diagnostic radiopharmaceuticals is enhanced or toxicity lessened by the co-administration of other drugs. For example, some patients (e.g., elderly, obese, those with orthopedic problems) might not be capable to undergo an exercise stress test prior to the administration of a radiopharmaceutical intended to visualize cardiac perfusion. Thus, dipyridamole, as mentioned earlier in this chapter, a vasodilator can be used pharmacologically as a substitute for the exercise stress test.

The short half lives of radiopharmaceuticals poses a special problem to the pharmacist in that the traditional pathways (e.g., drug wholesaler) to secure the drug might take longer than the lifetime of the drug. So, typically, the nuclear pharmacist will order the drug directly from the manufacturer, usually through overnight delivery. In addition, knowledge of calibration time, shipping/delivery schedules, and radioactive decay associated with the ordered radiopharmaceutical weigh heavily in the ordering process. Limited quantities of certain radiopharmaceuticals by manufacturers also plays a vital role in the attempt to obtain products.

Isotope storage areas, a laboratory for the manipulation and the preparation of the radiopharmaceutical dosage forms, a counting area for calibration of doses, and a treatment room are among the facilities necessary for this type of practice. In some hospitals, radiopharmaceuticals are dispensed by a knowledgeable hospital pharmacist skilled in working with radiopharmaceuticals. In the selection of a counting area in a hospital pharmacy practice, the location of X-ray equipment and other radiation sources must be considered to avoid the background in counting area be erratic or excessively high. With the advent of precalibrated dosage forms for a significant number of radiopharmaceuticals, elaborate facilities are not required for many diagnostic procedures.

Preparation of the Radiopharmaceutical

Compounding of the radiopharmaceutical can be a simple task (e.g., reconstituting reagent kits with Tc-99m sodium pertechnetate) to very complex tasks (e.g., operating a cyclotron). Aside from the typical compounding procedures with a normal prescription (e.g., receipt of order, validation, safety of dose, supplies/equipment to prepare), the preparation of a radiopharmaceutical is confounded by issues of radioactivity and chemical reactions.

The compounding of a radiopharmaceutical involves chemical reactions to label a molecule with a radionuclide. For most of Tc-99m labeled compounds, stannous chloride is used to reduce Tc(VII) pertechnetate to a lower oxidation state. This then is followed by chelation of the technetium atoms by multidentate ligands. For other radiopharmaceuticals, covalent bonding, transchelation, and coordination complexation reactions are utilized.

Expense, limited availability and shipping schedules dictate that radiopharmaceuticals be created on site using a cyclotron, particularly to PET. Because of this necessary path of preparation, these are usually more expensive than those purchased directly from the manufacturer. A significant number of radiopharmaceuticals use Tc-99m (in the form of sodium pertechnetate and sodium chloride [for isotonicity]). Tc-99m is formed by decay of molybdenum 99, a radioactive isotope of molybdenum obtained by neutron bombardment of molybdenum 98. Commonly, a generator or "cow" containing ^{99}Mo (half-life, 67 hours), produces the sodium pertechnetate Tc-99m at a rate that permits daily elutions of the generator. Other cylcotron-produced radiopharmaceuticals may be ordered for the next day (e.g., In-111, I-123, Tl-201)

A significant majority of radiopharmaceuticals are produced for parenteral administration. Thus, aseptic technique and methods must be maintained during the preparation of the radiopharmaceutical and when radiolabelling biological products (e.g., MoABs, peptides). Further, strict adherence to "universal precautions" and appropriate infection control handling are a necessity when radiolabelling patient blood cells from patients who are afflicted with blood borne pathogenic material (e.g., HIV, hepatitis).

Quality Assurance

To ensure the safe use of radiopharmaceuticals in patients, the pharmacist must carry out appropriate tests (e.g., chemical, physical, biological). USP Monographs dictate that radiopharmaceuticals meet specifications delineated including, radionuclide purity, radiochemical purity, chemical purity, pH, particle size, sterility, pyrogenicity (or bacterial endotoxin), and specific activity. When the pharmacist utilizes an already prepared and manufactured radionuclide these are assured by the manufacturer (e.g., Tl–201, I–123, I–131).

Radionuclide purity is the proportion of activity present as the stated nuclide. It can be measured by gamma-ray spectroscopy, half-life measurement and/or other physical measurements which help to detect the presence of extraneous nuclides. Examples of the lack of radionuclide purity are ^{198}Au contaminated with ^{199}Au or ^{99m}Tc contaminated with ^{99}Mo.

Radiochemical purity is the fraction of the stated radionuclide present in the stated chemical form. If there are nonradioactive contaminants, the radioactive drug may be radiochemically pure, but not chemically pure. Similarly, if there are small amounts of radioactive contaminants, the material may be chemically pure, but not radiochemically pure. Column or thin-layer chromatography are useful for purity determination.

Dispensing of a Radiopharmaceutical

A distinct difference with radiopharmaceutical dispensing compared to the traditional mode with which ordinary prescriptions are dispensed is that these never go directly to the patient. Rather they are provided to trained health care professionals at the hospital or the clinic and then administered to the patient. Also, because of the nature of the product, radiopharmaceuticals typically are dispensed in unit doses.

At the time the radiopharmaceutical is ordered, the dispensing pharmacist must ensure that the ordered dosage is safe for the patient. Thus, patient factors such as age, weight, surface area, and gamma camera sensitivity must be weighed and considered by the pharmacist with each order. Typically, too, prescriptions are ordered and shipped. Thus, radioactive decay considerations must be made to accommodate from when the radiopharmaceutical was prepared to the time it is ultimately administered to the patient. Because the product is a radiopharmaceutical, it is subject to special labelling requirements (e.g., Standard Radiation Symbol, "Caution—Radioactive Material"). Also, because the radiopharmaceutical is typically prepared as a parenteral dosage form precaution toward aseptic technique is a necessity.

Table 17.3   Concurrent Administered Drugs Known to Interfere with Tumor and Abscess Localization Scintigraphy

Interfering Drug	Effect on Image
Phenytoin	Localization of RP in the mediastinum & pulmonary hilar structures (in patients without clinical evidence of lymphadenopathy)
Amiodarone; Bleomycin; Busulfan; Nitrofurantoin; Bacillus Calmette-Guerin; Chemotherapy; Lymphangiographic Contrast Media; Addictive Drugs of Abuse	Diffuse pulmonary localization (sometimes local pulmonary uptake)
Metoclopramide; Reserpine; Phenothiazines; Oral Contraceptives; Diethylstilbesterol	Localization of RP in breast
Methotrexate; Cisplatin; Gallium Nitrate; Mechlorethamine HCl; Vincristine; Various Chemotherapeutic Agents; Iron	a) Increased skeletal uptake b) Increased renal elimination c) Decreased hepatic accumulation d) Decreased tumor or abscess uptake
Antibiotics (Clindamycin)	Localization of RP in bowel
Calcium Gluconate; IM injections	Soft tissue accumulation of RP
Ampicillin; Sulfonamides; Sulfinpyrazone; Ibuprofen; Cephalosporins; Hydrochlorothiazide; Methicillin; Erythromycin; Rifampin; Pentamidine; Phenylbutazone; Gold Salts; Allopurinol; Furosemide; Phenazone; Phenobarbital; Phenytoin; Phenindione	Increased accumulation of RP in the kidneys
Chemotherapeutic Agents; Antibiotics	Localization of RP in the Thymus

Distribution of Radiopharmaceuticals

Institutional procedures and policies dictate how a radiopharmaceutical is distributed within a health care facility. Generally, a lead-lined syringe container shipped in approved cases are used with appropriate identifying information. Local, state (e.g., State Board of Pharmacy), and federal (e.g., Department of Transportation, Nuclear Regulatory Commission) regulations are relevant when a radiopharmaceutical is distributed from a centralized nuclear pharmacy facility to another institution. Generally, these requirements relate to packaging, labelling, shipping papers, record-keeping, shipper and carrier licensing, and personnel training.

Health and Safety

The Nuclear Regulatory Commission establishes and enforces radiation safety standards (e.g., limits for radiation doses, levels of radiation in an area, concentrations of radioactivity in air and waste water, waste disposal, precautionary procedures) for the radiopharmaceutical compounding facility. Beyond the radiopharmaceuticals, related aspects of health and safety are a necessity. Hazardous chemicals (e.g., chromatography solvents) must be stored appropriately, handled safely, and disposed of using proper technique. Attention must also be paid toward the use of personal protective devices, containers, and to the physical environment in which the radiopharmaceuticals are prepared.

Table 17.4   Miscellaneous Brain Imaging Radiopharmaceuticals

Interfering Drug	Effect on Image
Cancer chemotherapeutic agents	Patchy increased uptake of RP as a result of chemoneurotoxicity
Corticosteroids	Decreased uptake into brain lesions
Psychotropic Drugs	Rapid accumulation of RP in nasopharyngeal area during arterial or capillary phase (cerebral radionuclide angiography)

Table 17.5   Concurrent Administered Drugs Known to Interfere with Myocardial Perfusion Scintigraphy

Interfering Drug	Effect on Image
Beta Blockers; Nitrates; and Calcium Channel Blockers	Decreases the number and size of exercise-induced Tl–201perfusion defects
Vasopressin	Appearance of myocardial defects in patients without coronary artery disease
Propanolol; Cardiac Glycosides; Procainamide; Lidocaine; Phenytoin; Doxorubicin	Decreased myocardial localization and increased liver localization

Provision of Drug Information and Consultation

It is very important that the nuclear pharmacist possess oral and written communications skills. His/her knowledge and expertise is only useful when it can be conveyed to an allied health professional, the patient, and the patient's care giver, among others. The nuclear pharmacist must be capable to answer inquiries and know where to find requested information.

The type of information provided can include, among others, the biological effects of radiation, radiation physics and radiation protection, radiopharmaceutical chemistry, radiopharmaceutical compounding and quality assurance, radiopharmaceutical products, diagnostic and therapeutic applications of radiopharmaceuticals, ancillary medications used to enhance radiopharmaceutical procedures, drug interactions associated with radiopharmaceuticals (Tables 17.3, 17.4, 17.5, 17.6), precautions associated with the use of radiopharmaceuticals[3], and regulatory requirements affecting the use of radiopharmaceuticals. This information can be used for educational purposes (e.g., allied health professionals, consumer groups), of organizational value (e.g., policies and procedures), and for diagnostic or therapeutic value in the pharmaceutical care patients.

Monitoring Patient Outcome

Patient safety and optimal patient outcomes are the goal of the nuclear pharmacist and a central tenet within pharmaceutical care. And, in that regard the nuclear pharmacist can be very instrumental in the contribution toward quality patient care through his/her activities. For example, the nuclear pharmacist can, among others:

- Develop institutional standards for the rationale and appropriate use of radiopharmaceuticals,
- Prospectively screen and review patient data to assure appropriate use of radiopharmaceuticals and ancillary medicines used to enhance their effect,
- Ensure that patients are selected appropriately for radionuclide therapy and monitored after therapy to prevent complications and/or intervene with necessary therapy(ies),
- Evaluate the safety and effectiveness of radiopharmaceuticals and ancillary medications,
- Ensure proper preparation of patients prior to the administration of the radiopharmaceutical and ancillary medications,
- Prevent, minimize, and/or rectify clinical problems associated with the use of radiopharmaceuticals and ancillary medications,
- Monitor patients for potential adverse effects following administration of a radiopharmaceutical or interventional medication,
- Discontinue potentially interfering medications before the nuclear medicine study, restarting them after the study, and appropriately managing the patient during their discontinuance,
- Ensure that patients with special needs, problems, or conditions (e.g., pregnancy, nursing mothers, dialysis patients, pediatric patients, geriatric patients) are given appropriate consid-

Table 17.6   Miscellaneous Renal Function Assessing Radiopharmaceuticals

Interfering Drug	Effect on Image
Iodinated Contrast Agents; Aminoglycosides	Decrease in effective plasma flow values; Decreased glomerular filtration rate
Cyclosporine; Cisplatin	Decreased urinary excretion; Decreased tubular function
Furosemide	Misleading renogram and flow curves resulting in false positive/negative studies
Probenecid	Decreased renal accumulation and accumulation

eration before, during, and after radiopharmaceutical administration,

- Ensure that information gained from the nuclear medicine procedure is considered during the development of the patient's therapeutic plan, and
- Perform and enhance the effectiveness of nuclear pharmacy procedures, including the administration of therapeutic or diagnostic radiopharmaceuticals and ancillary medications to the patient.

An example of a nuclear pharmacist intervention relates to the use of radiopharmaceuticals in a breast-feeding woman. Specifically, recommendations are made for the interruption of breastfeeding in patients who are undergoing a nuclear medicine diagnostic procedure. The nuclear pharmacist should review the patient data, especially if the woman is of childbearing age. These recommendations include the following:

- Breastfeeding should be noted in the patient history from the attending physician,
- A member of the interdisciplinary team should inquire about the patient's breastfeeding status and notify the nuclear physician when a patient is breastfeeding,
- Breastfeeding should be interrupted for the time radioactivity is known to appear in the breast milk, and
- Close contact with an infant should be restricted to 5 hours within 24 hours of the procedure for Tc-99m MIBI, Tc-99m labeled RBCs and I-131 (>3mCi) whether or not the mother is breastfeeding (14).

Indirectly, the nuclear pharmacist can provide clinical services that include consultation with other care givers (e.g., explain a nuclear medicine study), prepare institutional guidelines for the use of radiopharmaceuticals and ancillary medications, provide information and literature reviews related to specific questions or studies, formulate special drugs and/or dosage forms, and conduct drug use evaluation studies or drug use review (i.e., DUE, DUR).

References

1. Nickel RA. Radiopharmaceuticals. In: Early PJ, Sodee DB, eds. Principles and Practice of Nuclear Medicine. 2nd Edition. St. Louis, MO: Mosby, 1995 pp 94–117.
2. Newsline. Future of nuclear medicine, part 1: marketing research forecasts. J Nucl Med 1998;39(2):27N-33N.
3. Silberstein EB, Ryan J, the Pharmacopeia Committee of the Society of Nuclear Medicine. Prevalence of adverse reactions in nuclear medicine. J Nucl Med 1996;37(1):185–192.
4. Early PJ. Methods of radioactive decay. In: Early PJ, Sodee DB, eds. Principles and Practice of Nuclear Medicine, 2nd Edition. St. Louis, MO: Mosby, 1995 pp 23–49.
5. Shaw SM. Diagnostic imaging and pharmaceutical care. Am J Pharm Ed 1994;58: 190–193.
6. United States Pharmacopeia 23/The National Formulary 18, United States Pharmacopeial Convention, Inc., Rockville, MD, 1995, p. 2372.
7. Shaw SM. Nuclear pharmacy and radiopharmaceuticals. Hosp Pharm Times 1995;5HPT-15HPT.
8. Hoffman JM, Hanson MW, Coleman RE. Clinical positron emission tomography imaging. Radiol Clin North Am 1993;31(4):935–959.
9. Green MA, Welch MJ. Radiopharmaceuticals for positron emission tomography (PET). In: Early PJ, Sodee DB, eds. Principles and Practice of Nuclear Medicine, 2nd Edition. St. Louis, MO: Mosby, 1995 pp 739–751.
10. Romer W, Schwaiger M. Positron emission tomography in diagnosis and therapy monitoring of patients with lymphoma. Clinical Positron Imaging 1998;1 (2):101–110.
11. Park H-M, Duncan K. Nonradioactive pharmaceuticals in nuclear medicine. J Nucl Med Technol 1994;22 (4):240–248.
12. Nuclear Pharmacy Practice Guidelines, Section of Nuclear Pharmacy, American Pharmaceutical Association, Washington, DC, 1994.
13. Rhodes BA, Hladik WB III, Norenberg JP. Clinical radiopharmacy: principles and practices. Semin Nucl Med 1996;26(2):77–84.
14. Harding LK, Bossuyt A, Pellet S, Talbot JN. Recommendations for nuclear pharmacy physicians regarding breastfeeding mothers. Euro J Nucl Med 1995;22: BP17.

18

PRODUCTS OF BIOTECHNOLOGY

Chapter at a Glance

THE TERM *biotechnology* encompasses any technique that uses living organisms (e.g., microorganisms) in the production or modification of products. Historically, the classic definition of biotechnological drugs was that of proteins obtained from recombinant DNA technology. However, there is now a broader definition that encompasses the use of tissue culture, living cells, or cell enzymes to make a defined product. Foremost, recombinant DNA (rDNA) and monoclonal antibody (MAb) technologies are providing exciting opportunities for new pharmaceuticals development and new approaches to the diagnosis, treatment, and prevention of disease.

It is estimated that by the year 2000 biotechnological products will have a marked impact upon the practice of pharmacy (1). Research will continue to generate potent new medications that require custom dosing for the individual patient and concomitant pharmacist expertise in the use of, and familiarity with, sophisticated drug delivery systems.

The revolution in biotechnology is a result of research advancement in intracellular chemistry, molecular biology, recombinant DNA technology, genetics, and immunopharmacology. The first of these novel pharmaceuticals have been proteins, but eventually an increasing number will be smaller molecules, discovered through biotechnological based methods that will determine just how proteins work. Clearly biotechnology has established itself as a mainstay in pharmaceuticals research and development, and new products will enter the market at an increasing pace during the next decade of the new millennium.

The transition toward molecular medicine has already begun. As biotechnology advances, and growing numbers of cancer-related genes are identified and cloned, it is predicted that therapy with biotechnology products will eventually supplant chemotherapy as the first-line treatment for many malignancies. At the time of this writing, more than 100 gene-therapy trials are in progress, and conjugate molecules, genetically engineered for specific toxicity to cancer cells, are also entering clinical trials.

Growth in biotechnology products (including agricultural, diagnostic, environmental, and pharmaceutical products) was predicted to increase tenfold between the early 1990s and 2000. A total of 54 biotechnological-derived medications have been approved since human insulin, in 1982, became the first therapeutic recombinant protein drug. The commercial success of biotechnology has spurred the entry of many additional products into the development pipelines. Currently, 350 biotechnolog-

ical drugs are in various stages of development by over 140 pharmaceutical and biotechnological companies (2). It is anticipated that patients with hemophilia, serious sepsis infection, skin ulcers, rheumatoid arthritis, and a number of cancers will benefit over the next several years as drugs in clinical trials secure market approval. This abundant activity has grown out of entrepreneurism among many small, venture-funded, narrowly focused groups. Several of these small companies have by now prospered to the point of becoming fully integrated pharmaceutical companies. More than one-third of biotechnological drugs currently in clinical trials are being tested for the treatment of cancer, while 29 products are under development for HIV infection, AIDS, and AIDS-related diseases. Nineteen other biotechnological drugs are in development for autoimmune diseases (e.g., rheumatoid arthritis, lupus erythematosus).

Techniques Utilized to Produce Biotechnological Products

There are numerous techniques that are utilized to create biotechnological products. These include recombinant DNA technology, monoclonal antibody technology, polymerase chain reaction, gene therapy, nucleotide blockade or antisense nucleic acids, and peptide technology (3). The following section describes each of these techniques.

Recombinant DNA (rDNA)

DNA, deoxyribonucleic acid, has been called "the substance of life." It is DNA that constitutes genes, allowing cells to reproduce and maintain life. Of over 1 million kinds of plants and animals known today, no two are exactly alike; however, the similarity within families is the result of genetic information stored in cells, duplicated, and passed from cell to cell and from generation to generation. It is DNA that provides this continuity.

DNA was first isolated in 1869. Its chemical composition was determined in the early 1900s, and by the 1940s it had been proven that the genes within cell chromosomes are made of DNA. It was not until the 1950s, when James D. Watson and Francis H. C. Crick postulated the structure of DNA, that biologists began to comprehend the molecular mechanisms of heredity and cell regulation. Watson and Crick described their model of DNA as a double helix, two strands of DNA coiled about itself like a spiral staircase. It is now known that the two strands of DNA are connected by the bases adenine, guanine, cytosine, and thymine (A, G, C, and T). The order of arrangement of these bases with the two strands of DNA comprise a specific gene for a specific trait. A typical gene has hundreds of bases that are always arranged in pairs. When A occurs on one strand, T occurs opposite it on the other; G pairs with C. A gene is a segment of DNA that has a specific sequence of these chemical base pairs. The pattern constitutes the DNA message for maintaining cells and organisms and building the next generation. To create a new cell, or a whole new organism, DNA must be able to duplicate ("clone") itself. This is done through the unwinding and separation of the two strands and the subsequent attachment to each of new bases from within the cell according to the A-T/C-G rule. The result is two new double strands of DNA, each of the same structure and conformation.

DNA also plays an essential role in the production of proteins needed for cellular maintenance and function. DNA is translated to messenger RNA (ribonucleic acid), which contains instructions for the production of the 23 amino acids from which all proteins are made. Amino acids can be arranged in a vast number of combinations to produce hundreds of thousands of different proteins. In essence, a cell is a miniature assembly plant for the production of thousands of proteins. A single *Escherichia coli* bacterium is capable of making about 2000 proteins.

The ability to selectively hydrolyze a population of DNA molecules with a number of endonucleases promoted a technique for joining two different DNA molecules termed *recombinant DNA*. This technique utilizes other techniques (i.e., replication, separation, identification) that permits the production of large quantities of purified DNA fragments. These combined techniques, referred to as *recombinant DNA technology,* allow the removal of a specific piece of DNA out of a larger, more complex molecule. Consequently, recombinant DNAs have been prepared with DNA fragments from bacteria combined with fragments from humans, viruses with viruses, and so forth. The ability to join to different pieces of DNA together at specific sites within the molecules is achieved with two enzymes, a restriction endonuclease and a DNA ligase.

Through the process of recombinant DNA technology, scientists can utilize nonhuman cells (as a special strain of *E. coli*) to manufacture proteins identical to those produced in human cells. This process has enabled scientists to produce molecules naturally present in the human body in large quantities previously difficult to obtain from human sources. For example, approximately 50

cadaver pituitary glands were required to treat a single growth hormone-deficient child for one year until DNA-produced growth hormone became available through the new technology. Further, the biosynthetic product is more free of viral contamination than the previous cadaver source of the hormone. Human growth hormone and insulin were the first recombinant DNA products to become available for patient use.

DNA probe technology is a tool being utilized to diagnose disease. It utilizes small pieces of DNA to search a cell for viral infection or for genetic defects. DNA probes have application in testing for infectious disease, cancer, genetic defects, and disease susceptibility. Using DNA probes, scientists have acquired the capability of locating a disease-causing gene, which in turn can lead to the development of replacement therapies. In producing a DNA probe, the initial step involves the synthesis of the specific strand of DNA with the sequence of nucleotides that matches those of the gene being investigated. For instance, to test for a particular virus, first the DNA strand is developed to be identical to one in the virus. The second step is to tag the synthetic gene with a dye or radioactive isotope. When introduced into a specimen, the synthetic strand of DNA acts as a probe, searching for a matching or complementary strand. When located, the two hybridize, or join together. When the probe is bound to the virus, the dye reveals the location of the viral gene. If a radionuclide isotope was employed on the synthetic DNA strand, it will bind to the viral strand of DNA, and then reveal the virus through gamma-ray technology.

Monoclonal Antibodies

When a "foreign" body or antigen molecule enters the body, an immune response is initiated. This molecule may contain several different antigenic determinants and lines of β-lymphocytes will proliferate, each secreting an immunoglobulin (i.e., an antibody) molecule that fits a single antigenic determinant or part of it.

In contrast, monoclonal antibodies are produced as a result of perpetuating the expression of a single β-lymphocyte. Consequently, all the antibody molecules secreted by a series of daughter cells derived from a single, dividing parent β-lymphocyte are genetically identical. Through the development of hybridoma technology emanating from Kohler and Milstein's research (4), it became possible to produce identical, monospecific antibodies in almost unlimited quantities. These are constructed by the fusion of β-lymphocytes, stimulated with a specific antigen, with immortal myeloma cells (5). The resultant hybridomas can then be maintained in cultures and are capable of producing large amounts of antibodies. From these hybrid cells, a specific cell line or clone producing monospecific immunoglobulins can be selected.

A significant number of currently used antibodies belong to the immunoglobulin F (i.e., IgG) subclass. The IgG molecule has a molecular weight between 150 and 180 kD, consists of two heavy and two light polypeptide chains connected by disulfide bonds (Fig. 18.1). The heavy and the light chains can be divided into a variable and a constant domain. The constant domain amino acid sequence is relatively conserved among immunoglobulins of a specific class (e.g., IgGi, IgM). The variable domains of an antibody population are highly heterogeneous. It is the variable domain that gives the antibody its binding specificity and affinity. Thus, the antibody engineer must be cautious to maintain the tertiary structure and orientation of the complementary determining region.

Most of the monoclonal antibodies in clinical trials have been derived from mice, and patients exposed to them have developed human antimouse antibody (i.e., HAMA) responses. Thus, this has limited the number of treatments that patients can receive. Typically, patients develop detectable anti-

body responses against the foreign monoclonal antibody within 2–4 weeks. If the patient then receives additional doses of the antibody, a typical allergic reaction is elicited (i.e., chills, urticaria, wheezing) and the antibody is rapidly cleared from the serum. In response to this problem, antibody therapy now includes a variety of molecules apart from the conventional immunoglobulin molecule.

Recent advances in the understanding of immunoglobulin structure through three-dimensional studies using nuclear magnetic resonance and X-ray crystallography and increased computer-assisted molecular modeling capabilities, combined with the application of recombinant approaches has led to the evolution of a new class of antibody-like molecules or *man-made antibodies* (6). Consequently, chimeric and humanized antibodies have been constructed to overcome the lack of intrinsic antitumor activity and the immunogenecity of many murine monoclonal antibodies. These monoclonal antibodies retain the binding specificity of the original rodent antibody determined by the variable region, but can potentially activate the human immune system through their human constant region.

As an example, smaller fragments that contain intact immunoglobulin-binding sites, such as F[ab′]$_2$ and Fab′, do not contain the lower binding domain of the molecule (Fig. 18.2). A smaller-sized

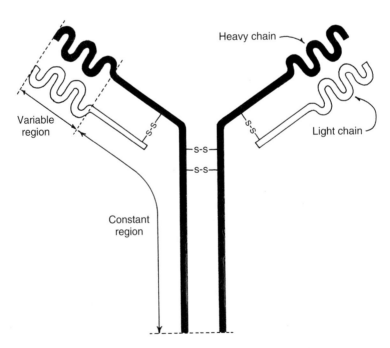

Fig. 18.1   *Basic shape of an immunoglobulin molecule akin to the class immunoglobulin G (IgG), a heterogeneous population of molecules sharing a Y-shaped structure composed of a heavy and light molecular chain linked by disulfied bonds (Illustration by Alan J. Slade).*

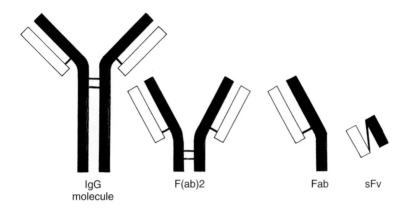

IgG
molecule   F(ab)2   Fab   sFv

Fig. 18.2   *Schematic depiction of an IgG molecule and its fragments (e.g., F[ab]2, Fab, sFv) (Illustration by Alan J. Slade).*

molecule will tend to be less immunogenic when administered systemically and is more likely to have a greater tumor penetration than a larger structure (7). Also, in diagnostic imaging applications, smaller fragments have demonstrated greater renal, biliary, and colonic uptake at 24 hours compared with the whole IgG, due to filtering by the kidneys and excretion via the biliary system of small protein compounds. All three smaller antibody forms have had success at detecting smaller (i.e., < 2 cm) lesions not seen on a CT scan and are superior to the IgC anti-carcinoembryonic antigen antibody.

Another example is the smaller Sfv molecule which contains the heavy and light chains of the binding sites joined by the shorter link (Fig. 18.2). These molecules also have been engineered to attach toxins, cytokines, radiolabeled elements, or genes, thus broadening their ability as delivery vehicles for cancer therapy.

Theoretically, when coupled with a drug molecule, radioactive isotope or toxin, a monoclonal antibody can target the desired cells or tissues with great precision. To date, however, the majority of monoclonal antibodies do not reach the target tumor cells (e.g., less than 0.1% locates in tumor tissue). There have been extensive descriptions of the barriers that impede antibody distribution within tumors. These include tortuous vasculature, increased hydrostatic pressure within the tumors, and heterogeneity of antigen distribution within tumors. Indeed, if antibodies do reach their intended target, there is little evidence that they can efficiently mediate *in vivo* antibody-dependent cytotoxicity. For this to occur, effector cells, such as macrophages, natural killer cells, or cytotoxic T-cells must be activated by the tumor.

Consequently, one advance has been the engineering and development of biospecific antibodies which consist of two antibodies with specificity for distinct antigens and immune effector cells. Bispecific antibodies can circumvent the T-cell receptor specificity for one antigen by binding to an activating epitope on the T cell. This provides the T-cell with an alternate specificity.

Another approach to activate the immune system is to link the antibody with a superantigen (e.g., staphyloccocal enterotoxin A). These toxins are capable of binding directly to macrophages and activating their action. For example, if the superantigen is linked to an antibody structure with specificity for a tumor-associated antigen, it targets the activated macrophage to the tumor cell. Both of these latter mentioned research approaches are undergoing Phase I studies at present.

Polymerase Chain Reaction

Polymerase chain reaction is a biotechnological process whereby there is substantial amplification (i.e., over 100,000-fold) of a target nucleic acid sequence (i.e., a gene). This enzymatic reaction occurs in repeated cycles of a three-step process. First, DNA is denatured to separate the two strands. Then a nucleic acid primer is hybridized to each DNA strand at a specific location within the nucleic acid sequence. Then, a DNA polymerase enzyme is added for extension of the primer along the DNA strand to copy the target nucleic acid sequence.

Each cycle duplicates the DNA molecules copied. This cycle is repeated until sufficient DNA sequence material is copied. For example, 20 cycles with a 90% success rate will yield a 375,000 amplification of a DNA sequence.

Gene Therapy

Gene therapy is a process in which exogenous genetic material is transferred into somatic cells to correct an inherited or acquired gene defect (8). Also, it is intended to introduce a new function or property into cells. These common and life-threatening diseases include cystic fibrosis, hemophilia, sickle cell anemia, and diabetes.

Scientific technology has developed safe and efficient means to transfer genes into cells. Consequently, a genetic and molecular delineation of the underlying pathophysiology of many of the primary immune deficiency disorders has occurred and gene-based therapy is now a viable option as long as the transferred genetic material can be delivered to the appropriate target cell or tissue.

Controversial ethical considerations over genetic intervention of germ line cells has fostered bioengineering to focus on gene therapy of somatic cells. Because somatic cells are end-stage, differentiated cells, research has examined the use of a "self renewing" stem-cell population for the therapeutic transfer of genetic material. Stem cells can self renew themselves, and the inserted gene will remain in place through subsequent generations of differentiated cells or tissue populations.

As an example, a patient's cells (e.g., T lymphocytes) are harvested and grown within the laboratory. The cells receive the gene from a viral carrier (e.g., Moloney murine leukemia virus) and start to produce the missing protein necessary to correct the deficiency. These cells with the extra functional gene are then returned to the patient, and the normal protein is produced and released, alleviating the disease.

The genetic cause of numerous primary immune deficiency disorders has been discovered and described. As a result, gene therapy can now be used as an alternative therapy, particularly in those patients in whom bone marrow transplantation may not be suitable (e.g., a bone marrow donor cannot be identified, the bone marrow preparative process carries substantial patient risk). The first primary immune deficiency disease defined was adenosine deaminase deficiency (ADA). The gene encoding for ADA is found on chromosome 20. Gene deletions and point mutations result in a loss or severe reduction in ADA enzymatic activity, leading to a clinical presentation of severe combined immunodeficiency disease (i.e., SCID), and often causing death in childhood or adolescence.

The first human protocol for gene therapy was performed in ADA deficient patients in 1990 at the National Institutes of Health. Since that time, several other primary immune deficiency disorders in which the genetic defect has been defined have been at least partially corrected by gene therapy using hemopoietic stem cells *in vitro*. For SCID and other diseases, gene therapy is life saving (8).

Nucleotide Blockade/Antisense

Nucleotide blockade and antisense technology focuses upon the study of function of specific proteins and intracellular expression. The sequence of a nucleotide chain that contains the information for protein synthesis is called the sense sequence. The nucleotide chain that is complementary to the sense sequence is called the antisense sequence. Antisense drugs recognize and bind to the nucleotide sense sequence of specific mRNA molecules, preventing the synthesis of unwanted proteins and actually destroying the sense molecules in the process.

The introduction of antisense nucleic acids into cells has provided new ideas to explore how proteins, whose expression has been selectively repressed in a cell, function within that cell. Another goal is to arrest the expression of dysfunctional messenger RNA or DNA and control disease processes. Antisense technology is part of a new approach termed *reverse genetics*.

Antisense RNA, for example, can be introduced into the cell by cloning technique. The specific gene of interest is cloned in an expression vector in the wrong orientation. Thus, a complementary m-RNA is created to match an abnormal m-RNA. Then when the two m-RNA strands complex together, this prevents translation of the m-RNA to form disease producing proteins. Anti-DNA strands also can be created to complex with DNA to form a triple helix. Oligonucleotides or short single strands of nucleic acids, instead of the full m-RNA also can be employed to block RNA expression. This form of biotechnology is being used for viral disease (e.g., herpes simplex, HIV) and cancer (i.e., oncogenes).

Peptide Technology

Peptide technology involves the screening for polypeptide molecules that can mimic larger proteins. This is intended to afford more simple products that can be more stable and easier to produce. These peptides can serve either as protein receptor agonists or antagonists.

Products of Biotechnology

Biotechnological drugs can be classified into major classes such as antisense, clotting factors, hematopoietic factors, hormones, interferons, interleukins, monoclonal antibodies, tissue growth factors, and vaccines. Biotechnological drugs are distinguished based on whether they are physiologic or nonphysiologic peptides, or whether they are new biotechnology products.

Physiological peptides can be further subdivided depending upon their intended use. For example, those for substitution include clotting factors, insulin, human growth hormone, and erythropoietin. Biotechnological products intended for therapeutic purposes in nonphysiological concentrations include interferons, cytokines, tissue plasminogen activator, and urokinase. Nonphysiological peptides include mutants of physiological peptides and include vaccines, thrombolytic agents and antithrombics.

The following descriptions by classification provide examples of products of biotechnology that have been approved by the FDA or are being developed for submission for approval (Table 18.1). Note that the section describing indication also lists in brackets for some biotechnology drugs/products proposed uses under the Orphan Drug Act. (The FDA Office of Orphan Products Development [OPD] provides an information packet that includes an overview of the FDA's orphan drug program, a brief description of the orphan products grant program and a current list on designated orphan products.)

Anticoagulant Drug

Lepirudin—Refludan

Lepirudin (rDNA), a recombinant hirudin derived from yeast cells, is a highly specific direct inhibitor of thrombin. It is the first of the hirudin class of anticoagulants. The polypeptide is composed of 65 amino acids and has a molecular weight of 6979.5 daltons. Natural hirudin is produced in trace quantity as a family of highly homologous isopolypeptides by the leach *Hirudo medicinalis*. Biosynthetic lepirudin is identical to natural hirudin except for substitution of a leucine molecule for isoleucine at the N-terminal end of the molecule and the absence of a sulfate group on the tyrosine molecule at position 63.

The activity of this anticoagulant is measured in a chromogenic assay. One antithrombin unit (ATU) is the amount of lepirudin that neutralizes one unit of WHO preparation 89/588 of thrombin. The specific activity of lepirudin is ≈16,000 ATU/mg. One molecule of lepirudin binds to one molecule of thrombin and blocks its activity.

Lepirudin is indicated for heparin-induced thrombocytopenia (HIT) and associated thromboembolic disease to prevent further thromboembolic complications. Of note is that the formation of antihirudin antibodies have been observed in approximately 40% of HIT patients treated with the drug. This ultimately may increase the anticoagulant effect of the lepirudin because of delayed renal elimination of active lepirudin-antihirudin complexes.

Initial dosage for anticoagulation in patients with HIT and associated thromboembolic disease is 0.4 mg/kg (≤ 110 kg) slowly IV (e.g., over 15–20 seconds) as a bolus dose followed by 0.15 mg/kg (≤ 110 kg/hr) as a continuous IV infusion for 2 to 10 days or longer if clinically necessary. The initial dosage depends upon the patient's weight and is valid up to ≤ 110 kg. For those who have weights >110 kg, the dosage should not be increased beyond the 110 kg body weight dose. The maximum initial bolus dose is 44 mg and the maximal infusion dose is 16.5 mg/hr.

Therapy with lepirudin is monitored using the aPTT (patient aPTT at a given time over an aPTT reference value, usually median of the laboratory normal range for aPTT). The patient's baseline aPTT should be determined prior to administration of the drug because lepirudin should not be initiated in patients with a baseline aPTT ratio of ≥ 2.5 to avoid initial overdosing.

Lepirudin powder for injection (Refludan), 50 mg, should only be reconstituted with Water for Injection, 0.9% Sodium Chloride Injection, or 5% Dextrose Injection. For rapid complete reconstitution, 1 mL of diluent is injected into the vial and the vial shaken gently. After reconstitution, a clear, colorless solution is obtained in no more than 3 minutes.

The reconstituted solution should be used immediately, and it remains stable for 24 hours at room temperature (e.g., during infusion). Prior to administration, it should be warmed to room temperature.

Antisense Drugs

Fomivirsen Sodium—Vitravene

Fomivirsen sodium injectable is an antisense drug that has been approved for the local treatment of cytomegalovirus (CMV) in patients with AIDS who are intolerant of or have a contraindication to other treatments for CMV retinitis. Also, it may be used in those instances where previous treatment for CMV retinitis failed.

Cytomegalovirus (CMV) is an extremely common virus which ultimately infects most people and remains latent (i.e., present but not active [akin

Table 18.1. Representative Biotechnology Products in Use in the United States

Generic Name	Trade Name (Manufacturer)	Indications [Proposed Use]*
Aldesleukin	Proleukin (Chiron)	Metastatic renal cell carcinoma/melanoma; primary immunodeficiency disease associated with T-cell defects
Alteplase	Activase (Genentech)	Ischemic stroke
Conjugate Vaccine-HibTITER	PedvaxHIB	Routine immunization of children 2 to 71 months of age against invasive diseases caused by *H. Influenzae* type b.
Efavirenz	Sustiva (DuPont)	For the treatment of HIV-1-infected individuals. Used in combination with other anti-HIV drugs (i.e., 2-, 3-, 4-drug combinations)
Epoetin alpha	Epogen (Amgen), Procrit	Certain anemias—chronic renal disease; AIDS; cancer chemotherapy [Anemia associated with end-stage renal disease or HIV infection or treatment; myelodysplastic syndrome; anemia of prematurity in preterm infants]
Filgrastim Granulocyte colony-stimulating factor (G-CSF)	Neupogen (Amgen)	To decrease the incidence of infection as manifested by febrile neutropenia in patients with non-myeloid malignancies receiving myelosuppressive anti-cancer drugs. To reduce the duration of neutropenia and neutropenia-related clinical sequela in patients with non-myeloid malignancies undergoing myeloablative chemotherapy followed by bone marrow transplant. [Severe chronic neutropenia (absolute neutrophil count <500/mm^3); neutropenia associated with bone marrow transplants; AIDS patients with CMV retinitis being treated with ganciclovir; mobilization of peripheral blood progenitor cells for collection in patients who will receive myeloablative or myelosuppressive chemotherapy; reduce duration of neutropenia, fever, antibiotic use and hospitalization following induction and consolidation for acute myeloid leukemia.]
Fomivirsen	Vitravene (Isis/Ciba)	Local treatment of cytomegalovirus (CMV) in patients with AIDS who are intolerant of or have a contraindication to other treatments for CMV retinitis or who have previously been unresponsive to other treatments for CMV.
Haemophilus b conjugate vaccine	Act-HIB (Connaught)	Routine immunization of children against invasive diseases caused by *H. Influenzae* type b.
Hepatitis B vaccine	Engerix-B (Smith Kline Beecham), Recombivax HB (MSD)	Hepatitis B prophylaxis
Human Growth Hormone	Protropin (Genentech), Humatrope (Lilly)	Human growth hormone deficiency in children
Human insulin	Humulin (Lilly), Rapid, Velosulin (Novo Nordisk)	Insulin-dependent diabetes mellitus
Imciromab pentetate	Myoscint (Centocor)	[Detection of early necrosis as an indication of rejection of orthotopic cardiac transplants]
Infliximab	Remicade (Centocor)	Active and fistulizing Crohn's Disease
Interferon a-2a	Referon A (Hoffman LaRoche)	Hairy cell leukemia, AIDS-related Kaposi's sarcoma
Interferon a-2b	Intron A (Schering-Plough)	Hairy cell leukemia; AIDS-related Kaposi's sarcoma; chronic hepatitis types B and C (non-A, non-B); condylomata acuminata
Interferon a-n3	Alferon N (Interferon Sciences)	Condylomata acuminata
Interferon B	Betaseron (Berlex)	Multiple sclerosis
Interferon y-1b	Actimmune	Chronic granulomatous disease
Muromonab-CD3	Orthoclone (Ortho), OKT 3 (Biotech)	Acute allograft rejection in renal transplant patients

continued

Table 18.1. Representative Biotechnology Products in Use in the United States

Generic Name	Trade Name (Manufacturer)	Indications [Proposed Use]*
Recombinant Factor VIII	Kogenate (Miles), Recombinate (Baxter)	Hemophilia A
Rituximab	Rituxan (IDEC/Genentech)	Treatment of patients with relapsed or refractory low-grade or follicular, CD20 positive, β-cell non-Hodgkin's lymphoma
Sargramostim (GM-CSF)	Leukine (Immunex), Prokine (Hoechst-Roussel)	Myeloid reconstitution after bone marrow transplantation [Leukine: Neutropenia associated with bone marrow transplant, graft failure and delay of engraftment, and for promotion of early engraftment; reduce neutropenia and leukopenia and decrease the incidence of death due to infection in patients with acute myelogenous leukemia]
Satumomab pendetide	Oncoscint CR/OV (Cytogen)	Detection of ovarian carcinoma
Somatropin	Genotropin (Genentech), Humatrope (Lilly), Norditropin (Novo Nordisk),	[Long term treatment of children with growth failure due to lack of adequate endogenous growth hormone secretion; growth failure in children with inadequate growth hormone secretion; idiopathic or organic growth hormone deficiency in children with growth failure; enhancement of nitrogen retention in hospitalized patients with severe burns; short stature in Turner's syndrome; adults with growth hormone deficiency]
Somatropin for Injection	Humatrope (Lilly), Nutropin (Genentech), Serostim (Seronol)	Long term treatment for growth failure in children who demonstrate a lack of endogenous growth hormone secretion. [Long term treatment of children with growth failure due to inadequate secretion of normal endogenous growth hormone; short stature in Turner's syndrome; growth retardation in chronic renal failure; catabolism/weight loss in AIDS; children with AIDS-associated failure to thrive including AIDS-associated wasting; replacement therapy for growth hormone deficiency in adults with epiphyseal closure.]
Tissue Plasminogen Activator (t-PA) (syn. Alteplase)	Activase (Genentech)	Management of acute myocardial infarct (AMI) in adults for the improvement of ventricular function following an AMI, the reduction of the incidence of congestive heart failure and the reduction of mortality associated with AMI. Management of acute ischemic stroke in adults for improving neurological recovery and reducing the incidence of disability. Management of acute massive pulmonary embolism (PE), for the lysis of acute PE, defined by obstruction of blood flow to a lobe or multiple segments of the lungs, and for the lysis of PE accompanied by unstable hemodynamics.
Tissue Plasminogen Activator (t-PA) [Non-glycosylated deletion mutein]	Retavase (Boehringer-Mannheim)	The management of AMI in adults for improvement of ventricular function following an AMI, the reduction of the incidence of congestive heart failure and the reduction of mortality associated with AMI.
Trastuzumab	Herceptin (Genentech)	Treatment of metastatic breast cancer or cancer that has spread beyond the breast and lymph nodes under the arm. Use can be alone in patients with primary failure with other chemotherapies or as a first-line treatment of metastatic disease when used in combination with paclitaxel (i.e., Taxol)

*Listing includes proposed uses for orphaned drugs in brackets [ ]. The Orphan Drug Act defines an orphan drug as a drug or biological product for the diagnosis, treatment, or prevention of a rare disease or condition. A rare disease is one which affects <200,000 persons in the US or one which affects >200,000 persons but for which there is no reasonable expectation that the cost of developing the drug and making it available will be recovered from sales of the drug in the US.

to chickenpox]). Although overt disease is uncommon in people with fully intact immune systems, CMV can be serious in those individuals with impaired immune systems. One of the most serious and debilitating CMV infections is CMV retinitis which results in a gradual destruction of the light-sensitive tissues of the eye which allows sight. CMV retinitis is the most common cause of blindness in persons with acquired immune deficiency syndrome (AIDS) and other immunosuppressed states.

Fomivirsen sodium, a phosphorothioate oligonucleotide, is administered by direct injection into the vitreous body (i.e., the transparent, gelatinous mass, filling the eyeball behind the lens) of the eye. This oligonucleotide is targeted specifically to the CMV genetic information so that it can shut down the CMV virus, but not interfere with the functioning of human DNA.

There are two induction intravitreal (i.e., into the eye under local anesthesia) doses of the drugs on days one and fifteen followed by a monthly intravitreal injection of 330 mcg. This is advantageous for the management of CMV retinitis because it obviates the need for IV therapies. Also, it potentially will offer avoidance of surgical implants and their associated complications, a decreased frequency of intravitreal injections compared to other antiviral compounds, and presents as a possible adjunct to oral ganciclovir therapy.

Efavirenz—Sustiva

Efavirenz is a non-nucleoside reverse transciptase inhibitor and the first anti-HIV drug to be approved by the FDA for once-daily dosing in combination with other anti-HIV drugs.

Clinical trials demonstrated that efavirenz reduces plasma viral RNA to below quantifiable levels in a majority of HIV-1-infected naive and treatment-experienced individuals in two-, three-, and four-drug combinations.

Efavirenz is available as an oral capsule and can be taken once a day with or without meals. However, it is advised that it not be administered with meals high in fat content. This drug-food interaction may increase the drug's systemic absorption.

Clotting Factors

Hemophiliacs suffer from internal bleeding because of a lack of clotting protein factors. Historically, their treatment has been infusions of protein derived from human blood. Now, through genetic engineering, factors can be created without using donor blood that produce more nearly contaminant-free products and therefore expose the patient to fewer contaminants.

Systemic Antihemophilic Factors— Kogenate, Recombinate

Recombinant antihemophilic factor (AHF) is indicated for treatment of classical hemophilia A, in which there is a demonstrated deficiency of activity of plasma clotting factor (factor VIII). Human recombinant AHF (rAHF) is a sterile, nonpyrogenic concentrate with biologic and pharmacokinetic activity comparable to that of plasma-derived AHF. Additional clinical trials are being conducted to determine whether antibodies to the recombinant product form more often than that with plasma-derived products (9).

The recombinant form contains albumin as a stabilizer, as well as trace amounts of mouse, hamster, and bovine proteins. These new products are made by modifying hamster cells through biotechnology processes so that they produce a highly purified version of AHF factor VIII (9).

Each vial of AHF is labeled with the AHF activity expressed in International Units (IU). The assignment of potency is referenced to the World Health Organization International Standard. One IU of factor VIII activity is approximately equal to the AHF activity of one mL of fresh plasma, and increases the plasma concentration of factor VIII by 2%. The specific Factor VIII activity ranges from 2 to 200 AHF IU per mg of total protein.

There is a linear dose-response relation with an approximate yield of a 2% rise in Factor VIII activity for each unit of Factor VIII/kg transfused. The following formulas provide a guide for dosing calculations:

$$\text{Expected factor VIII increase (in \% of normal)} = \frac{\text{Dose AHF/IU administered} \times 2}{\text{Body weight (kg)}}$$

$$\text{AHF/IU required} = \frac{\text{body weight (kg)} \times \text{desired factor VIII increase}}{(\% \text{ normal}) \times 0.5}$$

Kogenate is available in strengths of 250 IU (with 2.5 mL sterile water for injection provided as diluent), 500 IU (with 5 mL sterile water for injection provided as diluent), and 1000 IU (with 10 mL sterile water for injection provided as diluent). Each strength contains between 2 and 5 mmol of calcium chloride, 100–130 mEq/liter of sodium, 100–130 mEq/liter of chloride, 4 to 10 mg/mL of human albumin, and nanogram quantities of foreign protein (mouse, hamster) per IU. Kogenate is supplied in a single-dose vial, along with a suitable volume of diluent (Sterile Water for Injection, USP), a sterile filter needle, and a sterile administration set.

Recombinate is available in strengths of 250 IU, 500 IU, and 1000 IU, each with 10 mL sterile water for injection provided as diluent. Each strength contains 12.5 mg/mL of human albumin, 180 mEq/l of sodium, 200 mEq/l of calcium, and a small quantity of foreign protein.

Dry concentrates of rAHF should be stored between 2°C and 8°C, and the diluent protected from freezing. Kogenate, however, may be stored at room temperatures not exceeding 25°C for 3 months. After reconstitution, the solution should not be refrigerated.

The diluent and the dry concentrate should be brought to room temperature (approximately 25°C) prior to reconstitution. These may be allowed to warm to room temperature, or in an emergency situation warmed via water bath to a range of 30–37°C. Once reconstituted, the solution should not be shaken because this could cause the solution to foam. The reconstituted solution should be administered within 3 hours of reconstitution, and any partially used vial discarded. This preparation should be administered alone through a separate line, and without mixing with other intravenous fluids or medications.

Kogenate may be administered intravenously over 5 to 10 minutes, and Recombinate at a rate up to 10 mL per minute. The comfort of the patient should guide the rate at which the recombinant AHF is administered. If a significant increase in pulse rate occurs, the infusion should be slowed or halted until the pulse rate returns to normal. The risk of an allergic reaction to product proteins (mouse, hamster, bovine) may be present in the monoclonal antibody-derived and recombinant AHF products.

Colony Stimulating Factors

Colony stimulating factors (CSFs) are four glycoprotein regulators that bind to specific surface receptors and are able to control the proliferation and differentiation of marrow cells into macrophages, neutrophils, basophils, eosinophils, platelets, or erythrocytes (10, 11). These recombinant human CSFs have potential for wide use in the areas of oncology (e.g., chemotherapy-induced leukopenia, cancer patients having marrow transplants), inherited disorders (e.g., congenital neutropenia) and infectious

disease (e.g., AIDS) (12). Patients with low amounts of endogenous CSFs are prone to secondary infections because of diminished resistance associated with some forms of cancer or, more commonly, suppressed marrow function after the use of myelotoxic chemotherapy.

In the absence of pluripotent *stem cells* (an uncommitted cell with the potential to become any cell of the blood), the CSFs cannot be expected to stimulate cell formation and the development of neutrophils. Furthermore, it could be expected that the effectiveness of the CSFs be directly related to the absolute numbers of these potential target cells. For example, cancer patients with bone marrow severely depleted by chemotherapy may not respond as well to CSFs therapy as cancer patients with normal hemopoietic tissues.

If patients with neutropenia develop an infection, they will be unable to defend themselves against it because neutrophils are the body's initial defense mechanism. If neutrophils are absent, or in very low numbers, the classic signs and symptoms of infection (swelling, pain, redness, heat, purulent discharge) will be absent. Neutrophils cause these signs and symptoms, and if they are not present in sufficient numbers, only a fever—with or without sore throat—may signal a serious infection. Thus, a body temperature that exceeds 100.5°F is a serious occurrence in a patient who has undergone chemotherapy within the past 3–4 weeks.

Granulocyte Colony Stimulating Factor (G-CSF)—Filgrastim

Produced by recombinant DNA technology, this drug stimulates the production of neutrophils within the bone marrow. It is approved for chemotherapy-related neutropenia and is indicated (to decrease the incidence of infection, as manifested by febrile neutropenia) in patients with nonmyeloid malignancies who are receiving myelosuppressive anti-cancer drugs and exhibiting severe neutropenia with fever. This drug can also be used as an adjunct to myelosuppressive cancer chemotherapy to help speed the recovery of neutrophils after treatment and to reduce serious infection risk.

For chemotherapy-induced neutropenia, Filgrastim is administered intravenously (short infusion, 15–30 minutes), as a subcutaneous bolus or continuous intravenous or subcutaneous injection, in a starting dose of 5 mcg/kg once daily, beginning no earlier than 24 hours after administration of the last dose of cytotoxic chemotherapy. This regimen is continued for up to 2 weeks, until the absolute neutrophil count reaches 10,000/mm^3 following the *nadir* (the lowest neutrophil count, usually occurring 7–10 days after chemotherapy).

Filgrastim injection contains no preservative and should be stored between 2°C and 8°C. It is not to be frozen. Before use, the injection may be allowed to reach room temperature for a maximum of 24 hours, after which time it should be discarded. A clear, colorless solution, it should be inspected visually prior to injection. This product is supplied as a 1 mL or 1.6 mL, single-dose vial (Fig. 18.3).

Filgrastim is supplied in boxes containing ten glass vials, which are packaged in a gel-ice insulating container that has a temperature indicator to detect freezing. For convenience, and to minimize the risk of breakage, Filgrastim should be dispensed to the patient in its original packaging, and the patient instructed to refrigerate the product promptly after arriving home.

If the patient has to travel a considerable distance, and/or the outside temperature is high, it may be necessary to place the medication in a small cooler with a gel refrigerant (e.g., blue ice) for transport. It is suggested that the vials be wrapped in a towel to avoid direct contact between the product vials and the blue ice. The drug must be physically separated from the refrigerant to avoid the possibility of freezing. Dry ice should not be used because of the possibility of freezing the product through inadvertent contact.

It is conceivable that, when used as an adjunct to cancer chemotherapy, prescriptions for this product will be written for 7–10 vials. Indeed, patients may have extra vials of this product at home from previous courses of cancer chemotherapy. The pharmacist should question such patients about having any unexpired, properly stored, or unused vials remaining from the previous course of therapy. Filgrastim injection repackaged in 1 mL plastic tuberculin syringes stored at 2° to 8° remain sterile for 7 days.

Because granulocyte colony stimulating factor (G-CSF) is a protein, it is capable of being denatured if severely agitated. If the vial is shaken vigorously, the solution may foam or appear frothy, making its withdrawal difficult. Thus, the pharmacist should instruct the patient (or guardian) to avoid shaking the vial before use. If mistakenly shaken, the vial should be allowed to stand until the froth diminishes.

If it is necessary to dilute filgrastim, it may be diluted with 5% Dextrose Injection. When filgrastim is diluted to concentrations ranging between 5 and 15 mcg/mL, it should be protected from inadvertent adsorption to plastic materials by the addition of albumin (human) to a final concentration of 2 mg/mL. When diluted in 5% Dextrose or 5% Dextrose plus albumin, filgrastim is compatible with glass bottles, PVC and polyolefin IV bags and polypropylene syringes. Filgrastim should never be diluted with saline at any time as the product may precipitate.

The manufacturer of Filgrastim has developed a step-by-step guide to subcutaneous self-injection. However, the pharmacist should always emphasize the use of proper aseptic technique when preparing and administering the drug, to help avoid product contamination and possible infection.

Granulocyte Macrophage Colony Stimulating Factor (GM-CSF)—Sargramostim

Sargramostim is a recombinant human granulocyte-macrophage CSF produced by recombinant DNA technology in a yeast (*Saccharomyces cerevisiae*) expression system. GM-CSF is a hematopoietic growth factor that stimulates proliferation and differentiation of hematopoietic progenitor (i.e., precursor) cells into neutrophils and monocytes. It is a glycoprotein composed of 127 amino acids. The sequence of GM-CSF differs from the natural human GM-CSF at position 23, where leucine is substituted.

This drug is indicated for acceleration of myeloid (i.e., marrow) recovery in patients with non-Hodgkin's lymphoma (NHL), acute lymphoblastic leukemia (ALL), and Hodgkin's disease undergoing autologous bone marrow transplantation (a procedure in which the patient's bone marrow is removed, treated to destroy malignant cells, and

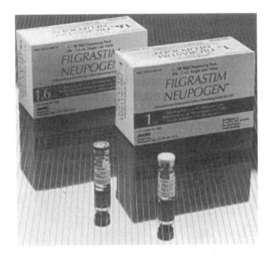

Fig. 18.3 *Example of the product package of Filgrastim (Courtesy of Amgen, Inc.).*

later reinfused into the patient). It is also indicated in bone-marrow-transplantation failure or engraftment delay (it takes between 3 and 4 weeks for the new marrow to begin to produce new white blood cells).

GM-CSF accelerates the engraftment process by promoting the production of white blood cells. Health care costs are controlled, because patients treated with it demonstrate significant earlier increases in WBC counts, a reduced need for antibiotics, and a shortened duration of hospitalization. For myeloid reconstitution after autologous bone marrow transplantation, it is administered in a dose of 250 mcg/m^2/day for 21 days as a 2-hour intravenous infusion beginning 2–4 hours after the autologous bone marrow infusion, and not less than 24 hours after the last dose of chemotherapy and 12 hours after the last dose of radiotherapy. For bone-marrow-transplantation failure or engraftment delay, the dose remains the same, but the duration is 14 days, again using a 2-hour intravenous infusion. The dose can be repeated after 7 days of therapy if engraftment has not occurred.

To avoid potential complications associated with GM-CSF in terms of excessive leukocytosis (i.e., WBC >50,000 cells/mm^3; ANC >20,000 cells/mm^3), a CBC with differential is recommended twice weekly during therapy. When the ANC is >20,000 cells/mm^3, the administration of GM-CSF should be interrupted or reduced by one half.

Sargramostim is manufactured as a powder for injection, lyophilized, in preservative-free, single-use vials of 250 mcg or 500 mcg. It is reconstituted with one mL of Sterile Water for Injection, USP (without preservative). The reconstituted solution should appear clear and colorless, and will be isotonic with a pH of 7.4 ± 0.3. During the reconstitution procedure, the Sterile Water for Injection, USP, should be directed at the side of the vial and the contents gently swirled to avoid foaming during dissolution. The product must not be shaken or vigorously agitated. The product can also be diluted for IV infusion in 0.9% Sodium Chloride Injection, USP. If the final concentration of GM-CSF is below 10 mcg/mL, human albumin (0.1%) should be added to the saline before adding GM-CSF. This addition prevents the adsorption of the drug to the components of the drug delivery system. To create a 0.1% albumin solution, the pharmacist should add 1 mg albumin (human) per 1 mL 0.9% Sodium Chloride Injection.

An in-line membrane filter for the IV administration of this drug should not be used. Further, in the absence of compatibility and stability informa-tion, other medications should not be admixed to infusion solutions containing sargramostim. Only 0.9% Sodium Chloride Injection should be used to prepare IV infusion solutions of the drug.

Because this product is preservative free, it should be administered as soon as possible, and within 6 hours following reconstitution or dilution for IV infusion.

Erythropoietins

Erythropoietin is a sialic acid-containing glycoprotein that enhances erythropoiesis by stimulating the formation of proerythroblasts and the release of reticulocytes from bone marrow. It is secreted by the kidney in response to hypoxemia and transported to the bone marrow through the plasma. It resembles an endocrine hormone more than any other cytokine (13).

Anemia (a deficiency of red blood cell production) is a frequent complication of cancer and cancer therapy. Although it is easily corrected through blood transfusions, erythropoietins are only available to treat the severest forms of anemia and not to maintain the red blood cell mass required for normal activity and well-being. As anemic patients with solid tumors often have lower serum levels of erythropoietin, correction of the erythropoietin deficiency through erythropoietin therapy may be as beneficial for these cancer patients as it has been for uremic patients (13).

Kidney disease also impairs the body's ability to produce this substance, and thus results in anemia. In the past, patients received blood transfusions. However, a problem with transfusions was possible exposure to infectious agents (hepatitis, HIV). An exciting alternative is the genetically engineered epoetin alpha, a drug capable of stimulating erythropoiesis. Although expensive (>$1000/month), it may prove beneficial for those patients who require extensive transfusions, because of the high cost of transfusions, the risk of infectious disease, and the consequent additional health care costs.

Epoetin Alfa—Epogen, Procrit

Epoetin alfa is a glycoprotein produced by recombinant DNA technology, and contains 165 amino acids in an identical sequence to that of endogenous human erythropoietin. This drug stimulates erythropoiesis by effecting the division and differentiation of committed erythroid progenitor cells. Erythropoietin also effects the release of reticulocytes from the bone marrow into the bloodstream, where these mature into erythrocytes. It is approved for anemia related to cancer chemotherapy, chronic dialysis, and AZT therapy.

Epoetin alfa stimulates erthropoiesis in anemic patients for dialyzed and nondialyzed patients. The first evidence of a response to this drug will be an increase within 10 days of the reticulocyte count. Coupled with this will be subsequent increases in the RBC count, hemoglobin and hematocrit, usually within 2 to 6 weeks. Once the hematocrit reaches the suggested target range (i.e., 30% to 36%), that level can be sustained in the absence of iron deficiency and concurrent illnesses by epoetin alfa therapy.

Epoetin alfa is administered intravenously or subcutaneously, in a dosage of 50–100 IU/kg body weight three times per week. It is given intravenously to patients with available intravenous access (e.g., patients who undergo hemodialysis), and either intravenously or subcutaneously to other patients. If after 8 weeks of therapy the hematocrit has not increased at least five to six points and is still below the target range of 30–33%, the dosage may be increased.

Epoetin alfa is available in 1 mL, nonpreserved, single-dose vials (Fig. 18.4) in varying strengths of 2000, 3000, 4000, 10,000 and 20,000 IU/mL. Each 1-mL vial contains human albumin, 2.5 mg, to prevent adsorptive losses. The product should be refrigerated at 2°C to 8°C, and protected from freezing. The vial of epoetin alfa, recombinant injection, should not be shaken because this may denature the glycoprotein and render it biologically inactive. Each vial should be used to administer a single dose only, and any unused portion of the solution must be discarded.

The 10,000 U/mL Injection is available in 2 mL multidose vials. These are preserved with 1% benzyl alcohol and contain 2.5 mg albumin (human) per mL. These vials should be stored at 2° to 8° after initial entry and between doses. These vials should be discarded 21 days after initial entry.

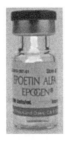

Fig. 18.4 *Example of the product Epogen (Courtesy of Amgen, Inc.).*

Epoetin alfa should not be administered in conjunction with other solutions. However, just before SC administration, the solution can be admixed in a syringe at a ratio of 1:1 with Bacteriostatic 0.9% Sodium Chloride Injection with Benzyl Alcohol 0.9%. The benzyl alcohol then acts as a local anesthetic that may ameliorate pain associated with SC injection.

Growth Factor

Endogenous platelet-derived growth factor increases the proliferation of cells that repair wounds and form granulation tissue. This factor promotes the chemotactic recruitment and proliferation of cells involved in wound repair and enhancing the formation of granulation tissue.

Becaplermin—Regranex

Becaplermin is a recombinant human platelet-derived growth factor (rhPDGF-BB) for topical adjunctive treatment of diabetic ulcers, a form of pressure ulcer, of the lower extremities that extend into subcutaneous tissue or beyond and having a sufficient blood supply. It is reasonable to assume that it might find utility as an adjunct to good pressure ulcer care.

Available in a 0.01% gel formulation, a measured quantity of gel is spread evenly over the ulcerated area to yield a thin, continuous 1/16 inch thickness over the ulcerated area. The prescribed, calculated length of the gel is placed onto a clean, firm, nonabsorbable surface (e.g., wax paper). Then, a clean cotton swab, tongue depressor, or similar aid applicator is used to spread the gel over the surface of the ulcer to obtain an even layer. The ulcer is then covered with a saline moistened gauze dressing.

After approximately 12 hours, the ulcer should be gently rinsed with saline or water to remove the residual gel and then covered with a saline-moistened gauze dressing without the gel for the remainder of the day. The next day, the process is repeated and performed continually until the ulcer has healed. The ulcer should demonstrate size reduction (about 30%) within 10 weeks time. If complete healing has not occurred within 20 weeks, the therapy should be reassessed. To facilitate patient acceptance and convenience, bedtime application can be considered.

Becaplermin gel must be refrigerated for stability, but need not be allowed to come to room temperature before it is applied. There is, however, a possibility the cold gel might cause discomfort when it is applied. The gel itself only has a expiration dating of nine months from the manufacture date, but because one tube lasts for about two to four weeks, pharmacists can dispense the gel up to one month prior to its expiration date.

Human Growth Hormone

The pituitary gland secretes human growth hormone (hGH), which stimulates an individual's growth. It is estimated that approximately 15,000 American children suffer from hGH deficiency, and consequently will not achieve normal height as an adult.

In the late 1950s, cadaver pituitaries were harvested to produce hGH and treat these deficient children. Besides the enormous expense, this method exposed the children to the risk of infection from viral contamination of the hormone (14). Genetic engineering now produces highly purified hGH.

Systemic Growth Hormone—Humatrope, Protropin

Somatrem (Protropin) is a biosynthetic, single polypeptide chain of 192 amino acids, produced by a recombinant DNA procedure in *E. coli* This drug has one more amino acid (methionine) than the natural occurring human growth hormone. Somatropin recombinant (Humatrope) is biosynthetically produced by another recombinant DNA process and possesses amino acid sequencing identical to the naturally occurring human growth hormone (i.e., 191 amino acids).

This hormone stimulates linear growth by affecting the cartilaginous growth areas of long bones. It also stimulates growth by increasing the number and size of skeletal muscle cells, influencing the size of organs, and increasing red cell mass through erythropoietin stimulation.

Somatrem for injection is initially administered intramuscularly or subcutaneously. The dosage is individualized at up to 0.1 mg/kg (i.e., 0.26 IU/kg) is administered SC or IM three times/week. The 5- and 10-mg, single-dose vials (Fig. 18.5) are reconstituted using standard aseptic technique with 1–5 mL of Bacteriostatic Water for Injection, USP (benzyl alcohol preserved) only. Because of the associated toxicity of benzyl alcohol in newborns, when administering to this patient population this product should be reconstituted with Water for Injection. The vial should then be swirled gently to dissolve the contents. If cloudy, the solution should not be used. When prepared with the manufacturer's provided diluent, the reconstituted solution

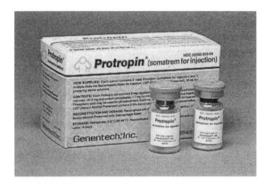

Fig. 18.5 *Example of the product Protropin (Courtesy of Genentech, Inc.).*

should be stored in the refrigerator and used within 14 days. When Water for Injection is used to reconstitute this product, each vial should only be used for one dose and the unused portion discarded.

Somatropin, recombinant, for injection, is administered subcutaneously in a dosage of 0.16 to 0.24 mg/kg body weight/week divided into six to seven SC injections. This drug is available in various strengths ranging from 1.5 mg (≈4 IU/mL) to 10 mg (≈30 IU/vial). As Genotropin, for example, the 5.8 mg Intra-Mix two-chamber cartridge (with preservative) is preassembled in a reconstitution device and co-packaged with a pressure release needle. The front chamber contains 1.5 mg of recombinant somatropin (approximately 4.5 IU), glycine, sodium dihydrogen phosphate anhydrous, and disodium phosphate anhydrous. The rear chamber contains 1.13 mL of water for injection. Depressing the stopper allows the two components to mix. If, however, the diluent and somatropin are in separate vials, aseptic technique must be used to add the desired amount of diluent (between 1.5 and 5 mL) provided by the manufacturer, or Sterile Water for Injection to a 5 mg vial. Like Somatrem, Somatropin is stable when refrigerated for up to 14 days following reconstitution with the diluent containing a preservative provided by the manufacturer. When Sterile Water for Injection is used to reconstitute this product, each vial should be refrigerated and used within 24 hours because there is no preservative.

Interferons

In 1957, two British scientists, Alick Isaacs and Jean Lindenmann, found that infected chick embryo cells released a naturally produced glycoprotein that allowed noninfected cells to resist viral infection. They named this factor *interferon*, because it appeared "to interfere with the transmission of infection." Later, these researchers demonstrated that interferon does not activate viruses directly, but rendered the host cells resistant to viral multiplication. Interferons exert virus-nonspecific but host-specific antiviral activity. By the mid-1970s, it appeared that interferon might also curtail the spread of certain types of cancer (e.g., small cell lung cancer, renal cell carcinoma, basal cell carcinoma).

As a class, interferons are a part of the large immune regulatory network within the body that includes lymphokines, monokines, growth factors, and peptide hormones. Interferons are classified into two types—type I interferons (alpha and beta), which share the same molecular receptor, and type II (gamma or immune), which has a different receptor (15).

Interferon beta-1b—Betaseron

Interferon beta-1b (IFNB) is a type I interferon made in *E. coli* using recombinant technology; it differs from natural interferon beta only by the substitution of a serine residue for a cysteine at position 17. This manipulation enhances the stability of the drug while retaining the specific activity of the natural interferon beta.

IFNB is effective in the treatment of relapsing-remitting types of multiple sclerosis, an inflammatory demyelinating disease of the CNS, in a dosage of 0.25 mg (8 mIU) injected subcutaneously every other day (15). This form of disease is characterized by recurrent attacks followed by complete or incomplete recovery (16).

The effectiveness of lower doses has not been documented and there is no evidence of efficacy when this drug is used for greater than two years

The lyophilized IFNB (Fig. 18.6), 0.3 mg (9.6 mIU), is reconstituted using a sterile syringe and needle to inject 1.2 mL of supplied diluent (sodium chloride, 0.54% solution) into the vial. The diluent should be added down the side of the vial and the vial then gently swirled, but not shaken, to dissolve the drug completely. After reconstitution with the accompanying diluent, the solution has a strength of 0.25 mg/mL. This product also contains dextrose and albumin (this adjuvant is often used in recombinant protein products to prevent adherence of the product to the glass vial, plastic tubing, or syringe). One mL of reconstituted solution is then withdrawn from the vial into a sterile syringe fitted with a 27-gauge needle and the drug is injected subcutaneously. For purposes of self-injection, the sites may include the arms, abdomen, hips, and thighs.

Because the product has no preservative, the vial is suitable for single use only. Before and after reconstitution, the product should be refrigerated. No more than 3 hours should elapse between reconstitution and use.

IFNB is currently distributed through a nationwide community pharmacy network called PCS

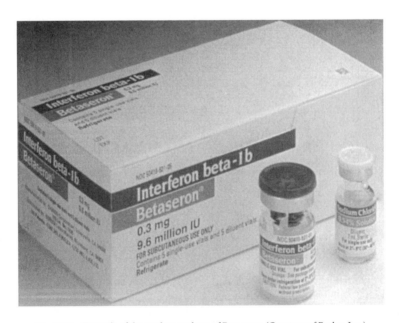

Fig. 18.6   *Example of the product package of Betaseron (Courtesy of Berlex, Inc.).*

Professional Service Network. The advantage of this system is that it eliminates the pharmacy's inventory and carrying costs, allows the IFNB patient to use a PCS prescription drug card, and pays the participating pharmacy a professional fee for each transaction (17). The cost of therapy is estimated to be approximately $1000/month.

Interferon beta-1a—Avonex

Interferon beta-1A was approved for use in multiple sclerosis therapy in 1996, three years after interferon beta-1B was approved. It is indicated for the treatment of relapsing forms of multiple sclerosis to slow the accumulation of physical ability and decrease the frequency of clinical exacerbations.

The dosage regimen of interferon beta-1A is 30 mcg IM administered once per week. The advantage compared to interferon beta-1B is less administration during the week. The lyophilized powder for injection is reconstituted with 1.1 mL of diluent and then swirled gently to dissolve the active ingredient. The prepared product should then be used as soon as possible, but no later than 6 hours after reconstitution if stored at 2° to 8°C.

Vials of interferon beta-1A must be refrigerated (2° to 8°C), and if refrigeration is not available, the product can be stored at 25°C (i.e., 77°F) for a period of up to 30 days.

Interleukins

Originally, these substances were thought to oversee interactions between white blood cells, key components of the immune system. Now, however, it is known that these substances affect a wider variety of cell types. Most clinical interest centers upon Interleukin-1 (IL-1), a substance secreted primarily by the monocyte/macrophage that activates T-cells and B-cells, and Interleukin-2 (IL-2), a substance secreted by the T-cell that supports the growth and differentiation of T-cells and B-cells. There are a total of 14 known interleukins.

IL-1 was discovered in 1972, and within 7 years its structure and function were delineated. It was first manufactured by recombinant-DNA technology in 1984. This substance is a key immune system regulator. It sets into motion a chain reaction that intensifies the immune response. IL-1 responds to the initial presence of an antigen. It activates T-cells to mature, proliferate, and produce other *cytokines* (a generic term for soluble substances produced by cells that communicate with other cells to trigger or suppress cellular activity after interaction with an antigen).

IL-1 also intensifies the production of collagenase, prostaglandins, and antibodies. Because of this activity, excess IL-1 is suspected to be behind many inflammatory disorders (collagenase breaks down connective tissue; prostaglandins are associated with inflammation). The cytokine may also be responsible for the fever, headache, fatigue, and weakness of influenza.

Interleukin-2 (IL-2), like other cytokines, was initially greeted with much enthusiasm. Since that time it has been found to be an essential component in the development of antigen-specific and antigen nonspecific immune responses, but has found few applications (18). Discovered in 1976, it became available through recombinant-DNA technology in 1984. When applied to white blood cells removed from patients, and then reinfused as "lymphokine activated killer cells" along with a booster injection of IL-2, spectacular remissions occurred in some patients with devastating conditions such as advanced malignant melanoma. Unfortunately, highly toxic side effects occurred because of a lack of knowledge of appropriate dosing. A combination of lower doses and physician experience managing its side effects will make IL-2 safer to use in the future.

Other interleukins are in the research pipeline. IL-11 is being investigated in vitro and in mice to stimulate platelet function. If successful, this substance could help counter the platelet-depleting effects of chemotherapeutic agents. IL-6 (synonymously known as beta-2 interferons) may also be a stimulator of platelet growth, and is being investigated as an antiproliferative treatment for breast, colon, and skin cancer.

Aldesleukin—Proleukin

Aldesleukin is synthetically produced by a recombinant-DNA process involving genetically engineered *Escherichia coli* containing an analog of the human interleukin-2 gene. An expression clone that encodes a modified human interleukin-2 results from genetic engineering techniques used to modify the human interleukin-2 gene. Aldesleukin differs from naturally occurring interleukin-2 in that it is not glycosylated because it is derived from *E. coli*, the molecule has no N-terminal alanine, and the molecule has serine substituted for cysteine at amino-acid position 125.

Designated an orphan drug, aldesleukin is approved for the treatment of metastatic renal carcinoma (about 10,000 cases diagnosed annually) in adults (over 18 years), melanomas, and primary immunodeficiency disease associated with T-cell defects. Currently, aldesleukin is being investigated in Phase II clinical trials for efficacy with zidovudine for human immunodeficiency virus (HIV) disease.

Because of its life-threatening toxicities (drug-related mortality rate is 4%), the physician should consider the benefit-to-risk ratio for the patient. The dosage of interleukin-2 is usually expressed in units of activity in promoting proliferation in a responsive cell line. Conversion to units from mg of protein varies, depending upon the source of interleukin-2. The strength and dosage of commercially available aldesleukin is expressed in International Units (IU). Eighteen million IU equals 1.1 mg protein.

For metastatic renal carcinoma, high-dose therapy involves an intravenous infusion over a 15-minute period, 600,000 IU/kg of body weight (i.e., 0.037 mg/kg body weight) every 8 hours for a total of 14 doses. Following a rest period of 9 days, the schedule is repeated for another 14 doses, for a maximum of 28 doses per course. The manufacturer of aldesleukin recommends that plastic bags be used as the dilution containers (as opposed to glass bottles and polyvinyl chloride bags) for more consistent drug delivery. In-line filters are not recommended for use during this drug's administration because of the risk of adsorption of aldesleukin to the filter.

Each aldesleukin for injection, single-use vial, contains 22 million IUs (1.3 mg of drug) and is reconstituted for intravenous or subcutaneous injection by adding 1.2 mL of Sterile Water for Injection to the vial. The diluent should be directed to the side of the vial and the contents swirled gently to avoid foaming. The resultant solution should be clear-and-colorless to slightly yellow and will contain 18 million IUs (1.1 mg) per mL. The vial should not be shaken. The appropriate dose is then withdrawn, diluted in 50 mL of 5% Dextrose Injection, and infused over a 15-minute period. Bacteriostatic Water for Injection, or 0.9% Sodium Chloride Injection, should not be used to reconstitute this product because of the increased aggregation of the product.

Because the vial has no preservative, the reconstituted and diluted solutions should be refrigerated. However, it should be brought back to room temperature prior to administration. Reconstituted solutions should be used within 48 hours.

Monoclonal Antibodies

Historically, monoclonal antibodies have found use in laboratory diagnostics, site-directed thera-pies, immunology, and home test kits (e.g., pregnancy, ovulation prediction). In the 1980s, monoclonals were expected to provide a tremendous potential for tumor therapy and immunomodulation. By coupling tracers and toxins to antibodies, tissue selective or cell specific targets can be attained. Despite intensive research and many promising results in the last decade, the number of monoclonals in clinical practice are rather limited.

As of March, 1997, there were only seven monoclonal antibody products licensed for *in vivo* use in the USA. There have been three reasons proposed for this low number (19). These include 1) insufficient characterization of the product and its performance *in vitro*; 2) inadequate preclinical testing, and 3) unrealistic expectations of clinical performance, leading to inadequately designed clinical trials (19).

Monoclonal antibodies are purified antibodies produced by a single source or clone of cells (20). These substances are engineered to recognize and bind to a single specific antigen. Thus, when administered, a monoclonal antibody will target a particular protein or cell having the specific matching antigenic feature. When coupled with a drug molecule, radioactive isotope or toxin, a monoclonal antibody theoretically, can target the desired cells or tissues with great precision. To date, however, the majority of the MoAb does not reach target tumor cells (less than 0.1% locates in tumor tissue).

Diagnostically, the specificity of monoclonal antibodies helps to detect the presence of endogenous hormones (e.g., luteinizing hormone, human chorionic gonadotropin) in the urine to establish the test results (21). They are also being used to detect allergies, anemia, and heart disease, and commercial monoclonal antibody diagnostic kits are available for drug assays, tissue and blood typing, and such infectious diseases as hepatitis, AIDS-related cytomegalovirus, streptococcal infections, gonorrhea, syphilis, herpes, and chlamydia. When covalently linked with radioisotopes, contrast agents, or anticancer drugs, monoclonal antibodies can be used to diagnose and treat malignant tumors (5).

Muromonab-CD3—Orthoclone OKT3

Muromonab-CD3 is a murine, monoclonal antibody that reacts with a T3 (CD3) molecule that is linked to an antigen receptor on the surface membrane of human T lymphocytes. Thus, it blocks both the generation and function of the T cells in response to antigenic challenge, and is indicated for the treatment of organ transplant rejection. Usually it is combined with azathioprine, cyclosporine, and/or corticosteroids to prevent acute rejection of renal transplants. Simultaneously, the amount of immunosuppressive drugs (e.g., azathioprine, prednisone) a patient must receive has been reduced, effecting better patient outcomes.

Muromonab-CD3 injection is administered by intravenous push over a period not less than 1 minute. For acute renal allograft rejection, it is given in a 5 mg/day dosage for 10 to 14 days. To decrease the incidence of reactions resulting from the first injection of muromonab, methylprednisolone sodium succinate, 8 mg/kg, should be intravenously administered 1–4 hours beforehand.

Muromonab-CD3 injection should be drawn into the syringe through a low-protein-binding 0.2–0.22 μm filter. Once withdrawn, the filter should be discarded and the needle for the intravenous bolus injection attached. Because the drug is a protein solution, it may develop a few fine translucent particles that do not affect its potency. This solution has no preservative, and thus the product must be used immediately upon opening and the unused portion discarded. As with other protein products, it must not be shaken.

Satumomab Pendetide—Oncoscint CR/OV Kit

OncoScint CR/OV-In (Indium In 111 satumomab pendetide) is a diagnostic imaging agent that is indicated for determining the extent and location of extrahepatic malignant disease in patients with known colorectal or ovarian cancer. Clinical studies suggest that this imaging agent should be used after completion of standard diagnostic tests, when additional information regarding disease extent could aid in patient management.

Satumomab pendetide is a conjugate produced from the murine monoclonal antibody, CYT-099 (Mab B72.3). MAb B72.3 is a murine monoclonal antibody of the IgG1, kappa subclass, which is directed to and localizes/binds with a high molecular weight, tumor-associated glycoprotein (TAG-72) that is expressed differentially by adenocarcinomas (22). (*Note:* Adenocarcinoma is a technical name for a malignant tumor derived from a gland or glandular tissue, or a tumor of which the gland-derived cells form gland-like structures.) In in vitro immunohistologic studies, MAb B72.3 has been reported to be reactive with about 83% of colorectal adenocarcinomas, 97% of common epithelial ovarian carcinomas, and the majority of breast, non-small-cell lung, pancreatic, gastric, and esophageal cancers evaluated.

OncoScint CR/OV is prepared by site-specific conjugation of the linker-chelator, glycyltryrosyl-(N,ε-diethylenetriaminepentaacetic acid)-lysine hydrochloride, to the oxidized oligosaccharide component of MoAb B72.3. Each OncoScint CR/OV kit contains all of the nonradioactive ingredients necessary to produce a single unit dose of OncoScint CR/OV-In for use as an intravenous injection. Each kit contains two vials. A single-dose vial of OncoScint CR/OV, formulated with Water for Injection, contains 1 mg of satumomab pendetide in 2 mL of sodium phosphate-buffered saline solution adjusted to pH 6 with hydrochloric acid. OncoScint CR/OV is sterile, pyrogen-free, clear, colorless, and may contain some translucent particles. A vial of sodium acetate buffer contains 136 mg of sodium acetate trihydrate in 2 mL of water for injection adjusted to pH 6 with glacial acetic acid. It is sterile, pyrogen-free, clear, and colorless. Neither solution contains a preservative. Each kit also contains one sterile 0.22 μm Millex GV filter, prescribing information, and two identification labels. The kit should be stored upright in a refrigerator (2°-8°C), but not frozen.

Proper aseptic technique and precautions for handling radioactive materials should be employed. Waterproof gloves should be worn during the radiolabeling procedure. Consistent with the instructions provided, the sodium acetate buffer solution must be added to the indium In-111 chloride solution to buffer it prior to radiolabeling satumomab pendetide. After radiolabeling with indium-111, the immunoscintigraphic agent, OncoScint CR/OV-In (Indium In 111 satumomab pendetide) is formed.

Rituximab—Rituxan

In November, 1997, Rituximab was the first monoclonal antibody approved to treat cancer. It is a chimeric human/murine MoAb directed against the CD20 antigen found on the surface of normal and malignant β-lymphocytes. The Fab domain of rituximab binds to the CD20 antigen on β-lymphocytes and the Fc domain recruits immune effector functions to mediate β-cell lysis *in vitro*.

Rituximab is utilized for the treatment of patients with relapsed or refractory low-grade or follicular, CD20 positive, β-cell non-Hodgkin's lymphoma. The recommended dosage is 375 mg/m^2 given as an IV infusion once weekly for 4 doses (i.e., days 1, 8, 15, 22). It may be administered in an outpatient setting.

The first infusion is administered at a rate of 50 mg/hr. Then, if hypersensitivity or infusion-related events do not occur, the infusion is escalated in 50 mg/hr increments every 30 minutes, to a maximum of 400 mg/hr. If hypersensitivity or infusion-related reactions (e.g., fever, chills, nausea, urticaria, fatigue, headache, bronchospasm) develop, the infusion is interrupted or slowed. These reactions generally present within 30 minutes to 2 hours of the first infusion. Subsequent infusions can be administered at a higher rate (i.e., 100 mg/hr), and increased by 100 mg/hr increments up to a maximum of 400 mg/hr as tolerated.

Premedication with acetaminophen and diphenhydramine may attenuate infusion-related events. Because hypotension may occur during infusion, consideration is suggested to withhold any antihypertensive medication(s) 12 hours prior to rituximab infusion.

Rituximab (as Rituxan) is available in 10 and 50 mL single-unit vials (10 mg/mL). The required amount of drug is withdrawn and diluted to a final concentration between 1 to 4 mg/mL into an infusion bag containing either 0.9% Sodium Chloride or 5% Dextrose in water. The bag is then gently inverted to mix the solution. Any unused portion of the injectable Rituxan is discarded.

Trastuzumab—Herceptin

In September, 1998, trastuzumab became the second monoclonal antibody approved to treat cancer. It is indicated for the treatment of metastatic breast cancer or cancer that has spread beyond the breast and lymph nodes under the arm. The drug is approved for use alone for certain patients who have attempted chemotherapy with little success or as a first-line treatment of metastatic disease when used in combination with paclitaxel (i.e., Taxol) in first-line metastatic breast cancer therapy patients whose tumors overexpress the HER2 protein overexpression.

Specifically, trastuzumab is a chimeric human/ murine MoAb that binds to the HER2 protein found on the surface of normal cells and plays a role in regulating cell growth. In the case of metastatic breast cancer cells, approximately 30% of tumors produce excess amounts of HER2. Thus, only those patients who have tumors with this characteristic have shown benefit to trastuzumab. It should only be used to treat tumors that have HER2 protein overexpression.

The labeling of trastuzumab contains a black box warning regarding risk of ventricular dysfunction and congestive heart failure. Thus, the patient receiving this medicine must be monitored closely.

The recommended intravenous loading dose is 4 mg/kg as a 90 minute infusion. The weekly maintenance dosage is 2 mg/kg over 30 minutes if the loading dosage was well tolerated. Herceptin is available in a 440 mg/21 mL multi-dose vial and can be administered in an outpatient setting.

Palivizumab—Synagis

Palivizumab is a humanized monoclonal antibody (IgG1k) produced by recombinant DNA technology, directed to the epitope in the A antigenic site of the F protein of respiratory syncytial virus (i.e., RSV). It is a composite of human (95%) and murine (5%) antibody sequences.

Palivizumab demonstrates neutralizing and fusion-inhibitory activity against RSV and thus is used therapeutically for the prevention of serious lower respiratory tract disease caused by RSV in pediatric patients. The safety and efficacy of this drug were established in infants with bronchopulmonary dysplasia (BPD) and infants with a history of prematurity ($\leq$ 35 gestational weeks).

Palivizumab is for IM use only and the single-use vials of the drug do not contain a preservative. The injection must be administered within 6 hours after reconstitution.

In prophylaxis studies of pediatric patients with BPD or prematurity, the proportions of subjects in either the placebo and palivizumab groups who experienced adverse side effects were similar. Adverse effects reported in >1% of the palivizumab group included cough, wheezing, asthma, dyspnea, and sinusitis, among others.

The recommended dosage of palivizumab is 15 mg/kg, intramuscularly in the anterolateral aspect of the thigh (preferable location). The use of the gluteal muscle is not advocated as a site of injection because of the risk of sciatic nerve damage. Patients, including those who develop an RSV infection, should receive monthly doses throughout the RSV season. The first dose is to be administered prior to the onset of the RSV season. In the northern hemisphere, the RSV season commences usually in November and lasts through April. However, given certain communities, this may be earlier or later.

Daclizumab—Zenapax

Daclizumab is an immunosuppressive, humanized IgG1 monoclonal antibody produced by recombinant DNA technology that binds specifically to the alpha unit 9Tac subunit) of the human, high affinity interleukin-2 (IL-2) receptor that is expressed on the surface of activated lymphocytes. Daclizumab is a composite of human (90%) and murine (10%) antibody sequences.

Daclizumab is indicated for the prophylaxis of

acute organ rejection in patients receiving renal transplants. It is used as part of an immunosuppressive regimen that includes cyclosporine and corticosteroids.

The typical adverse effects associated with the use of daclizumab were gastrointestinal disorders, including constipation, nausea, diarrhea, vomiting, and abdominal pain, among others. Other side effects include metabolic/nutritional effects (e.g., peripheral edema, fluid overload), CNS (e.g., tremor, headache, dizziness), and genitourinary (e.g., oliguria, dysuria, renal tubular necrosis).

The recommended dosage for daclizumab is 1 mg/kg IV, used as part of an immunosuppressive regimen. The calculated volume of daclizumab is mixed with 50 mL of Sterile 0.9% Sodium Chloride Injection and administered via a peripheral or central vein over a 15 minute period. The standard course of daclizumab therapy is five doses. The first dose is administered ≤24 hours before transplantation, and then the remaining four doses are given at intervals of 14 days.

Basiliximab—Simulect

Basiliximab is an Interleukin-2 (IL-2) receptor antagonist. It is an example of a chimeric (murine/human) monoclonal antibody (IgG_{1K}) produced by recombinant DNA technology. It functions as an immunosuppressive agent, specifically binding to and blocking the IL-2 receptor α-chain (IL-2Rα, also known as the CD25 antigen), which is selectively expressed on the surface of activated T-lymphocytes. This high affinity binding specificity of the drug to IL-2Rα competitively inhibits IL-2-mediated activation of lymphocytes, a critical pathway in the cellular immune response involved in allograft rejection.

Like daclizumab, basiliximab is indicated for the prophylaxis of acute organ rejection in patients receiving renal transplants. It is used as part of an immunosuppressive regimen that includes cyclosporine and corticosteroids.

Basiliximab demonstrates an adverse effect profile similar to daclizumab. Administration of this drug is centrally or peripherally intravenously only. The dilute reconstituted basiliximab (i.e., 20 mg/5 mL) is brought to a 50 mL volume with NSS or dextrose 5% and administered as an IV infusion over a 20 to 30 minute period.

The recommended regimen for an adult is two doses of 20 mg each. The first dose of 20 mg is administered within 2 hours prior to transplantation surgery. The second 20 mg dose is administered 4 days after surgery. For children and adolescents (i.e., 2 to 15 years of age), the recommended regimen is two doses of 12 mg/m² each, up to a maximum of 20 mg/dose. The schedule is the same as that for an adult.

Infliximab—Remicade

Infliximab is the only approved drug therapy specifically indicated for the treatment of fistulizing Crohn's disease. This monoclonal antibody binds and neutralizes tumor necrosis factor alpha (i.e., TNF-alpha). TNF-alpha is one of the primary cytokines that propagate the inflammatory response that is experienced by patients with Crohn's disease. Thus, infliximab reduces the intestinal inflammation indicative of this disease process.

Infliximab is administered in a dose of 5 mg/kg as a single intravenous infusion in those patients with moderately to severely active Crohn's disease. Patients with fistulizing Crohn's disease should receive an initial dose of 5 mg/kg followed by additional doses of 5 mg/kg at the second and sixth weeks following the initial infusion. Infliximab is supplied in single-use 20 mL vials containing 100 mg of the drug.

Infliximab has been associated with hypersensitivity reactions, e.g., urticaria, dyspnea, hypotension, and should be discontinued if severe reactions are experienced by and/or observed in the patient. Additionally, anti-TNF therapy may result in the formation of autoimmune antibodies and, rarely, in the development of a lupus-like syndrome. If a patient develops symptoms suggestive of a lupus-like syndrome and is positive for antibodies against double-stranded DNA, infliximab therapy should be discontinued.

The safety and effectiveness of infliximab therapy beyond a single dose have not been established for the treatment of patients with moderately to severe Crohn's disease or for continuation beyond the three administrations for the treatment of fistulizing Crohn's disease.

Tissue Plasminogen Activators

These are substances produced in small quantity by the inner lining of blood vessels and by the muscular wall of the uterus. Tissue plasminogen activators prevent abnormal blood clotting by converting plasminogen, a component of blood, to the enzyme plasmin. This latter substance breaks down fibrin, the main constituent of a blood clot.

Genetic engineering has prepared these substances artificially and these are used as *thrombolytic agents* (agents that dissolve blood clots).

They are used for conditions such as heart attack, angina, and occluded arteries. Unlike other antico-agulant drugs, tissue plasminogen activator acts only on the site of the clot.

Recombinant Alteplase—Activase

Alteplase, a tissue plasminogen activator produced by recombinant DNA, is used in the management of acute myocardial infarction (AMI), acute ischemic stroke, and pulmonary embolism (PE). It is a sterile, purified glycoprotein of 527 amino acids. It is synthesized using the complementary DNA (cDNA) for natural human tissue-type plasminogen activator obtained from a human melanoma cell line.

The biological activity of alteplase is determined by an in vitro clot lysis assay. The activity is expressed in International Units as tested against the WHO standard. Its specific activity is 580,000 IU/mg. Alteplase is an enzyme (i.e., serine protease) that has the property of fibrin-enhanced conversion of plasminogen to plasmin. It produces limited conversion of plasminogen in the absence of fibrin. When administered, alteplase binds to fibrin in a thrombus and converts the trapped plasminogen to plasmin. This initiates local fibrinolysis with limited systemic proteolysis.

Coronary occlusion due to a thrombus is present in the infarct-related coronary artery in approximately 80% of patients experiencing a transmural myocardial infarction evaluated within 4 hours of onset of symptoms. When administered into the systemic circulation at pharmacological concentrations, alteplase binds to fibrin in a thrombus and, as mentioned, converts the entrapped plasminogen to plasmin. This initiates the lysis of thrombi that are obstructing coronary arteries, thereby improving ventricular function and reducing the incidence of congestive heart failure.

The goal of the management of acute ischemic stroke is to improve neurological recovery and reduce the incidence of disability. Therapy with alteplase for this purpose must be within 3 hours after the onset of stroke symptoms and after exclusion of intracranial hemorrhage by a cranial computerized tomography (CT) scan or other diagnostic imaging procedure of sufficient sensitivity to detect the presence of hemorrhage.

Alteplase is indicated for the management of massive pulmonary embolism in adults, for the lysis of acute pulmonary emboli defined as an obstruction of blood flow to a lobe or multiple segments of the lung, and for the lysis of pulmonary emboli accompanied by unstable hemodynamics

(e.g., failure to maintain blood pressure without supportive measures). Unlabeled uses for alteplase are in patients with unstable angina pectoris where it may effect coronary thrombolysis and a reduction in ischemic events.

An appropriate volume of the accompanying sterile water for injection (without preservatives) is added to the vial containing the lyophilized powder (i.e., 20 mg or 50 mg) (Fig. 18.7). Reconstitution should be with a large-bore needle (e.g., 18 gauge) and the stream of Sterile Water for Injection directed into the lyophilized cake. A slight foaminess can be expected; when allowed to stand undisturbed, it should dissipate within several minutes. The resultant solution appears as a colorless-to-pale-yellow transparent solution having an approximate pH of 7.3 and containing 1 mg/mL.

There are no antibacterial preservatives in the product, so it should be prepared just before use. Because the alteplase possesses a large molecular size, it cannot easily diffuse across biological membranes and must be administered parenterally, usually IV. The solution may be used for direct intravenous administration within 8 hours following reconstitution when stored between 2° and 30° C. Before diluting or administering the product, it is necessary to inspect it visually for particulate matter and discoloration whenever the solution and container permit.

This product may be administered as reconstituted, i.e., 1 mg/mL. Or the reconstituted solution may be diluted further immediately preceding administration with an equal volume of 0.9% sodium chloride injection or 5% dextrose injection. Alteplase is stable for up to 8 hours in these solutions at room temperature and either polyvinyl chloride bags or glass bottles are acceptable. Light exposure has no influence upon stability.

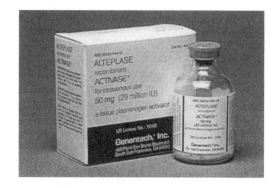

Fig. 18.7 *Example of the product package of Alteplase (Courtesy of Genentech, Inc.).*

Recombinant Reteplase—Retavase

Reteplase is a non-glycosylated deletion mutein of tissue plasminogen activator (tPA) containing 355 of the 527 amino acids of native tPA. It is produced by recombinant DNA in *E. coli*. Its mechanism of action is the same as alteplase.

Reteplase is indicated for the management of AMI in adults for the improvement of ventricular function following an AMI, the reduction of the incidence of congestive heart failure, and the reduction in mortality associated with an AMI.

Reteplase is for IV administration only. It is administered as a 10 + 10U double-bolus injection. Each bolus is administered IV over a 2 minute period. The second bolus is given 30 minutes after initiation of the first bolus injection. An important requirement is that the bolus injection is given via a line in which no other medication is being simultaneously injected or infused. If reteplase must be injected through an IV line containing heparin, the health professional should flush the line with Normal Saline or 5% Dextrose Solution prior to and after reteplase administration.

The lyophilized powder for injection of reteplase should only be reconstituted with Sterile Water for Injection (without preservatives) immediately before use. A colorless solution should be created containing 1 U/mL. A slight foaminess is not unusual at this point and allowing the solution to stand undisturbed for a few minutes will allow dissipation of any large bubbles.

Reteplase (as Retavase) is available in kits. Each kit contains a two single-use reteplase vials of 10.8 U (i.e., 18.8 mg), two single-use diluent vials for reconstitution (i.e., 10 mL Sterile Water for Injection), two sterile 10 mL syringes with 20-gauge needle attached, two sterile dispensing pins, two sterile 20-gauge needles for dosage administration, and two alcohol swabs.

Vaccines

Genetically engineered vaccines use a synthetic copy of the protein coat of a virus to "fool" the body's immune system into mounting a protective response. This avenue avoids the use of live viruses and minimizes the risk of causing the disease the vaccines were intended to prevent. Further, these vaccines will all but eliminate concern about the natural vaccine, which could be derived from blood-donor carriers who may harbor the AIDS virus.

The first genetically engineered vaccine for use in the United States was approved by the FDA in 1986 for hepatitis B, a widespread liver infection. This vaccine has now replaced the plasma-derived vaccine.

Hepatitis B Vaccine Recombinant—Engerix-B, Recombivax HB

The plasma-derived hepatitis B vaccine is no longer being produced in the United States, and its use is limited to hemodialysis patients, other immunocompromised patients, and persons with known allergies to yeast. Recombinant hepatitis B vaccine has demonstrated an ability to induce antibody-to-hepatitis B surface antigen (anti-HBs) that is biochemically and immunologically comparable to antibody induced by the plasma-derived hepatitis B vaccine. Studies demonstrate that the two are interchangeable in their use.

Hepatitis B recombinant vaccine is indicated for immunization of persons of all ages against infection caused by all types of hepatitis B virus. A dialysis formulation (Recombivax HB Dialysis Formulation) is indicated for immunization of adult predialysis and dialysis patients. The vaccine should be administered by intramuscular injection into the deltoid muscle (outer aspect of the upper arm) for the immunization of adults and older children. The anterolateral thigh is recommended for infants and younger children. For those patients with a risk of hemorrhage following IM injection, the vaccine may be administered subcutaneously, although the subsequent antibody titer may be lower and there may be an increased risk of a local reaction.

The vaccine is administered in a three-dose schedule, Recombivax HB (at 0, 1 and 6 months). Ideally, immunization with the vaccine for travelers should be 6 months before traveling to allow completion of the full three-dose vaccine series. However, if 6 months of time before travel is not possible, an alternative four-dose schedule, Engerix-B (at 0, 1, 2, and 12 months) may provide better protection if it can be completed before travel ensues. It is assumed that the four-dose schedule provides a more rapid induction of immunity. However, there is no demonstrated evidence that this schedule provides greater protection than the standard three-dose schedule.

Hemophilus b Conjugate Vaccine— HibTITER, PedvaxHIB, ProHIBiT

Hemophilus influenzae type b (syn. Hib) is a leading cause of serious systemic bacterial disease in the U.S. Among children, the most prevalent cause of *H. influenzae* meningitis is by the capsular strains of type b. In addition to meningitis, Hemophilus b is responsible for other numerous, invasive disease processes (e.g., epiglottitis, sepsis, septic arthritis, osteomyelitis, pericarditis).

Peak incidence of Hib occurs between the ages of 6 to 11 months of age. The incidence of the disease is also prevalent in populations at risk (e.g., daycare attendees, household contacts of cases, Native Americans, blacks, individuals with lower socio-economic status, antibody deficiency syndromes, sickle cell disease).

Hib conjugate vaccines use a new technology, i.e., covalent bonding of the capsular polysaccharide of *Hemophilus influenzae* type b to either diphtheria toxoid, diphtheria CRM_{197} protein or to an OMPC of *Neisseria meningitidis,* to produce an antigen which is postulated to convert the T-independent antigen into a T-dependent antigen. The protein carries both its own antigenic determinants and those of the covalently bound polysaccharide. Thus, the polysaccharide is theorized to be presented as a T-dependent antigen resulting in both an enhanced antibody response and an immunologic memory.

Data is not available regarding the interchangeability of Hib vaccines with regard to safety, immunogenicity or efficacy. Preferably, the same conjugate vaccine should be used throughout the course of immunization. However, it is likely that occasions will arise where the vaccine provider does not know which vaccine was previously used. Under these circumstances, it is prudent for vaccine providers to ensure that, at a minimum, an infant 2 to 6 months of age receives a primary series of three doses of conjugate vaccine.

PedvaxHIB is available as a powder for reconstitution and injection. It is reconstituted only with the aluminum hydroxide diluent that is provided. Once reconstituted, it should be stored in the refrigerator (2° to 8°) and discarded if not used within 24 hours. The reconstituted vaccine must not be frozen. HibTITER and ProHIBiT are available as injections in 1, 5, and 10 dose vials. The HibTITER multidose vials contain thimerosal (1:10000) as a preservative. The ProHIBiT is dissolved in sodium phosphate buffered isotonic sodium chloride solution.

Other Drugs

This section includes drugs that are not conveniently classified into the preceding categories of biotechnology drugs. Nonetheless, they are important for the pharmacist to know about.

Goserelin—Zoladex

Goserelin is indicated for palliative monotherapy of advanced prostatic carcinoma. It is a synthetic luteinizing hormone-releasing hormone (LHRH) analog. Administration of this drug stimulates the release of luteinizing hormone (LH) and follicle-stimulating hormone (FSH) from the anterior pituitary, which transiently increases testosterone concentrations in males. However, continual administration of goserelin in the treatment of prostatic carcinoma suppresses the secretion of LH and FSH, causes a fall in testosterone concentrations, and effects "medical castration." This drug offers an alternative treatment of prostatic cancer when *orchiectomy* (removal of one or both testes) or estrogen administration are not indicated or not acceptable to the patient.

In 1998, the FDA approved the combination of Zoladex (i.e., 3.6 and 10.8 mg goserelin acetate depots) and Eulexin (i.e., flutamide) for the management of locally confined stage B2-C prostate carcinoma.

Goserelin is also indicated for the management of endometriosis, for pain reduction/relief and reduction of endometriotic lesions during therapy. This drug has been demonstrated to be as effective as danazol in relieving the clinical symptoms (dysmenorrhea, dyspareunia, pelvic pain) and signs (pelvic tenderness) of endometriosis and decreasing the size of endometrial lesions. At present, the duration of therapy is recommended to be no longer than 6 months, because there are no clinical data on the effect of treatment of benign gynecological conditions with goserelin for periods greater than 6 months.

Goserelin is administered as a subcutaneous implant and, along with leuprolide acetate (Lupron Depot) was one of the first polymer systems to receive FDA approval for controlled release of a peptide. This drug is available in a 3.6 mg, biodegradable and biocompatible, sterile, white-to-cream-colored cylinder about the size of a grain of rice, which is implanted every 28 days into the upper abdominal wall (Fig. 18.8). The drug is dispersed in a matrix of D,L-lactic acid and glycolic acids copolymer. For additional information on this type of dosage form, the reader is referred to Chapter 19 (i.e., Novel Dosage Forms and Drug Delivery Technologies).

Leuprolide Acetate—Lupron

Leuprolide is a synthetic gonadotropin-releasing hormone (GnRH) analog. Like the naturally occurring luteinizing hormone-releasing hormone (LHRH), initial and intermittent administration of this drug stimulates the release of luteinizing hormone (LH) and follicle-stimulating hormone (FSH) from the anterior pituitary. Like goserelin, continuous administration of leuprolide suppresses the se-

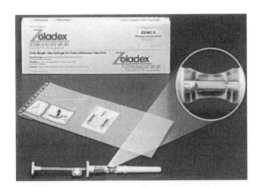

Fig. 18.8 *Example of the product package of Zoladex, which demonstrates the innovative delivery system for the continuous release of goserelin acetate from an injectable pellet (Courtesy of Zeneca Pharmaceuticals Group).*

cretion of LH and FSH, with a concomitant drop in testosterone concentrations and subsequent "medical castration."

The usual adult dose for prostatic carcinoma is a subcutaneous injection of 1 mg/day. There is also a once-a-month (every 28 to 33 days) depot, intramuscular injection. The 7.5 mg strength is used for prostatic carcinoma. The powder for intramuscular injection is reconstituted with a special diluent composed of D-mannitol, purified gelatin, DL-lactic and glycolic acids copolymer, polysorbate 80, and acetic acid.

Lupron should be refrigerated until dispensed, but patients may store the product at room temperature (no more than 30°C, or 86°F). The product should be protected from light and the vial stored in the carton until use. Following reconstitution, the suspension is stable for 1 day. However, because the product has no preservative, it should be discarded if not used immediately.

Recombinant Human DNase I—Pulmozyme

In 1989 the cystic fibrosis (CF) gene was discovered, and it has helped to lay the groundwork for new therapies to treat this disease, which is the most common fatal, genetically inherited disease affecting Whites. Cystic fibrosis transmembrane conductance regulator, the protein product of the CF gene, is defective in its ability to facilitate ion transport across the airway epithelial cells in the lung. This defective regulator allows excessive absorption of sodium and adequate amounts of chloride across the cell membrane. Consequently, water from the mucus of the lung gets absorbed into the cell and the mucus becomes dehydrated, resulting in a thick, tenacious mucus that accumulates in the small airways of the lung. This then leads to a domino effect of chronic infection and in-

flammation, followed by chronic lung disease, pulmonary hypertension, and heart failure.

DNase (recombinant human deoxyribonuclease I), or Dornase alfa, is a DNA enzyme indicated for the treatment of symptoms of cystic fibrosis (CF). This enzyme specifically cleaves extracellular DNA, such as that found in the thick, sticky, mucous secretions of CF patients.[23] As a result, airflow in the lung is improved and the risk of bacterial infection may be decreased. This drug offers hope for breaking the cycle of chronic lung infection and inflammation associated with CF disease, and it demonstrates no effect upon the DNA of intact cells.

DNase showed very successful efficacy data involving over 1100 patients in Phase II and Phase III testing. The drug improved the quality of life for the CF patient with mild to moderate pulmonary dysfunction by reducing the need for I.V. antibiotics, hospitalizations, and time missed from school, work, and everyday activities. The risk of respiratory infections was reduced by 27% for patients on 2.5 mg once daily in clinical trials, and hospital days were reduced from 7.6 days (untreated patients) to 6.2 days (for treated patients) (24).

Indicated to treat cystic fibrosis in patients age 5 years and older, DNase is available in 2.5 mL, single-use polyethylene ampuls for use with compressed air nebulizers (Fig. 18.9). Three nebulizer systems are recommended and the safety and efficacy of the administration of DNase with other nebulizer systems have not been demonstrated. Clinical trials have been performed with the Marquest Acorn II nebulizer; the Hudson T Updraft II nebulizer powered by a DeVilbiss Pulmo-aide Compressor; and the Pari LC nebulizer driven by the Pari Proneb Compressor. Each of these systems delivers approximately 25% of the dose.

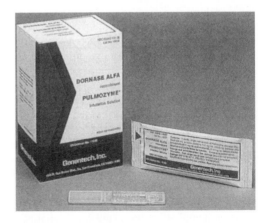

Fig. 18.9 *Example of the product package of Pulmozyme (Courtesy of Genentech, Inc.).*

Portable jet models and ultrasonic nebulizers should not be used to administer DNase. For example, the ultrasonic nebulizers may heat the protein enough to alter its structure. The portable jet nebulizers simply might not be capable of generating enough force or appropriate particle size to ensure optimal delivery of the drug into the lung.

To make administration efficient, it might be tempting to co-administer other compounds (e.g., albuterol, tobramycin) with DNase. However, no other medication should be mixed in the nebulizer system with this drug because the possibility exists that, with a pH change, an alteration of the DNase protein structure could occur. Bronchodilator and antimicrobial agents that are administered via nebulizer should be administered to patients sequentially, but not mixed together. To date, there is no literature that suggests the optimal sequence for all of these drugs to be administered.

The ampuls will have an 18-month expiration dating when stored in the refrigerator between 2° and 8°C and should be protected from light. The product cannot be exposed to room temperatures for more than 24 hours. The patient or caregiver should discard the solution if it is cloudy or discolored and should be told to make sure that the product is within the expiration dating on the amp. Unused amps should be placed in their protective foil pouches under refrigeration.

The Future of Biotechnology Products

The future will see the development of more protein-based pharmaceuticals as a result of modern biotechnologic strategies, including the development of "artificial" genes. These protein-based drugs will present unique challenges because of intrinsic instability, multifaceted metabolic properties, and limited gastrointestinal absorption (25). Their problems will include variable tissue penetration (because of the size of the molecules) and toxicity related to the stimulation of an immune or allergic reaction (25).

A distinct advantage of these biotechnological derived proteins over proteins from natural sources is enhanced purity. Hepatitis B virus and the human immunodeficiency virus (HIV) are capable of contaminating proteins and enzymes from human plasma. If their presence is known, they can be isolated or neutralized. However, sometimes their presence has been confirmed only after disastrous results. Products derived from recombinant technology will not have co-extracted contaminants.

Research is also directed toward the discovery of new methods of delivery for these agents. Delivery systems being explored include transdermal and nasal routes, other forms of injectables, and oral tablets for smaller proteins. Few protein biopharmaceutical products can be administered orally because of their instability in the strong acid environment of the stomach and the low systemic absorption through gastrointestinal mucosa. A challenge is to deliver regulatory proteins (e.g., insulin, growth hormone) to distant organs or tissue without biotransformation. One strategy that may bear fruit is encapsulating the protein-based compound in lipid complexes (liposomes). *Liposomes* are typically composed of some combination of phosphatidylcholine, cholesterol, phosphatidylglycerol, or other glycolipids or phospholipids. These are waterfilled, vesicular structures composed of several phospholipid layers surrounding an aqueous core, and with the outer shell capable of providing direction to specific target cells (e.g., tumors). Typically, liposomes will concentrate the drug in cells of the reticuloendothelial system of the liver and spleen, and will reduce drug intake in the heart, kidney, and gastrointestinal tract. The application of liposome-associated doxorubicin reduces cardiotoxicity, and liposome-associated amphotericin-B reduces nephrotoxicity and other adverse effects (26).

Liposomes are popular among particulate carriers because of their relatively low toxicity and the versatility of their release characteristics and disposition in vivo by changing preparation techniques and bilayer constituents. Depending upon their size, charge, and bilayer rigidity, among other characteristics, liposomes circulate only for a short period of time (minutes) in the circulation before degradation and uptake by macrophages of the mononuclear phagocyte system. Sometimes, their residence in the systemic circulation can be for hours (and even days) if they are stable and not recognized by macrophages as "foreign bodies."

Liposomes have been formulated to contain both the antibody fragment and active drug. For example, in a murine model, doxorubicin has been shown to be specifically targeted to a human breast cancer xerograft by such antibody-covered liposomes. For additional information on liposomes, the reader is referred to Chapter 19 (i.e., Novel Dosage Forms and Drug Delivery Technologies).

Insoluble polymers composed of polyethylene glycol can be utilized to form a protective sheath around a drug, thereby inhibiting its degradation (26). One application of this technology is for the delivery of enzymes that are rapidly cleared from body tissues and fluids. One PEG formulation of the enzyme adenosine deaminase (ADA) has been approved for patients suffering from severe combined immunodeficiency disease (SCID). This condition is caused by a lack of ADA enzyme in lymphocytic WBCs. The polymer affords "protected" delivery of the enzyme to restore lymphocyte function and immunoprotection.

A third strategy delivers extremely toxic proteins to tumor cells. In this prodrug approach, antibodies with specific sensitivities (e.g., monoclonal antibodies) are fused to toxic proteins (e.g., ricin, *Pseudomonas* exotoxin) and then administered intravenously (27). The fused protein is delivered directly to the specified cancer cells, where one released functional molecule can effect cell death. The most widely studied plant toxin is ricin, a natural product of beans from the plant *Ricinus communis* (28). An example of this strategy is Anti-B4-blocked ricin (Oncolysin B) being tested for B-cell leukemias and lymphomas. Ricin, with a protein structure and a molecular weight of 66 kD, has been the prime target for monoclonal antibody conjugation. This unmodified compound is extremely cytotoxic as it enzymatically blocks intracellular protein synthesis at the ribosomal level. It, as well as other immunotoxins, has demonstrated antitumor activity against cultured melanoma cells and melanoma tumors growing in mice. Unfortunately, to date these complexes still have limited target-cell specificity, and uptake/sequestration by the liver remains a problem. Further, once inside the cell, the toxin must translocate across membranes into the cytosol, where it can inhibit protein synthesis (28).

It is entirely feasible in the future that protein complexes will be engineered that combine a "transporting" protein with one that encodes the gene sequence to produce a therapeutic protein in the target tissue. In this instance, the gene will become functional only in certain tissue, with a resultant decrease in delivery to an unintended site.

There is also a growing knowledge base and research about signaling pathways. This has led to the creation of antibodies that target receptors or other molecules involved in the regulation of growth.

The future will also see the creation of more diagnostic products for "in home" testing. Monoclonal antibody-based diagnostic tests that are now restricted to physician use are under development for home testing. These include products for infectious disease processes (e.g., AIDS, chlamydia trachomatis, streptococcal throat infections). In addition, it is anticipated that monoclonal antibody-based tests will also be available to assay blood/plasma concentrations of a number of drugs (e.g., digoxin, phenytoin, theophylline).

To date, monoclonal antibodies have been used in home tests for confirmation of pregnancy or predicting ovulation. Quidel Laboratories has developed a monoclonal antibody product designed to detect pregnanediol glucuronide (a metabolite of progesterone) in female urine and to help avoid pregnancy (21). Levels of this substance fluctuate during the normal menstrual cycle (low in the follicular phase, high in the luteal phase). The self-test kit will enable a woman to monitor urine levels of pregnanediol to determine when fertilization is possible. A woman could then avoid intercourse during her fertile period and prevent the occurrence of pregnancy.

Several biotechnological drugs are being studied for the treatment of rheumatoid arthritis (RA), including monoclonal antibodies, recombinant interleukin-1 receptor antagonists, and a recombinant soluble tumor necrosis factor receptor. Also, the concept of activated T-cells initiating rheumatoid synovitis and maintaining chronic RA has focused new attention on specific pro-inflammatory cytokines such as IL-1 and TNF-α.

These cytokines are believed to be directly responsible for the clinical manifestations of rheumatoid arthritis, and therapies are being directed to specifically target these areas. TNF receptors, for example, are a naturally occurring counter-regulation mechanism to the activity of TNF. Levels of soluble receptors are elevated in plasma and synovial fluid samples of RA patients and patients with other autoimmune and inflammatory conditions. A recombinant human TNFR fusion protein (i.e., etanercept [Enbrelc], has been developed to neutralize TNF and is now undergoing clinical trials.

FDA Office of Biotechnology

In 1989, the FDA Office of Biotechnology was created. The office did not evaluate submissions to the FDA for approval of clinical investigations or for product marketing approvals; these functions are executed by the appropriate FDA Centers. Further, this office was not intended to perform laboratory research or mandate research priorities to the FDA centers. Instead, it was created to serve as a central coordinating, problem-solving, and advisory role within the Office of the Commissioner. It was to become an effective point of contact with the FDA for those outside of the agency on issues related to new biotechnology.

The FDA Office of Biotechnology had the following responsibilities: It,

1. was to advise and assist the Commissioner and other central officials about scientific issues related to biotechnology policy, direction, and long-range goals.
2. represented the Agency on biotechnological issues to other governmental agencies and intergovernmental groups, state and local governments, industry, consumer organizations, Congress, national and international organizations, and the scientific community.
3. provided leadership and direction on scientific and regulatory issues related to biotechnology. This is accomplished through an Agency-wide coordinating group (i.e., the Biotechnology Coordinating Committee) that promotes communication and consistency on biotechnology matters across organizational lines.
4. provided a problem-solving function for individuals, companies, associations, or organizations that have concerns, questions, or complaints about biotechnology policies or procedures, or about product jurisdiction or other aspect of product regulation.
5. coordinated and facilitated guidance on cross-cutting or controversial biotechnology program policies.

Unfortunately, the Office of Biotechnology is no longer in existence. In its place, six divisions relating to biotechnological products (e.g., Division of Monoclonal Antibodies) were created under the aegis of the Office of Therapeutics Research and Review, Center for Biologics Evaluation and Research of the Food and Drug Administration (19). This agency is located at 1401 Rockville Pike, Rockville, MD 20852–1448. Those in need of FDA documents can obtain them through the FDA CBER FAX Information System. This system can be reached at 1–888-CBER-FAX, or at 1–301–827–3844.

Patient Information from the Pharmacist

For those products that can be parenterally self-administered, the pharmacist should instruct patients in the use of aseptic technique. Appropriate verbal instruction that reinforces the printed information sheet should also be provided when the product requires reconstitution. It is desirable to perform the first injection under the supervision of an appropriately qualified health care professional to assure patient comprehension and understanding of technique. Some products (e.g., Betaseron) come with a training video that demonstrates reconstitution and self-administration techniques.

Patients who self-administer these products must be educated on how to prepare (Fig. 18.10) and give the injection and how to rotate injection sites (Fig. 18.11). Some products provide a schematic illustration of this on the patient information sheet. Patients should understand that changing sites each time helps avoid injection reactions and gives the site opportunity to "bounce back" from the previous injection. It is important that the patient understand not to administer an injection into the same area as the prior injection, nor within areas that are tender, red, or hard. The pharmacist should provide a method for the patient to record where previous injections have been made. One simple way is to suggest that the patient note the injection site on a calendar.

Patients should be advised about the proper disposal procedures for needles and syringes. In this day of the cost-conscious consumer, patients must be advised against reusing needles and syringes. A puncture-resistant container for disposal of used needles/syringes is very advantageous to provide the patient—along with instruction for the safe disposal of full containers.

The patient should understand that periodic injection-site reactions may occur during therapy. These may be transient (as in the case of interferon beta-1b) and not require discontinuation of the therapy. It is advisable, however, periodically to reevaluate patient understanding and use of aseptic self-administration technique and procedures.

It is very important for the patient to understand that these products should not be agitated or shaken. Otherwise, there is the possibility of product (protein) denaturation and resultant ineffectiveness. Much like the suspension forms of insulin, which should be rolled (or rotated) in the palms of the hands, these products should be gently swirled to dissolve their contents.

Whenever possible, pharmacists must emphasize the need for compliance with dosage regimens. Betaseron, for example, is administered every other day. A calendar reminder system might be helpful for a patient using this medication.

Pharmacist Self Help With Biotechnology Drugs

The advent of biotechnology drugs poses a real dilemma to some pharmacists. They may be reluc-

PREPARING THE INJECTION

1. Remove the needle guard of the 1 mL syringe and pull back the plunger to the 1 mL mark.

2. Insert the needle of the 1 mL syringe through the stopper of the vial of Betaseron solution.

3. Gently push the plunger all the way down to inject air into the vial (leave the needle in the vial).

4. Turn the vial of Betaseron (Interferon beta-1b) solution upside down.

NOTE: Keep the needle tip in the liquid.

5. Pull back the plunger to withdraw 1 mL of liquid into the syringe.

6. Hold the syringe with the needle pointing upward.

7. Tap the syringe gently until any air bubbles that formed rise to the top of the barrel of the syringe.

8. Carefully push in the plunger to eject ONLY THE AIR through the needle.

9. Remove the needle/syringe from the vial.

10. Recap the needle on the syringe.

NOTE: The injection should be administered immediately after mixing (if the injection is delayed, refrigerate the solution and inject it within 3 hours). Do not freeze.

11. Throw away unused portion of the solution remaining in the vial.

Fig. 18.10 *Preparing the Betaseron for injection (Courtesy of Berlex, Inc.).*

tant to stock these medications because of their high cost, their special storage and handling requirements, poor understanding of the drug's therapeutics (including side effects and counseling information required), and/or the difficult issue of reimbursement (29). These products also are comparably far more expensive than "ordinary" pharmaceuticals.

Unfortunately, pharmacists cannot assume that the responsibility for dispensing these products will automatically fall to them (1). Indeed, the profession's failure to accept responsibility for the radioactive pharmaceutical products used for diagnosis and treatment of disease has resulted in nonpharmacists managing them. Similarly, the profession was not positioned to accept responsibility for patient-controlled analgesia (see Chapter 8) and ultimately lost control to anesthesia depart-

ments in many hospitals. Although there are few biotechnological products for chronic conditions currently available in community pharmacies (except insulin, diagnostic tests, vaccines), drugs initially used exclusively in hospitals, as well as newly developed agents (e.g., Betaseron) will soon work their way into community practice (1).

It is advisable that pharmacists continue their education on these products, and there are numerous programs to do so. Some are available directly from the manufacturer or through professional associations (e.g., "Biotechnology Update," *Journal of the American Pharmaceutical Association*) and cover basic biotechnology and/or therapeutic applications of specific products. Pharmacists should realize that various manufacturers of biotechnology products and professional associations provide support services for the profession. Typically, manufacturer

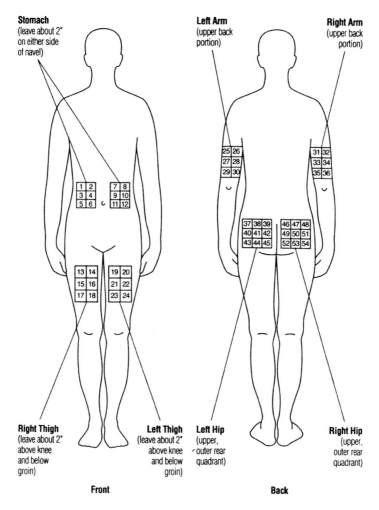

Fig. 18.11 *Schematic for rotation of injection sites (Courtesy of Berlex, Inc.).*

services fall into one of three broad categories—professional services, educational materials, reimbursement support. While the professional services may differ among companies, many have toll-free telephone numbers for obtaining information on biotechnology products.

Pharmacists should take advantage of these programs, realizing that complete knowledge of biotechnology drugs' manufacture is not necessary. Pharmacists should, however, understand protein chemistry (as it relates to drug stability and structure) and immunology. Many programs cover basic biotechnology, as well as therapeutic review of individual drugs. Programs can be very helpful—for example, a real danger with these products is that the pharmacist may confuse products with similar names. Many approved

and investigational interferons (alfa-n3, alfa-2b, gamma-1b, etc.) differ greatly in activity and indications for use (29).

That most biotechnological drugs must be administered parenterally poses a threat to some pharmacists, who are wary of this administration route and cognizant of their limitations/inability to counsel the patients in appropriate technique. Suffice to say, the pharmacist should assume the professional responsibility to secure educational materials (videotapes, print) from the manufacturer. For example, self-injection products contain instruction sheets that offer a step-by-step guide for preparing and administering the injection in the home.

Aside from being knowledgeable about such things as therapeutic use, side effects, precautions, and drug interactions, the pharmacist must also be able to identify monitoring parameters that need to be followed to ensure safety and efficacy.[30] For physiological peptide molecules used for substitution therapy (e.g., insulin, clotting factors, erythropoietin), therapeutic drug monitoring (i.e., measurement of serum drug concentrations) is not indicated because alternative methods are routinely available to assess the efficacy and toxicity of these compounds.[3] As an example, in IDDM patients, insulin is routinely monitored through the use of blood glucose measurements and glycosylated hemoglobin measurements. For clotting factors, their efficacy is assessed by measuring the specific factor being monitored or prothrombin time/partial thromboplastin time (i.e., PT/PTT).

The pharmacist should be aware of drugs that are administered in conjunction with these agents to reduce the incidence and severity of side effects (acetaminophen and indomethacin started immediately before aldesleukin therapy to reduce fever; methylprednisolone sodium succinate IV prior to first injection of muromonab-CD3).

Medical and product information services are available from the manufacturers for biotechnology drugs, just as for traditional drugs. In addition to answering conventional questions about drug use, indications, adverse effects, and so on, this service also helps answer difficult questions (e.g., what to do if a product requiring refrigeration has been left at room temperature for an extended period of time) and helps to facilitate quick replacement of defective products.

Reimbursement issues are not relevant here. However, it is important to realize that manufacturers do have support staff who will help the pharmacist deal with third-party payers, particularly if there is a reimbursement issue/problem. Manufacturer reimbursement assurance programs are designed to remove reimbursement barriers when reimbursement has been denied (e.g., if the drug has been used for an unlabeled indication or used in the home rather than in a hospital or physician's office). Many companies also have had a long-standing tradition of providing prescription medications free of charge to those who might not otherwise have access to necessary medicines. Physicians can secure these on behalf of their patients; the pharmacist can refer patients and their families to pharmaceutical companies who have cost-sharing or financial assistance programs. The Pharmaceutical Research and Manufacturers of America (PhRMA) has a directory of programs available for patients in need. Up-to-date information can be secured by a health care professional by calling the PhRMA (1–800-PMA-INFO) or through the Internet (www.pharma.org/patients).

References

1. Wade DA, Levy RA. Biotechnology: An opportunity for pharmacists. Am Pharm 1992;NS32(9):33–37.
2. Piascik P. Recent biotechnology drug approvals. JAPhA 1998;38 (4):502–505.
3. Wolf BA. Overview of therapeutic drug monitoring and biotechnologic drugs. Ther Drug Monit 1996; 18:402–404.
4. Kohler G, Milstein C. Continuous culture of fused cells secreting antibody of predefined specificity. Nature 1975;256:495–497.
5. Vermeij P, Blok D. New peptide and protein drugs. Pharm World Sci 1996;18 (3):87–93.
6. Peterson NC. Recombinant antibodies: Alternative strategies for developing and manipulating murine-derived monoclonal antibodies. Lab Anim Sci 1996; 46 (1):8–14.
7. Jurcic JG, Scheinberg DA, Houghton AN. Monoclonal antibody therapy for cancer. In: Pinedo HM, Longo DL, Chabner BA, eds. Cancer Chemotherapy and Biological Response Modifiers Annual 17. Elsevier Science B.V., 1997, pp. 195–216.
8. Ballow M, Nelson R. Immunopharmacology: Immunomodulation and immunotherapy. JAMA 1997;278 (22):2008–2017.
9. FDA Medical Bulletin. June 1993; 23(2):4.
10. Sahai J, Louis SG. Overview of the immune and hematopoietic systems. Am J Hosp Pharm 1993;50 (Suppl 3):S4-S18.
11. Metcalf D. The colony stimulating factors. Cancer 1990;65(10)2185–2195.
12. Blackwell S, Crawford J. Colony-stimulating factors: Clinical applications. Pharmacotherapy 1992;12(2, part 2):20S-31S.
13. Oettgen HF. Cytokines in clinical cancer therapy. Curr Opin Immunol 1991;3:699–705.
14. Bagley JL. Biotech. Am Druggist 1986;195(7):57–63.
15. Wordell CJ. Use of beta interferon in multiple sclerosis. Hosp Pharm 1993;28(8):802–807.
16. Piascik P. A new treatment for multiple sclerosis. Am Pharm 1993; NS33(12):25–26.
17. Piascik P. Administering betaseron for MS. Am Pharm 1994;NS34 (1):21–22.
18. Giedlin MA, Zimmerman RJ. The use of recombinant human interleukin-2 in treating infectious diseases. Curr Opin Biotechnol 1993;4:722–726.
19. Stein KE. Overcoming obstacles to monoclonal antibody product development and approval. Trends Biotechnol 1997;15(3):88–90.
20. Tami JA, et al. Monoclonal antibody technology. Am J Hosp Pharm 1986;43:2816–2826.
21. Newton GD. Monoclonal antibody-based self-testing products. Am Pharm 1993;NS33(9):22–23.
22. Berkower I. The promise and pitfalls of monoclonal

antibody therapeutics. Curr Opin Biotechnol 1996; 7(6):622–628.

23. Sindelar RE. Biotech products on the horizon. Am Pharm 1993;NS33(11):27–28.

24. Ramsey B. A summary of the results of the phase III multi-center clinical trial: Aerosol administration of recombinant human DNase reduces the risk of respiratory infections and improves pulmonary function in patients with cystic fibrosis. Pediatric Pulmonol 1993;9(suppl):12–153.

25. Reddy IK, Banga AK. Biotechnology drug delivery: Oral vs. alternate routes. Pharm Times 1993;59(11): 92–98.

26. Hudson RA, Black CD. Novel delivery for protein drugs. Am Pharm 1993;NS33(5):23–24.

27. Houston LL. Targeted delivery of toxins and enzymes by antibodies and growth factors. Curr Opin Biotechnol 1993;4:739–744.

28. Houghton AN, Coit DG. Therapy of metastatic melanoma with monoclonal antibodies. New Perspect Cancer Diagnosis Manage 1993;1 (3):65–70.

29. Piascik P. Getting information about biotechnology products. Am Pharm 1993;NS33(4):18–19.

30. Fields S. Dispensing biotechnology products. Am Pharm 1993;NS33(3):28–29.

Notes

1. The following reference is directed as a resource guide for faculty within schools/colleges of pharmacy: *Biotechnology Resource Guide*, L. Michael Posey, Editor, PCPS, Philadelphia, PA, 1992. Supported by Amgen Inc.

2. The Pharmaceutical Research and Manufacturers of America periodically disseminates *Biotechnology Medicines in Development*, which demonstrates biotechnology medicines that have reached the clinical marketplace or are currently in development. Those desiring to receive this regularly are asked to write to the Editor, Biotechnology Medicines in Development, Communications Division, Pharmaceutical Research and Manufacturers of America, 1100 15th Street, NW, Washington, DC 20005.

19

NOVEL DOSAGE FORMS AND DRUG DELIVERY TECHNOLOGIES

Chapter at a Glance

THIS CHAPTER discusses novel drug delivery systems that are modifications of those previously presented or do not really "fit" into categories in previous chapters. Dramatic changes have been introduced with new technology and new devices now on the market. In some cases, traditional capsules and ointments have been replaced by osmotic pumps, wearable ambulatory pumps, electrically assisted drug delivery and a host of other delivery methods based on various polymer technologies. Feedback mechanisms are now feasible where actual drug delivery may be a response to a sensor detecting variations in certain body chemicals with the resultant infusion of a drug to correct the imbalance.

These changes are coming about as new technologies are developed and to reduce the limitations of existing therapies. In some cases, the new drugs require new delivery systems as the more traditional systems are inefficient or ineffective; this may especially be true of some of the recombinant DNA and gene therapies of the future. We may soon be involved with manipulating genes as active drugs and as drug delivery systems. Some therapies may become very site-specific and require very high concentrations of drugs in certain select sites of the body, as more controlled drug delivery systems will be available in the very near future. Traditional oral medications may not be as effective in these cases.

New drug delivery system development is largely based on promoting the therapeutic effects of a drug and minimizing its toxic effects by increasing the amount and persistence of a drug in the vicinity of a "target" cell and reducing the drug exposure of "nontarget" cells. This is still largely based on Paul Ehrlich's "magic bullet" concept.

Benefits: New drug delivery systems can provide improved or unique clinical benefits, such as 1) improvement of patient compliance, 2) improved patient outcomes, 3) reduction of adverse effects, 4) improving patient acceptance of the treatment, 5) avoidance of costly interventions such as laboratory services, 6) allowing patients to receive medication as outpatients, and possibly 7) a reduction in the overall use of medicinal resources.

Mechanisms: Novel drug delivery systems can include those based on physical mechanisms and those based on biochemical mechanisms. Physical mechanisms, also referred to as controlled drug delivery systems, include osmosis, diffusion, erosion, dissolution and electrotransport. Biochemical mechanisms include monoclonal antibodies, gene therapy and vector systems, polymer drug abducts, and liposomes.

Therapeutic benefits of some of the new drug delivery systems include optimization of the duration of action of the drug, decreasing dosage frequency, controlling the site of release, and maintaining constant drug levels. Safety benefits include reducing adverse effects, decreasing the number of concomitant medications a patient must take, decreasing the need for interventions, and reducing the number of emergency department visits. Economic benefits of novel drug delivery systems include simplifying administration regimens, enhancing patient compliance and an overall reduction of healthcare costs.

Composition

Associated with the various mechanisms that are characteristic or the basis of the newer drug delivery systems, their composition can be quite variable; ranging from naturally-derived substances, such as gelatin and sugars, to the more complex polymers. New drug delivery systems also incorporate mechanical, electronic and computerized components.

The therapeutic efficacy of selected products can be enhanced and, in some cases, the toxicity can be decreased, by incorporating novel polymer technology. For example, degradable bonds can be used to attach an active drug to a synthetic or naturally occurring polymer. Upon delivery to the target site and in the presence of certain enzymes or through hydrolysis, etc., the product can be cleaved releasing the active drug at a specific site of action. Oral, topical, parenteral and implantable drugs can potentially be used with this approach.

A number of different release profiles using poly-

mers are possible as well as actual penetration into specific tissues and specific target sites selected. Potential problems of polymers, however, include 1) their high molecular weight may cause them to be very slowly excreted from the body, 2) due to their size, their permeability through various membranes may be slow, 3) immunologic or toxic reactions may occur, and 4) since they are complex, they may be labor-intensive and expensive to develop. Novel drug delivery systems will be discussed under the general categories of topical, oral, vaginal, implants, ophthalmics and parenterals.

Topical Administration

The basis for the development of transdermal drug delivery systems (patches) involves percutaneous absorption. The reader is referred to Chapters 9 and 10 for background information on transdermal systems and penetration enhancers. Novel topical systems include iontophoresis (IP) and phonophoresis.

Iontophoresis

Iontophoresis is an electrochemical method that enhances the transport of some solute molecules by creating a potential gradient through the skin tissue with an applied electrical current or voltage. It induces an increased migration of ionic drugs into the skin by electrostatic repulsion at the active electrode: negative ions are delivered by the cathode and positive ions by the anode. A typical iontophoresis device consists of a battery, microprocessor controller, drug reservoir and electrodes.

Advantages of IP include 1) providing for controlling the delivery rates (through variations of current density, pulsed voltage, drug concentration and ionic strength), 2) eliminating gastrointestinal incompatibility, erratic absorption, and first pass metabolism, 3) reducing side effects and interpatient variability, 4) avoiding the risks of infection, inflammation, and fibrosis associated with continuous injection or infusion, and 5) enhancing patient compliance with a convenient and non-invasive therapeutic regimen.

Disadvantages of IP can be skin irritation at high current densities; this can be eliminated or minimized by lowering the current for administration.

Iontophoresis is gaining increasing acceptance in the pharmaceutical industry with small, efficient iontophoretic patches projected to be on the market within the next few years. Miniaturization is now possible with smaller, more powerful batteries and electronics. The next generation iontophoresis patch may also include an electronic record of the date, time and quantity of each dose delivered; providing information for determining patient compliance. Currently, however, iontophoresis involves the use of an iontophoretic device attached to electrodes containing a solution of the drug.

As previously mentioned, iontophoresis involves the use of small amounts of physiologically acceptable electric current to move charged, or ionized, drugs through the skin. By placing an ionized solution of the drug in an electrode of the same charge and applying a current, the drug is repelled from the electrode into the skin. This method of drug delivery is not new but has been around for at least 100 years. Since the 1930s, iontophoresis of pilocarpine has been used to induce sweating in the diagnosis of cystic fibrosis. More recently, iontophoresis has been used in the topical delivery of fluoride to the teeth, dexamethasone as an anti-inflammatory into joints and lidocaine as a topical anesthetic. Drugs such as corticosteroids, nonsteroidal anti-inflammatory agents and anesthetics are commonly delivered via iontophoresis. Other drugs currently under study include a number of analgesics, nicotine, anti-AIDs drugs, and cancer drugs, insulin, proteins. Iontophoresis is also useful in veterinary medicine.

In the iontophoresis process, the current, beginning at the device, is transferred from the electrode through the ionized drug solution as ionic flow. The drug ions are moved to the skin where the repulsion continues moving the drug through whatever pathways are available, namely pores and possibly through a disrupted stratum corneum. The drug-containing electrode is termed the active electrode and the other electrode is the passive electrode, which is placed elsewhere on the body. Current densities up to 0.5 mA/cm^2 can be tolerated by the body with little or no discomfort. The larger the electrode surface, the greater the current the device must supply to provide a current density for moving the drug.

The delivery of a drug iontophoretically is quite complex, depending upon the interactions between the drug and the vehicle electrolyte or buffer, partitioning of the drug between the vehicle and the skin, and then diffusion through a highly heterogeneous membrane under the influence of both a chemical and electrical potential gradient.

The movement of ions across the skin is described by the relationship known as the Nernst-Planck equation:

$$J_i = -D_I \, dC_i/dx - z_i \, m \, F \, C_i \, dE/dx$$

where J_i = flux; D_i = diffusivity; dC_i/dx = concentration gradient; z_i = valence of the species

I; m = mobility; F = Faraday's constant; C_I = Concentration; dE/dx = electrostatic potential gradient.

Variables affecting the iontophoresis process include aspects of the current, the physicochemical properties of the drug, formulation factors, biological factors and electroendosmotic flow.

The *current* can be direct, alternate or pulsed and can have various waveforms, including square, sinusoidal, triangular and trapezoidal. There may not be much advantage to the more complex forms as direct current is most commonly used at this time.

Physicochemical variables include the charge, size, structure and lipophilicity of the drug. The drug should be water soluble, low-dose and ionizable with a high charge density. Smaller molecules are more mobile but large molecules are also iontophoresable.

Formulation factors include drug concentration, pH, ionic strength, and viscosity. Increasing drug concentration usually results in greater drug delivery to a certain degree. The inclusion of buffer ions in a formula will compete with the drug for the delivery current, decreasing the quantity of drug delivered, especially since buffer ions are generally smaller and more mobile than the larger active drug. The pH of solutions can be adjusted and maintained by larger molecules, such as ethanolamine:ethanolamine HCl rather than the smaller hydrochloric acid and sodium hydroxide. An increase in ionic strength of the system will also increase the competition for the available current, especially since the active drugs are generally potent and present in a small concentration as compared to these extraneous ions.

Biological factors involve the skin to which the electrodes are applied; its's thickness, permeability, presence of pores, etc.

Electroendosmotic flow results when a voltage difference is applied across a charged porous membrane, resulting in a bulk fluid flow which occurs in the same direction as the flow of counter-ions. This fluid flow can actually carry a drug with it into the skin, especially of positively charged, cationic, drugs. Neutral drugs can also be carried via electroendosmotic flow.

Iontophoretic devices have changed remarkably over the years, ranging from the galvanometers of the past to the small, specially designed units of today. Iontophoresis devices available from various companies are listed in Table 19.1.

Iontophoretic units of the future will soon be marketed in a size similar to the currently available transdermal patches. They will be slightly thicker to

Table 19.1.   Iontophoresis Equipment, Including Devices and Electrodes

Devices			*Electrodes*		
Company	*Brand Name*	*mA-min*	*Brand*	*Reservoir Comp.*	*Buffer System*
Empi, Inc. (St. Paul, MN)	Dupel	160	EBIE	Polyester fleece	Ion exch resin
Henley Healthcare (Sugarland, TX)	Dynaphor	manual	Iotrode	Cotton/Rayon	0.9% NaCl with 0.5% KHPO4-
Iomed (Salt Lake City, UT)	Phoresor II	80	Trans Q1/Q2 Trans QE	Hydrogel Hydrogel/Sponge	Ag+/AgCl Ag+/AgCl
LifeTech, Inc. (Houston, TX)	Iontophor PM/DX Microphor	150 80	Meditrode	Cotton/Rayon	0.9% Saline 0.5% KHPO$_4$
General Medical CO. (Los Angeles, CA)	Lectro Patch Drionic	Infinite Infinite	Lectro Patch Drionic	Polyester fleece Polyester fleece/wool	—
Wescor Inc. (Logan, UT)	Sweat-Chek	7.5	Pilogel discs	Gel reservoir	
Scandipharm (Birmingham, AL)	CF Indicator	160	Built-in	Hydrogel	Ag+/AgCl

accommodate the power source and small microprocessor controllers. The future may include IP patches capable of sampling and testing (e.g. glucose levels) and adjusting the delivery rate of a drug (e.g. insulin) all in the same IP system. It should be mentioned that reverse iontophoresis can be used to "extract" chemicals/drugs present in the body for testing. Many types of patches/electrodes may be available that require pharmacists involvement to add the drug prior to dispensing, as is done today in filling various reservoirs for parenteral administration. Drugs currently administered using iontophoresis are listed in Table 19.2.

A new iontophoresis system called Numby Stuff (IOMED) is used to achieve local anesthesia of the skin and is promoted as a "painless, needleless system."

Iontophoretic administration is also used in veterinary pharmacy, using drugs such as those listed in Table 19.3. Due to the difference in the size and anatomy of the animal patient, different electrodes may be required.

Phonophoresis

Phonophoresis (ultrasound, sonophoresis, ultrasonophoresis, ultraphonophoresis) is the transport of drugs through the skin using ultrasound; it is a combination of ultrasound therapy with topical drug therapy to achieve therapeutic drug concentrations at selected sites in the skin. It is widely used by physiotherapists. In this technique, the drug is generally mixed with a coupling agent, usually a gel but sometimes a cream or ointment is used, which transfers ultrasonic energy from the phonophoresis device to the skin, through this coupling agent. The ultrasonic unit has a sound transducer head emitting energy at 1 MHZ at 0.5 to 1 W/cm^2. Although the exact mechanism is not known, it may involve a disruption of the stratum corneum lipids allowing the drug to pass through the skin.

Originally, the drug-containing coupling agent was applied to the skin immediately followed by the ultrasound unit. Today, the product is applied to the skin and a period of time allowed for the drug to begin absorption into the skin; then, the ultrasound unit is applied. The ultrasound emitted from the unit is actually sound waves that are outside the normal human hearing range. As ultrasound waves, they can be reflected, refracted and absorbed by the medium, just like regular sound waves can. Consequently, these are factors that must be considered as affecters of phonophoresis efficiency.

Three effects that result from ultrasound include cavitation, microstreaming and heat generation. Cavitation involves the formation and collapse of very small air bubbles in a liquid in contact with ultrasound waves. Microstreaming, closely associated with cavitation, results in efficient mixing by inducing eddies in small volume elements of a liquid; this may enhance dissolution of suspended

Table 19.2. Drugs Used in Iontophoresis

Drug Solution	Concentration (%)	Use/Indication	Polarity
Acetic acid	2–5	Calcium deposits, calcified tendonitis	Negative
Atropine sulfate	0.001–0.01	Hyperhidrosis	Positive
Calcium chloride	2	Myopathy, myospasm, immobile joints	Positive
Sodium chloride	2	Sclerolytic, scar tissue, adhesions, keloids	Negative
Copper sulfate	2	Astringent, fungus infection	Positive
Dexamethasone Sodium phosphate	0.4	Tendonitis, bursitis, arthritis, tenosynovitis, Peyronie's Disease	Negative
Estriol	0.3	Acne scars	Positive
Fentanyl citrate		Analgesic	Positive
Fluoride sodium	2	Desensitize teeth	Positive
Gentamicin sulfate	0.8	Ear chronditis	Positive
Glycopyrronium bromide	0.05	Hyperhidrosis	Positive
Hyaluoronidase	150 units/mL solution	Absorption enhancement, edema, scleroderma, lymphedema	Positive
Idoxuridine	0.1	Herpes simplex	Negative
Iodine ointment	4.7	Sclerolytic, antimicrobial, fibrosis, adhesions, scar tissue, trigger finger	Negative
Iron/titanium oxide		Skin pigmentation	Positive
Lidocaine hydrochloride	4 (with or without epinephrine 1:50,000 to 1:100,000)	Skin anesthesia, trigeminal neuralgia	Positive
Lithium chloride	2	Gouty arthritis	Positive
Magnesium sulfate	2	Muscle relaxant, vasodilator, myalgias, neuritis, deltoid bursitis, low back spasm	Positive
Mecholoyl chloride	0.25	Vasodilator, muscle relaxant, radiculitis, varicose ulcers	Positive
Meladinine sodium	1	Vitiligo	Negative
Methylphenidate hydrochloride		Attention deficit disorder	Positive
Morphine sulfate	0.2–0.4	Analgesic	Positive
Pilocarpine hydrochloride		Sweat test for cystic fibrosis	Positive
Poldine methyl sulfate	0.05–0.5	Hyperhidrosis	Negative
Potassium iodide	10	Scar tissue	Negative
Sodium salicylate	2	Analgesic, sclerolytic, plantar warts, scar tissue, myalgias	Negative
Tretinoin		Acne scars	Positive
Water	100	Palmar, plantar, axillary hyperhidrosis	Post/Neg
Zinc oxide suspension	20	Antiseptic, ulcers, dermatitis, wound healing	Positive

drug particles resulting in a higher concentration of drug near the skin, for absorption. Heat results from the conversion of ultrasound energy to heat energy and can occur at the surface of the skin as well as in deeper layers of the skin.

The vehicle containing the drug must be formulated to provide good conduction of the ultrasonic energy to the skin. The product must be smooth and non-gritty as they will be rubbed into the skin by the head of the transducer. The product should be of relatively low viscosity for ease of application and ease of movement of the transducer head during the ultrasound process. Gels work very well as a medium. Emulsions have been used but the oil:water interfaces in emulsions can disperse the ultrasonic waves, resulting in a reduction of the intensity of the energy reaching the skin. It may also cause some localized heating. Air should not be incorporated into the product as air bubbles may disperse the ultrasound waves resulting in heating at the liquid:air interface.

Hydrocortisone is the drug most often administered in concentrations ranging from 1–10%.

Table 19.3.   Drugs Used in Veterinary Iontophoresis

Drug Solution	Commercially Available Concentration (mg/mL)	Total Quantity used in a 6 mL Electrode (mg)	Polarity Used
NSAIDS			
Phenylbutazone	200	1200	Negative
Flunixin meglumine	50	300	Negative
Ketoprofen	100	600	Negative
CORTICOSTEROIDS-ANTI-INFLAMMATORY AGENTS			
Dexamethasone sodium phosphate	2 or 4	12 or 24	Negative
Betamethasone	4	24	Negative
Prednisolone sodium succinate	10 or 50	60 or 300	Negative
ANTIBIOTICS			
Gentamicin sulfate	50 or 100	300 or 600	Positive
Amikacin sulfate	50	300	Positive
Ceftiofur sodium	50	300	Negative
LOCAL ANESTHETICS			
Ldiocaine hydrochloride	20	120	Positive

*Adapted from Product Information 801419 Rv., B:, Empi, Inc., St. Paul, MN., 1996

Oral Administration

Rapid-Dissolving Tablets

A relatively new entry into the market place is the new "rapidly dissolving tablets" (RDTs). The original "fast-dissolving tablets" are the molded tablets for sublingual use. These tablets generally consisted of active drug and lactose moistened with an alcohol-water mixture to form a paste. The tablets were then molded, dried and packaged. For use, they were simply placed under the tongue to provide a rapid onset of action for drugs such as nitroglycerin. Also, they have been used for drugs that are destroyed in the gastrointestinal tract and were administered sublingually for absorption that would minimize the first-pass effect, such as testosterone.

The new "rapidly dissolving tablets" are designed for orally administered drugs for patients that have difficulty swallowing standard tablets/capsules, such as children and the elderly. These RDTs are more convenient to carry and administer than an oral liquid. There currently are no standards that define a "rapidly dissolving tablet" but one that could be considered would be a tablet that disintegrates/dissolves within approximately 15–30 seconds in the mouth; anything slower than about 15–30 seconds would not really be categorized as "rapidly" dissolving.

In addition to the advantages listed above, there are a number of disadvantages and difficulties associated with formulating RDTs, including drug loading, taste masking, friability, manufacturing costs and stability of the product.

Drug loading involves the incorporation of the drug into the dosage form. Some RDTs are made as blanks to which a drug is "postloaded" or added after the blank is made. Generally, the drug is in solution form and is added to the tablet where the solvent then evaporates. It is also possible for the drug to be added as a dry powder electrostatically at this stage. Most drugs, however, are incorporated into the tablets during the manufacturing process.

Taste masking poses numerous challenges for RDTs. Since the drug product dissolves in the mouth, any taste of the drug must be covered, either by a flavoring technique or by micro- or nanoencapsulation. The product also should be nongritty, necessitating very small particle sizes if microencapsulation is used.

Friability is an inherent problem in RDTs. For a product to instantly dissolve, is may be quite friable. To make it less friable, then the disintegration/dissolution time may be increased. A balance generally must be achieved between friability and speed of disintegration/dissolution.

Lyophilized Foam

The first entry into this field was the Zydis delivery system. The tablets are prepared by foaming a mixture of gelatin, sugar(s), drug, etc. and pouring the foam into a mold. The mold also serves as the unit-dose dispensing package. The foam is lyophilized and the tablets in the mold are packaged. This system is the fastest on the market as the tablets will dissolve in a matter of a few seconds when placed on the tongue. One disadvantage of this method is that tastemasking can be a problem since the drug is incorporated during the formation of the tablet itself. Another difficulty is that these tablets are sometimes difficult to remove from the packaging, since they are soft and one should not press on the dosage unit to remove it, but should peel off the material exposing the tablet in its mold. A commercial example is the Dimetapp Cold & Allergy Quick Dissolve Tablets. The tablets contain phenylpropanolamine hydrochloride 6.25 mg, brompheniramine maleate 1 mg, aspartame, FD&C Blue 2, FD&C Red 40, Flavors, Gelatin, Glycine and Mannitol (1).

Claritin (loratadine) rapidly-disintegrating tablets (Reditabs, Schering Corporation) contain 10 mg of micronized loratadine in a base containing citric acid, gelatin, mannitol and mint flavor; the Zydis technology. It disintegrates within seconds after being placed on the tongue, with or without water. Claritin Reditabs have been shown to provide at least equivalent pharmacokinetic parameters as compared to the traditional tablets; in some cases the Reditabs provided greater C_{max} and AUC values. Claritin Reditabs are blister package-formed tablets that should be stored in a dry place, between 2 and 25°C. They should be used within 6 months of opening the protective laminated foil pouch containing the blister cards of tablets; each foil pouch contains one blister card containing 10 individually sealed tablets (2).

Compression

Another method of preparation is using standard tableting technology with a composition that will enhance fluid uptake and tablet disintegration/dissolution. For example, superdisintegrants incorporated with a small quantity of effervescent material will lead to an intermediately fast disintegration. The tablets are compressed a little thinner in geometry than standard tablets to allow for a larger surface area being exposed to the saliva in the mouth. Upon placement in the mouth, the disintegrant starts wicking water into the tablet. The effervescent materials start dissolving and aid in the breakup process. This continues until the tablet has disintegrated.

An example product is Tempra Quicklets containing 80 mg of acetaminophen. These tablets also contain aspartame, citric acid, D&C Red No. 27 Lake, FD&C Blue No. 1 Lake, Flavor, Magnesium stearate, mannitol, potassium carbonate, silicon dioxide and sodium bicarbonate. These tablets are somewhat slower than the Zydis tablet taking about 30–45 seconds for completion, unless some tongue pressure is used. These tablets are packaged in a firm molded plastic package to prevent breakage (3).

Osmotic Pump

Numerous drug delivery devices now use osmosis as the driving force. The Alzet (Alza osmotic minipump) is used in research laboratories to provide constant-rate delivery and preprogrammed delivery of a drug. It consists of a flexible impermeable diaphragm surrounded by a sealed layer containing an osmotic agent that is enclosed within a semipermeable membrane. A tube or catheter (stainless steel or polyethylene) is inserted into the inner chamber from which the drug is channeled. When the unit is subjected to an aqueous medium, the water flows through the rate-controlling semipermeable membrane and dissolves the osmotic agent, which provides the pressure on the flexible lining and forces the drug through the tube or catheter. The unit can be presterilized and prefilled using a filling tube.

With the Alzet pump, the drug reservoir is a liquid solution inside a collapsible, impermeable polyester bag coated with a layer of an osmotically active salt. It is sealed within a rigid structure coated with a semipermeable membrane. As the salt dissolves, it creates an osmotic pressure gradient, the drug compartment is reduced in volume forcing the drug solution out. The delivery rate can be changed by changing the drug concentration. The Acutrim product containing phenylpropanolamine is an example product that is used as an appetite suppressant in weight-control programs (4).

Fentanyl Lollipops

The fentanyl Oralet (Abbott Laboratories) is a bullet-sized red "lollipop" that is used to relax a patient and block pain; it is used as a preoperative sedative indicated for sedation/analgesia prior to diagnostic or therapeutic procedures in hospital settings. After sucking on the raspberry flavored lollipop, the fentanyl is absorbed into the bloodstream with an onset of action of about 10 minutes. The Oralet produces a light "conscious sedation" and only relaxes the child. Its effects wear off quickly which decreases the risk of complications that stronger sedatives may cause. One concern that has been expressed is that the product looks and tastes like candy and may be accidentally ingested by a child. This is handled by special child-resistant packaging for the product. An overdose is not too likely as the child will become sleepy, fall asleep and stop licking the sucker (5).

The fentanyl Actiq (manufactured by Anesta Corporation and distributed by Abbott Laboratories) is a raspberry lollipop that differs from the fentanyl Oralet. It is a sugar-based lozenge on a stick and contains fentanyl citrate. It is an off-white color and the stick bears a large "Rx" mark. Actiq is the first product specifically designed to aid in controlling "breakthrough" pain experienced by cancer patients. It is indicated only for the management of breakthrough cancer pain in patients with malignancies that are already receiving and who are tolerant to opioid therapy. Breakthrough cancer pain occurs in about 50% of all cancer pain patients and is a component of chronic cancer pain that is particularly difficult to treat due to its severity, rapid onset and frequent unpredictability. The lollipop provides almost immediate relief as the drug starts being absorbed in the oral cavity and starts to work within minutes; its effects last for only about 15 minutes but that is usually long enough to relieve breakthrough pain. The concern expressed about this product being accidentally used by children is addressed by special packaging that requires scissors to open (6).

Vaginal Administration

Intravaginal Drug Delivery System

Vaginal administration of drugs, especially hormones, has several advantages, including self-insertion and removal and continuous drug administration at an effective dose level and better patient compliance. The continuous release and local absorption of drug minimizes systemic toxicity that may result from oral peak and valley drug administration.

In a polymeric vaginal drug delivery system, such as a medicated, resilient vaginal ring, shown in Figure 19.1 or a copper-containing intrauterine contraceptive device, the drug may be uniformly distributed throughout the polymeric matrix. Upon administration and when in contact with vaginal fluids, the drug will slowly dissolve and migrate out of the device. Drug inside the device will diffuse towards the surface along a concentration gradient resulting in a long-acting drug delivery system.

Intrauterine Progesterone Drug Delivery System

The Progestasert System (Alza Corporation) shown in Figures 19.2 and 19.3 slowly releases an average of 60 µg of progesterone per day for a period of 1 year after insertion. The continuous release of progesterone into the uterine cavity provides a local rather than a systemic action. Two hypotheses for the contraceptive action have been offered:

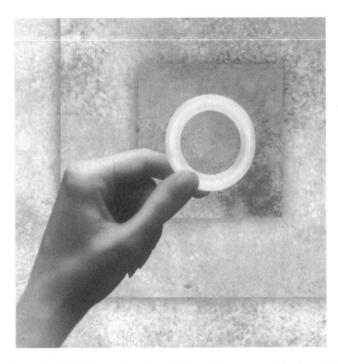

Fig. 19.1   *The Estring (Pharmacia & Upjohn), a polymeric vaginal drug delivery system. (Courtesy of Pharmacia & Upjohn).*

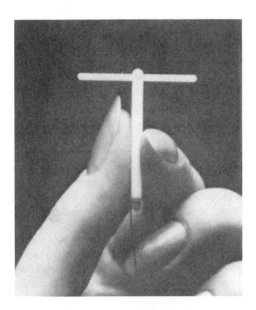

Fig. 19.2 *Progestasert Intrauterine Progesterone Contraceptive System enables the prevention of pregnancy in women for a year or more after each insertion. This small, flexible unit releases the natural hormone progesterone directly into the uterus. (Courtesy of Alza Corporation).*

progesterone-induced inhibition of sperm capacity or survival; and, alteration of the uterine milieu so as to prevent nidation. The intrauterine device contains 38 mg of progesterone, a much smaller amount than would otherwise be taken by other routes over a year period for the same purpose. The intrauterine device is replaced annually for the maintenance of contraception (7).

The Progestasert is a T-shaped, polymeric, progesterone-containing device that continuously delivers 65 μg of progesterone per day for one year. This provides contraception without the need for daily self-medication and has the advantages of 1) using a natural hormone, 2) no estrogens, 3) using a T-shaped delivery device to assure comfort, safety and retention, minimizing mechanically-induced irritation, and 4) the hormonal action is confined to the uterus.

The device contains 38 mg of progesterone suspended in silicone oil; barium sulfate is added to make it radiopaque. The EVA membrane surrounding the drug core controls the rate of drug release. Titanium dioxide is added to the EVA for a white color. At the end of one year, the device will contain approximately 14 mg of progesterone; the excess being required to maintain the thermodynamic activity of the drug reservoir.

Dinoprostone Vaginal Insert

Dinoprostone (Cervidil, Forest Pharmaceuticals, Inc.) is a thick, flat, polymeric slab, rectangular in shape enclosed in a pouch of a knitted polyester retrieval system. The polymeric, hydrogel slab is buff colored, semitransparent and contains 10 mg of dinoprostone. The retrieval system is in the shape of a long knitted tape that is used to retrieve, or remove, the unit after the dosing interval is completed. The product is designed to release dinoprostone in vivo at a rate of about 0.3 mg/hour. The unit contains 10 mg of dinoprostone in 236 mg of a cross-linked polyethylene oxide/urethane polymer slab that measures 29 mm by 9.5 mm and is 0.8 mm thick. When placed in a moist environment, the unit absorbs water, swells and releases dinoprostone.

It is indicated for the initiation and/or continuation of cervical ripening in patients at or near term when there is medical or obstetrical indication for labor induction.

The product is dosed at 10 mg of dinoprostone (1 unit) inserted vaginally and removed upon onset of active labor or 12 hours after insertion. After administration, the patient should remain supine for 2 hours, but may be ambulatory after that time.

This product should be stored in a freezer between -20 and -10°C (-4 and 14°F); it is packaged in foil and is stable in the freezer for a period of three years. After opening and upon exposure to humidity, it is hygroscopic and the release characteristics of the dinoprostone may be altered if improperly stored (8). An example is shown in Figure 19.4.

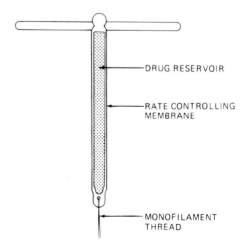

Fig. 19.3 *Schematic of the Progestasert intrauterine drug delivery system. (Courtesy of Alza Corporation).*

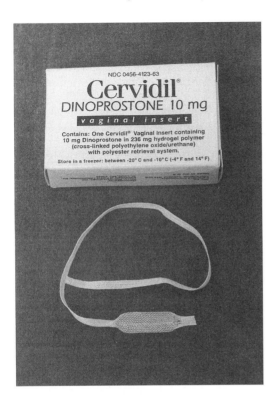

Fig. 19.4 *Cervidil (dinoprostone) vaginal insert. The polymeric slap, containing the dinoprostone, is encased in a pouch of a knitted polyester delivery and retrieval system. (Courtesy of Forest Pharmaceuticals, Inc.).*

Urethral Administration

Alprostadil Urethral MicroSuppository

The MUSE (alprostadil) urethral microsuppository is a single-use, medicated transurethral system for the delivery of alprostadil to the male urethra. The drug is suspended in a polyethylene glycol 1450 excipient and is formed into a medicated pellet, or microsuppository, measuring 1.4 mm in diameter by 3 mm or 6 mm in length. Available strengths are 125, 250, 500 and 1000 μg per unit. The microsuppository resides in the tip of a tran-slucent hollow applicator. It is administered by inserting the applicator tip into the urethra after urination. The pellet is delivered by depressing the applicator button. The polyethylene glycol 1450 vehicle will dissolve in the available fluid releasing the drug for absorption. The applicator system is composed of medical grade polypropylene; each system is individually foil-packaged. The MUSE microsuppository is indicated for the treatment of erectile dysfunction.

Implants

Implants are defined as sterile, solid drug products made by compression, melting or sintering processes. They generally consist of the drug and rate-controlling excipients.

Levonorgestrel Implant

The "Norplant" device consists of levonorgestrel incorporated into a medical-grade silastic material measuring about 34 mm long. For administration, six capsules are placed subdermally, within one week of the onset of menses, into the inner portion of the upper arm in a fan shape. This is done through a 5 mm incision and the drug delivery is designed to last approximately 5 years. The Norplant device has been shown to be an excellent contraceptive with a significantly lower pregnancy rate then the copper-based IUD. Movement of the capsules within the implanted site have been minimal. Removal of the device due to side effects has been primarily related to bleeding irregularities (9).

Gliadel Wafer Implant

Gliadel Wafer (polifeprosan 20 with carmustine implant), shown in Figures 19.5 through 19.7, is a sterile, off-white to pale yellow wafer approximately 1.45 cm in diameter and 1 mm thick. Each wafer contains 192.3 mg of a biodegradable polyanhydride copolymer and 7.7 mg of carmustine. Polifeprosan 20 consists of poly[bis(p-carboxyphenoxy) propane: sebacic acid] in a 20:80 molar ratio and is used to control the local delivery of carmustine, which is distributed uniformly throughout the copolymer matrix.

Gliadel is designed to deliver the carmustine directly into the surgical cavity created when a brain tumor is resected, with numerous wafers being used depending upon the desired dose. When exposed to the aqueous environment in the resection cavity, the anhydride bonds in the copolymer are hydrolyzed, releasing the carmustine, carboxyphenoxypropane and sebacic acid. The active drug, carmustine, is released from the wafer and diffuses into the surrounding brain tissue, producing an antineoplastic effect by alkylating DNA and RNA.

In three weeks, more than 70% of the copolymer degrades; with carboxyphenoxypropane being eliminated by the kidney and sebacic acid being metabolized by the liver and expired as carbon dioxide.

Each wafer contains 7.7 mg of carmustine and

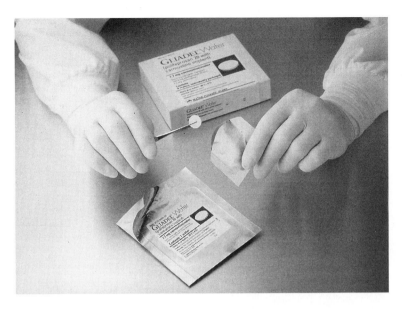

Fig. 19.5 *Gliadel Wafer (polifeprosan 20 with carmustine implant) and packaging components. (Courtesy of Guilford Pharmaceuticals).*

when eight wafers are used (the recommended dose), a dose of 61.6 mg is delivered. The wafers are supplied in a single dose treatment box containing eight individually pouched wafers. Each wafer is double pouched in foil. The inner pouch is sterile; upon removing the outer foil pouch in an aseptic working environment, the inner pouch is treated as a sterile item. Gliadel wafers must be stored at or below -20°C.(10)

Zoladex Implant

Zoladex (goserelin acetate implant, Zeneca Pharmaceuticals) is a sterile, biodegradable product containing goserelin acetate, equivalent to 3.6 mg of drug, designed for subcutaneous injection with continuous release over a 28 day period. Goserelin acetate is dispersed in a matrix consisting of D,L-lactic and glycolic acids copolymer

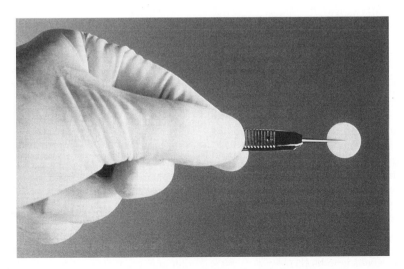

Fig. 19.6 *Gliadel Wafer removed from sterile foil pouch in preparation for implantation. (Courtesy of Guilford Pharmaceuticals).*

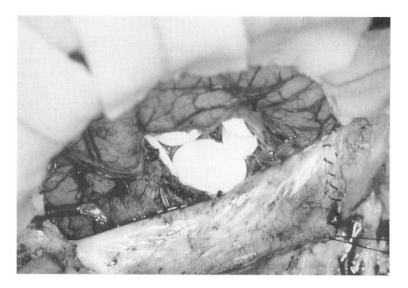

Fig. 19.7   *Gliadel Wafer implanted into the brain. (Courtesy of Guilford Pharmaceuticals).*

(13.3–14.3 mg/dose) containing less than 2.5% acetic acid and up to 12% goserelin-related substances. It is a sterile, white to cream colored 1 mm diameter cylinder, preloaded in a special single use syringe with a 16 gauge needle. The unit is packaged in a sealed, light and moisture proof, aluminum foil laminate pouch containing a desiccant capsule.

Zoladex is indicated for a number of disorders, including the palliative treatment of advanced carcinoma of the prostate offering an alternative treatment of prostatic cancer when orchiectomy or estrogen administration are not indicated or unacceptable to the patient. It is also used in the treatment of endometriosis and advanced breast cancer.

The product is administered subcutaneously into the upper abdominal wall using aseptic technique. The product should be stored at room temperature and should not exceed 25°C.

Zoladex is also available as Zoladex 3-Month, containing the equivalent of 10.8 mg of goserelin. The base consists of a matrix of D,L-lactic and glycolic acids copolymer (12.82–14.76 mg/dose) containing less than 2% acetic acid and up to 10% goserelin-related substances and presented as a sterile, white to cream colored 1.5 mm diameter cylinder, preloaded in a special single-use syringe with a 14-gauge needle and overwrap, as previously described. This preparation is designed for administration every 3 months (11).

Implanted Pumps

The DAD (Medtronic) is a sophisticated implant delivery device that can be programmed from outside the body. It consists of a titanium housing containing a 20 cm^3 refillable reservoir, an electronic control module, a battery and a peristaltic drive pump that delivers the program rate with an accuracy of +/- 15%. It is implanted and an attached catheter is routed to the site of administration. The reservoir is refilled or evacuated by percutaneous insertion of a syringe-mounted hypodermic needle that is inserted through a self-sealing septum. Numerous different drugs can be used as the titanium and silicone components are inert. The unit has a "low battery" alarm, "low reservoir volume" alarm, and a "memory error" alarm. The unit delivers at rates from 0.025 to 0.9 mL/hour constant or in single or multiple boluses. The unit can be reprogrammed via a radio wave-like telemetry link using an office-based programming system. The system has security codes and a strong magnetic field produced by the programming wand is required for the program to be changed. The unit can be implanted during outpatient surgery (12).

Fluorocarbon Propellant Pump

The Infusaid (Infusaid Inc.) constant-rate pump requires no external energy. It consists of a hollow titanium disk that is divided into two chambers by a freely moving titanium bellows. The drug solution is contained in the inner chamber separated from a fluorocarbon liquid that exerts a vapor pressure well above atmospheric pressure at body temperature. The drug chamber is filled by injection of the drug thorugh the skin and a self-sealing silicone rubber and Teflon septum. This pressure caused by the fluid being injected expands the fluid chamber and compresses the fluorocarbon chamber. Then, as the fluorocarbon vaporizes and compresses on the fluid chamber, the drug solution is forced through the fine-bore Teflon tubing. The restricted size of the Teflon capillary tubing serves to regulate the flow of solution from the device. Flow rates of 1 to 5 mL/day are usual and the actual drug delivery rate can be altered by changing the concentration of drug placed in the device. Heparin and insulin are examples of drugs that have been delivered via this pump.

Patients using the Infusaid pump should avoid prolonged hot baths, prolonged direct exposure to the sun, rough contact sports such as football and deep sea or scuba diving, as these activities may alter the pressure inside the unit resulting in a change in the delivery rate of the drug.

Ophthalmics

Pilocarpine Ocusert

Pilocarpine is available in a membrane-controlled reservoir system that is used in the treatment of glaucoma, called the Ocusert (Alza Corporation), previously introduced in Chapter 8. Pilocarpine is sandwiched in between two ethylene-vinyl acetate membranes. Also contained is alginic acid, a seaweed carbohydrate, that serves as a carrier for pilocarpine. The small, clear device has a white annular border made of ethylene-vinyl acetate copolymer impregnated with titanium dioxide (pigment) that makes it easier for the patient to visualize. The Ocusert is placed in the cul-de-sac where it will float with the tears. The pilocarpine will diffuse from the device and exert its pharmacological effect.

The tear fluid penetrates the microporous membrane, dissolving the pilocarpine. The release rate of pilocarpine is in the range of 20 or 40 μg/h for four to seven days. One advantage to this system is enhanced compliance as the patient does not have to remember to instill the drops and they do not experience the blurred vision or slight discomfort that occurs when applying drops to the eyes.

The release rate of pilocarpine from the EVA system is:

$$dm/dt = \frac{ADK\Delta C}{h}$$

where dm/dt is the release rate; D is the diffusion coefficient of the drug in the membrane; K is the partition coefficient that is the ratio of drug concentration at equilibrium inside the membrane to that outside the membrane; ΔC is the difference of the drug concentration between the inside and the outside walls of the membrane; A and h are the area and thickness of the system, respectively.

Under routine conditions, the concentration of the drug in the tears is negligible (2–3 μg/mL) compared to that inside, which is basically the solubility of the drug, so the equation can be rewritten as:

$$dm/dt = \frac{ADKS}{h}$$

The systems are designed to release at 20 or 40 μg/hour for one week. Over a weeks time, the total drug released by the system is 3.4 or 6.7 mg, for the 20 or 40 μg/hr units, respectively. The units contain either 5 mg or 11 mg of drug initially, and the units are designed to retain about 40% of the initial quantity of drug to provide for a constant delivery rate as well as a safety margin of an extra days delivery of drug.

Parenteral Administration

Infusion pumps consist of mechanical pumps, closed- and open-loop systems, programmable and manual systems, implantable and external systems, syringe pumps, piston pumps, peristaltic pumps, balloon pumps, gas pressure pumps, portable infusion pumps, and other controllers.

Intravenous Controllers and Infusion Pumps

Generally, almost half of drugs administered in hospitals and with home healthcare patients involve parenteral drugs. With the transition of the healthcare setting tending more towards homecare, there was a need for devices that would better control drug administration. Computer technology has been the basis for a large number of microprocessor driven devices that have been recently introduced to the market. Also, a number of unique pumps involving elastomeric balloons are in use as well as units that can deliver multiple solutions simultaneously or in a predetermined sequence. Most of the units are external controlling volumes of drugs ranging up to several liters and some are internal implanted pumps, where the volume is smaller and is administered over a period of time ranging from a few hours to a few days.

An *intravenous solution controller* depends upon gravity to provide the driving force for delivery of the solution. Flow regulation may be controlled by an electronic/optical counting of drops. Other controllers may depend upon flow restriction through an orifice. Variables involved may include the height of the solution and the solution viscosity.

The *infusion pump* uses positive pressure to move the solution through the tubing into the patient. Pumps in this category include peristaltic pumps, syringe pumps, cassette systems and elastomeric pumps.

Peristaltic pumps are usually either rotary cam driven or a linear peristaltic design using fingerlike projections to move the fluid down the line as each projection squeezes the tubing in sequence. These devices generally use either a reservoir bag or cassette containing the drug. The size of the bag or cassette determines the quantity of drug to be delivered. An advantage to using a bag reservoir, is that the reservoirs can be easily changed without interrupting the flow of medication to the patient. Generally, these devices are accurate to approximately +/− 10%. Examples of these devices are shown in Figure 19.8.

Syringe pumps involve the administration of a drug solution placed in a standard syringe. The syringe is inserted into a motor-driven device (gear or screw-driven) that will intermittently or continuously drive the plunger forward delivering the drug to the patient. The speed of movement of the motor dictates the rate at which the drug is delivered. Higher concentrations at slower rates can provide for continuous drug delivery over a prolonged period of time. One disadvantage of these devices is the volume of the syringe determines the quantity of drug delivered and the time required for administration. These devices generally deliver at about +/−5% accuracy.

Cassette systems are designed to be filled and attached to an electronic infuser. After administration is complete, the cassette is discarded and a new one put in its place. The shape of many of these cassettes makes it feasible for them to be contained in a small pouch the patient can wear and carry on routine daily activities.

Examples of drugs that are commonly administered using syringe, peristaltic or cassette infusion devices include antibiotics, oncology agents and analgesics. Many pumps are designed for patient controlled analgesia (PCA) where a baseline level of an analgesic may be delivered but a bolus can be administered upon demand by the patient, with a maximum level programmed in over a set time period that cannot be exceeded.

Elastomeric reservoir pumps are probably the simplest that are in use. They are filled with a set volume of solution, for example 50, 100 or 200 mL, and clamped. They can be stored until ready to use, depending upon the stability of the individual drugs. For use, they are attached to the catheter and the clamp opened starting fluid flow. The fluid flow is governed by a flow restrictor and most of these devices deliver the drug over a relatively short period of time of one to a few hours. Flow may be variable, however, depending upon temperature and fluid viscosity. These devices are often used for products where a defined quantity of drug is to be administered within a set period of time and not necessarily for drugs where a certain blood level must be maintained. They are widely used for antibiotics. It isn't unusual to require several of these devices daily but they do allow for ambulatory administration. After use, the devices are discarded. Elastomeric reservoir pumps are commonly used for antibiotics.

Liposomes

Liposomes are composed of small vesicles of a bilayer of phospholipid encapsulating an aqueous space ranging from about 0.03 to 10 μ in diameter. They are composed of one or many lipid membranes enclosing discrete aqueous compartments. The enclosed vesicles can encapsulate water-

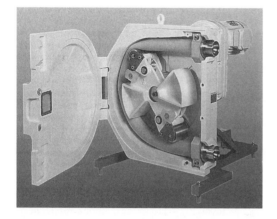

Fig. 19.8 *Watson-Marlow/Bredel 800 Series Peristaltic Pump. (Courtesy of Watson-Marlow/Bredel Pumps).*

soluble drugs in the aqueous spaces and lipid-soluble drugs can be incorporated into the membranes. Liposomes can be administered parenterally, topically, by inhalation or possibly by other routes of administration. Currently available products are administered parenterally.

The following is an oversimplification but will serve to illustrate the preparation of liposomes. Prepare a solution of a lipid (lecithin) in an organic solvent (acetone, chloroform) in a beaker. Allow the solvent to evaporate leaving a thin film of the lipid on the walls of the container. Add an aqueous solution of the drug to the beaker and place it in an ultrasonic bath. As the lipid is displaced from the beaker walls, it forms either spheres or cylinders while trapping the aqueous solution inside. The liposomes can then be collected, sized and used.

Numerous configurations are possible for liposomes, including spheres and cylinders. Spherically-shaped liposomes can be unilamellar (only one layer) or multilamellar (many layers). They are often given the designation as LUV (Large Unilamellar Vesicles), SUV (Small Unilamellar Vesicles and MLV (Multi Lamellar Vesicles). The smaller vesicles, or liposomes, generally range in size from 0.02 μm to 0.2 μm and the large vesicles from about 0.2 μm to over 10 μm. The MLVs may have an onion skin type structure of several layers.

The phospholipids composing liposomes are amphipathic, possessing both a hydrophilic or polar head and a hydrophobic or nonpolar tail. This is similar to the HLB and wedge orientation theories of emulsification. The hydrophobic tail is composed of fatty-acids containing generally 10 to 24 carbon atoms and the polar end may contain phosphoric acid bound to a water-soluble portion; the composition may vary considerably. Lecithin (phosphatidylcholine) is a backbone structure that has been studied extensively. When these phospholipids are exposed to water and "line up", they will do so in a manner that the fatty-acid tails associate together as the lipophilic phase and the polar head groups associate towards the bulk water phase. Depending upon the "system" and the water solubility of the drug, the drug may be located in the aqueous compartments (if water soluble) or within the lipophilic bilayers (if oil soluble).

Some liposomes are unique because they can be selectively absorbed by tissues rich in reticuloendothelial cells, such as the liver, spleen and bone marrow. This can serve as a targeting mechanism but it also serves to remove liposomes from the circulation rather rapidly. In order to extend the half life of liposomes in the body, "stealth liposomes" have been developed by coating the liposomes with materials, such as the polymer polyethylene glycol, enabling liposomes to evade detection through the components of the body's immune system. This extends their half life and may also alter their biodistribution.

Advantages of liposomes include the following: 1) Liposome-encapsulated drugs are delivered intact to various tissues and cells and can be released when the liposome is destroyed, enabling site-specific and targeted drug delivery, 2) Liposomes can be used for both hydrophilic and lipophilic drugs without the need for chemical modification, 3) Other tissues and cells of the body are protected from the drug until it is released by the liposomes, thus decreasing the drug's toxicity, and 4) The size, charge and other characteristics can be altered depending upon the drug and the intended use of the product.

Disadvantages of liposomes include their tendencies to be taken up by cells of the reticulendothelial system and the slow release of the drug when the liposomes are taken up by phagocytes through endocytosis, fusion, surface adsorption or lipid exchange.

Many advances have been made in liposome preparation including composition, sizing, classification and enhancing stability. Stability has been a problem but stable liposomes can now be prepared. Liposomes have been investigated for a number of years as potential drug delivery systems and now are on the market.

One product is Abelcet Injection (The Liposome Company, Inc,). It is a sterile, pyrogen-free suspension for intravenous infusion consisting of amphotericin B complexed with two phospholipids in a 1:1 drug-to-lipid molar ratio. The two phospholipids, L-α-dimyristoylphosphatidylcholine (DMPC) and L-α-dimyristoylphosphatidylglycerol (DMPG) are present in a 7:3 molar ratio. The product is yellow and opaque in appearance with a pH in the range of 5–7. The formulation, per mL, is provided as:

Amphotericin B USP	5 mg
L-α-dimyristoylphosphatidylcholine	3.4 mg
L-α-dimyristoylphosphatidylglycerol	1.5 mg
Sodium Chloride USP	9 mg
Water for Injection USP, qs	1 mL

The product contains the following bolded note:

NOTE: Liposomal encapsulation or incorporation in a lipid complex can substantially affect a drug's functional properties relative to those of the unencapsulated or nonlipid-associated drug. In addition, different liposomal or lipid-complexed products with a common active ingredient may vary from one another in the chemical composition and physical form of the lipid component. Such differences may affect functional properties of these drug products (13).

Amphotec (Amphotericin B Cholesteryl Sulfate, Sequus Pharmaceuticals, Inc.) is a sterile, pyrogen-free, lyophilized powder for reconstitution and intravenous administration. It is a 1:1 molar ratio complex of amphotericin B and cholesteryl sulfate that, upon reconstitution, forms a colloidal dispersion of microscopic disc-shaped particles. Each 50 mg single dose vial contains amphotericin B, 50 mg; disodium edetate dihydrate, 0.372 mg; lactose monohydrate, 950 mg; and hydrochloric acid, qs. The 100 mg single dose vial contains amphotericin B, 100 mg; sodium cholesteryl sulfate, 52.8 mg; tromethamine, 11.28 mg; disodium edetate dihydrate, 0.744 mg; lactose monohydrate, 1900 mg; and hydrochloric acid, qs.

Amphotec is indicated for the treatment of invasive aspergillosis in patients where renal impairment or unacceptable toxicity precludes the use of amphotericin B deoxycholate in effective doses and in aspergillosis patients where prior amphotericin B deoxycholate therapy has failed.

The drug is reconstituted with Sterile Water for Injection by rapidly adding the water to the vial; it is shaken gently by hand, rotating the vial until all the solids have dissolved. The fluid may be opalescent or clear. For infusion, it is further diluted in 5% dextrose injection. The product should not be reconstituted with any fluid other than Sterile Water for Injection; do not reconstitute with dextrose or sodium chloride solutions. Also, for further dilution, it should not be admixed with sodium chloride or electrolytes. Solutions containing benzyl alcohol or any other bacteriostatic agent should not be used as they may cause precipitation. An in-line filter should not be used and the infusion admixture should not be mixed with other drugs. If infused using a y-injection site or similar device, flush the line with 5% dextrose injection before and after infusion of Amphotec.

After reconstitution, the drug should be refrigerated and used within 24 hours; do not freeze. If further diluted with 5% dextrose injection, it should be refrigerated and used within 24 hours (14).

DaunoXome (daunorubicin citrate liposome injection, NeXstar Pharmaceuticals, Inc.) is an aqueous solution of daunorubicin citrate encapsulated with liposomes composed of distearoylphosphatidylcholine and cholestrol (2:1 molar ratio), with a mean diameter of about 45 nm (range from 35 and 65 nm). The lipid to drug weight ratio is 18.7:1 (total lipid:daunorubicin base), equivalent to a 10:5:1 molar ratio of distearoylphosphatidylcholine:cholesterol:daunorubicin.

DaunoXome is formulated to maximize the selectivity of daunorubicin for solid tumors *in situ*. The liposomal formulation helps to protect the daunorubicin from chemical and enzymatic degradation, minimizes protein binding and generally decreases uptake by normal tissues.

The product should be diluted 1:1 with 5% dextrose injection prior to administration. Each vial contains the equivalent of 50 mg daunorubicin base at a concentration of 2 mg/mL after preparation; it is recommended to be diluted to 1 mg/mL for administration. The only fluid recommended for preparation is 5% dextrose injection; it must not be mixed with sodium chloride solution or solutions containing benzyl alcohol or any other solution. An in-line filter should not be used for the intravenous infusion of DaunoXome. The final product is a red translucent dispersion of liposomes that does scatter light but it should not be used if it appears opaque or has precipitate or foreign matter in it. It should be stored in a refrigerator (2–8°C; 36–46°F), do not freeze, and protect from light (15).

Doxil (doxorubicin HCl liposome injection) is doxorubicin hydrochloride encapsulated in STEALTH liposomes for intravenous administration. The product is provided as a sterile, translucent, red liposomal dispersion in 10 mL glass, single use vials; each vial containing 20 mg of doxorubicin HCl at a concentration of 2 mg/mL and a pH of 6.5. The STEALTH liposome carrier consists of N-(carbamoyl- methoxypolyethylene glycol 2000)-1,2-distearoyl-sn-glycero-3-phosphoethanolamine sodium salt (MPEG-DSPE), 3.19 mg/mL; fully hydrogenated soy phosphatidylcholine (HSPC), 9.58 mg/mL; and cholesterol, 3.19 mg/mL. Each mL also contains approxmiately 2 mg of ammonium sulfate, histidine as a buffer; hydrochloric acid and/or sodium hyroxide for pH adjustment, and sucrose for tonicity. Over 90% of the doxorubicin is incorporated into the STEALTH liposomes.

Stealth liposomes are specially formulated to circulate in the body "undetected" by the mononuclear phagocyte system for a prolonged circulation time of about 55 hours. This is accomplished by pegylation, or binding methoxypolyethylene glycol on the surface of the liposomes. These liposomes are small, in the range of 100 nm in diameter.

Doxil must be diluted in 250 mL of 5% dextrose injection prior to administration; once diluted it should be refrigerated and administered within 24 hours. It should not be mixed with any other diluent or any preservative-containing solution. It should not be used with in-line filters. The product is not a clear solution but a red, translucent liposomal dispersion. Unopened vials should be stored in a refrigerator but freezing should be avoided; even though short term freezing (less than one month) does not appear to adversely affect the product.(16)

References

1. Package Insert. Dimetapp Cold & Allergy Quick Dissolve Tablets, Whitehall-Robins Healthcare, Madison NJ.
2. Physicians' Desk Reference, 52nd ed., 1998, Montvale NJ, Medical Economics Company, Inc., pp 2613–2615.
3. Package Insert. Tempra Quicklets, Bristol-Myers Products, New York NY.
4. Product Literature. Alza Corporation, Palo Alto CA.
5. Package Insert. Fentanyl Oralet, Abbott Laboratories, North Chicago IL.
6. Product Information, Fentanyl Actiq, Abbott Laboratories, North Chicago IL.
7. Product Literature, Alza Corp., Palo Alto CA.
8. Physicians' Desk Reference, 52nd ed., 1998, Montvale NJ, Medical Economics Company, Inc., pp 945–947.
9. Ibid., pp 3085–3089.
10. Ibid., pp 2365–2367.
11. Ibid., pp 3194–3198.
12. Product Information. Medtronic Inc., Minneapolis MN.
13. Physicians' Desk Reference, 52nd ed., 1998, Montvale NJ, Medical Economics Company, Inc., pp 1516–1517.
14. Ibid., pp 2764–2768.
15. Ibid., pp 1807–1810.
16. Ibid., pp 2768–2771.

Appendix I

SYSTEMS AND TECHNIQUES OF PHARMACEUTICAL MEASUREMENT

A KNOWLEDGE and application of the systems of pharmaceutical measurement are essential to the practice of pharmacy. Whether applied to the compounding and dispensing of prescriptions in the community pharmacy, the filling of medication orders in the institutional pharmacy, or the large-scale industrial manufacture of pharmaceuticals, quantitative accuracy is of prime importance in the preparation of safe and effective medications.

Pharmaceuticals prepared industrially undergo rigid in-process controls and final product assays to assure conformance with the applicable standards for drug content. Prescriptions and medication orders filled extemporaneously in the community and institutional pharmacy usually lack the advantage of control by assay, and thus the pharmacist must be absolutely certain of the accuracy of all calculations and measurements employed. Calculations should be double-checked by the pharmacist and whenever possible by a colleague. The importance of accurate calculations and measurements cannot be overstated. For example, an error in the placement of a decimal point represents a *minimum* error of a factor of ten and if applicable to the active ingredient, a critical drug underdosage or overdosage results.

The pharmacy student must have a working knowledge of the systems of pharmaceutical measurement, their application in pharmaceutical calculations, the factors used for conversion between the systems, and the proper techniques of weighing and measuring.

Systems of Pharmaceutical Measurement

Although pharmacy has moved toward the exclusive use of the metric system, two other systems of measurement occasionally may be encountered, namely the *apothecary system* and the *avoirdupois system.* The metric system includes units or weight, volume and linear measure; the apothecary system includes units of weight and volume; and the avoirdupois systems includes only units of weight. The metric system has replaced the apothecary system in virtually all pharmaceutical measurements and calculations, although some use remains, as common reference to the dose of thyroid in terms of *grains,* an apothecary system unit. The avoirdupois system is the *common* commercial system of weight used in the United States. It too is being replaced by the metric system but at a much slower pace. The avoirdupois system is encountered by the pharmacist in the purchase of bulk chemicals and other items packaged and sold by the ounce or pound.

The Metric System

The metric system is the most widely used system in pharmacy. It is the system used in the USP/NF, by the federal Food and Drug Administration, in manufacturers' labeling of pharmaceutical products, and in most physicians' writing of prescriptions and medication orders.

In the metric system, the *gram* is the main unit of weight, the *liter* the main unit of volume, and the *meter* the main unit of length. Subunits and multiples of these basic units are indicated by the prefix notations and symbols shown in Table A-1.

In pharmacy, the most commonly used metric units are:

units of weight, expressed in terms of the kilogram (kg), gram (g), milligram (mg), or microgram (μg).
units of liquid measure, expressed in terms of the liter (L) or milliliter (mL).

Table A.1.   Metric System Unit Prefixes*

Multiplication Factor	Prefix	Symbol	Term (USA)
1 000 000 000 000 000 000 = 10^{18}	exa	E	one quintillion
1 000 000 000 000 000 = 10^{15}	tera	T	one quadrillion
1 000 000 000 000 = 10^{12}	giga	G	one trillion
1 000 000 000 = 10^{9}	mega	M	one billion
1 000 000 = 10^{6}	kilo	k	one million
1 000 = 10^{3}	hecto	h	one thousand
100 = 10^{2}	deka	da	one hundred
10 = 10	peta	P	ten
0.1 = 10^{-1}	deci	d	one tenth
0.01 = 10^{-2}	centi	c	one hundreth
0.001 = 10^{-3}	milli	m	one thousandth
0.000 001 = 10^{-6}	micro	μ	one millionth
0.000 000 001 = 10^{-9}	nano	n	one billionth
0.000 000 000 001 = 10^{-12}	pico	p	one trillonth
0.000 000 000 000 001 = 10^{-15}	femto	f	one quadrillionth
0.000 000 000 000 000 001 = 10^{-18}	atto	a	one quintillionth

*Adapted from *Metric Editorial Guide,* 4th Ed., American National Metric Council, Washington, D.C., 20005. The table is based on The International System of Units ("SI," from the French "Le Systeme International System of Unites"), as modified for use in the United States by the Secretary of Commerce.

units of linear measure, expressed in terms of the meter (m), centimeter (cm), or millimeter (mm).
units of area measure, expressed in terms of the square meter (m^2) or square centimeter (cm^2).

The "metric weight scale" in Figure A-1 is in-tended to depict the relationship between the units of weight in the metric system and to demonstrate an easy method of converting from one unit to another (1).

In the example shown, 1.23 kilograms (kg) are to be converted to grams (g). On the scale, the gram position is three decimal positions from the kilogram position. Thus, the decimal point is moved three places toward the right. In the other example, the conversion from milligrams (mg) to grams (g) also requires the movement of the decimal point three places, but this time to the left. The same method may be used to convert metric units of volume or length.

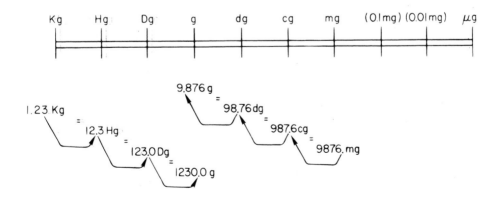

Fig. A.1   *Metric weight scale.*

Table of Metric Weight

1 kilogram (Kg or kg) = 1000.000 grams
1 hectogram (Hg or hg) = 100.000 grams
1 dekagram (Dg or dg) = 10.000 grams
1 gram (Gm, gm or g) = 1.000 gram
1 decigram (dg) = 0.100 gram
1 centigram (cg) = 0.010 gram
1 milligram (mg) = 0.001 gram
1 microgram = 0.000,001 gram
  (µg or mcg)
1 nanogram (ng) = 0.000,000,0001 gram
1 picogram (pg) = 0.000.000.000.001 gram

or

1 gram = 0.001 kilogram
 = 0.010 hectogram
 = 0.100 dekagram
 = 10 decigrams
 = 100 centigrams
 = 1000 milligrams
 = 1,000,000 micrograms
 = 1,000,000,000 nanograms
 = 1,000,000,000,000 picograms

Table of Metric Volume

1 kiloliter (Kl or kl) = 1000.000 liters
1 hectoliter (Hl or hl) = 100.000 liters
1 dekaliter (Dl) = 10.000 liters
1 liter (L or l) = 1.000 liter
1 deciliter (dl) = 0.100 liter
1 centiliter (cl) = 0.010 liter
1 milliliter (mL) = 0.001 liter
1 microliter (µL) = 0.000,001 liter

or

1 liter = 0.0001 kiloliter
 = 0.010 hectoliter
 = 0.100 dekaliter
 = 10 deciliters
 = 100 centiliters
 = 1000 milliliters
 = 1,000,000 microliters

Table of Metric Length

1 kilometer (Km or km) = 1000.000 meters
1 hectometer (Hm) = 100.000 meters
1 dekameter (Dm) = 10.000 meters
1 meter (M or m) = 1.000 meter
1 decimeter (dm) = 0.100 meter
1 centimeter (cm) = 0.010 meter
1 millimeter (mm) = 0.001 meter
1 micrometer (µm) = 0.000,001 meter
1 nanometer (nm) = 0.000,000,001 meter

or

1 meter = 0.001 kilometer
 = 0.010 hectometer
 = 0.100 dekameter
 = 10 decimeters
 = 100 centimeters
 = 1000 millimeters
 = 1,000,000 micrometers
 = 10,000,000,000 nanometers

The Apothecary System

The apothecary system provides for the measurement of both weight and volume. The tables of the system are presented below.

Table of Apothecaries' Fluid Measure

60 minims (m) = 1 fluidrachm (f₃) *
8 fluidrachms = 1 fluidounce (f℥)*
  (480 minims)
16 fluidounces = 1 pint (pt)
2 pints (32 fluidounces) = 1 quart (qt)
4 quarts (8 pints) = 1 gallon (gal)

Table of Apothecaries' Measure of Weight

20 grains (gr) = 2 scruple (Э)
3 scuples (60 grains) = 1 drachm (₃)
8 dram (480 grains) = 1 ounce (℥)
12 ounces (5760 grains) = 1 pound (℔)

The Avoirdupois System

The avoirdupois system is used in commerce to supply bulk chemicals and other items by weight, in ounces or pounds (e.g., epsom salts).

The "grain" represents the same weight in the apothecary and avoirdupois systems. However, the "ounce" and the "pound" in the two systems differ in the number of grains contained per unit; i.e., the apothecary ounce contains 480 grains whereas the avoirdupois ounce contains 437.5 grains and the apothecary pound contains 5760 grains whereas the avoirdupois pound contains 7000 grains. It also should be noted that the symbols for the ounce and pound are different in the two systems.

Table of Avoirdupois Measure of Weight

437.5 grains (gr) = 1 ounce (oz)
16 ounces (7000 grains) = 1 pound (lb)

NOTE: * When there is no doubt that the material referred to is a liquid, the *f* is usually omitted from this symbol. *Drachm* is also spelled *dram*.

Intersystem Conversion

A pharmacist may convert the weight, volume, or dimensions of length from one system to another through the use of intersystem conversion factors. Depending upon the circumstances and requirements or accuracy, conversion factors of different exactness may be used. The following is a table of the factors commonly used in prescription practice. They are exact equivalents which have been rounded off for practical application. Exact equivalents, utilized in the conversion of specific quantities in pharmaceutical formulas, may be found in the USP.

Useful Conversion Equivalents of Weight

1 g	= 15.432 gr
1 Kg	= 2.2 Avoirdupois lb
1 gr	= 0.0648 g or 64.8 or 65 mg
1 ℥	= 31.1 g
1 oz (Avoir)	= 28.35 g
1 lb (Apoth)	= 373.2 g
1 lb (Avoir)	= 453.6 or 454 g

Useful Conversion Equivalents of Volume

1 mL	= 16.23 minims
1 minim	= 0.06 mL
1 fℨ	= 3.69 mL
1 f℥	= 29.57 mL
1 pt	= 473 mL
1 gal (U.S.)	= 3785 mL
1 gal (British Imperial)	= 4546 mL

Conversion Equivalents of Length

1 inch = 2.54 cm
1 meter = 39.37 inches

Today there are very few occasions in which intersystem conversion is needed, owing to the almost exclusive use of the metric system in both product formulation and prescription compounding. However, when conversion is necessary or desired, it is a simple matter of selecting and applying the appropriate intersystem conversion factor.

For example, if one wishes to determine the number of milliliters present in 8 fluid ounces of a liquid, the conversion factor that most directly relates milliliters and fluid ounces is selected. That factor is one fluidounce = 29.57 mL; thus 8 fluidounces contain 8 × 29.57 mL, or 236.56 mL.

Another example: how many 30 mL containers may be filled from 10 gallons of a formulation? One gallon is equivalent to 3785 mL. Thus 10 gallons have 10 × 3785 mL, or 37,850 mL. By dividing this total number of milliliters by 30 mL, the number of containers that may be filled is found to be 1,261.

Another example: how many ½ grain tablets may be prepared from 1 kilogram of a drug substance? Since one grain is equivalent to 64.8 mg, ½ grain is equal to 32.4 mg. One kilogram is equal to 1000 g, or 1,000,000 mg. Since 32.4 are required for one tablet, dividing 1,000,000 mg by 32.4 mg shows that 30,864 tablets may be prepared.

A final example: if a transdermal patch measures 30 mm square, what is this dimension in inches? The conversion factor, 1 inch equals 2.54 cm, may be expressed as 1 inch equals 25.4 mm. Thus, by dividing 30 mm by 25.4 mm/inch, one finds the patch is 1.18 inches square.

Quantitative Product Strength

The quantitative composition of certain pharmaceuticals, particularly liquids and semisolid dosage forms, often is expressed in terms of the *percentage strength* of the active, and sometimes inactive, ingredients. For some dilute solutions, the strength may be expressed in terms of its *ratio strength.* For most injections, many oral liquids, and some semisolid dosage forms, the quantity of active ingredient commonly is expressed on a weight (of drug) per unit volume basis, as "milligrams of drug per milliliter" (of injection or oral liquid), or on a weight (of drug) per unit weight of preparation, as "milligrams of drug per gram" (of ointment). The strength of solid dosage forms is given as the drug content (e.g., 5 mg) per dosage unit (e.g., tablets and capsules).

Percent, by definition, means parts per hundred. In pharmacy, percentage concentrations have specific meanings based on the physical character of the particular product or formulation. That is:

Percent weight-in-volume. Expressed "% w/v," this defines the number of grams of a constituent in 100 mL of a preparation (generally a liquid);

Percent volume-in-volume. Expressed "% v/v," this defines the number of milliliters of a constituent in 100 mL of a preparation (generally a liquid); and,

Percent weight-in-weight. Expressed "% w/w," this defines the number of grams of a constituent in 100 g of a preparation (generally a solid or semisolid, but also for liquid preparations prepared by weight).

Thus, a 5% w/v solution or suspension of a drug contains 5 g of the substance in each 100 mL of product; a 5% v/v preparation contains 5 mL of the substance in each 100 mL of product; and, a 5%

w/w/ preparation contains 5 g of the substance in each 100 g of product.

In the manufacture or compounding of pharmaceutical preparations, the pharmacist may (1) calculate the strength of an individual component in a product, or (2) calculate the amount of a component needed to achieve a desired percentage strength.

For example, what is the percentage strength, w/v, of a solution containing 15 g of drug in 500 mL? Since, by definition, percentage strength is parts per hundred, we simply need to determine how many grams of drug are present in each 100 mL solution. Solving by proportion: 15 g/500 mL = (x) g/100 mL, the answer is 3 g, and thus the solution is 3 % w/v in strength.

Other examples: 3 mL of a liquid in a liter of solution represents 0.3% v/v; 4 g of drug in 250 mL represents 1.6% w/v; and 8 g of drug in 40 g of product represents 20% w/w.

How many grams of drug are needed to prepare 400 mL of a 5% w/v preparation? In w/v problems, the specific gravity *of the preparation* is assumed to be the same as water (sp. gr. 1.0) and thus 1 mL is assumed to weigh 1 g. Therefore, in the problem example, the 400 mL is assumed to weigh 400 g; and, 5% of 400 g = 20 g, the amount of drug needed.

A v/v problem example: How many mL of a liquid are needed to make one pint of a 0.1% v/v solution? One pint contains 473 mL and 0.1% of that is 0.473 mL, the answer.

A w/w problem example: How many grams of zinc oxide powder should be used in preparing 120 g of a 20% w/w ointment? Twenty percent of 120 g is 24 g, the answer.

Ratio strength is sometimes used to express the strength of, or to calculate the amount of, a component needed to make a relatively dilute preparation. Compared to percentage strength designations, for example, a 0.1% w/v preparation (0.1 g per 100 mL) is equivalent to 1 g per 1000 mL, and may be expressed as a ratio strength of 1:1000 w/v. Ratio strength expressions utilize the w/v, v/v, and w/w designations in the same manner as percentage strength expressions, for example:

> A *1:1000 w/v preparation of a solid constituent in a liquid preparation* = 1 g of the solid constituent in 1000 mL of preparation;
> A *1:1000 v/v preparation of a liquid constituent in a liquid preparation* = 1 mL of constituent in 1000 mL of preparation; and
> A *1:1000 w/w/ preparation of a solid constituent in a solid or semisolid preparation* = 1 g of constituent in 1000 g of preparation.

A ratio strength calculation example: what is the ratio strength of 6000 mL of solution containing 3 g of drug? Whenever possible, it is preferable for ratio strengths to be expressed as 1: In this example, if 3 g of drug are in 6000 mL of solution, 1 g of drug would be contained in 2000 mL, and thus the ratio strength of 1:2000 w/v. Sometimes the answers do not come out as evenly; for example, what is the ratio strength of 0.3 mL of a liquid in a liter of solution? In this instance, there would be 0.3 mL in 1000 mL, equivalent to 3 mL in 10,000 mL, or a ratio strength of 3:10,000 v/v, or 1:3, 333.3 v/v.

Another ratio strength calculation example: How many grams of drug are needed to make 5 L of a 1:400 w/v solution? By definition (of 1:400 w/v), there would be 1 g of drug needed for each 400 mL of solution. Since 5 liters, or 5000 mL, of solution are to be prepared, the amount of drug required is found by solving 1 g/400 mL = (x) g/ 5000 mL, or 12.5 g, the answer.

Rather than being expressed in terms of percentage strength or ratio strength, the strength of some pharmaceutical preparations, particularly injections and sometimes oral liquids, is based on drug content per unit of volume, as "mg per mL." Thus flexibility in dosing can be achieved by administering the volume of preparation that contains the desired dose.

Reducing and Enlarging Formulas

In the course of pharmaceutical manufacturing, and in professional practice activities, it is often necessary to reduce or enlarge a pharmaceutical formulation in order to prepare the desired amount of product. A standard manufacturing formulation, or *master formula,* contains the quantitative amounts of each ingredient needed to prepare a specified quantity of product. When preparing other quantities, larger or smaller, the *quantitative relationship* of each component to the other in the formula must be maintained. For example, if there are 2 g of ingredient A and 10 mL of ingredient B (among other ingredients) in a formula for 1000 mL, then there needs to be 0.2 gram of ingredient A and 1 mL of ingredient B used when only 100 mL, or 1/10 of the formula, is prepared. If, on the other hand, a formula is to be enlarged—for example, from a liter (1000 mL) of product to a gallon (3785 mL)—the amount of each ingredient required would be 3.785 times that needed to prepare the liter of product.

In these examples the quantity of product prepared is reduced or enlarged, but the quantitative relationship between each ingredient and the product strength remains unchanged.

Dosage Units

Drug dosage is selected by the prescriber based upon clinical considerations and the characteristics of the pharmacologic agent. Dosage forms (tablets, injections, transdermal patches) are used to administer the drug to the patient. Solid dosage forms, such as tablets and capsules, are generally prepared in various strengths to allow flexibility in dosing. The desired dose for a drug prepared in a liquid dosage form may be provided by the volume administered. For example, if a liquid dosage form contains 5 mg of drug per milliliter, and if a dose of 25 mg of drug is desired, 5 mL of the liquid may be administered. Commercially manufactured products are formulated to provide the drug in dosage forms and amounts convenient for administration. In instances in which the desired dosage or dosage form is commercially unavailable, the pharmacist may be called upon to compound the desired preparation.

Common Household Measure

Liquid and powdered medications which are not packaged in unit dose systems are usually measured at home by the patient with common household measuring devices as the teaspoon, tablespoon, and other utensils. Although the household teaspoon may vary in volume capacity from approximately 3 to 8 mL, the American Standard Teaspoon has been established as having a volume of 4.93 ± 0.24 mL by the American National Standards Institute. For practical purposes, most pharmacy practitioners and pharmacy references utilize 5 mL as the capacity of the teaspoon. This is approximately equivalent to 1⅓ fluid drams although physicians commonly utilize the dram symbol (3) to indicate a teaspoonful in their prescription directions to be transcribed by the pharmacist to the patient. The tablespoon is considered to have a capacity of 15 mL, equivalent to three teaspoonfuls or approximately one-half fluid ounce.

Occasionally the pharmacist will dispense a special medicinal spoon which the patient may use in measuring this medication. These spoons are available in half-teaspoon, teaspoon, and tablespoon capacities. Some manufacturers provide specially designed devices to be used by the patient in measuring medication. These include specially calibrated droppers, oral syringes, measuring wells or tubes, and calibrated bottle caps. In health care institutions, disposable measuring cups and unit-dose containers are commonly employed in administering liquid medication. Examples of measuring devices are shown in Fig. A-2.

Techniques of Pharmaceutical Measurement

Weighing and the Prescription Balance

In weighing materials, the selection of the instrument to use is based on the amount of material involved and the accuracy desired. In the large scale manufacture of pharmaceuticals, large industrial *scales* of varying capacity and sensitivity are employed, and later, highly sensitive analytical balances are utilized in the quality control and analytical work.

In the hospital and community pharmacy, most weighings are made on the *prescription balance.* Two examples of these balances are shown in Figure A-3. Prescription balances are termed *Class III* (formerly Class A) balances, which meet the prescribed standards of the National Institute of Standards and Technology. Every prescription department is required by law to have a prescription balance. The sensitivity of a balance is usually represented by the term *sensitivity requirement* (SR) which is defined as the maximum change in load that will cause a specified change, one subdivision on the index plate, in the position of rest of the indicating element(s) of the balance. The *sensitivity requirement* (SR) is determined in the following manner: (1) level the balance, (2) determine the rest point, (3) place a 6-mg weight on one of the empty pans, (4) the rest point is shifted *not less than* one division on the index plate. The entire operation is repeated with a 10-g weight placed in the center of each balance pan. A Class III balance has an SR of 6 mg with no load as well as with 10 g on each pan. This means that under the above conditions, the addition of 6 mg of weight to one pan of the balance will disturb the equilibrium and move the balance pointer one division marking on the scale.

The USP directs that to avoid errors in weighing of 5% or greater, which may be due to the limits of accuracy of the prescription balance, one must weigh a minimum of 120 mg of any material in each weighing (5% of 120 mg being the 6 mg SR or error inherent with the balance). If a smaller weight of material is desired, it is directed that the pharmacist mix a larger, calculated weight of the ingredient (120 mg or over), dilute it with a known

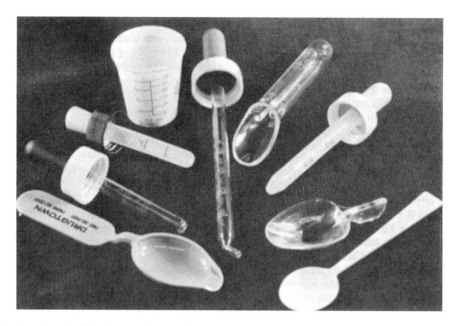

Fig. A.2 *Examples of medicinal spoons of various shapes and capacities, calibrated medicine droppers, or an oral medication tube, and a disposable medication cup.*

weight of an inert dry diluent (as lactose), mix the two uniformly, and weigh an aliquot portion of the mixture (again 120 mg or over) calculated to contain the desired amount of agent. The Class III balance which has a capacity of 120 g should be used for all weighings required in prescription compounding.

Weights

Today, pharmacies usually have a metric set of weights. Some commercial weight sets contain both the metric and apothecaries' systems of weights in a single container. Prescription weights meet the National Bureau of Standards' specifications for analytical weights. Metric weights of 1 g

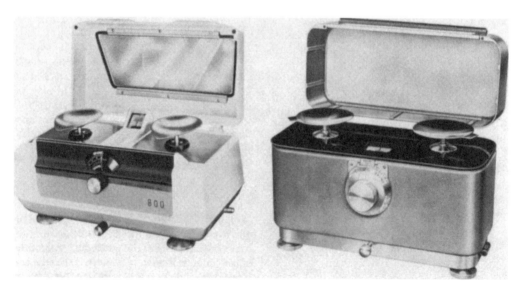

Fig. A.3 *Examples of commonly used Class III prescription balances. On left is the Troemner Model 800 Prescription Balance (Courtesy of Henry Troemner, Inc.); on right, the Model DRX2 Torsion balance (Courtesy of Torsion Balance Company.)*

and greater, and apothecaries' weights of 1 scruple and greater, are generally conical in shape with a narrow neck and head which allows them to be easily grasped and picked up with small forceps. Most of these weights are made of polished brass, with some coated with nickel or chromium or other materials to resist corrosion. Fractional gram weights are made of aluminum and are generally square-shaped and flat with one raised end or corner for picking up with the forceps (Fig. A-4). Apothecaries' weights of one-half scruple are frequently coin-shaped brass and those of 5 grains and less are usually bent aluminum wires, with each straight side representing 1 grain of weight. The half-grain weight is usually a smaller gauge wire bent in half.

To prevent the deposit of moisture and oils from the fingertips being deposited on the weights, all weights should be transferred with the forceps provided in each weight set.

Care and Use of a Prescription Balance

First and foremost, the prescription balance should be located in a well-lighted location, placed on a firm, level counter approximately waist-high to the operator. The area should be as free from dust as is possible and in an area that is draft-free. There should be no corrosive vapors present nor high humidity or vibration. When not in use, the balance should be clean and covered with the balance cover. Any agent spilled on the balance during use should be wiped off immediately with a soft brush or cloth. When not in use, the balance should always be maintained with the weights off and the beam in the fixed or locked (arrested) position.

Before weighing an article, the balance must be made level. This is accomplished with the leveling screws on the bottom of the balance, according to the instructional materials accompanying the balance. The balance should be level, front-to-back and side-to-side, as indicated by the leveling bubble of the balance.

In using a prescription balance, neither the weights nor the substance to be weighed should be

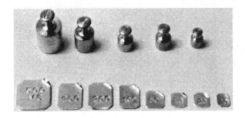

Fig. A.4 *Examples of some metric weights, showing their shape and markings.*

placed on the balance while the beam is in the *un*arrested position and free to oscillate. Before weighing, powder papers of equal size should be placed on both pans of the balance and the equilibrium of the balance tested by releasing the arresting knob. If the balance is unbalanced due to differences in the weight of the powder papers, additional weight may be added to the "light pan" by adding small tearings of powder papers. When balanced, the balance is placed in the arrested position and the desired weight added to the right-hand pan. Then, an amount of substance, considered to be approximately the desired weight, is carefully placed on the left hand pan, with the assistance of a spatula. The beam should then be slowly released by means of the locking device in the front of the balance. If the substance is in excess, the beam is fixed again and a small portion of the substance removed with the spatula. The process is continued until the two pans balance, as indicated by central position of the balance pointer. If the amount of weight on the balance is initially too little, the reverse process is undertaken. The powder paper used on the left hand pan, intended to hold the substance to be weighed, is usually folded either diagonally or with the edges of the sides folded upwards to contain the material being weighed.

In transferring material by spatula, the material may be lightly tapped from the spatula when the correct amount to be measured is approached. Usually this is done by holding the spatula with a small amount of material on it in the right hand, and tapping the spatula with the forefinger. As material comes off the spatula, the left hand is working the balance arresting mechanism and the status of the weight observed alternately with the tapping of the spatula. Most balances have a "damping" mechanism which slows down the balance oscillations and permits more rapid determinations of the balance or imbalance positions of the pans.

Once the material has been weighed, the balance beam is again put in the fixed position and the paper holding the weighed substance carefully removed. If more than a single weighing is to be performed, the paper is usually marked with the name of the substance it holds. After the final weighing, all weights are removed with the forceps and the balance cleaned, closed, and the balance cover placed over the balance.

Most prescription balances contain built-in mechanisms whereby external weights are not required for weighings under 1 gram. Some balances utilize a rider, which may be shifted from the zero position toward the right side of the balance to add increments of weight marked on the scale in 10-mg units, up to 1 g. Another type of balance uses a centrally located dial, calibrated in 10-mg units, to add weight up to 1 gram. Both types of devices add the weight internally to the right-hand pan. In each case, the pharmacist may use a combination of the internal weights and external weights in his weighings. For instance, if 1.2 g are to be weighed, the pharmacist can place a 1-g weight on the right hand pan and place the rider or adjust the dial to add 0.2 g additionally. Care must always be exercised to bring the rider or dial to zero between weighings to avoid the inadvertent weighing of rider- or dial-amounts on subsequent weighings.

Most weighings on the prescription balance involve the weighing of powders or semisolid materials, as ointments. However, liquids may also be weighed through the use of tared (weighed) vessels of appropriate size, by placing the liquid inside of the vessel. The pharmacist must always be certain that he has accounted for the weight of the vessel in calculating the amount of liquid weighed.

Materials should never be "downweighed;" that is, substances should never be placed on the pan with the balance in the unarrested position forcing the pan to drop suddenly and forcefully as the ex-

cess material is placed on it. The sudden slamming down of the pan can do serious damage to the balance, affecting its sensitivity and the accuracy of subsequent weighings.

The two most popular types of prescription balances are the compound lever balance and the torsion balance. The former type operates through the use of a series of knife edges held in delicate contact and suspension. The torsion type operates on the tension of taut wires, which when twisted through the addition of weight, tend to twist back to the original balance position. The compound level principle is the basis for the Troemner balance and the torsion principle is applied in the Torsion Balance (Fig. A-3).

Measuring Volume

The common instruments for pharmaceutical measurement are presented in Figure A-5. Two types of graduates are used in pharmacy, those which are *conical* in shape and those which are *cylindrical.* Cylindrical graduates are generally calibrated in metric units, whereas conical graduates may be graduated in both the metric and apothecary units' dual scale) or with a single scale of either

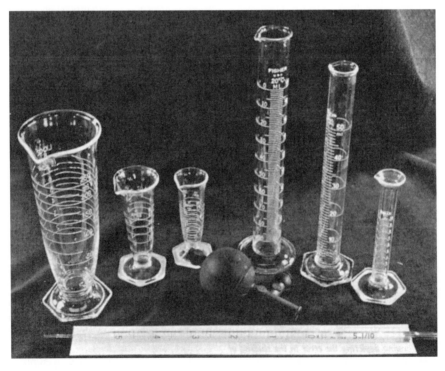

Fig. A.5   *Typical equipment for the pharmaceutical measurement of volume. On the left are conical graduates and on the right, cylindrical graduates. In the front is a pipet for the measurement of small volumes. Behind the pipet is a pipet filler, used instead of the mouth to draw acids and other dangerous liquids into the pipet.*

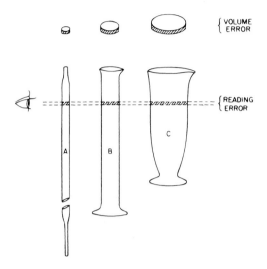

Fig. A.6 *Drawing showing the difference in the volume-error occurring with the same reading-error in measuring devices of different diameters.*

of the systems. Graduates of both shapes are available in a wide variety of capacities, ranging from 5 to 1000 mL or more. Most graduates in use are made of a good quality, heat-treated glass, although graduates of polypropylene are also available. In measuring small volumes of liquids, as less than 1.5 mL, the pharmacist should utilize a pipet as the one shown in Figure A-5. The bulk-like device shown with the pipet is a pipet filler, used for drawing acids or other toxic solutions into the pipet without the necessity of using the mouth. The device, without being removed from the pipet, also allows for the accurate delivery of the liquid.

In measuring volumes of liquids, the pharmacist should select the measuring device most appropriate to the volume of liquid to be measured and the degree of accuracy desired. It should be recognized that in measuring liquids, the more narrow the column of liquid, the more accurate is likely to be the measurement. Figure A-6 demonstrates this point. A reading error of the same dimension will produce a small volume-error when using a pipet, a greater volume-error when using a cylindrical graduate, and the greatest volume-error when using a conical graduate. The greater the flair in the design of the conical graduate, the greater is the volume-error due to an error in reading.

In reading the level of liquid in a graduate, it is important to recognize the error which could result due to the error of parallax. Figure A-7 depicts this point. A liquid in a graduate tends to be drawn to the inner surface of the graduate and rises slightly

against that surface and above its true meniscus. If one measured looking downward, it would appear as though the meniscus of the liquid is at this upper level, whereas it is slightly lower, at the actual level of the liquid within the center of the graduate. Thus, measurements of liquids in graduates should be taken with the eyesight level with the liquid in the graduate.

If a pharmacist was in error in his reading of a graduate, the *percentage of error* of his measurement would be affected by the volume of liquid that he was measuring. According to the USP, an acceptable 10-mL graduate cylinder with an internal diameter of 1.18 cm contains 0.109 mL of liquid in each 1 mm of column. A reading error of 1 mm in magnitude would cause a percentage error in the measurement of only 1.09% when 10 mL were being measured, 2.18% when 5 mL were being measured, 4.36% when 2.5 mL were being measured, and 7.26% when 1.5 mL were being measured. It is apparent that the greatest percentage error occurs when the smallest amount is being measured. Thus, the rule of thumb for measuring liquids in graduates is that a graduate should be used having

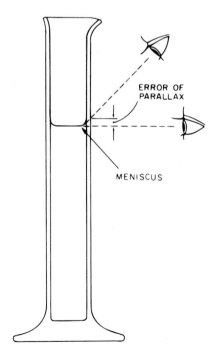

Fig. A.7 *Drawing depicting the error in the reading of the meniscus of a liquid in a graduate cylinder when the reading is made from above the level of the liquid rather than at the same level.*

a capacity *equal to or just exceeding* the volume to be measured.

According to Goldstein and Mattocks, (2) based on a deviation of 1 mm from the mark and an allowable error of 2.5%, the smallest amounts that should be measured in the following size cylindrical graduates having the stated internal diameters are as follows:

Graduate Cylinder Size	Internal Diameter	Deviation in Actual Volume	Minimum Volume Measurable
5 mL	0.98 cm	0.075 mL	3.00 mL
10 mL	1.18 cm	0.109 mL	4.36 mL
25 mL	1.95 cm	0.296 mL	11.84 mL
50 mL	2.24 cm	0.394 mL	15.76 mL
100 mL	2.58 cm	0.522 mL	20.88 mL

For a 5% error, the minimum volumes measurable would be one-half of those stated. It is apparent that for accuracy, one should not select a graduate for use when the measurement involves utilization of only the bottom portion of the scale.

In using graduates, the pharmacist pours the liquid into the graduate slowly, observing the level as he proceeds. In measuring viscous liquids, adequate time must be allowed for the liquid to settle in the graduate, as some may run slowly down the inner sides of the graduate. It is best to attempt to pour such liquids toward the center of the graduate, avoiding contact with the sides. In emptying the graduate of its measured contents, adequate drain time should be allowed.

When pouring liquids from bottles, it is considered good pharmaceutical technique to keep the label on the bottle facing upwards; this avoids the possibility of any errant liquid running down over the label as the bottle is righted after use. The bottle orifice should be wiped clean after each use.

References

1. Stoklosa MJ, Ansel HC. Pharmaceutical calculations. 10 ed. Baltimore: Williams & Wilkins, 1996.
2. Goldstein SW, Mattocks AM. How to measure accurately, J Am Pharm 1951; 23:421.

Index

Page numbers in *italics* indicate figures; numbers followed by "t" indicate tables; numbers followed by "c" indicate Physical Pharmacy Capsules.